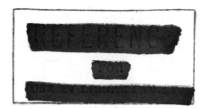

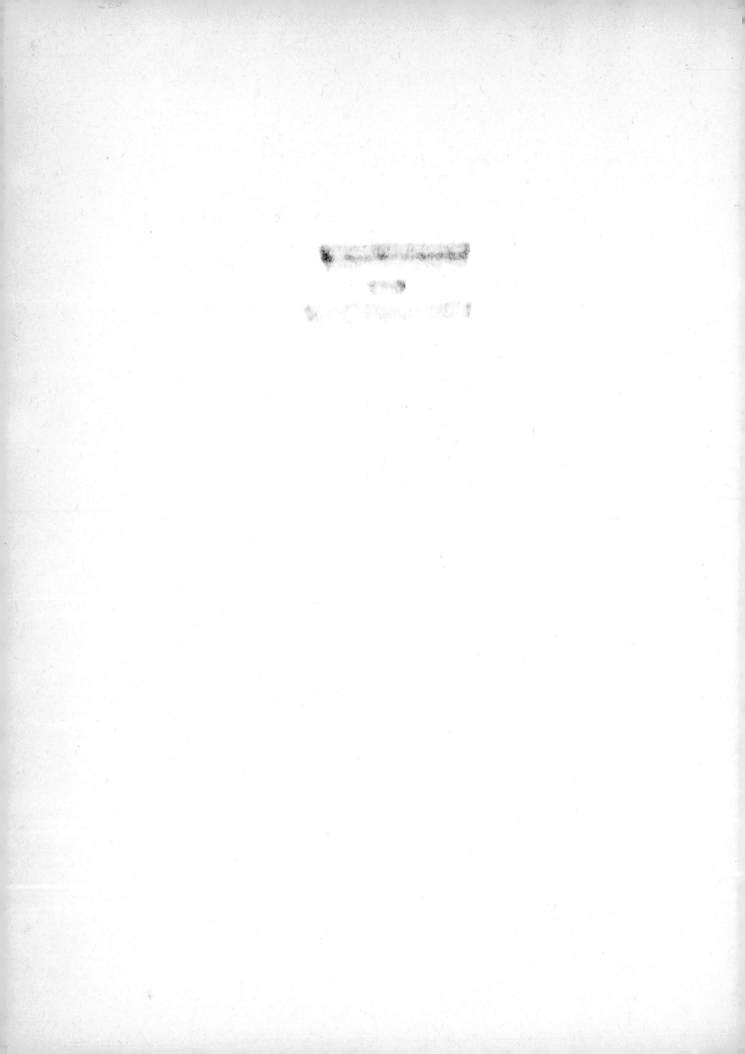

ORGANIZING FOR HEALTH CARE

SOURCE 3

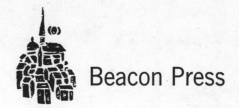 Beacon Press

Copyright © 1974 by Source, Inc.

Library of Congress catalog card number: 74-254

Beacon Press books are published under the auspices
of the Unitarian Universalist Association

Simultaneous publication in Canada by Saunders of Toronto, Ltd.

Published in simultaneous hardcover and paperback editions

International Standard Book Numbers: 0-8070-2178-4
0-8070-2179-2 (pbk.)

9 8 7 6 5 4 3 2 1

ORGANIZING FOR HEALTH CARE

A TOOL FOR CHANGE

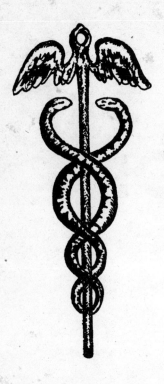

TABLE OF CONTENTS

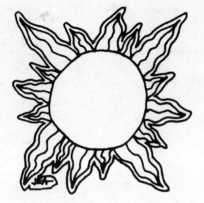

INTRODUCTION

The purpose of Source Catalog is to assist the people challenging outmoded and oppressive institutions. Our role is locating resource tools (groups, strategies, books, films, and tapes) that will further enable organizations to redesign communities to meet the needs of all people. The catalog does this in four ways: first by clarifying a few of the mechanics and roots of oppression; second by outlining visions of new social/political/economic systems; next suggesting strategies and programs which can begin to move people from what is to what can be; and finally by describing organizations and resources presently working in all the above areas.

CATALOG STRUCTURE AND MECHANICS

The "PROBLEM" . . . in each section is a relatively brief overview of how a particular aspect of the health system operates. This is intended to put the struggle of the organizations described in the section in a working context; materials from which we took our indictments in most cases were from the groups described in the section. By no means a complete analysis, the problem highlights basic contradictions.

The "PLATFORM" . . . is an outline of some of the goals different organizations are working toward to change the health system. They are interim demands around which organizing work can begin, plus a few visions for building new institutions.

The "PROGRAM" . . . lists some of the many tactics and methods used by groups fighting around these issues. It is organized, for the most part, in ascending complexity of action to offer alternative forms of action, not to suggest priority or a necessary order.

GROUPS. . . in the catalog, like an iceberg's tip, are merely the surface of an immense health movement in America. Its strength cannot be judged by the quantity here or even the

FOREWORD

The process of learning the truth about the health system in this country is jolting and depressing. Many of us have grown up trusting that doctors and hospitals are basically there to help us. The idea that hospitals would turn away an injured person without money is hard to accept. Even for those of us who didn't have the money and were turned away, it is hard to believe that a doctor would deliberately perform an unnecessary operation, or prescribe a drug without knowing all the dangers. There are a lot of ideas floating around about how to change the health system; a lot of politicians and government officials who say they have the answers. But when it comes down to it, the health system reflects the way our society is structured. As long as serving people is secondary to making money, the basic problems of health care will not change. This is not a new idea in the US. There was a Popular Health Movement back in the 1830's and 40's, a "radical assault on medical elitism and an affirmation of the traditional people's medicine." ("WITCHES, MIDWIVES, AND NURSES") This was when doctors were just beginning to establish their monopoly on medical knowledge, making it illegal for anyone without formal training to use their knowledge about their bodies to help someone else.

Today the control of health care delivery has shifted from the private practitioner (though his/her role cannot be discounted) to what has become one of the largest and fastest expanding industries in the country. The high cost and low quality care we face is not the result of a disorganized "non-system," as some reformers would have us believe. It is "quality," for many significant forces and actions go unrecorded. We could not be a complete directory. Some group write-ups will inevitably be incomplete, outdated, or inaccurate. We have categorized many groups with various approaches and experience that can be learned from. Our purpose is to suggest a broad range of possible actions while putting them in the context of far reaching social change.

BOOKS. . . were chosen and annotated as sources of more complete or specific information than we are able to cover in the catalog. Our main criteria for including books was our judgement of their worth in aiding work in a community. Hopefully more and more books in the future will be suggested by you—the people who need them and use them. Not all prices are listed, and some are very expensive. Ask your local library to find the book for you through their resources or inter-library loans. These loans can be extended to make all libraries in your state open to you. Legal journals can generally be found in university libraries. A few of the books and magazines will be in medical school libraries.

FILMS AND TAPES. . . are a dependable means for bringing people together, raising consciousness, providing income, and spreading the word; however, unlike our book research, our film research was not extensive. The films and tapes with longer reviews were ones we've seen or were recommended by reliable people. But most of the reviews are taken from PR blurbs.

CONTENTS. . . the catalog was designed to put people in touch with projects and resources and to encourage the building of creative new working relationship among people. Group listings have addresses and usually phone numbers; resources have publishers' or distributors' names and addresses. Individual people's names have not been included except when necessary in the address because our struggle is not built on personalities.

The cross-referencing in sections is very important to note since so many concepts in health are interrelated. Cross-referencing was a way of saving space through avoiding repetition.

When contacting groups, try to include stamps for return information, and when calling for information or to see if a visit is possible, don't call collect; groups that don't rely on big funding sources must be supported by the people's ideas, energy—and money, when we have it.

Due to what is called the "paper shortage," the paper companies have raised the price of all grades of paper and have stopped carrying the cheapest grades. Thus, a month before our deadline, we found out that the price would be doubled. This trend has ominous implications for radical and subsistance publishers. In the future Source will be reevaluating the whole idea of catalogs, since high prices will exclude many of the people we hope to reach.

It's hard for us to think of the catalog without thinking about what was cut. Our space constraints were rigid and some sections were cut to less than half their original size—a painful process. There are many good groups and resources that could not be included.

What you have in your hands is the result of many dreams, disappointments and lost sleep. It is not a Sears Catalog of emotionless products designed by technicians, but a revolution in action. If we are helpful, tell us how; if we aren't, tell us why and what might be better. Source is a book now, but you are the real source. In the struggle. . .

the source collective.

rather the result of a highly organized and effective system—one based on making money for the providers of health care, not on keeping the people of this country healthy. The hospitals and medical centers which form the central core of this complex make huge amounts of money from our inflated health care costs. Support industries like insurance, drug, and supply companies all profit tremendously from their relationship to the institutions. Banks also reap immense profits from the selling of medical care, through investment into the system, interest on loans, etc., while construction companies are making a killing from the excess expansion of the industry. The funds going into these profits are diverting needed resources away from good preventive and ambulatory care.

The government, too, has been instrumental in this whole process. It has cut off millions of dollars of social welfare funds within the past two years, and has poured millions of dollars into private industry to pick up its abandoned health projects. These subsidies have happened with little overview and poor, unenforced regulations on how public money was to be spent.

The providers' monopoly on health education and skills is almost as great as their monopoly of facilities. Most of us are pitifully ignorant about our own bodies, having been taught that this knowledge is the exclusive domain of professionals with years of training. We are denied a voice in the

decisions that affect our health care, let alone control of health facilities. If this is to change, we must begin to challenge our internalized attitudes and values that tell us to rely on "experts" rather than trusting our own feelings and experiences.

In researching this catalogue, we have discovered a growing anger among the victims of this "illness" care system, as people become aware of the profit motive behind it. We have seen the strength of old people, women, workers, students, Third World people, and the middle class as they strive to gain control over their own bodies and the health care resources in their communities. The challenge has come in a number of ways. Whole communities are building coalitions to challenge hospital policy and establish community-controlled clinics as an alternative to impersonal government or provider-sponsored ones. Women across the country are joining a growing self-help movement based on a rejection of White, male, professional domination of medical knowledge about women's bodies.

Institutions are being challenged directly by both the workers and patients, while health science students are fighting the senseless regimentation of their minds. Old people, mental patients, prisoners, workers faced with occupational disease, and Third World people are demanding their rights and learning new ways of working with and helping one another. The catalogue hopes to give a sense of the spirit of the fight, as well as practical ways each of us can join in.

COMMUNITY HEALTH ORGANIZING

PROBLEM

All our lives, we have heard the claim that US citizens are the healthiest, best-cared-for people in the world. For most of us, this is simply not true. Health care in this country is both inaccessible and cripplingly expensive. Even those of us who can summon up the strength, determination, and financial resources required to locate health care find that our needs are not being met by the present health care delivery system.

People seeking health care face a maze of fragmented, specialized services. At best there is a demoralizing array of different offices, doctors, and labels, sometimes widely separated. At worst, specialization focuses on specific problems to the detriment of the whole person. One doctor puzzled for months over the deterioration of a woman patient's kidney. Only after it had been removed did he learn that another doctor (a heart specialist) had been giving her medicine known to be hard on the kidneys.

The pervasive specialization of medicine extends to government programs, confronting those who depend on them with a frustrating jig-saw puzzle of partial responses to their needs. One rural health worker condemns government programs that "may be concerned with contraception,. . .but cannot pay to keep [a woman] alive by excising her cervical cancer, so that she can survive to enjoy the benefits of planning her family."

Along with fragmentation goes mystification—the assumption that only the doctor understands anything about the patient's situation, that only the doctor is capable of such understanding. Patients rarely receive explanations of their condition, or of the various options for treatment. Most doctors prefer to imply that their knowledge is complete and there is no element of gamble or trial-and-error. Patients are treated as children. This is especially true of Third World people and women. A medical system dominated by White male doctors cannot avoid reflecting the racism and sexism of the culture. The problems of non-English-speaking people are especially acute, since many facilities do not provide translators, even in areas where

many people speak Spanish or other languages. For example, a Spanish-speaking mother, taking an injured child to the emergency room of a large city hospital, was repeatedly shifted to the end of the line while an interpreter was sought in another part of the hospital. By the end of the day, no interpreter had been found; she was told to take the child home and return the next day if she wished.

For many, rural people and the urban poor in particular, health care is not only inadequate but physically out of reach. Those facilities that do exist are understaffed and over-crowded. Milwaukee County Hospital is one example. The only source of medical care for tens of thousands of poor and working people, it is sixteen miles outside the city—often an hour and a half bus ride away. In Louisiana, community workers are struggling to organize local health centers for sugar cane workers. Though the state has a network of charity hospitals, most cane workers have neither automobiles nor money for other transportation, so medical care remains totally inaccessible. A county hospital in Portland, Oregon not long ago had a six month waiting list for appointments at the psychiatric clinic, a four month wait at the eye clinic, and a three month wait at the hematology (blood) and neurology (brain and nervous system) clinics. Working people may lose a half-day or full day's work in reaching a doctor's office or clinic and waiting their turn; the lost pay adds to the already heavy expense. Poor people may arrive at a public clinic at 9 in the morning and be seen by a harried doctor at 5 pm—or be told to return the next day.

Even when modern, well-staffed and equpped facilities are located near areas of need, there is no guarantee that health care will be provided. Hospitals are often more interested in teaching and research than providing basic patient care. Their funds go toward prestigious and "professionally interesting" specialties rather than the major needs of community people. In the present system, such priority decisions belong entirely to the hospital; the community has no voice at all. Thus, as The American Health Empire points out, "in a city studded with major hospitals, the person with multiple bullet wounds or a rare and fatal blood disease stands a far better chance of making a successful medical 'connection,' than the person with stomach pains, or the parents of a feverish child."

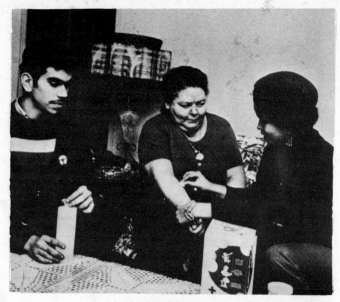

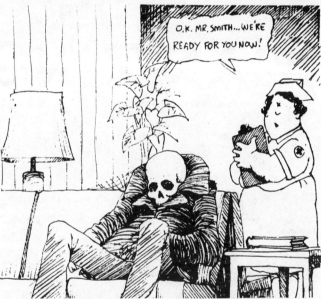

O.K. MR. SMITH...WE'RE READY FOR YOU NOW!

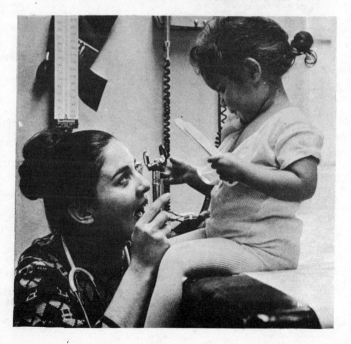

The situation is made worse by the shortage of doctors and other health personnel, and their concentration in affluent areas. On Chicago's wealthy North Side, one medical building has more doctors than the entire West Side ghetto of 300,000 people.

But even when health care is physically available, the cost puts it out of many people's reach. The average cost of a day in a US hospital doubled between 1962 and 1970. Prices for medicine, laboratory work, and doctor's visits have followed not far behind. Today, even middle class families are financially devastated by one serious illness. As medical costs rise, insurance costs skyrocket; more and more people find themselves caught without health coverage— too poor to pay health bills or rising insurance rates, too rich for Medicaid, too young for Medicare. Those supposedly covered by government programs may find legislatures (in New York in 1968, for example) reacting to rising medical costs by slashing Medicaid funding, leaving the poor to fend for themselves.

As costs rise, more and more people must turn to public health facilities for low cost or free care. So the waiting time gets longer, the doctors more brusque, and the treatment more inadequate. All pretense of early treatment of preventive health disappears; only crisis care is available, and the emergency room becomes the primary source of health care for many people. For others, in rural areas or some cities, even that much is simply not to be found.

The present health care system is concerned with symptoms of illness, not with the conditions that create good health. As long as people are trapped in situations harmful to their physical and emotional well-being, this curative approach will be inadequate. City dwellers breathing polluted air, children in houses covered with lead paint, poor people with no money for nutritious food need a change in their living conditions, not a doctor's prescription.

Recognition of the failings of the health system leaves most people with a feeling of helplessness. It is a system directed by professionals and large, prestigious institutions. Patients are not expected to provide any input beyond sick bodies and cold cash. Doctors and health institutions are in most cases resistant to the mildest forms of consumer participation, not to mention control of health facilities by the communities they supposedly exist to serve.

All these problems extend far beyond the local community. The exclusive nature of the medical profession is involved; the training provided in medical schools and the process of selecting students; the banks, drug companies and builders who profit from hospitals and other health institutions; federal policy and those who influence it.

But it is in local communities that work for change must begin—where people are directly confronted with the realization that, although the health industry is organized to efficiently produce profits, this country has no effective system of providing decent health care.

3

PLATFORM

A SYSTEM OF CONTINUOUS PREVENTIVE HEALTH CARE MUST BE ESTABLISHED BY:

1. Revamping federal food programs to provide community access to nutritious foods without additives.
2. Sending out mobile clinics or teams to do door-to-door well-baby care and well-person care, including periodic screenings, physical exams, and immunizations.
3. Establishing community health education programs through local organizations, clubs, schools, and workplaces. These programs should discuss physical and mental needs and functions in a clear, complete way, including such topics as sex, nutrition and drugs.
4. Providing community outreach workers, particularly in isolated rural areas, to train families in nutrition, child care, sanitation, and basic home health care: first aid, care for common ailments, etc.
5. Beginning the struggle against environmental health hazards such as lead paint poisoning, air and water pollution.

COMPREHENSIVE, UNFRAGMENTED, PERSONALIZED HEALTH CARE MUST BE MADE ACCESSIBLE TO ALL COMMUNITY MEMBERS BY:

1. Providing health care to all people regardless of income.
2. Establishing medical teams of health personnel who are non-judging and receptive to the individual's needs, life-style, and problems. They should also be committed to changing the causes of ill health rather than just treating symptoms.
3. Fully explaining all medical procedures and, when more than one course of treatment is available, respecting the patient's right to an informed choice.
4. Giving each community member the right to choose her/his own medical team and health center.
5. Monitoring health care delivery through statistics, patient criticism, and regular staff and staff-community meetings; setting up advocacy programs in health centers. Advocates should also accompany patients to the hospital, if necessary.

6. Providing mobile medical teams for rural areas equipped for rough travel and emergencies.
7. Providing mobile medical teams for urban areas to care for elderly, handicapped, and those too sick for travel but who don't require hospitalization.
8. Establishing a network of centrally-located urban and rural community health centers.
9. Providing a physician or medical team at each center available at all times for emergency care.
10. Developing a crisis hotline for community members which can handle counseling, emergency, and informational calls, including hospital referrals.
11. Providing support, personnel, supplies, equipment, and back-up services for community health centers from local hospitals, medical schools, and other health institutions.
12. Providing regular staff people who share the languages and culture of the community.
13. Providing staff people whose attitudes are non-sexist, non-racist, and non-elitist.
14. Providing neighborhood day care centers to allow adults to use health care facilities.

COMMUNITY-WORKER CONTROL OF HEALTH CARE SERVICES AND DELIVERY MUST BE ESTABLISHED BY:

1. Electing consumer-worker boards of directors for health centers with the power to make policy and monetary decisions: staff elected from among all those employed at the center, by all those employed; consumers elected from among community members using the center or in the area served by the center.
2. Hiring health workers from working class, low-income, and minority communities wherever and whenever possible; training unskilled community members to fill positions from outreach workers to doctors and administrators; forcing local health training schools to draw students from working class, low-income, and minority communities.

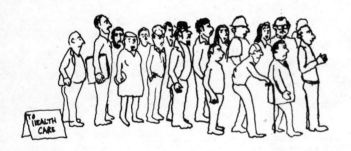

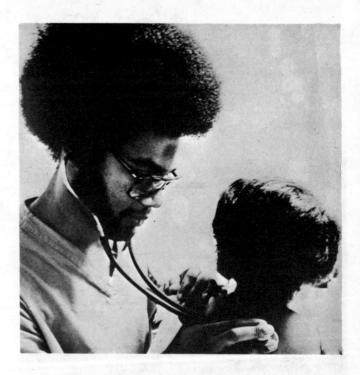

PROGRAM

BROADEN community support and participation:
—use local media to publicize results of your research (which should be on-going) or put out your own publication
—call public meetings in the community
—plan larger demands and actions around your priorities, such as emergency room care, etc.—keep in mind that individual projects can reinforce each other
—meet with health facility staff and workers to gain support from them—two against one is always better, and besides, health workers' and patients' suffering often stem from the same source.

MOVE on your demands: which programs you choose, or which come first, will depend on the conditions of the community and the concerns of its people
—fight for hospital and government funding to pay for mobile units and paid staff to continue screening programs in communities
—publicize the results of these programs and push for follow-up treatment—for example, in lead paint poisoning, fight for a system of half-way houses as a temporary measure to protect children from returning to an infected environment, and push for enforcement of housing codes
—organize your own community clinic—use it to challenge the existing system by demonstrating the needs that the system does not meet and by pressuring hospitals for back-up services—use it as a model of personalized, comprehensive health care in a radical context by training community people in basic health skills, by including programs on health politics, by operating collectively, by challenging sexist, racist, and professional attitudes in the clinic and by providing care free or on a pay-as-you can basis
—organize a patient/hospital advocate program for those in the community forced to visit clinics and hospitals
—demand that local care facilities include transportation costs when computing fees; develop transport systems for rural areas and isolated urban neighborhoods
—elect a community board to represent you and demand that members be given equal place on existing health facility boards of directors
—study the cost and quality of treatment at local out-patient departments, Health Maintenance Organizations, private practices, free clinics—publish the results for the community
—demand the hiring of community people to act as translators in health facilities
—begin a food campaign—work to increase participation on the local food stamp program—push schools, child care centers, and community houses to institute free meal programs

RESEARCH Your community:
—do surveys to learn what issues people feel most strongly about—collect community grievances and document abuses in the local health institutions—determine the need for health services not currently provided for
—locate local health education and preventive medicine programs
—find the number and types of health care services available in the community and who controls them
—unravel the local power structure—who is on the board of directors of health facilities, pharmaceutical companies and insurance companies; who are the politicians, businesspeople, and professionals influential in the area and why
—document the extent of malnutrition and delve into the local administration and abuses of federal food programs
—research patients' rights and learn your community's most pressing concerns. (See also Hospitals section.)

ORGANIZE:
—hold a gathering of local community people (you should have a few staunch supporters already, drawn from your work)
—exchange ideas and information on your research
—start with projects that are within your abilities; a success in the beginning will raise morale and help build a strong group. For example: organize a health fair to bring together community members. Distribute information, and do necessary preventive health screening and testing—use it to educate the community—push health facilities to follow up on the needs your research uncovered—start a hotline or create a directory to give people the necessary information on what services are available—their cost and quality.
—begin a food campaign—work to increase participation on the local food stamp program—push schools, child care centers, and community houses to institute free meal programs for children, group and delivered meals for the elderly and ill
—organize a food co-op—use it to buy in bulk, as an alternative to the high-priced items in the supermarket—begin teaching people about nutrition and the dangers of most food additives

CONTINUE planning:
—work towards full community/worker representation on all health facility policy boards
—fight for training programs for community members as health personnel and for hiring of staff from among the community (see Health Personnel and Training)
—fight for stronger environmental pollution laws and demand better enforcement of present laws
—demand a network of community clinics offering comprehensive medical services
—institute and enlarge health education and preventive medicine programs for schools, homes and workplaces

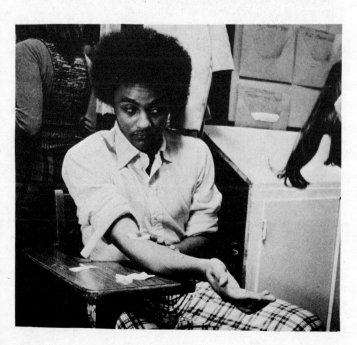

RESEARCH AND ORGANIZING

The first step in challenging the present health system is understanding how it functions in our local communities. It is important to know who is on the Board of Directors of the local clinic or hospital—and more important to know how wealthy those people are, how they make their money, what other boards they sit on, what interests they represent. The number of contractors or hospital supplies manufacturers on a hospital board, for example, may be very educational. Laws and the violation of laws need to be checked out—from local ordinances on lead paint to federal regulations requiring community representatives on the boards of government-funded projects. Research in the form of surveys and digging out official statistics can clarify community needs while a close look at the local government power structure can help determine tactics and pressure points. Solid research should undergird every stage of an ongoing organizing effort.

Often, too, research results can be publicized through both radical and regular public media. Let the community know about corruption, apathy, conflicts of interest, profit margins and neglected human needs. Power-holders have good reason to be leary of publicity that exposes their shenanigans. Publicity hampers their ability to maneuver, opens the possibility of legal challenges, and by raising community ire lends energy to organizing. It removes the mask of respectability worn by politicians and—especially—by the health care industry, and so paves the way for change.

This section focuses on resources for local community research. Projects researching specific issues such as insurance or drug companies are listed in the following chapters.

Finding Community: A Guide to Community Research and Action, W. Ron Jones. James E. Freel and Assoc., 577 College Ave., Palo Alto, CA 94306, 1971. 217 pp. $4.95 . . .assails the manipulations of urban corporate enterprise in selling practices and credit abuses, corporate medicine, the police, the warfare economy, housing. Well researched indictments introduce each section, followed by action investigation guides and readings on alternative institutions that answer the problems raised by the old. A good reader in local institutional muckraking.

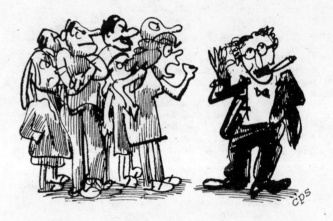

Where It's At: A Research Guide for Community Organizing, Jill Hamberg. New England Free Press, 60 Union Square, Sommerville, MA 02143, 1967. 91 pp. $.95. . .explains where to learn the why's, who's, and wherefore's of local government, business, and industry and of health legal and welfare systems. The health section gives an excellent outline of questions to ask, resources, and general directions for communities organizing around health. A good guide to discovering the hidden super-powers ruling your community. Two other New England Free Press articles are also included in the packet: "The Care and Feeding of Power Structures," by Jack Minnis, and "Researching the Governing Class of America: a Guide to Sources."

Studying Your Community, Roland L. Warren. Free Press/ MacMillan, 866 Third Ave., New York, NY 10022, 1955. 385 pp. $2.95. . .an exhaustive aid for the organizer or journalist undertaking a "total" community study—including how to conduct a community survey and a smattering of example charts and maps. References to books and organizations and up to 200 prying questions in each chapter, are leads to uncovering the functions of housing, communications, economic life, etc. Though devoid of any political context, " Studying Your Community" is without question, the most comprehensive book in its field for lay people. It is applicable to "highly urban as well as highly rural communities."

NACLA Research Methodology Guide, North American Congress on Latin America, PO Box 57, Cathedral Park Station, New York, NY 10025, 1970. 72 pp. $1.00 . . .recommends power-structure research to those without power in order to identify the people and institutions which make our lives intolerable, locate weak points in the system, and suggest a strategy for resistance. NACLA urges the study of Political Parties, Corporations, the University-Military—Industrial Complex, Police, The Health Industry, and Imperialism. We need to understand the structures we're fighting—a valuable tool.

Organizing requires a whole range of skills. There is the initial process of defining needs, drawing a group together, and building people's confidence in their ability to make change. There are technical skills ranging from bookkeeping to fundraising or writing a press release. There is the challenging task of choosing tactics, evaluating their success, and developing new ones when necessary.

The last ten years has produced many resources that allow us to draw on the combined knowledge and creativity that make successful organizers. The resources in this section are packed with tips on everything from running a meeting to negotiating with local power structures. Group dynamics, tactics from demonstrations to elections and court-cases, and the personal insights of long-time community workers are all included. Such resources are one of the prime ways the movement can share its strengths and cut down on the repetition of old mistakes.

ORGANIZERS BOOK CENTER . . . distributes by mail the books listed on these pages, as well as other, more specific organizing material. A spin-off of Source, OBC exists to make organizing resources more widely known and available. Other books carried cover such areas as cable TV, tenant organizing, community schools, and women's organizing. Write for listings. Contact ORGANIZERS BOOK CENTER, PO Box 21066, Washington, D.C. 20009, (202) 387-1145.

The Organizer's Manual, O.M. Collective. Bantam Books, 666 Fifth Ave., New York, NY 10019, 1971. 368 pp. $1.25
. . . an all-round organizing tool touching on almost every question a project or issue organizer could have—from the details of putting out a leaflet to using establishment struc-

How People Get Power: Organizing Oppressed Communities for Action, Si Kahn. McGraw-Hill, New York, NY, 1970. 128 pp. $2.45. . .speaks directly to the organizer in a rural community. The organizer can be effective only when the poor become their own leaders. "How People Get Power" gives a step by step progression from the time the organizer analyses and enters a community, develops the poor people's organization and introduces various power tactics, until she or he finally leaves satisfied that the community can direct and handle its new power. Unusually insightful.

The Organizer's Library Series, Southern Conference Educational Fund, Inc. 3210 W. Broadway, Louisville KY 40211, 1967. About 85 pp. $2.75. . .a classic set of seven pamphlets that have guided groups from the draft movement to recent political collectives. Titles include "Getting and Keeping People Together;" "The Care and Feeding of Power Structures Revisited;" "How to Put Out Community Newspapers;" "How to Negotiate;" and three others.

Dynamics of Group Action, D.M. Hall. The Interstate, Danville, FL, 1964. 243 pp. $4.75
. . .a guide to effective intra-group relations: "The success of any group will depend on individual abilities but it will also depend upon how skillful it becomes in solving its problems and in regulating, strengthening, and perpetuating group interactions." "Dynamics of Group Action" tackles What Holds Us Together, Problem Solving Steps, and Group Maturity. Any group, from the PTA to a political collective will recognize some of the personalities and problems described here, and can learn from the advice it gives.

tures. Encompasses self-education; building alternative structures (youth services, medical clinics, etc.); forms of group action; legal and medical protection; and suggestions on constituency organizing. Designed for persons committed to long term political/social/economic change. Given the number of topics discussed, coverage is sometimes limited, but it offers an exciting array of ideas.

Rules for Radicals: A Pragmatic Primer for Realistic Radicals, Saul Alinsky, Vintage, 201 E. 50th St., New York, NY 10022, 1971. 196 pp. $1.95
..."The Prince" was written by Maciavelli for the Haves on how to hold power. "Rules for Radicals" is written for the Have-Nots on how to take it away." Throughout the book is advice: "Remember: once you organize people around something as commonly agreed upon as pollution, then an organized people is on the move. From there it is a short and natural step to political pollution, to Pentagon pollution." Alinsky mixes his experiences and the experiences of other famous and infamous organizers into a flowing text for "realistic radicals."

Storefront Organizing: A Mornin 'Glories' Manual, Sam W. Brown, Jr. Pyramid Publishers, 9 Garden St., Moonachie, NJ 07074, 1972. 142 pp. $1.45. . .is especially important for those organizing in urban areas around mass appeal issues or electoral candidates. Covers storefront organizing, fundraising, the press, canvassing, and Election Day, and each section communicates valuable tricks of the trade proven by the experience of an organizer who has "been there" in campaigns for peace, McCarthy, and others. It has the best material we have seen on fundraising without depending on foundations, large corporations, or the government.

The Community Activist's Handbook: A Guide for Citizen Leaders and Planners, John Huenefeld. Beacon Press, 25 Beacon St., Boston MA 02108, 1970. 160 pp.
. . .how to make a community campaign—whether project-oriented or electoral—dramatic, suspenseful, and fun. A high degree of organization, pre-planning, and creativity are the ingredients of such programs.

A Public Citizen's Action Manual, Donald Ross, Grossman Publishers, 625 Madison Ave., New York, NY 10019, 1973. 237 pp. $1.95
. . .About 35 different ways to get involved are discussed, from citizen hearings, to occupational safety and health projects; from investigating sex discrimination in employment agencies to tax action and consumer protection. The issues behind each project are outlined and tactics briefly reviewed. The book ends by describing the Citizen Action Group, an organization of full-time professionals, volunteers and on-the-job citizens protecting the public interest.

Contemporary Films, McGraw Hill, Princeton Rd., Hightstown, NJ 08520; 828 Custer Ave., Evanston, IL 60202; 1714 Stockton St., San Francisco, CA 94133

"People and Power," 17 min. b&w 1968 $12.00 Conflict and controversy are an integral part of Saul Alinsky's approach to organizing communities. Here he talks about his philosophy and the dynamics of organization.

"A Continuing Responsibility," 42 min. b&w 1968 $16 As demonstrated by the Woodlawn Organization in Chicago, Saul Alinsky's technique creates on-going organizations firmly rooted in the community.

COMMUNITY CLINICS AND HEALTH CENTERS

In many communities the institutions and personpower for the delivery of health care do not exist. Often people must travel far from home to find the care they need. Finding facilities where health personel are helpful and unpatronizing is even more of a problem, especially in low-income areas.

Community clinics and health centers are a step towards a solution to this problem. They cover a wide spectrum from free clinics to health centers offering family care, but the concept common to all of them is local control. The well-being of the people, not the profits of individuals, is the motivating force behind community clinics, because they are controlled by the people they serve. Although people differ on how much control workers should have in making policy decisions, eventually the division between community member and health worker can be eliminated by training and hiring health workers from the community.

There are many benefits inherent in community/worker controlled health facilities. Care is more readily accessible because facilities are located within easy reach of all community members and because the patronizing racist and sexist attitudes that often discourage people from seeking care can be dissipated. Outreach work, preventive screening and health education is easier to deliver because a whole geographic area is involved and because workers are natives of area: when they try to teach their neighbors about health, they have the advantage of being accepted, of knowing how to speak without using medical jargon, and of understanding the many barriers to good health that exist in the culture and environment of the area.

A community/worker controlled health center, however, is not easy to create. In many communities there is already a clinic which is controlled by the local government or hospital. In this situation, people must demand more community representation in decision-making, more training programs to distribute skills to community members, and more hiring of those in the community who already have skills. Thus clinic workers and community members must join together to take control of the clinic into their own hands.

In communities where there is no health facility, people must either demand help in building one from the local health department or hospital, or rely on other outside help. Free clinics often rely on sympathetic health workers and private organizations to volunteer time, equipment, and money. Often, though, this dependence becomes a trap. Volunteers need have no commitment to the clinic; they may be unreli-

able or hold patronizing attitudes and the community is helpless to control them; after all, they are offering their help as a favor. Since volunteers must support themselves through other jobs, clinics that rely on them are limited in the hours they can operate. Funding from foundations, grants, and the government may tend to limit the clinic by consciously or unconsciously influencing its attitudes and political stands. Many clinics, however, have developed good relationships with progressive church affiliates and private foundations, finding this type of funding to be an adequate short-term financing plan.

Some communities have arranged for financing through patient payments, either as a fee or donation, through third-party payments such as Medicaid and Blue Cross, or on a monthly pre-payment basis (see also "pre-paid plans" under Health Planning section). This arrangement allows the center to pay its staff and remain open for as long as necessary. It also leaves the center free to challenge local health facilities and do political education without fear that funding will be withdrawn. However, in poor communities people often cannot pay even low health fees and eventually the community is forced whether to fight for government funding with "no strings attached" or to subsidize the poor by charging others more. Part of the solution to this problem is for people to take more control of their local government. Then they can put their tax monies into those areas most important to the community, such as health.

Some serious political criticisms have been levelled against community clinics and health centers, particularly those that are content to provide services, rather than seeing the clinic as a step towards a more total change in the health system. Rather than moving towards a strong position for demanding and fighting for a community health facility that meets the needs of the community and which is supported by money already taken out of the community (like taxes), these clinics patch people up until their next sickness, making no demands upon health care delivery system, but instead relieve some of the pressures on the health institutions by doing their job for them. Such clinics and health centers often do not even provide preventive health education, not to mention political education. Such a facility is serving a need in the community, but when it closes because its doctors are unable to come that night or because its funding source has run dry, the community is no closer to obtaining good medical care than it was before. Meanwhile doctors who volunteer at the clinic continue their lucrative small private practices, maintaining traditional doctor-staff-patient roles.

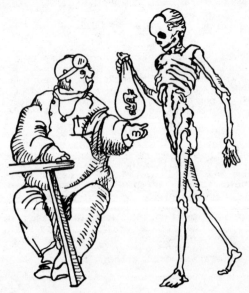

The question of who controls a community clinic is of major importance. While the community must have a major degree of control over policies, the amount of input health workers have in these decisions is debatable. Some clinics prohibit workers from being members of decision-making bodies, feeling that many health workers are "professionals" whose interests conflict with those of the community. They believe that the health workers who could contribute most to policy decisions are those working directly with patients, but that most of those workers are native to the community and are therefore already represented on the community board. Many clinics, are controlled only by those working and contributing to the facility. The feeling in these clinics is that concerned community members will give their time to the clinic and will earn the right to participate on a policy board by showing that they have a real commitment to the community. Ideally, a large proportion of the workers in a community health care center should be community members whose main interests are in delivering good health care. Yet many health workers will still be drawn from outside the community and in many cases the ideas of health workers will conflict with those of community representatives. These facts make a strong case for both workers and community input into all decisions relevant to the community health center.

A new health center can demonstrate to people what good health care should be; it may be a necessity for keeping the community alive while pushing for change of the whole system, but it should never be an end in itself. Behind community-care is hospital care and more specialized regional care; these too must be made more responsive to the needs of the people. There also remain the fee-for-service professionals, the big drug industries, and the medical supply companies which can force the price of health care to rise out of the reach of the community no matter how care is financed. Building a community health facility is only the beginning.

NATIONAL FREE CLINIC COUNCIL...acts as a funding channel and information disseminator, and an educational resource for free clinics. Most of their funds come through the National Institute of Mental Health and the White House Special Action Office for Drug Abuse Prevention, and are earmarked for outstanding drug abuse programs. They feel that federal funds do not limit a project any more than foundation funds and have participated in federally sponsored National Drug Abuse Council conferences, and in the Federation of Concerned Drug Abuse Workers. Another recent project was a national conference on free clinic health to discuss national legislation and problems on local levels. In the future they plan to obtain federal funds for general free clinic use on the basis that free clinics function as "total human service/care agencies." Contact NATIONAL FREE CLINIC COUNCIL, 1304 Haight St., San Francisco, CA 94117, 415-864-6232.

SOUTH WEST FREE CLINIC COUNCIL...was formed a year ago to meet the regional needs that clinics in the area felt could not be resolved by a national organization. The Council is a loose-knit coalition of clinics from Louisiana, Arkansas, Texas, Oklahoma, New Mexico, Arizona, and Nevada. One current project is a directory of the forty clinics in the Southwest, compiling information on each one's relationship with its community. A training program is being established to exchange workers so that each clinic benefits from others' experiences. HEW's Task Force on Youth has given some technical assistance. SWFCC also helps individual clinics to get needed supplies. SWFCC represents an encouraging step in maintaining the decentralized nature of free clinic services. Contact SWFCC, c/o Ted Ochs, 1130 N. Rampart St., New Orleans, LA 70116, 504-524-1446.

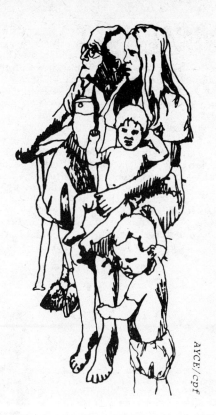

AYCE/cpf

POOR AND WORKING CLASS CLINICS

TWENTY-SEVENTH STREET PEOPLE'S FREE HEALTH CENTER . . . is a three-year-old health service in a low-income, working class neighborhood of Milwaukee. It is a family clinic for a stable patient group with heavy emphasis on education, preventive care, and the politics of health delivery in the city. Open one night a week and two Saturdays a month, the clinic offers screening for high blood pressure and VD, and runs special gynecological and weight-watchers clinics. The small staff strives to share skills and eliminate traditional hierarchies. They are in the process of starting a dental clinic. Twenty-seventh Street was instrumental in forcing the re-opening of the Downtown Medical Services, the only city health facility in this section of Milwaukee, and has been active in the City-Wide Health Consumers Coalition. They are fighting for free screening and testing in local hospitals, hiring of interpreters and more consumer participation in health delivery. Contact TWENTY-SEVENTH STREET PFHC, 1409 N. 27th St., Rm. 204, Milwaukee, WI 53208, (414) 344-5141.

PEOPLE'S FREE CLINIC/BURLINGTON. . .began in August, 1971, when a group of people who believe in free, high-quality personalized health care for all came together to make changes in the health care system. The clinic's all-volunteer staff of forty stresses health education, preventive care, and lobbying to obtain more responsive care from other institutions. They also run about two six-month paramedic training programs each year. Since the clinic is in a fairly low-populated area, they have more time than most city clinics to do in-depth patient care and education. BirthWork, which operates out of the clinic, educates and gives pre-natal care to pregnant women planning on home birth. A Birth-Work person is also present at the delivery. Open three nights the People's Free Clinic serves up to 60 people each week. Contact PEOPLE'S FREE CLINIC, 260 North St., Burlington, VT 05401, (802) 864-6309.

NEAR WEST SIDE PEOPLE'S FREE CLINIC . . . started out as part of West Side Citizens for Better Health, Inc., (WSCBH) as an alternative to the bureaucratic, professionally controlled city health care clinic. The staff was drawn out of the community when possible, and clinic decisions are made in joint staff/community meetings. Patients' advocates on the staff act as liasons between medical professionals and the patient and do lab work. Some are trained by a feminist collective to do birth control and abortion counseling. Two nights a week the clinic is open by appointment and on Wednesdays there is either a specialty clinic (podiatry, gynecology, orthopedics) or a well-person clinic staffed by RNs and nurse practitioners. All clinic-prescribed x-rays, labwork, and medicines are donated by a nearby hospital. The clinic hopes to force local and city hospitals to establish a network of neighborhood health satellites backed by area health centers and staffed by paid advocates and nurse practitioners. Contact NWSPC, 1965 West 44th, Cleveland, OH 44113, (216) 281-4242.

er projects center around the red tape of hospitals. At a local children's hospital emergency room the clinic pressured for the establishment of sliding scale payments on people's first hospital visits. The hospital had been charging a flat fee for first visits and waited until second visits to establish sliding scale fees. Contact FEHC, 2751 N. Wilton, Chicago, IL 60614, 312-750-9408.

FAIR HAVEN COMMUNITY HEALTH CENTER...is located in a low-income inner city neighborhood of New Haven. A group of community residents founded the clinic in 1971 as an alternative to the inaccessible health system of New Haven. They have a large volunteer staff plus workers paid by VISTA, OEO, National Free Clinic Council, and other sources. The clinic's goal is to be a primary health care center, including necessary transportation, language translation, screening programs, and preventive health education. Policy is set by a board composed of patients, staff and community people. Contact FHCHC, 388 Grand Ave., New Haven, CT 06513, 203-777-3704.

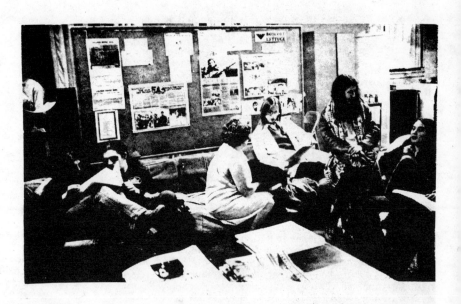

FRITZI ENGLESTEIN HEALTH CENTER...is in Lincoln Park, a low-income White and Chicano area of Chicago, and grew out of the struggle between a community group called Concerned Citizens of Lincoln Park, and a local hospital. When the hospital received urban renewal land for expansion, the community group demanded an area free clinic in return. The hospital finally agreed to the program, sending in doctors and nurses to supplement community volunteers and backing the clinic with lab and x-ray services. There have been serious conflicts since then, but the community group kept the pressure on. In 1972, the clinic became a program of a new Chicago political organization, Rising Up Angry. Operating three nights a week, the clinic offers general medical services and some lab work with funds from Medicaid and Medicare and the proceeds from dinners, fairs, and dances. The staff is all volunteer and includes an active patient advocate system. Recognizing the importance of environment in health, the clinic did a major project on lead paint poisoning and housing, modeling their program on the limited Chicago Board of Health program. This demonstrated how many cases had been untouched, and it forced the Board of Health to expand its program. They also successfully challenged the inadequate Board policy on analyzing house paint for lead content. Oth-

CHICO NEIGHBORHOOD HEALTH CENTER...began in 1972 as a city-funded free clinic for students at nearby University of California at Davis. However, as the staff became more aware of the needs of the Chico community and the problems created by the county closing down its public health hospital and health center, they began to actively discourage student use and to build community support. The Center is now open on weekdays, offering primary health care in the following areas: TB, VD, and Rubella testing, general medical care, birth control counseling, obstetrics, a family clinic with pediatrics, and pregnancy counseling. If a pregnant woman wants an abortion, she is referred to the Oakland Feminist Women's Health Collective; those who continue their pregnancy are sent to a local obstetrician. Right now only some of the staff are paid but the Center will be employing three full-time doctors with University and foundation funding in the fall. Their goal is to pay all their workers and to encourage more community people to join the staff which functions as a collective. The Center focuses on serving low-income people of Chico's south side. They publicize their services in free TV spots, at PTA meetings, and through school nurses. Currently operating on city revenue sharing funds, they will be trying for county money soon, as well as HEW grants. Contact CHICO NEIGHBORHOOD HEALTH CENTER, PO Box 3222, Chico, CA 95926, 916-345-9104.

THIRD WORLD CLINICS

BENITO JUAREZ PEOPLE'S HEALTH CENTER...was started in 1970 by community residents and young professionals to provide primary health care to their low income Chicano area. Open three days a week, and staffed by 8-10 volunteer doctors, nurses, and patients' advocates, the center provides most routine laboratory work, a pharmacy, and a well-baby clinic for about 150 patients a week. In order to "educate the people while challenging the system," the clinic teaches simple testing and translates health information into Spanish. Patients' advocates take each person's history, act as interpreters, and accompany patients to the hospital if necessary. This practice gained the clinic a measure of recognition from Cook County Hospital; though formerly quite unresponsive, the hospital offered to hire three people from the center to set up an advocate system for the hospital. The center now

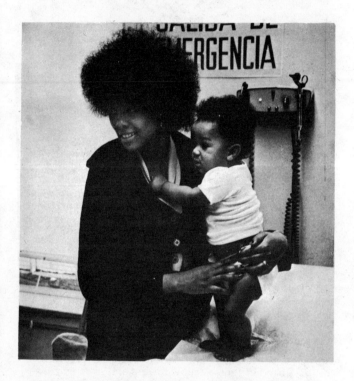

hopes to work out a referral system with the hospital. As with many all-volunteer clinics, rapid staff turnover is one of their worst problems. But they are more fortunate than most in terms of funding: demonstrations aimed at HEW and the University of Illinois during the election year of '72 brought them enough HEW funds to keep going for 2 more years. Contact BENITO JUAREZ PEOPLE'S HEALTH CENTER, 1831 S. Racine Ave., Chicago, IL 60608, 312-733-4381.

GEORGE JACKSON FREE CLINIC. . .was opened in 1971 as a program of the San Francisco Black Panther Party. Seven doctors and 10-15 other professional and community members volunteer their time to staff the clinic, providing pediatrics, VD, and general medical services. They are beginning hypertension screening on an outreach basis, but their main thrust is sickle cell anemia testing and counseling. By creating a comprehensive medical clinic, the Panthers hope to expose the contradictions between racist attitudes and treatment in the established health care delivery system and the personal treatment of a human-oriented health care system. The long-range goal is to get people to speak out against this contradiction and demand their human rights. Contact GEORGE JACKSON FREE CLINIC, 3236 Adeline, Berkeley, CA 94703, (415) 653-2534.

NORTH EAST NEIGHBORHOOD ASSOCIATION HEALTH CENTER...is a vigorous community-initiated and community-controlled project, in existence since 1966 and still growing. Located in a ghetto area about 75% Puerto Rican, with a sizeable minority of Blacks and a scattering of Jews, Poles, and other Whites, the NENA Center grew out of a harsh awareness of the inaccessability of health care. A transit strike in '66 left Lower East Side residents effectively cut off from Bellevue Hospital, the only source of general medical care for the area. Instances resulting from the lack of transportation, such as the near-death of a child during an asthmatic attack, roused community anger, which found focus in a determination to have health facilities available in their own community. Today, the Center is governed by a health council, elected every two years by the patients. Their family enrollment plan for families with young children reflects their emphasis on childhood as the time when most attention is needed. The Center staff of 45 is divided into teams, consisting of a doctor, a pediatrician, a nutritionist, and social workers; each team is responsible for the continuing care of 250 families apiece. There is also a basic health clinic where general practitioners see up to 300 patients a day. Dental screening is provided, as well as routine dental work, such as fillings, and fluoride treatments for children under 5. Their outreach program includes education and annual home visits to all patients, and they do VD screening and hold sex education seminars weekly. The Center's ambulance and two station wagons are available for night-time emergency services. Now two-thirds funded by HEW, they hope to become more self-sufficient through Medicaid and other sources including sliding scale payments by patients who can afford it. The NENA Center exemplifies the problems of trying to provide more humane and responsive care with limited resources: the small building is constantly crowded; the continual pressure of the people's needs can leave clinic workers harried and unresponsive at times in spite of the general sense of commitment and pride in the clinic. The NENA Center is trying to deal with these problems by expanding their program. Having won use of a city-owned lot, they are trying to raise money to erect a new mini-hospital—enabling them to see twice as many patients and to provide some in-patient care. A satellite clinic in a nearby storefront is another important new project. Contact NENA HEALTH CENTER, 42 Avenue C, New York, NY 14303, 212-677-5040.

We are trying to provide medical care and create challenge to the social system which causes these problems. We cannot have good health if we cannot feed our families. . . Good health does not come out of a bottle of vitamin pills, it comes from food on the table and good working and living conditions.

—Benito Juarez People's Health Center

SOUTH-END HEALTH CENTER...in Boston was conceived by an area businessperson who saw the need for good, community based health care. The center is based in a low-income, mainly Black and Puertoriqueno neighborhood where a great deal of "urban removal" (of poor people to make room for white professionals) is occurring. The community has grown very strong through a variety of housing fights; it solidly controls its health center. All policy is set by a community board in open meetings. Although staff members cannot be board members, the ties between staff and community people appear to be very strong. Many of the staff members are drawn from the community; for example, the ex-director of dental care was a welfare mother who learned administrative skills through her work in the center. The center staff are all paid; the community feels volunteers are generally unreliable. Also, a dependence upon volunteers takes away the community's ability to control the attitudes and behavior of center workers. The center turned down an offer from Boston University hospitals to put residents in the clinic due to this feeling and to the fact that BU makes no effort to draw students from the surrounding community. Because of the center's decision, BU lost a $100,000 grant. Contact SOUTH-END HEALTH CENTER, 65 West Brookline, Boston, MA 02130, 617-266-6336.

GARDNER COMMUNITY HEALTH CENTER...began in 1972 as an all-volunteer, community-controlled clinic in a mostly Chicano inner city neighborhood. They now provide services for more than 300 patients per month. They have 1½ paid doctors and several part-time volunteer doctors, but much of the work is done by nurse practitioners and by medical assistants that they train themselves. Services include general medical, laboratory, and x-ray; all aspects of the clinic are bilingual. The county hospital does back-up work; good relations have been worked out with the staff there, in spite of the administration's negative attitude. The Center has explored a variety of funding sources, including the National Free Clinic Council and the Neighborhood Youth Corps, and they recently won revenue sharing money from the county government. The hospital administration opposed funding the clinic, but a letter-writing and community pressure campaign, backed by the clinic's reputation and credentials, won out. Not trusting the continuance of county funding, the Health Center plans to move toward self-sufficiency through third party payments and patient payments based on a sliding scale. They will do patients' advocacy when abuses come to their attention; for example, they went to the hospital Board of Supervisors to get changes in the emergency room's treatment of poor people. Contact GARDNER COMMUNITY HEALTH CENTER, 325 Willow St., San Jose, CA 95110, 408-998-2264.

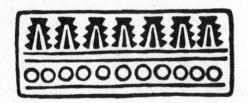

AMERICAN INDIAN FREE CLINIC . . . drew upon the California Regional Medical Program to fund a health service for the largest urban Indian population in California. At first the clinic served only as an information and referral service, but monies from the National Free Clinic Council and support from the local community allowed the clinic to grow into a source of primary health care. Most of the staff is volunteer, but there are three paid Native American staff members and a nutritionist. Contact AIFC, 329 East Roscrans, Compton, CA 90221, (213) 537-0103.

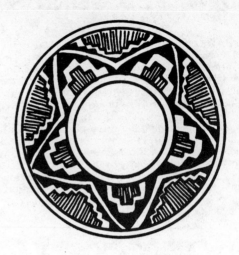

NATIVE AMERICAN HEALTH CLINIC. . .serves the needs of Native Americans in the San Francisco Bay area. The clinic has a full-time paid staff of doctors, nurse, nutritionists, outreach workers, and others. Funding comes from the county, HEW, and the US Department of the Interior Bureau of Indian Affairs. In addition many patients have Medical (California Medicaid), since once an Indian has left the reservation, the US government no longer provides her/him with health care. The clinic has a training program for community members; many housewives have already become inservice workers, doing clerical and outreach jobs. In the Bay areas where Native Americans cannot reach the clinic easily, a team of health workers gives care. Once a month a community meeting is held for health education. Through the California Urban Indian Health Council and contact with Native American Studies Programs, the clinic is helping to establish a resource library of traditional Indian medicine which will be presided over by a medicine man. Contact NAHC, 56 Julian St., San Francisco, CA 94103, 415-863-8111.

SALUD DOYLE COLONY...has been operating in the low-income Chicano community of Porterville for two years. The clinic is run by eight staff members—five of them Chicanos, seven of them Spanish-speaking. All receive the same pay based on size of family, and they make policy decisions as a collective. The aim of the clinic is to be a primary health care center delivering "quality medical care at the lowest cost possible," including follow-up care and screening as well as out-patient care. Through the California Welfare Department Medi-screen Program, the clinic has established a complete physical for all youth under 21. Fees are charged on a sliding scale of $4-$7. Contact SALUD DOYLE COLONY, 1243 E. Date St., Porterville, CA 93257, 209-781-4835.

PEOPLE'S HEALTH CENTER...has served the South Bronx community for four years. It began through group efforts, funded by loans from a local agency and from individuals. They now have their own small building with room for three dentists and three physicians. Income from third party payments such as Medicaid, and small payments from those who can afford them help the Center survive; the staff operates collectively and are all paid the same salary. Patients from the community make up the Board of Directors. The Center staff offers a six-week training course for dental and medical assistants and a three-month program to train community residents to recognize and deal with such common problems as high blood pressure, diabetes, and first aid. Those trained then work at the Center and in their local neighborhoods. The Center also aims to educate the community about the failings of the health system as a whole. They held a health fair combining education with screening for lead paint poisoning, hypertension, and sickle cell anemia. Although many people had high lead levels in their blood, the local public health department could not be convinced to act. In the future, the Center hopes to hold more health fairs and they are beginning a dental check-up program in the public schools. Contact PEOPLE'S HEALTH CENTER, 438 Claremont Parkway, New York, NY, 212-583-8010.

BOSTON CHINESE COMMUNITY HEALTH SERVICES...
operates as a primary health care delivery clinic for general medical care. Doctors from Chinese and western backgrounds serve as volunteers at the clinic along with a paid staff of nurses and community health aides. The aim is to acclimate the many Chinese immigrants to western health care, and to act as advocates for change in the present system of health care so that it accounts for many traditional Chinese beliefs. Bilingual outreach workers and clinic staff explain the differences between traditional Chinese medicine and western medicine to both patients and other health institutions, working on extending the accessibility of care in the community through extensive referrals and by encouraging people to join Medicaid/ care and other health insurance programs. Eventually the Clinic hopes to move into the health center in a school complex that is now in process and establish itself as a permanent part of the community. Contact BCCHS, 197-199 Harrison Ave., Boston, MA 02111, 617-482-7555.

CHINATOWN HEALTH CLINIC...grew from the Chinatown Health Fair, where 2500 community residents were screened in December, 1971. The clinic now provides ten hours of general medical services per week, as well as health education, screening and referral for non-English speaking patients. The paid staff are a coordinator and an outreach worker. Fifty volunteer staff, including ten MDs, saw over 2000 patient visits last year. A recent success of the clinic was pressuring local hospitals to hire 120 bilingual workers. In the future they would like to see teams trained for para-legal and para-medical work. Contact CHINATOWN HEALTH CLINIC, 22 Catharine St., New York, NY 10002, 212-732-9545.

In Portland, Oregon, many private doctors refuse to treat Medicaid patients. As a result, the city's poor must get their medical care at the county hospital on 'Pill Hill', a base for three hospitals, on one of the highest hills in southwest Portland. For some in the city, Pill Hill is as far as 30 miles, several bus rides, and hours away. When asked why the county did not establish decentralized clinics, the dean of the University of Oregon Medical School replied that it would be 'inconvenient for medical students' to have to travel away from Pill Hill.
—Heal Yourself

YOUTH AND
STREET PEOPLE CLINICS

Many of the free clinics across the country grew out of the counter-culture and student community during the late 60's and early 70's. Some have continued to serve primarily young people -- often in urban areas with many students, drop-outs and transient youth. Other clinics have consciously worked to broaden the community they serve and to become focuses of education and change. The groups below illustrate some of the range of forms free clinics have taken.

PEOPLE'S CLINIC/BOULDER...was begun three and a half years ago as a response to the influx of transients and street-people. The clinic now sees a majority of Boulder residents. Its purpose is to serve anyone who prefers the clinic atmosphere or who does not have money for private health care. An important part of their philosophy is that medical and psychological counseling is an integral part of medical care— and the beginning of preventive medicine. They are working to serve a broader section of the community and to expand their services to include geriatrics and crisis intervention care. Presently they hold seven separate clinics a week—including general medicine, VD, and women/pediatrics clinics staffed only by women, including the doctors. The clinic also holds health classes for staff and community members. Three full and two part-time paid people and 40-50 volunteer doctors, nurses, and community people make up the staff. With funding from the National Free Clinic Clearinghouse the clinic is creating a Jail Counseling Program. Contact PEOPLE'S CLINIC, 999 Alpine, Boulder, CO 80302, (303) 449-6050.

BERKELEY FREE CLINIC, INC...began during the agitation over the People's Park when those assaulted by the police were refused care at local hospitals. Since then the clinic has become an emergency first aid center during days with primary health services available Monday-Friday evenings. On Wednesdays the clinic offers Women's and pediatrics services run by the Berkeley Women's Health Collective. Dental care, psychological counseling, and a rap program are also available through the week. Since many of the programs are run by health workers trained at the clinic, the clinic is trying to alter the state para-medic bill which licenses only graduates

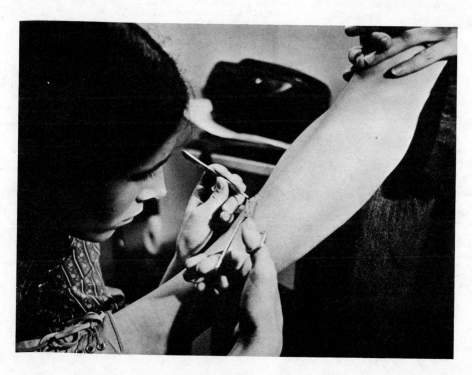

of university programs. Most of the staff is also volunteer, but the clinic hopes to get more public funds to pay all staff members. Last year they applied for a grant from the county government, but the money was offered only under the condition that the county have access to clinic files. The clinic held a public meeting generating a great deal of publicity, and forced the county to give them the money without any conditions. Contact BERKELEY FREE CLINIC, 2339 Durant, Berkeley, CA 94704, 415-548-2570.

WASHINGTON FREE CLINIC...has been serving the Washington DC community for about five years. Open in the evenings, the clinic has a weekly women's night run by a separate collective; there are also paraprofessional women's gynecological teams each night. A gay men's VD collective does VD screening on Saturdays. The clinic has a 10-week training program for its paraprofessionals and is governed by a community board. Funded mostly by donations, the clinic turned down funding from the National Free Clinic Council because they felt there were too many strings attached. When it began, WFC was concerned with providing a service, but it is now doing political and personal health education. A newsletter is in the planning stages, and they have made several videotapes on health issues such as diaphragm fitting and VD. Contact WASHINGTON FREE CLINIC, 1556 Wisconsin Ave., NW, Washington, DC 20007, (202) 965-5476.

HEALTH EMERGENCY AID DISPENSARY...began almost four years ago, filling the gap and ignorance regarding young people's health care, especially preventive care. As in other cities, members of the alternative community in New Orleans are seen as "transient undesirables" and are systematically excluded from existing social services. HEAD has sought to meet both the emergency and educational needs of youth, offering preventive care and regular medical services four nights a week. The all-volunteer staff of 49 people trains interested patients to assume clinic duties. The clinic also acts as a first aid station during each Mardi Gras, and trains over 100 street medics in advanced first aid and cardiopulmonary resuscitation. The medics provide a presence at police barricades and on police buses. This year the street medic program will continue after carnival time to cover rock concerts. Because the city and state officials recognize HEAD as one of the few services trusted by the youth population, they have provided funds for a doctor to treat VD two nights a week. (It was just recently that Louisiana law was changed to permit the treatment of minors with VD.) HEAD has been active in the independent South West Free Clinic Council, and recently put out an excellent Mardi Gras survival book. (See Emergency resources.) Contact HEAD, 1038 Esplanade Ave., New Orleans, LA 70116, 504-524-9314.

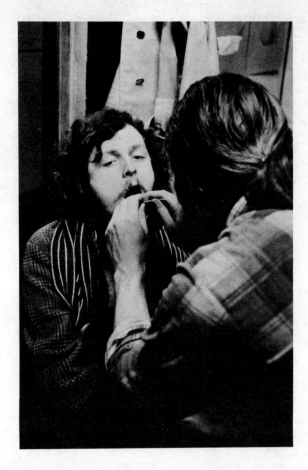

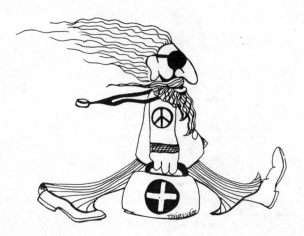

WHITEBIRD SOCIO-MEDICAL AID STATION...started in 1969 as a drug crisis center, but the counseling and emergency service has evolved into a wide range of community health services. Whitebird is now open 5 days a week, including special clinics for women, pediatrics, and VD cases, and maintains a 24 hour hotline. Twenty-seven paid staff and 100 volunteers serve over 400 people a week in direct medical care, crisis intervention, and on-going counseling. When Whitebird staff refer people to other agencies, patients' advocates are provided to accompany them. A community change workgroup at Whitebird stresses the connection between health and other socialist concerns. Whitebird may become a health co-op, asking a small membership fee to provide comprehensive, preventive care for a stable community. Contact WHITEBIRD, 341 E. 12th St., Eugene, OR 97402, 503-342-8255.

FREE MEDICAL CLINIC OF GREATER CLEVELAND... has grown during its 3-year existence from a youth-oriented drug education and treatment center to a general medical clinic striving for adequate, comprehensive, free care. The clinic has a volunteer staff of over 100 professionals, paraprofessionals, and trained community workers. Twelve mental health workers are paid by a grant from the Cuyahoga County Mental Health and Retardation Board, and a grant from the Robert Wood Johnson Foundation funds regular dental clinics. The clinic staff hopes to force surrounding institutions to take on their functions; meanwhile, they watch-dog local hospitals through a patient advocacy program and present educational programs in local schools and on local media. Some staff members are preparing malpractice suits against two regional abortion clinics, known to be low quality, and many are supporting the push for the Kennedy-Griffith National Health Insurance Bill. Fighting local anti-abortion legislation is another clinic concern. Contact FREE MEDICAL CLINIC OF GREATER CLEVELAND, 2039 Cornell Rd., Cleveland, OH 44106, 216-721-4010.

FREE PEOPLE'S HEALTH CLINIC/ANN ARBOR...was founded in January 1971 to serve the youth community's needs for an alternative health care institution. They do not attempt to meet all the demands for adequate health care which are not being met by the established medical facilities, but "serve as a model of the direction we believe health care delivery should be moving in." The clinic and the community joined together to fight the move of a local hospital from the community. The hospital still plans to move, but the clinic and the community have begun to recognize the need for a community organization. The clinic is open three nights a week for community patients only; they ask the local student population to use the University health center. They have a 24 hour answering service and a volunteer staff at close to 50, with one full-time and two part-time paid staff members to initiate community liaisons and political education programs. Their "medical mediators" hotline and newsletter document hassles with the health care delivery system. They also have hospital advocates to accompany patients referred to the local hospitals and patient advocates to assist and follow-up the clinic patients. The presence of hospital advocates during the doctor's examination has been prevented at the doctor's discretion in many hospitals, but the FPHC hopes to challenge this in court in the near future. Last year the City Council voted $20,000 of its revenue sharing funds to the FPHC for direct health care. The county also pays for the clinic's birth control and venereal disease treatment, tests, and supplies. Contact FREE PEOPLE'S HEALTH CLINIC, 225 East Liberty St., Ann Arbor, MI 48108, (313) 761-8952.

THE BRIDGE, INC. (BRIDGE OVER TROUBLED WATERS) ...operates a medical van five nights a week to bring free medical care to the youth and street people of Boston and "stimulate... them to move in their positive life directions." Doctors, nurses, and streetworkers staff the van, giving both medical and psychological help, including referrals to legal, employment, social welfare, and other resources. The van also has a dental staff and a four-chair dental clinic. Although the major emphasis of Bridge is to offer support to youth, they also "encourage established institutions to become more responsive to the needs of young people." Contact THE BRIDGE, INC., 1 Walnut St., Boston, MA 02108, 617-227-7114.

DENTAL CLINICS

VERMONT DENTAL CARE PROGRAM...is six mobile units which provide statewide comprehensive dental care for anyone under 21. Each unit is staffed by a full-time dentist, a part-time hygienist, and two dental assistants who are usually housewives from the local community with some background in dental care. The unit locates in an area for 3 to 4 months, where concerned community people and two volunteer college students do publicity and outreach, and coordinate transportation for the children. Now in its second year of operation, the program is almost self-supporting through sliding scale fees and third party payments such as Medicaid, Head Start, and the state of Vermont "Tooth Fairy" act which subsidizes poor children. Many private dentists have objected to the program and assert that they are taking care of dental needs. However, statistics prove them wrong: although the dentists in the program represent only 2% of the dentists in the state, they see 25% of the state's Medicaid patients. They have educated people to their need for and right to health care, and have helped sign up many new people for Medicaid and food stamps. The program's emphasis on children precludes treating adults except in emergency situations, but each unit makes referrals to medical and dental professionals. Contact VERMONT DENTAL CARE PROGRAM, Montpelier, VT, 05602, (802) 223-6355.

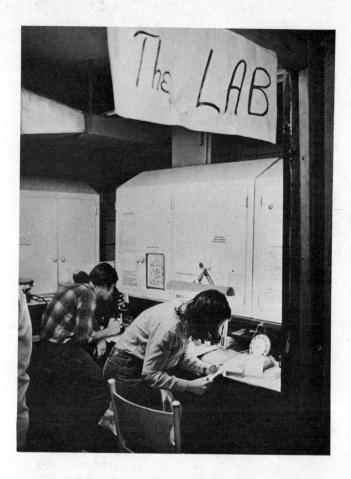

PEOPLE'S DENTAL SERVICE...was originally part of the Young Great Society Medical Center, which is now defunct. One man operates the service, providing all types of dental care at a cost based on income. He works at bridging the gap between professional and patient by eliminating the title of "Doctor" and the intimidating white coat, and teaching people to evaluate the dental care they receive. He refuses to overschedule patients or to act as a paternalistic bill collector. A year ago he helped a patient sue the city of Philadelphia for dental malpractice. More recently he has been speaking to groups and schools, and working to set up an oral hygiene program for preventive dentistry. Contact PDS, 1006 S. 46th St., Philadelphia, PA 19104, 215-387-1096.

LOWER CHATTAHOOCHEE COMMUNITY ACTION AGENCY MOBILE DENTAL CLINIC...is a self-contained dental office on wheels. During the past three years the clinic has done both rural and urban work, beginning with low-income rural school children, then moving to the Muskogee County Headstart Center in Columbus, and now returning to rural schools. The goal of the program is to take dental care directly to those who need it and who would probably never see a dentist otherwise. In Columbus the clinic trailer was parked outside the HeadstartCenter and carried on an extensive program for the children as the dentist gradually became an accepted friend and neighbor. In the rural areas the clinic is also located outside a school which supplies electricity, and water, while other children from other schools are scheduled for appointments and bussed in. Eventually the clinic plans to serve adults as well as children and has taken the first step towards this by applying for Medicaid certification. Contact LCCAAMDC, 900 Linwood Blvd., Columbus, GA 31901, (404) 324-2148.

icans (from a reservation 45 miles north). The paid staff of 10 includes two doctors, one dentist and community people trained at the clinic. Funding comes from sliding scale payments, some donations, medicaid/care, and the Migrant Health Act. Many of the local people who are seasonal farmworkers have been able to qualify for assistance under the act as it is interpreted in New Mexico. Contact LA CLINICA DE TIERRA AMARILLA, Tierra Amarilla, NM 87575 (505) 588-7252 or 588-7425.

NATIONAL FARMWORKERS HEALTH GROUP (NFHG)

. . . was created in 1970 to coordinate the United Farm Workers health plan. Under the Robert F. Kennedy Farm Workers Medical Plan employers pay 10 cents per worker/hour to cover the expenses of operating four clinics in California: Delano, Calexico, Sanger and Salinas. Staffed by MDs, nurses, aides, counselors, and others, the clinics provide complete ambulatory services (including dental and OB/GYN) as well as maintain an active outreach program of preventive and educational services in farmworkers' homes and labor camps. All clinic workers are paid the same salary. Much of the health work is done by community workers trained in anatomy, first aid, basic patient screening skills (history taking and blood pressure measurement), diet, diabetes, pre-natal care and more. There are special classes for expectant parents. The clinics use a problem-oriented medical record system and encourage routine screening and check-ups, especially to detect such common diseases of farmworkers as TB and other respiratory problmes. Contact NFHG, Box 131, Keene, CA 93531, (805) 822-5571.

RURAL CLINICS

MUD CREEK HEALTH PROJECT... began in 1972 when a group of poor mountain people from the Eastern Kentucky Welfare Rights Organization (EKWRO) joined together to bring better health services to their community. With money donated from private sources, supplies from hospitals and friends, and local labor, they opened a clinic that is now self-sufficient. Services are open to all, but the clinic is controlled by low-income people. Operating six days a week, the project provides general ambulatory medical care, with a complete battery of screening tests (EKG, chest X-ray, hearing, pap smears, etc.) for all patients during their first year. Nurses make frequent home visits to check on patients and teach about diet and drugs. Recently people from the Mud Creek Project were involved in a suit filed by EKWRO and other groups against the Internal Revenue Service to protest giving tax exempt status to private non-profit hospitals who refuse to serve patients with no money. The Washington D.C. District Court ruled in EKWRO's favor, but the IRS is taking the case to the U.S. Court of Appeals. Mud Creek Health Project is interested in hearing from health personnel who want to work in the clinic or anyone with money to donate, but discourages curious correspondence which burdens the already over-worked staff. Contact MUD CREEK HEALTH PROJECT, c/o Eula Hall, Craynor, KY 41614.

MARTIN LUTHER KING, Jr. MEMORIAL CLINIC... opened in fall, 1973 and serves a poor, virtually all-Black and densely populated rural area of small family plots. The project really began in 1972 by four women fed up with a racist and inadequate medical system. Disillusioned by the limitations and waste of government poverty programs, they decided to ignore government funding and rely on their own resources. They completed work on an unfinished house in return for a year's use of it, rounded up an all-volunteer staff (including two doctors, two registered nurses, and three nurses aides), and collected donations to pay for operating costs. They have several rural health aides, whose goal is to do community outreach work. Staff training emphasizes preventive medicine: pre-natal care, testing for common ailments such as high blood pressure, teaching about sanitation, nutrition, and such frequent problems as hook worm. Prevention is particularly important in an area where poverty and scarcity of health services combine to ensure that people rarely see a doctor before they are seriously ill. The national office of Vietnam Veterans Against the War has given the clinic support. Contact Martin Luther King, Jr., Memoral, c/o Cheryl Buswell Robinson, Rt. 1, Box 125a, Browns, AL 36724, (205) 996-3971.

LA CLINICA DE TIERRA AMARILLA... serves the people of a mountain community in northern New Mexico, where family income averages about $2000 per year, and unemployment is higher than 60% in the winter. La Clinica was started by a community organization, La Cooperativa, which also runs a legal office, silkscreen workshop, auto shop, child care project, and family rights program. The members of La Cooperativa elect the clinic's Board of Directors. The clinic serves mostly Chicanos, with some Anglos, and Native Amer-

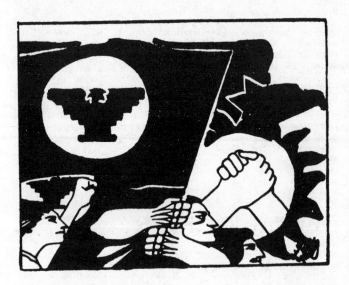

DELTA COMMUNITY HOSPITAL AND HEALTH CENTER

. . . were formerly two separate facilities funded by OEO which merged in 1972 and are now HEW funded. DCHHC serves four rural counties in Mississippi. Their emphasis on regular check-ups and health education has substantially affected the infant mortality rate in the area. For example, in Coahoma County the "infant mortality rate showed a drastic decline from 65.1/1000 births in 1966 to 36.9 in 1970, coinciding almost exactly with the extension of the Delta Community Hospital services to Coahoma County residents." As one patient with hypertension remarked: "If it wasn't for the Center and the hospital, for these folks right here, I'd be dead years ago." The outpatient services include prenatal care, OB/GYN, nutrition, environmental education, X-rays, and lab services. DCHHC is controlled by a board of community people, health professionals, and business people. Contact DCHHC, Mound Bayou, MS 38762 (601) 741-2151.

CLOVERFORK CLINIC. . .is the only health facility to serve a community of 9,000 scattered over a 23-mile area in an isolated valley of Harlan County, Kentucky. Cloverfork provides ambulatory care, including dental work and emphasizes prevention; they show films and slides on health education in the lobby. Their two doctors and three nurse practicioners operate a team, while speech therapists, mental health workers and others make weekly visits from a nearby town. Cloverfork has a home health unit which does outreach work and limited emergency services—fortunately there is a large hospital 10 or 15 miles away that can provide more extensive emergency care. The worst problem so far has been lack of space ("we've outgrown our breeches!") and the fact that they are a demonstration project of the Appalachian Regional Commission with their last grant year staring this June. But the people of Cloverfork do not intend to abandon the clinic. Although they may have to cut back on some of their services, they already have begun applying to foundations and have a pledge of money from the University of Kentucky. (Some medical students from UK will be taking their residencies at Cloverfork.) Cloverfork is controlled by a board of community members. Contact CLOVERFORK CLINIC, Evarts, KY 40828 (606) 837-2108.

MOUNTAIN COMPREHENSIVE HEALTH CORPORATION
. . .Serves 86,000 people of four rural counties in Southeastern Kentucky. Currently they have three primary care centers, including one mobile unit, although soon they will have five permanent centers with outreach workers and a transportation system. Their mobile dental unit travels to schools in the area. Because of its excellent reputation, the corporation has never had to pay for land. Some has been donated by school boards and local governments; in one town, the people went out and raised $5000 for land. A 17-member Board (including 8 consumers) from the four counties makes policy decisions. Fees come from Medicare/caid, sliding scale payments, and United Mine Workers of America. Contact MCHC, Central Office, Begley Bldg., E. Main St., Hazard, KY 41701, (606) 439-1314.

HOT SPRINGS HEALTH PROGRAM. . .is comprised of three small clinics in rural North Carolina offering outpatient medical and dental services; one of the clinics has a separate dental facility. Each clinic is headed by a nurse-practitioner with a full-time physician and pharmacist dividing their time among the three places; since there are no drug stores in the area the pharmacist distributes medication. The other health aides and staff are all hired from the local communities. Hot Springs has free transportation services and does health education, diagnosis and screening in the local schools. The 20-person governing board is locally elected. Hot Springs' main problem is that they are a demonstration project of Appalacian Regional Commission (ARC) in the third year of a maximum five-year grant. They hope for revenue-sharing funds, but are certain that their services will be limited when the grant is gone. As a result of the Hot Springs success in pro-

viding primary care, the North Carolina governor recently agreed to give financial support to fifteen other new nurse-practitioner clinics. Contact HOT SPRINGS HEALTH PROGRAM, Box 68, Hot Springs, NC 28743 (704) 622-7311.

BLACK BELT COMMUNITY HEALTH CENTER. . .is currently being constructed by community people of Epes, Alabama. This is a project of the Federation of Southern Co-ops, which formerly had HEW health money and was providing outpatient care for over 10,000 people. But since the grant was not renewed, community people are donating their time to build a clinic to serve about 3,000 people in the rural county when completed in July. Two physicians have been recruited who will be paid through third party payments, Medicaid/care and fees-for-service, when possible. Meanwhile they are applying to foundations for funding. Contact BLACK BELT COMMUNITY HEALTH CENTER, Federation of Southern Co-ops, P.O. Box 95, Epes, AL 35460 (205) 652-5181.

CLINIC RESOURCES

BOOKS

<u>Assessment of Medical Care for Children,</u> Institute of Medicines, National Academy of Sciences, available from Printing and Publishing Office, 2101 Constitution Ave., NW, Washington, DC 20418, 1974. 231 pp.
...shows the range in quality of health care received by children in different facilities in Washington, DC. Comparing the incidence of middle-ear infection, hearing loss, anemia and visual disorders, the results show much higher disease rates in the poor and those using public clinics. Good indictive material.

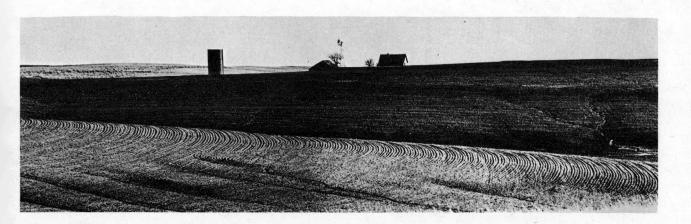

The Tooth Trip: An Oral Experience, Thomas McGuire, DDS, Random House/Bookworks, 1972. 233 pp. $3.95.
...an instructive "people's guide" to preventive dentistry. The author emphasizes healthful measures to prevent the source of dental disease: poor nutritional habits, and to initiate dental care in your home. Explains tooth decay and self-examination, and follows into such subjects as emergencies, care of children's teeth, and the effect that drugs have on the mouth. "A Manual for Survival in the Dental Office," one of the chapters, discusses procedures used in the dentist's office and what the patient should watch for. This book recognizes that the key to improved dental health is not necessarily fluoride, nor filling teeth, but lies in developing educative materials in nutrition.

Understanding Dentistry, Minna Lantner and Gerald Bender, DDS. Beacon Press, 1969. 214 pp. $6.00
...written for the patient, this book thoroughly explains all aspects of dentistry: general information on the teeth and mouth; advice on care of teeth and preparing for a child's first visit; with a large portion devoted to "what a patient might expect"—from the dentist's office and equipment to all possible dental work that might be performed. Well illustrated.

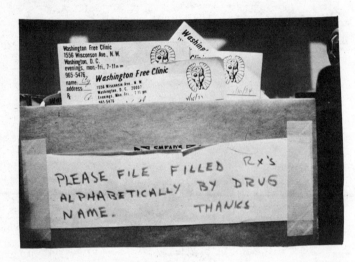

PAMPHLETS AND ARTICLES

Community Health Centre Handbook, Stanley Cornfield, Community Health Centre Group, Room 211, 455 Spadina Ave., Toronto 4, Ontario, Canada, 1972. 34 pp. $1.50
...an enthusiastically recommended tool for community health organizers. It outlines the issues to be considered when setting up a community health center with useful accounts of individual Canadian clinics—where they got funding, how they were started, the services provided and problems they faced.

"Organizing a Community Around Health," Ana Dumois, SOCIAL POLICY, 901 N. Broadway, White Plains, NY 10603, Jan/Feb 1971. pp. 10-14
... describes how a Lower East Side community organized to work for a neighborhood health center. The people succeeded in starting the center but not without considerable struggles with public agenices and various professionals. They learned that it was necessary to "use the 'inside' politics of health as well as the political process in order to get serious negotiation."

Sometimes its just impossible for me to get to the hospital for medicine since I can't even pay for the bus.
—diabetic Mexican-American woman
Heal Yourself

"Storefront Clinics: Activist Fad or Workable Health Care System," MEDICAL WORLD NEWS, available from MCHR, PO Box 7155, Pittsburgh, PA 15213, 1971. 7 pp.
...a rather limited but informative article on neighborhood health centers: funding problems, such as the difficulties in trying to stay free from constricting government financing; professional resistance to working in "makeshift" facilities; and problems inherent in community control and doctor accountability. The article gives a good idea of the issues facing people setting up a clinic; unfortunately, it represents storefront medicine as an extension of the present system rather than a way to challenge it.

Nothing to Smile About: A Report on the Dental Health of Vermont's Children, Jay Breines, Director, Vermont Public Research Group, 26 State St., Montpelier, Vermont, 05602, 1972. 22 pp. $1.00. Free to PIRG members.
...speaks out against the lack of dental care in a state where one person out of five is missing at least half of his/her teeth. The problem hits children particularly hard: half of the elementary school children have "teeth requiring extraction or extensive restorative procedures." VPIRG offers a plan for a state-wide children's dental health program with suggestions for monitoring and financing.

"A SHOPPER'S GUIDE TO DENTISTRY," Herbert Dennenberg, available from Consumer Insurance, 873 National Press Building, Washington, DC 20004, 1973. 23 pp. $1.00
...guide to dentistry, designed especially for Pennsylvania residents. This is written in the form of do's and don'ts involving billing procedures, explanation of treatments, preventive training and more.

FILMS AND TAPES

Solidarity Films, 2490 Challing Way, Rm. 207, Berkeley, CA 94704

> **"People's Health Film,"** still in production
> This film will deal with how the medical/drug industry in a profit-motive society oppress people. It will examine groups who are fighting the health care system; they are setting up alternatives while struggling to change the existing institutions.

NBC Educational Enterprises, 30 Rockefeller Pl., New York, NY 10020

> **"Health on Wheels,"** 14½ min. b&w $6.00
> Shows the operation of a mobile unit used to screen members of a community in order to detect chronic diseases.

Great Atlantic Radio Conspiracy, 2603 Talbott Rd., Baltimore, MD 21216
> **"Free Clinics",** 30 min. $2.50 for individuals, $5.00 for others. A good overview of free medical clinics. The tape begins with an analysis of what's wrong with the present health care system, including high costs and fragmentation of care. It then moves on to a general discussion of what free clinics are working for (health care as a right, community-worker control of health institutions), and interviews a woman from a Baltimore free clinic. The tape recognizes that clinics must combine political education with their services to avoid perpetuating the system. Ultimately clinics are seen as a "mild anesthetic for a chronic injury... Bad health care is the symptom of a pathological society. The pathology is located in its political economy. It is a disease called state capitalism and major surgery is in order."

PREVENTIVE HEALTH CARE

Nearly 11,000 women die each year of cervical cancer—a disease which can be cured if detected in its early stages through a simple five minute PAP test. Another 700,000 people die of heart disease, and 40,000 of diabetes; these diseases can also be controlled or eliminated in most cases. 26.1 million Americans are either undernourished or malnourished and therefore doubly susceptible to disease and death. Young children develop sudden convulsions and die, leaving distraught parents who never noticed the chips of poisonous lead-based paint the child ate; and if they did notice, did not know the danger.

Many deaths, diseases and handicaps could be avoided through regular physicals, screening, testing and immunizations. Yet preventive care is the most ignored form of health care, because it is the least profitable. In our health system, where in the past, preventive care has been minimal at best, screening an entire community for hypertension, diabetes, or anemia could take months or even years and would involve an initial outlay of millions of dollars—dollars which go out of the health industries' pockets instead of in. Our present health system is set up so that curative health care costs the provider less and brings in more money at a faster rate. Curative care is also more prestigious. Medical students are taught how to treat diseases; "this, they are told, is a big challenge—the diagnosis and successful handling of disorders with its logical sequel, the dramatic surgical repair of diseases or injured bodies." (How You Can Get Better Medical Care for Your Money). Most health insurance plans pay for doctor's office visits when the patient is sick, but do not cover diagnostic tests or regular medical and dental check-ups, thereby discouraging people from seeking them.

Those who challenge this system by trying to take control of and maintain their own bodies find themselves foiled by inadequate or unreliable information, whether from the AMA or from slick health food stores.

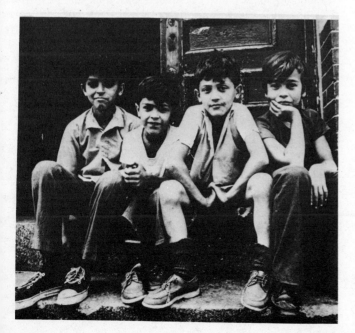

School health programs provide only half-truths, if they provide any information at all. And asking the doctor why or how you got sick and how to prevent it results in a frustrating "medi-code" answer as s/he rushes off to the next patient. Thus profit and professionalism present enormous obstacles to the foundation of preventive health care—health education.

But the largest barrier to establishing a system of preventive health care is the radical nature of the project. Practicing preventive medicine means recognizing and eliminating the basic roots of much disease: the poverty that keeps us from buying the food that we need, or seeing the health worker who could help us; the inadequate education which leaves us ignorant of our bodies and their signs of ill health; and the inadequate system for health care delivery which ignores health problems until they become major crises.

SCREENING AND TESTING

Regular health screening is the best way to find disease early before it spreads or causes damage. Health screening involves both medical history and a number of simple laboratory tests. Common tests include a hematocrit (finger-stick blood test for anemia which is also used in lead poisoning tests), a blood count (over-abundance of red or white cells can indicate infection), a test for blood sugar, a TB test, an electrocardiogram for heart disease, a urinalysis, and a PAP test for women. Other important tests are VD and strep throat cultures, sickle cell anemia testing, vision, and hearing tests.

Many communities and workplaces offer mobile units which do "multi-phasic screening." This involves a battery of tests covering all aspects of health. However, such units are often available only to affluent neighborhoods and eliminate poor people and welfare recipients by charging a fee, requiring daytime appointments, and making referrals to private physicians. In most cases, they do not try to provide any health education or work to combat professionalism. Often the unit will not come into a community without strong indication that the community will respond. This practice immediately eliminates those areas where people have never seen a doctor and must be sought out and convinced that the mobile unit can be the beginning of help. Mobile units can also be used as an excuse for not creating true outreach programs for the poor and isolated. Just setting up the personnel and facilities for a community screening program does not produce one; publicity and door-to-door canvassing are necessary to inform and interest people in the project.

The federal government, under the Social Security Administration and the Public Health Service, funds a number of screening programs. The most outstanding is the Social Security Act which requires an early periodic screening, diagnosis, and treatment program in all states for children under 21 who receive Medicaid Funds. This means not simply doing tests on a child when s/he is ill, but also actively bringing community children to health centers to be screened. Often this provision is ignored, yet demanding its enforcement could bring screening programs to many children and eliminate diseases which physically and mentally cripple them.

The government funds lead poisoning and venereal disease detection programs through the Public Health Service. However, this funding is channelled through state and local public health departments and often times much of it never makes it to the community level, having been spent on administrative salaries higher up. Most cities provide public VD clinics, but the waiting time is long, the treatment impersonal, the location often inaccessible. In some cases, Third World people, women, and gays are discriminated against or verbally abused, especially if they are minors. Funding for lead

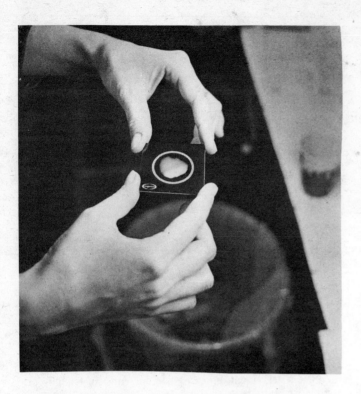

was designated by federal law to start by July 1973. The committee found that the health department and the social services department had never heard of the program. At this point they began holding meetings to force the departments to implement EPSDT. Initially the departments would only come to separate meetings so that they could verbally place responsibility on each other. However the departments finally agreed to joint meetings, and the EPSDT program was implemented for children under two in August. When the committee sent four young adults to the clinic to demand their screening, they were refused; but the four were sent back after Labor Day, and the clinic expanded its program to take care of them. Since then, the committee has forced the expansion of the program from one clinic location to other clinics of various types. They are currently pushing the health department to start an extensive advertising campaign. Contact DURHAM EARLY SCREENING COMMITTEE, c/o Operation Breakthrough, PO Box 1470, Durham, NC 27702, 919-477-7327.

THE CHILDREN'S DEFENSE FUND...is a major component of the Washington Research Project, a public interest law firm. WRP, in conjunction with National Welfare Rights Organization, did much of the preliminary research and confronting of the Department of Health, Education, and Welfare to force the implementation of the EPSDT program. The Children's Defense Fund now monitors many of those programs and helps community groups work out the many problems inherent in the state programs. They do so by connecting local community groups with local providers through contacting known groups such as welfare rights organizations and helping them make a directory of local, state, and federal health officials. When necessary they help the groups bring law suits against state or local providers. Their emphasis is on showing the community the "how-to's" specific to their area. Contact THE CHILDREN'S DEFENSE FUND/WASHINGTON RESEARCH PROJECT, 1763 "R" St., Washington, DC 20009, 202-483-1470.

COMMUNITY ACTION COMMITTEE TO FREE METRO DC OF VENEREAL DISEASE...was set up in late spring of 1972 to enlist community support from the most radical groups to the most capitalistic, in the fight against gonorrhea and syphillis. The Committee distributed information on VD throughout the summer, climaxing in a treatment week in October. 52 temporary clinics were set up to handle as many people as possible, particularly asymptomatic women. During this time, a VD hotline was also established. Although the committee is officially defunct, the Hotline continues to operate with grants and donations. Workers are paid, preferably inner city Black high school students. Contact VD HOTLINE, 202-VD2-7000.

HEALTH FAIR/VOLUNTEERS IN MISSION. . .is dedicated to developing the community's awareness of the fundamental need for health care. The program operates in rural areas of Oklahoma, Arkansas, Ohio, Oregon, and New York. Volunteer health teams travel from town to town, setting up facilities in neutral community places, such as a church or school, where the doctors, dentists, nurses, and others do simply diagnostic tests and educate community members on health: "what is a blood pressure?"; "why do you need protein?" "what is the difference between normal and abnormal health?" The Fair remains for about a week, attracting as many people as possible, then moving on. The program's goal, which has been achieved in many areas, is to make people willing to seek out and demand health care facilities in their communities. The program has sparked new clinics and greater cooperation among existing clinics. Contact VOLUNTEERS IN MISSION, United Presbyterian Church, 475 Riverside Dr., New York, NY 10027 (212) 870-2801.

CITIZENS' COMMITTEE FOR CHILDREN OF NEW YORK, INC...is a community organization whose members serve as advocates on the behalf of children. The committee is mon-

poisoning can be obtained by non-profit organizations, but this entails incorporating. Demanding that the state, city, and local hospitals fund the project, or, better yet, design and carry it out under community guidance is more productive both for the community morale, and for the program.

In a community where health care is scarce or inaccessible, screening programs have a special importance. Health fairs or one-problem screening projects like lead paint poisoning cover large portions of the community, uncover many problems, and educate many people. Many of the groups listed under Health Education will be happy to supply testing equipment and sometimes personnel, although most communities prefer to hand-pick their professionals, choosing those who lack racist, elitist and sexist attitudes, and who have a desire to demonstrate how health care should be delivered. The location of the fair can be a church, a park, a school, or even a street. Screens and trailers create examing rooms, equipment can be borrowed or donated, and educational aids can be homemade. Local groups can be involved through skits, displays, and fund-raising. If testing is too complex a project, it can be eliminated in favor of education and community involvement, factors which can lead to the creation of a strong community health coalition.

The importance of community health screening, however, is not simply education. The fact that a community can organize itself and control its own care, even if for a limited time, is a direct challenge to the existing health system and an encouragement to the community to make more demands. Many community clinics grew out of health fairs and screening projects. They are a beginning, helping people to discover the importance of their bodies and the power to control them.

DURHAM EARLY SCREENING COMMITTEE...is a coalition of community groups and individuals including the Durham Welfare Rights Organization, a community action agency, the Durham Medical Committee for Human Rights, and two Durham health committees. The coalition began late in the spring of 1973 when it became obvious that the local health department was not going to implement the Early Periodic Screening, Diagnosis, and Treatment program (EPSDT), which itoring the implementation of the EPSDT program in New York state, working with city, state, and federal officials on implementation plans, and monitoring the health professionals through on-site visits. The project committee's goal is to educate the community on EPSDT services that should be available and to help press for and monitor these services. Contact CITIZENS' COMMITTEE FOR CHILDREN OF NEW YORK,INC., 2 Park Ave., New York, NY 10003, 212-725-7940.

MONTANA STATE DEPARTMENT OF HEALTH...has a multi-phasic screening program for adults designed specifically to meet the needs of a rural, under-doctored population, and is a model of the kind of screening that states should provide. The screening unit, consisting of health personnel from various fields, comes into communities by request. Community members help the staff find a facility for the unit to work in and disseminate information on the program. Equipment, supplies, and personnel are supplied by the screening unit for testing anemia, diabetes, hearing problems, and much more. The staff also takes a comprehensive, personal health history of each patient, making referrals when necessary. Referrals are followed up by a return postcard system; when the postcard is not returned after some time has elapsed, a public health nurse visits the person. The staff also does follow-up educational work. Atlhough they charge $3 per person for screening, the state absorbs the cost when an individual cannot pay. Contact MONTANA STATE DEPARTMENT OF HEALTH AND ENVIRONMENTAL SCIENCE, St. John's Hospital, Helena, MT 49601, 406-449-2544.

PEOPLE'S COALITION AGAINST LEAD POISONING . . . organizes against lead paint poisoning in hopes of raising a challenge to the profit-at-any-cost logic of American capitalism. The local media has given sympathetic coverage to their criticisms of the city's "exemplary" anti-lead poisoning law (which it never intended to enforce); student volunteers have done a lot of research on slum ownership patterns and the failure of city policies. They have never backed down from the position that the lead poisoning problem can only be dealt with when tenants organize to take control of the landlord's property. Hence, their education work has been mostly in support of tenant organizing. They are also organizing food co-ops to build a more collective community consciousness. Contact PEOPLE'S COALITION AGAINST LEAD POISONING' c/o St. Stephen's Church, 13th and Parks, St. Louis, MO 63104, (314) 531-3479.

HARTFORD COMMUNITY RENEWAL TEAM . . . is composed of community members working out of the Hartford City Health Department in conjunction with the University of Connecticut Medical School. The Team conducts lead paint poisoning surveys and screening in nursery schools, daycare centers, and homes on all children under five, and a community organizer does speaking engagements in local schools. When a child's blood lead level is elevated above 40, s/he is referred to a local clinic and followed for six months. The home is inspected by the city housing department and when paint lead content is over 1% the landlord must make repairs within 90 days. Many families have been relocated to public housing but two major problems have been encountered: the protests of extended families over separation and the replacement of high lead paint content by high lead absorption from traffic fumes. Contact HARTFORD COMMUNITY RENEWAL TEAM, University of Connecticut Medical School, 1 Holcomb St., Hartford, CT 06112, (203) 243-2531.

BALTIMORE CITY HEALTH DEPARTMENT . . . runs a multi-faceted lead poisoning case-finding and housing inspection program. They have a walk-in screening clinic to test children who have no regular source of medical care, and hospital workers are trained to look for symptoms of lead poisoning in children admitted to the hospitals for other causes. If they are found to have high lead levels, the Health Department has the authority to inspect their house, take paint samples, test all other children in the house and get the courts to order repairs if there is danger of further poisoning. Though the law only requires repair of single apartments and now whole buildings, courts have been fairly good about enforcing it. Because the Health Department inspects and the Department of Licenses and Inspections enforces the law, there have been some lags in repairs, but a whole system of half-way houses for poisoned children has been established to keep them from returning to poisoned environments. Another system has been worked out whereby families with poisoned children get first priority on public housing openings. Contact BALTIMORE CITY HEALTH DEPARTMENT, 250 Lexington St., Baltimore, MD 21202, (301) 752-2000.

RESOURCES

"HEALTH FAIR REPORT," Dr. Kenneth Tittle, Volunteers in Mission, The Division of Voluntary Service, The United Presbyterian Church in the USA, 475 Riverside Dr., Room 1133, New York, NY 10027, 1971. 10 pp. Free
...tells what to consider when organizing a health fair: what the coordinator should do, the role of the doctor, what services to offer, who to involve. Asserts that the doctor must take direction from community people. Good resource.

HEALTH RIGHTS NEWS, Medical Committee for Human Rights, 542 S. Deaborn St., Chicago IL 60605, December 1971. 11 pp. $5/year
. . . this issue of HRN has 4 excellent articles on different aspects of the lead poisoning issue. In each one the political analysis comes through strong and clear: the victims of lead paint poisoning hold "no political power, while the primary offenders [are] wealthy, corporate, political. Why should the city enforce a law which is burdensome to the very power interests it is wedded to—real estate firms, banks, savings and loan companies, insurance companies?" The accounts of struggles in various cities are frustrating, inspiring, undoubtedly a must for anyone concerned with this problem in his/her community.

"HANDBOOK FOR THE PREVENTION OF LEAD POISONING IN CHILDREN," Robert Klein, MD, Citizens' Committee to End Lead Poisoning and the Lead Poisoning Prevention Center, Boston City Hospital, Boston, MA. 27 pp. $1.21
. . . a great little pamphlet with details on where to look for lead paint, screening methods and costs, treatments, and house inspection. One very helpful section lists some common evasive arguments used by landlords and local officials when pressured by citizen groups to remove lead paint from houses.

"LEAD POISONING," Medical Committee for Human Rights, c/o Louise Rice, 65 Chestnut St., Cambridge, MA 02139, 1971. 12 pp. $.54
. . . brief account of Boston MCHR's work around the issue of lead poisoning. Summarizes the major purposes in dealing with this issue, how to start fighting the problem, and a description of a Massachusetts bill on lead poisoning. The pamphlet is concise, and pragmatic, geared towards encouraging other communities to fight this health hazard.

"Landlord's Free Breakfast For Children Program", American Independent Movement Newsletter, 148 Orange St., New Haven, CT, available from Louise Rice, 65 Chestnut St. Cambridge, MA 02139, Nov. 1969. 4 pp. $.18
. . . exposes the extent and dangers of lead paint poisoning in and around New Haven, Conn. The main article reports on a workshop sponsored by area residents and attended by the State Commissioner of Health and two major landlords. Participants discuss a rent strike, although "Many of the families in danger of lead poisoning are on welfare. The Welfare Department passed a ruling on October 1, saying that if a welfare family does withhold rent, the department will send rent money directly to the landlord involved and bypass the family."

NUTRITION

" . . . In the wealthiest nation in the history of the world, millions of men, women, and children are slowly starving . . . teachers report children who come to school without breakfast, who are too hungry to learn, and in such pain that they must be taken home or sent to the school nurse . . . doctors personally testify to seeing case after case of premature death, infant deaths, and vulnerability to secondary infections all of which were attributable to or indicative of malnutrition . . . the aged living alone, subsist on liquid foods that provide inadequate sustenance." ("Hunger USA", Citizen's Board of Inquiry into Hunger and Malnutrition in the United States.)

No human being can be healthy without good food. Trips to the doctor are futile for people who can't afford a decent diet. Yet even those in the US who can pay for food are spending more and eating more poorly. In 1968, a United States Department of Agriculture survey found that only 50% of the families questioned had a "good" diet and this figure had declined from earlier ones. "This is the age when manufacturers pay 5 cents for the package for a breakfast cereal and 4 cents to the farmer for the ingredients . . . " (Great American Food Hoax)

Many low income Americans are forced to depend on government food programs to survive. But these programs are designed not to serve the needs of people, but rather to serve the needs of national agriculture policy. "That policy, as led by the Department of Agriculture and Congressional committees and sub-committees of agriculture and agricultural appropriations, is dominated by a concern for maximizing agricultural income, especially within the big production categories . . . almost never does our agricultural policy take a direct concern with the interests of consumers and, certainly, not of poor consumers." (Hunger USA)

Federal food programs come in three major types: I. direct distribution of food, as in the Supplemental Food Distribution Program for Mothers and Children; 2. sale or distribution of vouchers used, like money to buy food, as in the Food Stamp Program; 3. reimbursement of an organization or institution for food it buys and serves, as in the School Lunch and Breakfast Program. Often a program is a combination of types as in the Special Food Service Program where institutions are eligible for both food and reimbursement; programs are also eligible for Non-Food Assistance Programs, which helps pay for equipment, however, no assistance is available for labor costs. This fact tends to keep these programs out of reach of community

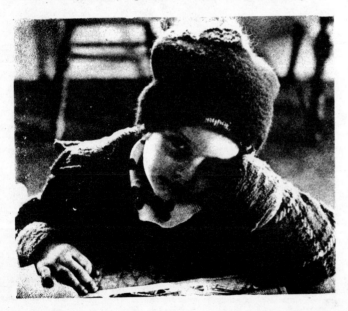

groups whose members must work full-time and in the control of large, corporate, foundation-funded, voluntary groups or of local government bureaucracies.

Some federal feeding programs are administered directly through the Food and Nutrition Services of the Department of Agriculture (USDA); most are administered through the state government, or one of its branches, subsidized by the USDA. Yet all communities and individuals have certain rights under the federal feeding programs. Every child has a right to a School Lunch and Breakfast Program in her/his school. Special Food Service Programs are available to day care centers, summer recreation programs and neighborhood centers. Anyone with a low-income (presently $178 per month for one person) or on welfare is eligible for food stamps. Finding your way through the morass of legalities is not easy, but many of the groups listed here offer help and information on your rights in the federal feeding programs.

Having the money to buy food does not guarantee a decent, healthy diet. Most American adults have very limited knowledge of basic nutrition requirements and food producers make no effort to increase the consumer's knowledge of the food's nutrients. Food production has moved from small family operations to a $110 billion industry, with annual advertising expenditures totaling $3 billion. Increasingly , the money that you spend in the supermarket goes for fancy packaging, research into chemical concoctions of limited nutritional value, and slick advertising campaigns to trick you into buying more and more. Companies are putting unnecessary, non-nutritious, and sometimes even dangerous additives into foods to make them more attractive, longer lasting, and more profitable.

The Food and Drug Administration (FDA) is responsible for protecting the quality of food although, in fact, it does far more to protect the food industry than the consumer. It is no coincidence that 22 of the top 53 officials at FDA have worked for regulated food or drug industries or organizations catering to them. For example, Dr. Virgil Wodicka, Director of the Bureau of Foods, has worked for Ralston-Purina; Libby, McNeill & Libby; and Hunt-Wesson. "The top officials (of FDA have) spent a cumulative total of 180 years in industry, as compared to 63 years on college campuses." No FDA official has work experience with a consumer group.

But the monstrous food industry is being attacked. Public interest groups are exposing the collusion between the FDA, USDA and the capitalist agricultural system. Food cooperatives offer an alternative through bulk buying, elimination of the profit motive, and a consciousness of which foods are nutritionally sound. Co-ops which expand into anti-profit warehouses and trucking companies further lower costs and eliminate the middle person processes of agri-biz.

FOOD RESEARCH AND ACTION CENTER. . .is a vigorous, hard-working group serving as a litigation and organizing resource in the area of federal food programs. The Center has won two cases before the Supreme Court on the food stamp act and many cases before district courts, including one of the USDA's inaction in establishing the supplemental feeding program, WIC (Women, Infants, and Children); they have also won many cases on the refusal of public schools to implement school lunch programs. Two current projects are a national food stamp campaign to increase participation in the program and to force new counties to establish programs, and a nutrition program for the elderly. FRAC has published some excellent studies on food programs, as well as much "how-to" literature. Contact FRAC, 25 West 43rd St., New York, NY 10036 (212) 354-7866.

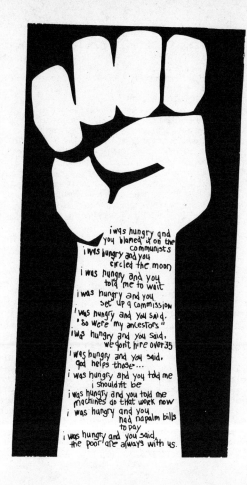

i was hungry and
you blamed it on the
communists
i was hungry and you
circled the moon
i was hungry and you
told me to wait
i was hungry and you
set up a commission
i was hungry and you said,
"so were my ancestors"
i was hungry and you said,
we don't hire over 35
i was hungry and you said,
god helps those...
i was hungry and you told me
i shouldn't be
i was hungry and you told me
machines do that work now
i was hungry and you
had napalm bills
to pay
i was hungry and you said,
the poor are always with us.

THE CHILDREN'S FOUNDATION...provides technical assistance to communities to organize, build, and up-date child feeding programs. The Foundation has worked on school lunch and breakfast programs with the Welfare Rights Organization; on food for daycare, Headstart, and residential child-care programs; on the US Department of Agriculture supplemental food programs for women, infants, and children. They helped build Hunger Task Forces as part of the Mass Alliance Against Hunger, and their organizers have worked in migrant farmworker camps and on Oklahoma Indian reservations, where CF revealed blatant misuse of federal funds, precipitating a Justice Department investigation of the situation. The Foundation also investigates low-income and working-class poor communities to implement food programs. Teaching communities the basic organizing skills necessary to achieve and exercise their rights is a major goal. Their long-range commitment is to creating self-sustaining communities with the power to control themselves. This power will be amassed by buying out major food companies and destroying their monopoly over people. Contact CF, 1028 Connecticut Ave., Suite 614, Washington DC 20036, 202-296-4451.

It seems that the advertising budget for General Mills is larger than the entire budget for the Food and Drug Administration, which is supposed to regulate foods and drugs. Which should make it of no surprise that the Betty Crocker Butter Pecan Cake Mix was approved by the hard-working bureaucrats who run the FDA—even though the mix contains neither butter nor pecans.
—FOOD CO-OP NOOZ

COMMUNITY NUTRITION INSTITUTE ... "develops service programs and provides information on food and nutrition to state and federal agencies, industry, community groups and concerned citizens." CNI produces a weekly newsletter, CNI WEEKLY REPORT, on all areas of research, legislation, and action in nutrition. They also sponsor conferences on nutrition and feeding programs, and work with community groups on instituting feeding pro-

grams on nutrition for the elderly. The program began under a grant from the Office of Economic Opportunity, one of the conditions being that CNI must periodically submit its weekly report to the OEO Office of Health Affairs for prior review. The groups cooperated well for two years, but when OEO made some major censorship attempts in March 1973, CNI renounced their grant. Contact CNI, 1910 "K" St., NW, Washington, DC 20006, 202-833-1730.

BOSTON FOOD CO-OP. . .is a non-profit bulk buying store committed to an alternative way of providing food. The co-op has a double operation, selling to ten neighborhood co-ops and 4000 members. All members make a monthly work commitment, pay a one-time membership fee, and go through orientation sessions on capitalism, sexism, and racism. The co-op has ten different committees dealing with such concerns as personnel, correspondence, employment, the elderly, day care, nutrition, and their newsletter. They are trying to start day care centers, and are developing a program for using members' skills for the benefit of the community. Contact BOSTON FOOD CO-OP, 12 Babbit, Boston, MA 02215, (617) 267-9090.

PEOPLE'S WAREHOUSE. . .grew out of the North County co-op Food Store which evolved from a bulk buying project. The People's Warehouse is run collectively by a staff working for subsistence salary that comes from a 10% mark-up on the food. The warehouse is also connected with an anti-profit trucking company and trades with other warehouses in Ann Arbor, Madison, Seattle, and Rochester. Any non-profit or anti-profit group which encourages neighborhood or community participation can buy from the warehouse. Eventually the staff hopes to see the local community control all aspects of food production and distribution in its area on an anti-profit basis, and become physically involved in every aspect of farm production. Contact PEOPLE'S WAREHOUSE' 123 East 26th St., Minneapolis, MN 55415 (612) 824-2634.

WASHINGTON FOOD FEDERATION. . .is a loose organization of four Washington food co-ops. All four co-ops are united in their belief in the need for an alternative to the large agricultural corporations which put dangerous additives into food for the sake of profit. The Federation is presently involved in creating a community warehouse which can act as a distributor for the co-ops; they may eventually contract with local small, organic farmers to create a self-reliant food system in the DC area. A mill and bakery are already being set up in the warehouse. Co-ops belong to the Federation/Warehouse must be anti-profit, collectively run, and community owned. Other co-ops may buy from the warehouse as long as they do not resell the food at a profit. Contact WASHINGTON FOOD FEDERATION, c/o Community Warehouse, 2010 Kendall NE, Washington, D.C. 20002 (202) 832-4517.

PROJECT GREEN POWER. . .is conducted by a group of approximately 100 adult and young volunteers. They have cultivated ten acres at Weston College and plant a variety of vegetables. From July through October the weekly harvest is distributed through outlets in the city, such as settlement houses, providing fresh vegetables for approximately 500 people. The outlets pay Weston $1 per crate of produce and give the food away free or charge a very small amount. As the project has grown, some of the low-income city people who were receiving the food have begun working the land themselves to feed their families. The Project hopes this trend will continue. Contact PROJECT GREEN POWER, 650 Boston Post Rd., Weston, MA 02193, (617) 893-5775.

CONSUMER'S FOOD COUNCIL. . .in Portland is basically a group of suburban residents concerned about food supplies and the agricultural industries' effect on the environment (including pesticides). The group set up a statewide coalition for truth in labeling and is currently pushing the legislature to pass a law on unit pricing and ingredient labeling. Working with the Oregon Student Public Interest Research Group to study current problems in food and agriculture, such as the effect of the energy crisis, is another project. The Council publishes a newsletter, and in the past it has helped pressure state legislation on 'open-dating'—an uncoded date beyond which the food is not good for sale or consumption. The goal of the Council is to create an awareness of the adverse effects which the agricultural industries have on the environment and to encourage citizen participation in governmen decisions affecting food and agriculture. Contact CONSUMER'S FOOD COUNCIL, 1734 NW Aspen, Portland, OR 97210 (503) 223-1614.

OPERATION BABY FOOD. . .provides supplemental baby food, vitamins, and formula to infants newborn to age two. For over a year, Marillac House attempted to sub-contract with the USDA to sponsor the infant supplemental feeding program; however, the project was limited to serving only about 5,000 needy infants on Chicago's south side. No provision was made for equally needy west side infants. Private donations by church and school groups and a substantial donation from the North Suburban "Walk for Development" of the American Freedom from Hunger Foundation in May 1970 enabled the agency to provide supplemental packages of formula, vitamins, and baby food to over 100 needy infants. These infants have been recruited by outreach social workers or have been referred by medical social workers, Board of Health nurses, or Public Aid workers. Additionally, for three summers, the Marillac Social Center has provided breakfast for needy children through funds from the special lunch program of the USDA. Contact OPERATION BABY FOOD/MARILLAC SOCIAL CENTER, 2822 W. Jackson, Chicago, IL 60612 (312) SA2-7440.

AMERICAN FREEDOM FROM HUNGER FOUNDATION . . .has worked with such groups as the Southern California Free Clinic Council, the American Indian Movement, and the Peace Corps. The Foundation sponsors workshops and conferences in population and development, and leadership training for young organizers. They also help groups raise money through "Walks for Development" in which people plan long hikes and get sponsors to pay for each mile they walk. The goal of the Foundation is to help others feed themselves: they support an internationalist perspective on hunger and underdevelopment, and have funded liberation groups in Mozambique and Angola. Contact AMERICAN FREEDOM FROM HUNGER FOUNDATION, 1100 17th St., NW, Suite 701, Washington, D.C. 20036, (202) 254-3487.

FOOD PROJECT. . .provides a meal at a reduced cost or free to anyone in need. The program is sponsored by the congregation of the University Lutheran Chapel and is funded by the City of Berkeley and the US Department of Agriculture food program. It has four paid staff, three street people and one student, plus many volunteers. The staff makes an effort to reach out to people, counseling them and making referrals on jobs, welfare, medical and legal aid. Contact FOOD PROJECT, University Lutheran Chapel, 2425 College Ave., Berkeley, CA 94704 (415) 843-6230.

FOCUS: HOPE. . .administers the Detroit food prescription program, the largest in the country. This program is a component of the Women, Infants, and Children Supplemental Feeding Program of the USDA. To receive extra food, the mother must get a prescription from a doctor, usually through the Detroit infant and maternity clinics. She is then driven to the Focus: Hope center by a volunteer, where she turns in her prescription for a variety of foods: canned meats, dried milk, peanut butter, infant formula, and canned juices. The center volunteers also give demonstrations, recipes, and educational information on nutrition and cooking. Contact: Focus: Hope, 1123 Oakman Blvd., Detroit, MI 48238 (313) 833-7440.

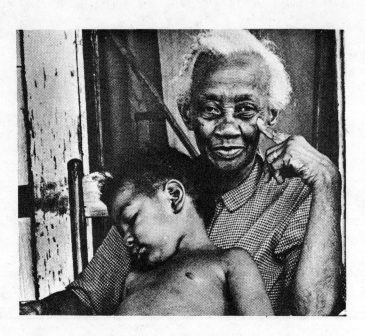

I like to think of Harriet Tubman.
Harriet Tubman who carried a revolver,
who had a scar on her head from a rock thrown
by a slave-master (because she
talked back), and who
had a ransom on her head
of thousands of dollars and who
was never caught, and who
had no use for the law
when the law was wrong,
who defied the law. I like
to think of her.
I like to think of her especially
when I think of the problem of
feeding children.

The legal answer
to the problem of feeding children
is ten free lunches every month,
being equal, in the child's real life,
to eating lunch every other day.
Monday but not Tuesday.
I like to think of the President
eating lunch Monday, but not
Tuesday.

RESOURCES

BOOKS

__Hunger USA__, Report by the Citizens' Board of Inquiry into Hunger and Malnutrition in the United States. Beacon Press, 25 Beacon St., Boston, MA 02108, 1968. 96pp. $1.95
. . .powerful expose of the extent of malnutrition and starvation in the US. In a sweeping indictment that is still applicable 6 years later, it condemns the Department of Agriculture's commodity distribution program and food stamp program for serving the agribusiness at the expense of the poor. Includes dramatic testimony from poor people throughout the country relating stories of days with little or no food, lack of money to buy foodstamps, babies and children slowly dying of malnutrition. The switch from a commodity distribution program to foodstamps results in far greater hardships in areas where the food stamp office is only open one or two days per month, and grocers raise prices the day stamps are issued. Many families lack even the money to buy foodstamps. Concludes with positive recommendations for changing the food commodity, food stamp and school lunch programs, consumer education, and public assistance.

__Hunger USA Revisited__, Citizens' Board of Inquiry into Hunger and Malnutrition in the United States, Southern Regional Council, Inc., 52 Fairlie St., NW, Atlanta, GA 30303, 1972. 52 pp. Free
. . .once again federal, state and local governments, particularly the US Department of Agriculture, are found guilty of insensitivity to the poor, bureaucratic bungling, rigidity, and political expediency. Early in 1969, President Nixon was quoted as saying in regards to food programs: "You can say that this administration will have the first complete, far-reaching attack on the problems of hunger in history. Use all the rhetoric, so long as it doesn't cost any money." Concludes with a strong statement in favor of cash disbursements rather than foodstamps, thus allowing people the opportunity to divide their income as they choose.

__Sowing the Wind__, Harrison Wellford. Bantam Books, 1973. 384 pp. $1.95
. . .hard-hitting attack on the food industry with emphasis on meat, poultry and pesticides. A Report for the Center for Study of Responsive Law on Food Safety and the Chemical Harvest, it delves into the politics behind legislation, degree of enforcement and consumer involvement. Detailed and factual. Highly recommended, but don't read it just before you plan to eat. . .it takes your appetite away.

__The Great American Food Hoax__, Sidney Margolius. Walker and Co., 720 5th Ave., New York, NY 10019, 1971. 216 pp. $5.95
. . .first-rate discussion of the $110 billion food industry, exploring why consumers pay more for less nutritional value. While sympathizing with small farmers and consumers, the author pins the blame on processors, packagers, distributors, advertisers, and the USDA. His description of the close relationship between government and the food industry is an eye-opener: "In effect, the USDA has become the Pentagon of the food industry. . . . When President Nixon took office, Bryce Harlow, the Washington lobbyist for Procter & Gamble, joined the White House staff. There was an even trade. Mike Manatos, administrative assistant to both President Johnson and President Kennedy, joined Procter & Gamble's Washington office." Recommended for groups organizing around nutrition and consumer issues—and for anyone trying to eat sanely at reasonable prices.

In eighteen months General Foods spent a cool 5.4 million dollars to promote Cool 'n Creamy.

—The Great American Food Hoax

__Consumer Beware: Your Food and What's Been Done to It__, Beatrice Trum Hunter. Simon and Schuster, New York, 1971. 442 pp.
. . .top notch expose of the food industry, with sections on the effects of advertising, how producers reduce the nutritional value of common foods, and more. "Consumer-hypnosis is never ending: soft background music, pleasant lighting, free cheese clube
sant lighting, free cheese cubes. . .and other snacks, a soft-drink bar, electric fans wafting baking smells from class side ovens, aerosprays filled with coffee or chocolate aromas. Reveals the extent to which commercial farmers raise unhealthy food because it is cheaper and easier. "Currently 90% of all commercial chickens are raised with arsenic in their feed. . . .pesticides continue to contaminate meat and run especially high in fat." Documented and detailed, this book is strongly recommended for consumer advocacy groups and consciencious shoppers.

__Out to Lunch, A Study of USDA's Day-Care and Summer Feeding Programs__, Food Research and Action Center, 25 W. 43rd St., New York, NY 10036, 1974. 94 pp. $2.00
. . . a look at the Special Food Service Program for Children. Set up to provide free and low cost meals for children not in school (too young or on summer vacation), the program has been consciously undermined by the USDA and federal government. Funds go unappropriated as restrictions and bureaucracy grow. Concludes with a score of recommendations on improving food programs for children.

__The Chemical Feast__, James S. Turner. Grossman Publishers, 44 W. 56th St., New York, NY 10019, 1970. 274 pp. $.95
. . .a Ralph Nader Study Group Report on the Food and Drug Administration's food protection efforts. The book highlights 3 major danger areas: the increasing number of chemicals in the food supply, the existence of undernutrition, and food poisoning hazards related to new food production methods. FDA's attitude has always been that the food industry (now reaching conglomerate size) is willing and able to provide the safest, highest-quality food possible. Thus, FDA simply accepts the research done by the food industry, resulting in low quality and dangerous food for the consumer. Calls for major organizational changes in FDA and offers legislative goals.

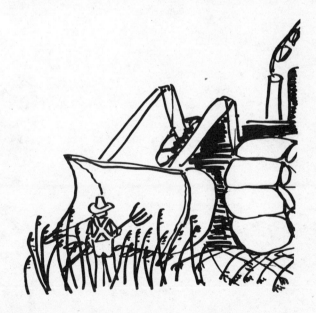

Today the government pays $4 billion yearly not to grow food, but most of this money ends up in the farm corporations; the largest 5% of farms get more cash subsidies than the smallest 60%, so the government is actually helping these corporations to drive the small farmer bankrupt. Surplus food purchases—buying surplus crops that would normally glut the market—amounts to another giveaway to Oscar Meyer, Ralston Purina, Swift, Dole, and others who share more billions each year.

—from Dave Hereth/LNS

If We Had Ham, We Could Have Ham and Eggs. . .If We Had Eggs—A Study of the National School Breakfast Program, Food Research and Action Center, 25 W. 43rd St., New York, NY 10036, 1972. 145 pp. $2.00
. . .an evaluation of the National School Breakfast Program which provides free or low-cost breakfasts for hungry children through the US Department of Agriculture. This study documents the importance of breakfast for all children, and reveals improved attendance, behavior, alertness, and classroom performance in schools that implemented the program. USDA regulations and restraints have severely inhibited the use of the program, however; in 1971, Congress was forced to pass a joint resolution ordering USDA to correct proposed new regulations restricting availability of funds and preventing new schools from entering the program. With its useful appendices covering the Statute, statistics on state participation in the program, and more, this study is a valuable piece of ammunition for those fighting to widen the scope of the Breakfast Program.

Diet for a Small Planet, Frances Moore Lappe. Ballantine Books, 101 5th Ave., New York, NY 10003, 1971. 301 pp. $1.25
. . .sound and basic guide to nutritous eating, with a wealth of information on protein, meat, sane eating habits, nutritive value of common foods. The author believes that mean consumption in the US is unnecessarily high: "Although North Americans comprise only 7% of the world population, we consume 30% of the world supplies of food of animal origin." She gives statistical back-up to the belief that malnutrition in the world could be wiped out through changes in US food consumption. Contains over 130 pages of recipes and menus which maximuze protein intake and facilitate low-cost, high-value eating.

PAMPHLETS AND ARTICLES

"YOUR GUIDE TO THE FOOD STAMP PROGRAM," Jay Lipner and Jeff Kirsch, Food Research and Action Center, 25 W. 43rd St., New York, NY 10036, 1974. Free
. . .detailed, practical tool for anyone dealing with the food-stamp bureaucracy. Includes a specific explanation of all rights under foodstamps, who is eligible, how to apply, how to compute the price of stamps and more. First class resource for community groups and individuals.

"THE REVISED SCHOOL BREAKFAST PROGRAM," Suzanne Vaupel, Food Research and Action Center, 25 W. 43rd St., New York NY 10036, 1973. 16 pp. Free
. . .useful guide for setting up a free or reduced cost school breakfast program. A step-by-step explanation of how to rally community support, approach the school board, and maintain momentum. Explains what is legally required and offers sample fliers, agendas for preparation of meetings and a section on "how to fight the 'We can't because. . .' Problem".

The Foodmakers, Center for Science in the Public Interest, 1779 Church St., NW, Washington, DC 20036. 7 pp. $.50
. . .a must for groups trying to understand the food industry. Reveals the advertising budget of leading food producers, executive salaries and the range of their products. "Coca Cola and Pepsi Cola each spend $37 million a year to promote their. . .products; in 1971, General Foods spent $4 million to promote Jell-o. General Foods spent as much on advertising as the whole state of Nevada spent on all its public schools."

"A GUIDE FOR FOOD PROGRAMS IN MONTGOMERY COUNTY," Nutrition Services, Montgomery County Health Department, Rockville, MD, 1973. 41 pp.
. . .covers food stamps, free school breakfast and lunch programs, additional public assistance for expectant women, meals on wheels and emergency food grants. Each section covers the program's purpose, who is eligible, when and where to apply, fair hearing procedures, and more. Prototype guide to one county's resources; well worth preparing in your own community.

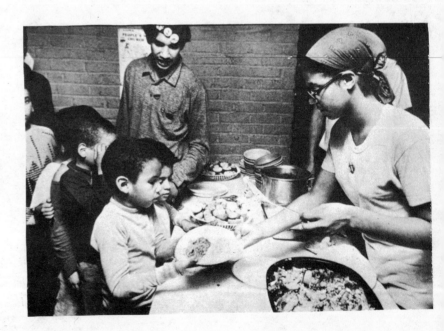

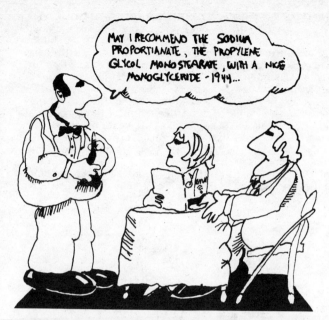

May I recommend the sodium proportianate, the propylene glycol monostearate, with a nice monoglyceride - 1944...

"**Feeding Ourselves,**" Berkeley Women's Health Collective, 2214 Grove St., Berkeley, CA 94704, 1972. 32 pp. $.35
. . .detailed, informative "people's" guide to nutritious eating. Covers how the digestive system functions (with diagrams), essential nutrients (fats, proteins, vitamins, minerals), specific diets and dieting, food for pregnancy and babies, how to conserve time and money, cooking tips, and an excellent bibliography. Chapter one is a first-rate political discussion of the $125 billion food industry: lack of power and initiative of the FDA, over-use of chemical preservatives, emphasis on appearance rather than quality, etc. "The government pays billions of dollars to keep land out of production (35 million acres in 1968) and destroys food, keeping food supply low and the prices and profits high. . .The total food packaging bill in 1968 was 3.19 billion dollars, three times the bill for welfare. . . . Every year we each eat an average of three pounds of chemical additives, chemicals they add to our food during processing." Well worth reading and distributing at neighborhood clinics and centers.

PERIODICALS

NUTRITION ACTION, Center for Science in the Public Interest, 1779 Church St., NW, Washington DC 20036. Free
. . .a bi-monthly resource aimed at developing a more political understanding of nutrition problems. "In the past, professionals have too often focused on modifying the dietary habits of a few individuals rather than on modifying corporate and government policies which shape those habits." Articles cover current local and national issues, on-going projects, program ideas, job announcements and information on Center for Science in the Public Interest undertakings.

CONSUMER PROTECTION REPORT, Center for Study of Responsive Law, Box 19367, Washington, DC 20036. $3.50/year . . . the latest investigative reporting on the food industry. The emphasis is on national issues but local struggles are also covered. Worthwhile resource.

FEED THE KIDS: IT'S THE LAW, The Children's Foundation, 1028 Connecticut Ave., NW, Washington DC 20036 Free
. . .bimonthly newsletter relating current events in the area of child nutrition. Focus is on changes in legislation as well as local programs.

CNI Weekly Report, Community Nutrition Institute, 1910 "K" St., NW, Washington, DC 20006. $10-$20/year
. . .the latest news in the food field, with an emphasis on changes in government programs. Analysis of legislation and regulations is specific and aimed at people actively involved in nutrition and food distribution programs.

FOOD CO-OP NOOZ, American Friends Service Committee, Room 370, 407 S. Dearborn St., Chicago IL 60605. $1/year
. . .facilitates the formation of co-ops, cooperation between co-ops and a political understanding of the co-op movement. Articles cover regional news, the politics of food (agribusiness, land issues, etc.), nutrition, co-op models and theory and announcements. A national food co-op directory is also available.

FILMS AND TAPES

University of California Extension Media Center, Berkeley, CA 94720

"**South: Health and Hunger,**" 23 min. b&w 1969 $12
Documents inadequate nutrition, lack of water, and shortage of medical facilities for Black people in Deep South.

"**To Feed the Hungry,**" 45 min. cl. 1969 $32
Documents extent of urban hunger caused by poverty in Chicago. Describes effects of hunger on the health of children, adults, and the elderly.

Audio-Visual Center, Indiana University, Bloomington, IN 47401
"**Hunger In America,**" 51 min. cl. $19.00
Presents evidence that 10,000,000 Americans go to bed hungry every night from "gut hunger" accompanied by malnutrition. Indicts the Department of Agriculture for its inadequate programs.

HEALTH EDUCATION

Understanding our own bodies is the first step in controlling the health care that we receive and the environment in which we live. Much of the health professionals' power over us comes from knowledge: they spent years learning about medicine or dentistry or whatever while we know nothing. Patients' feelings of inferiority in the face of this knowledge allow health professionals to get away with charging outrageous prices, writing unnecessary prescriptions, performing unnecessary operations, and, ultimately deciding who should live and who should die.

Although lack of time may prevent us from learning as much as health workers, we can certainly learn enough about our bodies to recognize and seek treatment for common diseases. Schools and youth groups should be sources of honest, complete information for children and teenagers—information on sex, drugs, mental illness, and venereal diseases in particular. Venereal disease, which can cripple and kill, is an epidemic in the US today, yet three states still have laws against classes in sex education where facts about VD, its causes, its effects, and its transmission can be taught. Many more schools either treat health education as peripheral material, thus conveying to students that it is unimportant, or else they limit the teaching to half-truths and personal opinions, leaving students unable to make their choices concerning sex and drugs.

Once out of school, individuals face mass markets of books, health care gadgets and products, over-the-counter drugs, health care plans, and nutrition fads. Swamped in advertisements with no knowledge upon which to base a decision, they are forced to believe either the ads or a doctor, in a society where the two are often in collusion (witness the recent rash of diet books by MDs). Others, too poor to join the consumerism are simply stranded, aware that their bodies have certain needs, but unable to fulfill them. Nutrition, hygiene, neurosis, and amphetamine are fancy words without meaning to many people whose ignorance makes them exceptionally gullible to the intimidation of doctors and government officials.

Creating programs in health education is not simple. Many community clinics have educational programs for patients, workers, and community; others have outreach workers who teach hygiene, home health care, and nutrition. Community groups can hold educational meetings and push for better school health programs. Laws like the VD education laws that deny us the knowledge to control our bodies must be eliminated; for knowledge, like health care in general, is our right.

The following groups are somewhat limited in their usefulness. They are, for the most part, very well funded conventional service organizations that do not in any way challenge the economic or political reasons behind poor health care in this country. But they are a source of information and statistics; some of them will provide community groups with resources for special projects such as health fairs.

COMMUNITY HEALTH EDUCATION PROJECT ...
is a project of the American Public Health Association through HEW funding. There are three components of the project: a technical assistance program in which health education workers were placed in four existing neighborhood health centers; an inter-organizational task force set up to draw health education organizations into some type of co-ordinating body; and a resource document project which studies successful health education programs and is compiling a listing of helpful projects, programs, books, films, tapes, etc. Contact CHEP/APHA, 1015 18th St., NW, Washington, DC, 20036, (202) 467-5062.

NATIONAL OPERATION VENUS PROGRAM...is a program of a Catholic youth organization in Philadelphia. Its goal: to "bring a new light to the VD problem." Since then it has expanded amazingly to some nine other cities. The program has two major activities: education and transportation to treatment. Volunteer students staff a toll-free number Hotline 24 hours a day, distribute stickers and cards, and provide the transportation for those needing it. Contact NATIONAL OPERATION VENUS PROJECT, 1620 Summer St., Philadelphia, PA 19103, 800-567-6969

NATIONAL SEX FORUM...grew out of a 1962 conference of clergy and laypeople concerned with sexuality. The conference established a commission to develop educational models and published materials. They also make extensive use of audio and video resources. Although their major work is group counseling, they are trying to develop a low-cost self-help program. "The Forum takes an esthetic view of human sexuality, emphasizing both the value of sexuality and of proficiency rather than constraint." Contact NATIONAL SEX FORUM, 540 Powell St., San Francisco, CA 94102, 415-989-6176.

INSTITUTE FOR FAMILY RESEARCH AND EDUCATION
..."is devoted to the strengthening of the American family" through pushing parents to communicate with their children about human development and sexuality. The Institute has two sub-divisions: the Family Planning and Population Information Center and Ed-U-Press. In the past they have published five comic books geared towards teaching adolescents about sex, birth control, VD, drugs, and nutrition, and they are now producing a sixth on alcoholism. Although they are admittedly conservative, their past publications, newsletters, and resource guides have been straightforward and well-written. Facts About Sex for Today's Youth, their book for young people, is probably the first to use Black and other minorities among its illustrations. Contact IFRE, Syracuse University, College for Human Development, 760 Ostrum Ave., Syracuse, NY 13210, 315-476-4584.

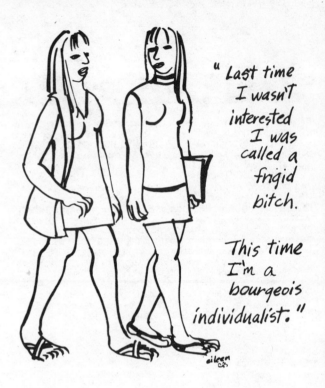

" Last time I wasn't interested I was called a frigid bitch.

This time I'm a bourgeois individualist."

SEX INFORMATION AND EDUCATION COUNCIL OF THE US...was founded in 1964 by a group of professionals, including physicians, sex educators, and social workers who feel that preventive medicine, rather than remedial help, is the key to problems in understanding human sexuality. They conduct conferences and workshops, and serve as a clearinghouse for sex education materials and programs, helping others to build their own programs. SIECUS REPORT is their bi-monthly newsletter of developments and resources in sex education. Contact SIECUS, 1855 Broadway, New York, NY 10023, 212-581-7480.

AMERICAN HEART ASSOCIATION...does education and research on heart disease and heart attacks. One third of their total budget goes to research and another third to publicity and administration, but they still spend $8 million on community services and $6 million on public education. Their health education program includes speakers, films, pamphlets, and periodicals; they also provide community and individual services such as rehabilitation, referrals, and some help in organizing campaigns against strep throat, since strep leads to rheumatic, which can cause heart damage. State and city AHA agencies are autonomous and choose their own programs. Contact AHA, 44 E. 23rd St., New York, NY 10010, 212-477-9170.

AMERICAN CANCER SOCIETY...is a private organization working to control and eradicate cancer. The Society is involved primarily in education, but also supports research and runs rehabilitation and aid programs for cancer patients. Pamphlets, films, speakers, and exhibits are provided on request. Contact the local chapter listed in your phone book, or ACS, 219 E. 42nd St., New York, NY 10017, 212-867-3700.

RESOURCES

BOOKS

The Well Body Book, Mike Samuels, MD, and Hal Bennett, Random House/Bookworks, 1409 Fifth St., Berkeley, CA 94710, 1973. 350 pp. $5.95
...the best of a recent barrage of home medical handbooks. A very supportive, reassuring and relaxing book to read, it combines aspects of Eastern philosophy with Western medicine, describing "how to do a complete physical exam, how to diagnose common diseases, how to practice preventive medicine, and how to get the most from your doctor." The back cover says "look inside for ways to help overcome your fear of disease and enjoy your body more;" the authors live up to that promise through a realistic and sensitive view of how much a layperson can care for his/her body and when a doctor is needed as a resource person. Makes for educational and very pleasurable reading.

An Everyday Guide To Your Health, David Stuart Sobel and Faith Louise Hornbacher, Grossman Publisher, 625 Madison Ave., New York, NY 10022, 19 . 192 pp. $4.95
...tells how to take the time to be kind to your body. The book promotes health of the whole person through relaxation, laughter, good eating habits, sensitivity to body rhythms, and creating healthy environments. Graphics are pleasant, often instructive. This is recommended as an introduction to a more total approach to health than many people are accustomed.

The Complete Reference Book on Vasectomy, Michael Greenfield, M.D., and William M. Burrus, Avon Books, 959 Eighth Ave., New York, NY 10019, 1973. 253 pp. $1.65
...a persuasive and informative guide to male sterilization. The authors discuss the history of vasectomy, sperm banks, and machismo, as well as personal accounts of the operation. For the most part they seem to be men who are fighting traditional sex roles, although there are a few statements meant to reassure men that make a feminist cringe: "One might say ...that this operation now restores manliness in a sense, for it gives a man a chance to control his own and his mate's child-bearing destiny." The appendix of vasectomy clinics and resources is useful.

PAMPHLETS AND ARTICLES

"VENEREAL DISEASE," Health Organizing Collective of NY Women's Health and Abortion Project, 36 W. 22nd St., New York, NY 10010, 1971. 8pp.
...a political discussion of VD, particularly Gonorrhea. "No one in authority was ready to put money into researching and eliminating a disease which most severely affected poor (White, Black and Brown) people... As long as we have racism, sexism, a profit-making health care system, and an uninformed, moralistic public, we will continue to have terrible health problems such as uncontrolled gonorrhea." Covers symptoms (and lack of), testing, diagnosis, effects of gonorrhea, treatment, funding for research, and lack of preventive care.

Today's VD Control Problem: 1973, American Social Health Association, New York, NY 10019, 1973. 62 pp. $2.00
...outstanding collection of statistics, charts, and tables as well as an evaluation of recent national campaigns against VD. Includes information of public funds available for fighting VD, effectiveness of the Model Cities Program's publicity on VD, and more.

"VD CLAPTRAP," Ed-U-Press, 760 Ostrum Ave., Syracuse, NY 13210, 1972. 16 pp. $ .25
...introductory material in comic book form, geared to teenagers. Ms. Wanda Lust and Captain Vee-dee-o zap the Kling-on invaders as well as myths about VD. Their exploits on Venus provide some down-to-earth information on how to get VD, how to get rid of it, and how to prevent it. Effective and well-presented.

Venereal Diseases: the Silent Menace, Abe A. Brown and Simon Podair. Public Affairs Pamphlets, 381 Park Ave., S., New York, NY 10016, 1970. 20 pp. $ .35
...one in a series of pamphlets published by the Public Affairs Committee, founded to "educate the American public on vital economic and social problems" through a series of pamphlets. The pamphlet is short and factual; it gives definitions, erases misconceptions, explains causes and suggests controls. The conclusion is succinctly stated: "VD can be controlled only if we recognize it for what it is—a serious symptom of public apathy." Contains listing of books and films. Good beginning resource for educational work.

"A BASIC LIST OF SEX EDUCATION AND POPULATION RESOURCE IDEAS," Prepared by Institute for Family Research and Education, Syracuse University, 760 Ostrom Ave., Syracuse, NY 13210, 1974. 11 pp. Free
...lists national organizations, federal programs on family planning, films, publications, books designated for parents, students, and adolescents, and general resource books. Some of these resources are very useful.

"The Houston Story: A Vasectomy Service in a Family Planning Clinic," FAMILY PLANNING PERSPECTIVES, 515 Madison Ave., New York, NY 10022, July 1971. pp. 46-49
...Factual account of the creation and operation of a vasectomy clinic. The clinic was a direct result of concern over the safety of birth control pills and the effectiveness of other

methods. Details prior attitudes of area doctors towards vasectomy (fear of malpractice suits, religious and personal hesitations) and specifics on how the clinic functions. Eight pictures show exactly how a vasectomy is performed. This is an excellent resource for groups starting a clinic or wishing to explain the operation to potential patients.

"PHYSICAL FACTS OF SEXUAL INTERCOURSE," Minnesota Women's Counseling Service, 808 E. Franklin, Minneapolis, MN 55404 1971. 5 pp. $.10
. . .straightforward description of the four physical phases of intercourse: excitement, plateau, orgasm and resolution. Using Masters and Johnson as a reference, the article dispels the myths of female frigidity and the vaginal orgasm. Offers basic facts with a blatant feminist perspective.

"THE MYTH OF THE VAGINAL ORGASM," Anne Koedt, Minnesota Women's Counseling Service, 808 E. Franklin, Minneapolis, MN 55404, 1969. 5 pp. $.15
. . .a brief history of the sexual oppression of women by Freudian thought and belief in the vaginal orgasm. Explains the physiological fallacy of vaginal orgasm and male fear of the clitoris. Acceptance of the clitoral orgasm makes men dispensible, thus male psychologists perpetuate the myth. Good feminist introduction to female sexuality.

"TEN HEAVY FACTS ABOUT SEX," Sol Gorden and Roger Conant, Ed-U-Press, 760 Ostrum Ave., Syracuse, NY 13210, 1972. 8 pp. $.25
. . ."that your friends don't know, that your parents didn't tell you, that your doctors and counselors ain't talkin' about, that your school is steppin' light around." Covers sexuality, VD, birth control methods, and abortion through comix and text. Written for teenagers; good for youth and free clinic waiting rooms.

"PROTECT YOURSELF FROM BECOMING AN UNWANTED PARENT" Sol Gorden and Roger Conant, Ed-U-Press, 760 Ostrum Ave., Syracuse, NY 13210, 8 pp. $.25
. . .much the same as "TEN HEAVY FACTS ABOUT SEX" (same formate, some overlap of information) with more detail on sexual relationships, pregnancy, and birth control methods. Urges those who do decide to be heterosexually active to protect themselves from unwanted pregnancy and VD.

"POLITICS OF GONORRHEA," Sharon Rozan and Michael Liebowitz. Available from Louise Rice, 65 Chestnut St., Cambridge, MA 02139, 1971. 22 pp. $1.00
. . .a fine pamphlet documenting both the severity of the gonorrhea epidemic in the US and the inadequacy of present attempts to stop it. Emphasizing that "our present American health system is not capable of dealing with the gonorrhea problem," the authors call for the training of paramedics for massive screenings of possible gonorrhea carriers, especially women (since their symptoms often go undetected).

FILMS AND TAPES

Texture Films, 1600 Broadway, Room 604A, New York, NY 10023
    "How About You?" $35 (sale: $290.00)
    Records high school students involved in rap sessions with several women counselors about sex and birth control.

Audio-Visual Center, Indiana University, Bloomington IN 47401
    "Three R's. . .and Sex Education," 60 min. b&w $13.50 (sale: $265)
    Explores the many opposing feelings and ideas on teaching sex education in schools. Shows a bitter campaign against sex education in Cedar Rapids, Iowa.

EMERGENCIES

Emergency medical care is something that most people don't think about until they find themselves on their way to the emergency room. At that point they are totally vulnerable in a situation where the lack of an essential piece of equipment, the mistakes of an untrained, over-worked attendant, or a delay of several minutes can mean the difference between life and death. In the U.S., 115,000 people die each year from accidents and more than 50 million are injured. There is little data available to indicate how many injuries are needlessly compounded or how many deaths could have been avoided, but it is clear that the components of an effective emergency medical system are missing in most parts of the country. The government reports that only 20% of ambulance personnel have received emergency care training up to the level of national standards and only one-third of hospital emergency rooms are adequately equipped and staffed.

The first connection between the person in need and proper medical care is usually the telephone. Often there is no central place to call for emergency medical assistance and

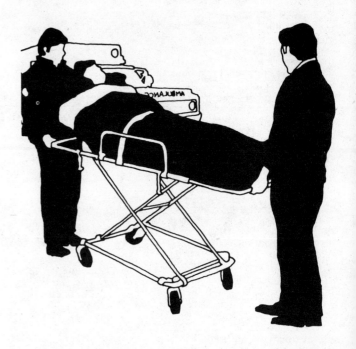

The Ambulance Association of America has estimated that 25,000 persons are permanently injured or disabled every year by untrained ambulance attendants and rescue workers.
—Emergency Health Services

the operator who receives the call has limited knowledge of how to handle the request. Many cities are putting in the 911 telephone system so that citizens can dial that number, preferably toll-free, for police, ambulance and firefighters. This is certainly more efficient, but bring up questions such as: Who runs the 911 system—police, firefighters or community people? This is particularly important if the 911 system is to be computerized (a demonstration project is going on in Alameda County, California to explore this possibility). Will the same computer handle law enforcement data and emergency location data? What other information will be computerized? If the computer is to identify the telephone number and location of callers, will unlisted numbers be identified? Will computerized 911 be abused to violate civil liberties? When private ambulance services are available, who decides which company should pick up the patient—and make the money? All these questions have serious political implications.

After the initial call for help, the next step is the dispatching of the ambulance which may be controlled by volunteers, the police or fire department, although the latter are generally overloaded with other responsibilities. Or it may be controlled by a profit-making company. A private ambulance service may not make pick-ups in low-income areas, and may refuse to pick up those who can't pay in advance. Even if a person has the money, s/he may receive low quality care en route to the hospital. Only two states have laws regulating ambulance services and the vehicles themselves are often not built for the high speeds and frequent stops they must endure. Working under conditions that "demand long hours of grim, depressing work for incredibly low wages" (PIRG in Michigan), attendants and drivers usually have a high turnover rate and inadequate training. Only 15% of ambulances are able to communicate by radio with hospital emergency departments.

The typical emergency room is truly the "back door" of the hospital: crowded, understaffed, poorly designed, and underequipped. Patients complain of overcharging and receiving substandard care from inexperienced interns who usually understand English only and have no interpreters available. Sometimes those who can't pay are turned away at the door or interrogated about credit and insurance before receiving treatment. It is not uncommon for group practices to lease emergency rooms; the doctors involved are not accountable to the hospital administration and generally make more money than those on the hospital staff. In California there are documented cases of doctors leasing emergency rooms and then further increasing their profits by selling patients to hospitals, often for unnecessary treatment. Since few medical schools offer specialized training in emergency care, it is not surprising to find aggravated injuries and needless deaths caused by neglect and professional incompetence. Even Dr. Walter C. Bornemeir, AMA president in 1971, admitted that "It has been said facetiously but perhaps with some truth, that there are a great many perfectly competent physicians who, when faced with an emergency outside of their special field, are little more effective in helping the victim than a well-trained Boy Scout." Because the emergency room is one of the least prestigious and most frustrating parts of the hospital, personnel tends to move to other department quickly.

The emergency medical technicians and staff have their own complaints; since two-thirds of all cases coming in are not true emergencies, the number of patients is unnecessarily large and conditions crowded. Poor people who have no other transportation to medical facilities take up needed ambulance space and time. Often they do not need emergency services, but they do need medical care; the emergency room is the only place they can get it, since they lack access to regular medical check-ups, private doctors, and clinics that are open only while they are at work. Middle class people are also forced to use the emergency room as back-up service when their doctors are unavailable (i.e., on weekends, summer months and late evenings).

What is bad in the cities is usually worse in the country, where hospitals are few and accidents may go undiscovered for long periods of time. Until recently, many rural area ambulance servicers were provided by funeral homes; recent federal legislation on ambulance regulations has resulted in the discontinuation of funeral home ambulance services, leaving the area even worse prepared than before to deal with emergencies.

Thus, the right to decent medical care is routinely denied in the ambulance and in the emergency room. There are obvious first steps that must be taken if the situation is to be alleviated. Ambulance attendants should be required to undergo a uniform training program, and should be better paid

with shorter work shifts. Ambulance regulations should be more strict in the areas of equipment and design. Communication between a well-trained dispatcher and ambulance, and between the ambulance and the emergency room technician can facilitate more efficient care. And since firefighters and police are often the first on the scene of an accident, many lives can be saved if they are trained to provide more than the most elementary first aid before the ambulance carries.

Area-wide planning and regionalization of hospitals is being implemented in some cities and can improve emergency care. This means that all hospitals would provide basic emergency care with some also offering specialized treatment for unusually critical cases, such as severely burned patients. Emergency cases would go to the nearest hospital and then, after receiving preliminary treatment, some patients would be sent to a hospital offering the necessary specialty. This saves money and resources as well as improving the quality of care in unusual and critical cases.

The situation in the emergency room itself can be improved if the hospitals will provide a 24-hour outpatient clinic with free non-emergency transportation so that only true emergencies go to the emergency room. The emergency room should be adequately staffed by personnel (including doctors) who are specially trained in providing emergency care. Interpreters should be provided for non-English-speaking patients and all bills, treatments and tests should be thoroughly explained. No one should be asked about money before receiving treatment.

It seems highly unlikely that hospitals will improve emergency services on their own initiative but there are various ways community people can push them along. One method is to set up a complaint and information table in the hospital to find out specific incidences and common problems. Do a case review of deaths en route to and in the emergency room—how many can be avoided? Find out about your state's regulations involving emergencies and see who's responsible for enforcing them and how effective they are. The local Public Interest Research Group may be of help or a patient's rights group may want to organize around emergency rooms.

Emergency medical care is a crucial problem that is all too often ignored. There is very little work going on in the area that has real consumer participation. The group write-ups that follow show a few different trends and approaches to emergency care on a local and state level.

SEVEN AREAS COUNCIL FOR HEALTH EMERGENCY SERVICE ASSOCIATION... began in 1972 when people in the Deckers Valley region of West Virginia started getting together for health sound-offs. It soon was clear that ambulance services were a major gripe. The city ambulance service was restricted to certain city boundaries, the one private purveyor demanded $30 before picking people up, and the local mortician had discontinued his ambulance service. So some people of Rockforge began working to establish a community based, community controlled volunteer service for the 75,000 residents of the seven town area. The ser-

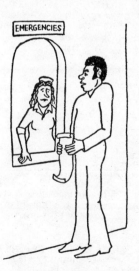

"I BLED ON THIS FORM. MAY I HAVE ANOTHER?"

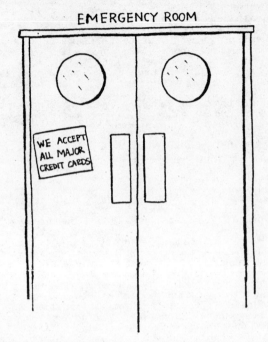

EMERGENCY ROOM

WE ACCEPT ALL MAJOR CREDIT CARDS

vice is just getting off the ground and is based on subscriptions: $15 per family per year covers as many runs as are needed. This should pay for about 25% of the cost. The rest will be covered by a federal grant and county money, so they will be able to serve those who cannot pay. About 20 people ranging in age from 17 to 81 operate the service, each working three or four hours a week. They are being trained as emergency medical technicians, will do maintenance on the ambulance, collect subscription money, and are building a center for the ambulance to work out of. This exceptional group is governed by an elected board of directors and is in the process of buying their first ambulance. Contact SEVEN AREAS COUNCIL FOR HEALTH EMERGENCY SERVICES, Rockforge Neighborhood House, Rockforge, WV 26505, (304) 292-3286.

MEDICAL COMMITTEE FOR HUMAN RIGHTS. . . provides medical presence in potential and actual emergency situations, such as Wounded Knee, Mardi Gras, and various demonstrations. The level of involvement varies from chapter to chapter. To find your closest chapter, contact MCHR, P.O. Box 7155, Pittsburgh, PA 15213, (412) 682-1200.

DIVISION OF EMERGENCY MEDICAL SERVICES AND HIGHWAY SAFETY. . .in Illinois has developed a total state-wide emergency service system that is the best in the country. The Division has developed training and education courses for doctors, nurses and ambulance attendants, as well as developing radio equipment enabling ambulances to communicate with hospitals and other ambulances. But the key to Illinois' success is regionalization and categorization of hospitals around the state, carefully planned to provide a center for every 25-mile radius. All hospital emergency rooms in the state are coordinated on a local, area-wide and regional level. The regional trauma centers are the most specialized, with sophisticated equipment and highly-trained staff. In extreme cases, helicopters are used to transport patients from local or area-wide centers to the regional. Illinois has received a federal grant to help pay for emergency services and develop public education programs. Contact DIVISION OF EMERGENCY MEDICAL SERVICES AND HIGHWAY SAFETY, Illinois Department of Public Health, 1825 W. Harrison St., Chicago, IL 60612, (312) 793-3880.

US DEPARTMENT OF TRANSPORTATION. . . offers a number of training courses for emergency medical technicians and traffic law enforcement officers. For information on teaching aids and course guides, contact US DEPARTMENT OF TRANSPORTATION, National Highway Traffic Safety Administration, Rescue and Emergency Medical Services Division, 400 7th St., SW, Washington, D.C. 20590, (202) 426-9650.

RESOURCES

BOOKS

State Statutes on Emergency Medical Services, US Department of Health, Education and Welfare. Available from US Superintendent of Documents, US Government Printing Office, Washington, D.C. 20402, 1972. 192 pp.
. . . a summary of all state legislation pertaining to emergency medical services, as well as the highlights of the acts in each state. Ends with a model act for emergency medical services.

The Ambulatory Care Program: A Manual for Consumers, Margaret F. McCann, Community Health Institute, 55 W. 44th St., New York, NY 10036, 1974. 50 pp. $3 for consumers, $5 for providers

. . . "designed to help consumers participate actively on Ambulatory Care Services Advisory Committees." in New York City. This useful manual tells how the committee can best use its power to promote accountability of the hospital to the community, giving specific guidelines for out-patient departments and emergency rooms, while also emphasizing the responsibility of the committee to find out the health needs of the community. Written in a straightforward and interesting style, this book is a fine model for any community health organization, with a good glossary of unfamiliar terms at the end.

PAMPHLETS AND ARTICLES

They're Supposed to Save Your Life: An Evaluation of the Private Ambulance Industry in Michigan, Michael B. Peisner and R. Eldridge Hicks, Public Interest Research Group in Michigan, 615 East Michigan Ave., Lansing, MI 48933, May 29, 1973. 89 pp. $.75
. . . a shocking expose of the ambulance industry. In their relentless pursuit of the facts, the authors lay down horror story upon horror story. For example, the regulations for ambulances in Michigan are so vague that a VW station wagon can legally be used. According to one former ambulance attendant and Red Cross instructor, "Under present laws and regulations in Michigan, a Boy Scout with an advanced first aid merit badge. . . and $225 can start his own ambulance business." Factual, concise, well-documented, this report is an excellent model for other groups investigating the issue of emergency medical care.

"THE HERRICK STRUGGLE: ORGANIZING ISSUES," Nancy Green, available from Robert Boesch, 209 W. 97th St., New York, NY 10025, April, 1972. 8 pp. Free
. . . the story of an MCHR attempt to improve emergency room care at Berkeley's Herrick hospital. MCHR had community support and managed to force Herrick to institute new billing policies which do not require cash or proof of insurance before treatment, but they made some crucial mistakes, discussed here in terms of goals, strategy, and basic analysis. Very important resource.

"The State of Emergency Medical Services Under the Highway Safety Act, or Don't Be Caught Dead in an Ambulance," Susan Grossman Alexander, CLEARINGHOUSE REVIEW, National Clearinghouse for Legal Services, Northwestern University School of Law, Abbott Hall, 710 N. Lake Shore Dr., Chicago, IL 60611, June, 1971. pp. 72-74
. . . discusses the Highway Safety Act of 1966 which "requires that each state have a highway safety program meet-

ing certain uniform standards promulgated by the Secretary of the Department of Transportation (DOT)." This includes 16 standards for emergency medical services that focus on highway accidents, but will improve emergency care for everyone. As of March, 1971, no state had received an "A" rating for their emergency plan. The DOT has the option of cutting off Federal highway funds to states that do not meet the Highway Safety Act's requirements. The author, a staff attorney for the National Legal Program on Health Programs of the Poor, is interested in the possibility of aggrieved individuals starting litigation against states where the emergency plan is substandard by the guidelines of this act. The article is slightly outdated but still very valuable.

THE THREE FUNCTIONS OF THE EMERGENCY ROOM— A PLEA FOR THE PATIENT," Louise Lander, Health Law Project, University of Pennsylvania Law School, 133 South 36th St., Philadelphia, PA 19174, 1972. 52 pp. $2.00 on a sliding scale
. . . an excellent analysis of the emergency room in its three functions: trauma center, family doctor, and medical back-up. Most professional groups and government agencies are concerned with improving the emergency room in its trauma center function but are not dealing with the other demands the public makes on it. Lander sees the solution in consumer control of health care delivery, so that the family doctor and medical back-up functions will be filled through "group practices, satellite clinics, neighborhood health centers, and outreach programs by health care teams." She also suggests ways to improve the emergency room as a trauma center through protection of patients' rights, better organization and departmental status for the emergency service.

ACCIDENTAL DEATH AND DISABILITY: THE NEGLECTED DISEASE OF MODERN SOCIETY, Division of Medical Sciences, National Research Council, 2101 Constitution Ave., NW, Washington, D.C. 20418, 1970. 38 pp. Free
. . . points out the failings and inadequacies of US emergency medical services. This excellent study outlines specific areas of failure, the results in terms of cost, deaths and disabilities, as well as recommendations for change.

"First Aid for Activists," in Beat the Heat: A Radical Survival Handbook, Berkeley International Liberation School, Ramparts Press, Box 10128, Palo Alto, CA 94303, 1972. pp. 169-241. $2.45
. . . was written collectively by nurses, doctors, and medics, many of them active in Medical Committee for Human Rights. It is a well-illustrated guide to street medicine, emphasizing that the information presented is only useful if practiced under knowledgeable supervision. A brief introduction to physiology, diagnosis and treatment, and recommendations for medical preparation in collective living are presented in an informal style. There are a few questionable recommendations (such as telling raped women to ask for the "morning-after" pill), but this is a basically worthwhile book.

"Medical Problems of Civil Disorders: Organization of a Volunteer Group of Health Professionals to Provide Health Services in a Riot," Arthur Frank and other members of the Metropolitan Washington Chapter of MCHR, NEW ENGLAND JOURNAL OF MEDICINE, available from MCHR, 2506 Cliffbourne Place, Washington, D.C. 20009, January 30, 1969. pp. 247-253
. . . an excellent article giving strategies and considerations for people practicing street medicine during demonstrations and riots. Obviously the authors have had a lot of experience in the area; they tell how to organize the original group of volunteers, set up headquarters, broaden community contacts, and choose proper supplies. Also covers the care of the injured in jails and hospitals, establishing refugee centers and spreading medical information. An outstanding pragmatic guide.

EMERGENCY MEDICAL SERVICES COMMUNICATIONS SYSTEMS, U.S. Department of HEW Health Services and Mental Health Administration, Division of Emergency Health Services, 5600 Fishers Lane, Rockville, Maryland 20852, August, 1972. 38 pp. Free
. . . deals with some of the major considerations in planning Emergency Medical Services Communications Systems: how will ambulances be dispatched, who provides EMS transportation services, will there be a central dispatch for the entire area, etc. The pamphlet also describes 911 briefly.

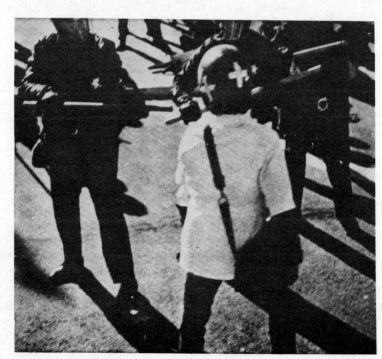

GAY RESOURCES

Gay people are consistently ridiculed and discriminated against by a frightened and ignorant "straight" society whose rigid male&female roles they threaten. Legally they are selectively persecuted (homosexuality is still officially illegal in all but 8 states) and denied human respect and basic rights. In the area of health, gay people face overwhelming problems. For instance, doctors seldom check gay men for anal or oral VD, although both can cause serious illness. Gay hospital patients are often ignored by attendants and professionals who are afraid to touch them; documented cases exist of patients dying as a result of this neglect. A less dramatic but more common problem faced by sexual minorities (gay people, transexuals, and transvestites) is being treated by doctors with whom open, honest communication is impossible. And in one major eastern city the gay doctors who do exist routinely charge more than straight doctors.

Psychiatric care, when sought, is often very destructive. Lesbians are driven to shrinks by gynecologists who tell them they are "sick, but young enough to change"; male psychiatrists' "therapy" is often to proposition them. The resulting frustration can help push gay people into dependencies on drugs and alcohol.

Gay people are coming together to confront the oppressive attitudes of straight society. They are organizing switchboards, rap groups, counseling services and making referrals to gay and non-offensive doctors. Gay organizations have recently been successful in their demands for gay advocates in health institutions; several groups have formed to halt the increase of VD in the gay community and many free clinics offer special services one night a week for gay people. In addition, some lesbians are forming self-help groups. As the gay health movement grows, two major focuses can be identified: those challenging the health profession from the outside through law suits, etc. and those organizing caucuses of gay nurses, medical students and other health workers from within.

GAY NURSES ALLIANCES. . .consists of caucuses of gay nurses in 6 states as well as individuals throughout the country. Formed in August, 1973, the Alliance, which includes men and women, works to protect the rights of gay nurses and to improve the way gay people are treated by all health professionals. Many of the organization's struggles have centered around the American Nursing Association (ANA); currently they are working to guarantee gay representation on ANA's Task Force For Affirmative Action (which is supposed to represent the interests of minorities). The Alliance is also organizing support in the National League of Nursing for their proposal that nursing schools discuss gayness as a lifestyle in community medicine courses rather than an issue in mental health. GNA has also been instrumental in helping gay nurses who have had their licenses suspended because of their sexual orientation regain the right to practice. Contact Gay Nurses Alliance, P.O. Box 5687, Philadelphia, PA 19129.

"NINE ONE-ONE/THE EMERGENCY TELEPHONE NUMBER: A HANDBOOK FOR COMMUNITY PLANNING," Executive Office of the President, Office of Telecommunications Policy, for sale by the Superintendent of Documents, US Government Printing Office, Washington, D.C. 20402, 1973. 62 pp. $1.35
. . . a handbook "to assist communities in the implementation of 911 service." 911 is easy to dial and remember, gives fast access to emergency services and is especially beneficial to travelers who need help in a strange town. This handbook tells in some detail the problems a community must work out before implementing 911: location of answering center, selection of agencies to be included in the emergency services, the area to be served and more. This handbook is a pretty complete guide to 911, although it does not discuss computerized 911 systems.

"Dial 911," ROLLING STONE, 625 Third St., San Francisco, CA 94107, May 14, 1974. p. 11
. . . brief discussion of the possible ways in which computerized 911 systems may violate civil liberties.

MEDICAL REQUIREMENTS FOR AMBULANCE DESIGN AND EQUIPMENT, National Research Council, National Academy of Sciences, Division of Medical Science, available from Superintendent of Documents, U.S. Government Printing Office, Washington, D.C. 20402, 1970. 23 pp. $.25
. . . guidelines for automotive designers and manufacturers as to what an ambulance must be if it is to provide safe emergency care. Good resource for those concerned with promoting state legislation for ambulance design.

Newsreel, 26 W. 20th St., New York, NY 10011

"Cyclone," 20 min. b&w $20
Ravaged by hurricanes and floods, Cuba mobilizes her forces to save lives, salvage belongings, and bring food and medical aid to the hurricane victims.

"Medical Committee for Human Rights," 15 min. b&w $25
The film shows the committees role during the long strike at San Francisco State College and the need for tactical knowledge of first aid as our struggle intensifies.

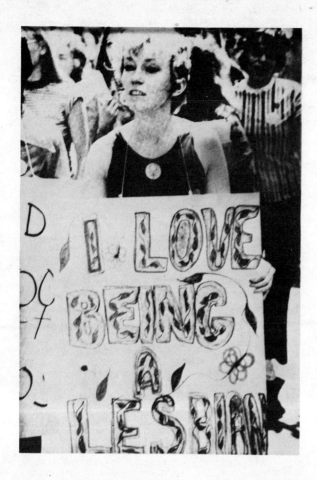

GAY MEN'S HEALTH PROJECT... operates a V.D. diagnostic clinic. Run collectively by and for gay men, the clinic is open two nights a week and sees up to 30 people each evening. Although the clinic can not provide direct treatment, it does make referrals. The project grew out of a gay counseling-coffeehouse collective whose members were approached by a city V.D. control worker to do a seminar on gay V.D. problems. Currently, the clinic receives medical supplies from the city and other expenses are paid from patient donations. A 60 page booklet covering all aspects of V.D. in gay people is to be published soon by the project. Contact Gay Men's Health Project, 247 W. 11th St., New York, NY 10014, (212) 691-6969.

GAY MEN'S V.D. COLLECTIVE... began in September, 1973 by a small group of gay men who were disturbed by the rapid rise of V.D. in the gay community. They have set up a V.D. testing and treatment program every Saturday afternoon using the facilities of the Washington Free Clinic. The collective sees 10-15 patients each weekend and is also responsible for training screeners for the clinic's nightly testing and treatment program. Further, they are involved in writing articles in community papers and developing educational projects. Contact Gay Men's V.D. Collective, c/o Washington Free Clinic, 1556 Wisconsin Ave., NW, Washington, D.C. 20007, (202) 965-5476.

HOMOPHILE COMMUNITY HEALTH SERVICE... began in 1972 with a staff of 5 and has since grown to 40 people. Client fees, private donations, and church grants fund the Service, which provides all types of counseling therapy, education, and social work. The staff teach courses on homosexuality at nearby universities, and many universities and colleges place student interns at the Service. They soon hope to have their own Institute of Homophile Studies. Contact Homophile Community Health Service, Rm 403, 419 Boylston St., Boston, MA 02116, (617) 266-1950.

ASSOCIATION OF GAY PSYCHOLOGISTS... was founded at the 1973 American Psychological Association convention. The more than 150 lesbian and gay male members insist ""that homosexuality be viewed as a viable alternative lifestyle rather than as a sickness". They are pressuring the APA to support the right of lesbian mothers to rear their own children, to eliminate all forms of discrimination against gay people and to remove homosexuality from the list of official psychiatric disorders. Recently APA reclassified homosexuality as a "sexual deviation" rather than as a "sickness." AGP recognizes that many gay people have been unjustly told by psychologists that they are bad or crazy. Tactics of AGP include creation of a speakers bureau, representation at national conferences and visiting lectureships. Contact AGP, c/o Dr. Mark Freedman, 1111 Jones St., No. 9, San Francisco, CA 94109, (415) 776-8842.

GAY COMMUNITY SERVICES CENTER... is a widely known, active organization offering psychological and informational help to the gay community. The center was founded by gay men and women in 1971, and is supported by donations. Services are given in a "non-judgemental and supportive atmosphere" and include such projects as a 24-hour hotline, awareness, consciousness-raising, and lesbian mother discussion groups, a drug/alcohol abuse program, a welfare rights group, transvestite and transexual counseling, temporary food and housing, VD and women's clinic and much more. The prisoner, parole and probation program provides counseling and supportive services to gay inmates and parolees. A representative of the Center is present daily at the Los Angeles sentencing and probation programs for sexual minorities. The Center also has a booklet on gay health in the process of being published. Staff is mainly volunteer, with a core group of paid workers. Contact Gay Community Services Center, 1614 Wilshire Blvd., Los Angeles, CA 90017, (213) 482-3062.

SEATTLE COUNSELING SERVICE... started in 1968, and is the oldest mental health agency for sexual minorities in the U.S. A small professional staff, paid at a subsistence level, is assisted by many paraprofessional volunteers, with all workers participating in collective decision-making. The Service is funded by the County Board of Mental Health, and offers crisis intervention counseling over the phone, as well as in-person individual and group-counseling. Although the group has no political line, many of the workers consider themselves close to the ideas of radical therapy. Fees are based on a sliding scale and no one is turned down for services. They also work with the straight community, from police recruits to social workers, to help them understand the problems of gayness. Contact: Seattle Counseling Service, 1720 16th Ave., Seattle, WA 98122, (206) 329-8708

GENERAL GROUPS

LESBIAN RESOURCE CENTER... part of the University YWCA programming, it is totally staffed by volunteers and coordinated by the Y staff. A Survival file, small library, speakers bureau, small rap groups, counseling and information on homophile organizations in the Seattle area are available over the phone or in person. For more information contact: Lesbian's Resource Center, 4224 University Way, NE, Seattle, WA 98105, (206) 632-4747.

NATIONAL GAY STUDENT CENTER... "is currently compiling a list of gay student groups, gay studies course syllabi and information on campus problems." Welcoming input from campuses on any of the above, the Center, which is a project of the National Student Association, also publishes a bimonthly newsletter, "Interchange", available for $3 yearly. Though not an official Center project, the coordinator is compiling information on lesbian health problems. For a listing of the Center's resources or more information, contact NGSC, c/o NSA, 2115 S. St., NW, Washington, D.C. 20010, (202) 265-9890.

DAUGHTERS OF BILITIS. . . began in 1955 as a women's organization dedicated to seeking rights for Lesbians. In the 1960's DOB expanded to include the struggle for the rights of all women. Presently they offer rap sessions for older gay women, for lesbian mothers and on being gay. Local chapters frequently do referrals, counseling, and consciousness-raising, as well as sponsoring speaker bureaus and serving as educational and civil rights organizations. Contact: Daughters of Bilitis, 419 Boylston St., Boston, MA 02116, (617) 262-1592.

MATTACHINE SOCIETY. . . is the oldest gay organization in the country and serves both men and women. Their services include making referrals, educating the public, and acting as an information center for gay people. Lawyers try to get victims of antiquated sex laws off with the least amount of publicity and embarrassment, and help gays who are being blackmailed. Since no federal law prohibits discrimination based upon sexual preferences, the Mattachine Society is working for the passage of such legislation. They have offices in Washington, D.C., Chicago, and New York City. Contact Mattachine Society, 243 W. 5th Ave., New York, NY 10016, (212) 262-1592.

SWITCHBOARDS

PHILADELPHIA GAY SWITCHBOARD, 1735 Naudine St., Philadelphia, PA 19146, (215) 978-5700.

GAY INFORMATION OF SAN DIEGO, 2250 B St., San Diego, CA 92102, (714) 232-1411.

CHICAGO GAY SWITCHBOARD AND INFORMATION SERVICE, Beckman House, 3519 N. Halsted, Chicago, IL 60657, (312) 929-HELP.

GAY HOTLINE OF BOSTON, HUB, 419 Boyleston St., Room 509, Boston, MA 02116, (617) 354-1555.

ANN ARBOR GAY HOTLINE, 530 S. St., Room 325, Ann Arbor, MI 48103, (313) 761-2044. Daily 6-10.

SAN ANTONIO GAY SWITCHBOARD, Gay Community Services, San Antonio Free Clinic, 1136 W. Woodlawn, San Antonio, TX 78201, (512) 733-7300. Daily 7am to 11 pm.

NEW ORLEANS GAY SWITCHBOARD, 832 Governor Nichols, New Orleans, LA 70116, (504) 586-0217. Wed/Th/Fri, 5-11 pm.

DC GAY SWITCHBOARD, 1724 20th St., NW, 20009, (202) 387-3777.

GAY SWITCHBOARD OF NEW YORK, 247 W. 11th St., 10014, (212) 924-4036.

RESOURCES

BOOKS

The Gay Militants, Donn Teal. Stein and Day, Briar Cliff Manor, New York, 10510. 1971. $7.95
. . . an encyclopaedia-type chronical of the gay movement. Full of quotes from gay activists and publications, descriptions of demonstrations and historical background.

> *. . . She has taken a woman lover*
> *whatever can we say*
> *she walks around all day*
> *quietly, but underneath it*
> *she's electric;*
> *angry energy inside a passive form.*
> *The common woman is as common*
> *as a thunderstorm.*
> *--Judy Grahn*

Sappho Was A Right-On Woman, a Liberated View of Lesbianism, by Sidney Abbott and Barbara Love, Stein and Day, Briarcliff Manor, NY 10510, 1972, 251 pp., $1.95
. . . an honest and compelling account of the Lesbian experience, including the role and responsibility of the gay activist. The authors conclude: "Lesbians are providing women with the psychological breathing space to invent themselves. They are helping to make it impossible to brush aside the importance of women who insist on total autonomy."

We see that it is not Lesbianism that makes some Lesbians prone to alcoholism, suicide, or drug abuse: it is the self-degradation our society went to such pains to teach us, and which is hammered into us not only by the overwhelming force of public opinion, but specifically by lost jobs, lost homes, and -- if we are mothers -- by lost children.

--Sappho Was A Right-On Woman

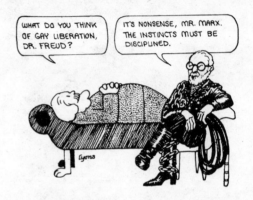

Homosexual Liberation: A Personal View, John Murphy. Praeger Books, P.O. Box 1323, Springfield, MA 01101, 1971. 182 pp. $5.95
. . . personal account of the author's experience as an active member (though decidedly not a "heavy") of New York's Gay Liberation Front (GLF). Includes a good review of contemporary literature's attitude toward homosexuality, as well as the author's experience with consciousness-raising.

Lesbian/Woman, Del Martin and Phyllis Lyon. Bantam Books, Inc., 666 5th Ave., New York, NY 10019, 1972. 310 pp. $1.50
. . . deals with the questions and fears of the heterosexual reader, yet is unyielding in its demands for change. Two strong, sensitive women with 20 years of experience in the lesbian movement tell the emotional hardships that lesbians have endured as workers, wives, mothers, and women.

Because Mourning Sickness Is a Staple In My Country, distributed by "Ain't I A Woman?", P.O. Box 1169, Iowa City, IA 52240, 1974. 52 pp. $.25
. . . "collection of poems by workingclass dykes who have been going through changes." Raw and powerful.

Homosexual: Oppression and Liberation, Altman, Outerbridge and Dienstfey. Dutton Books, 201 Park Ave. South, New York, NY 10003. 1971. 256 pp. 6.95
. . . the first politically developed book on gay liberation. It is an excellent response to the questions, "What are the politics of gay liberation? Why is it revolutionary?" Deals with Marxism-Leninism, youth culture, Marcuse, feminism and more.

Rubyfruit Jungle, Rita Mae Brown, Daughters, Inc., Plainfield, VT 05667, 1973. 217 pp. $3.00
. . . the tough, insightful, adventurous tale of a poor but gutsy girl working out her identity (of which gayness is an integral part) in the Amerikan 50's and 60's. Inspiring.

Edward The Dyke and Other Poems, by Judy Grahn and the Women's Graphics Collective, 5251 Broadway, Oakland, CA 94618, 1972. 86 pp. $1.25
. . . a very special collection for all feminists, written with humor, anger and refreshing clarity. Sprinkled with fine illustrations and suffused with a strong sense of self, the book explains: "The subject of lesbianism/ is very ordinary; it's the question/ of male domination that makes everybody/ angry."

Amazon Expedition, a lesbian feminist anthology, edited by Berkby, Harris, Johnston, Newton and O'Wyatt, Times Change Press, c/o Monthly Review Press, 116 W. 14th St., New York, NY 10011, 1973. 93 pp. $1.75.

PAMPHLETS AND ARTICLES

"Men And Our Bodies," BROTHER, April 1973,
. . . is an entire issue written for gay and straight men. Topics range from male sexuality to V.D. Included is an article on the facts and history of circumcision, a discussion of the effects of work on men's bodies, and an article on how gay men make love. Also contains poetry, drawings, and photographs.

"Bottoms Up", GAY SUNSHINE, Spring 1974
. . . "an indepth look at V.D. and your asshole." This excellent article covers types of V.D. seldom mentioned elsewhere: anal warts, anal syphlis, and gonorrhea, fissures, abscesses, and fistulas, herpes, and prostrate and sphincter problems. It discusses some preventive measures such as cleanliness, self-examination, periodic testing, and communication between partners.

"V.D. In Women," GAY LIBERATOR, April, 1974, reprints 25 cents
. . . is a short article on gonorrhea in gay women; syphilis is not covered because it is relatively easy to detect. Contained are descriptions of the gonococcus organism, the symptoms in women, ways of transmitting the disease, what tests are most effective, and possible treatments for the disease. Also mentioned are precautions women should take to insure confidentiality when treated.

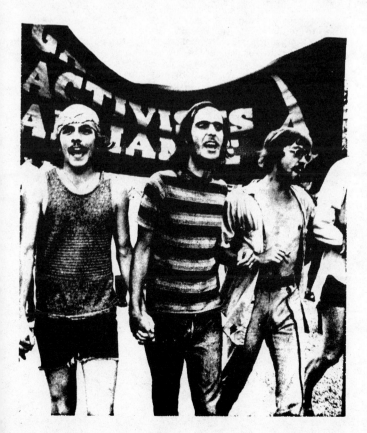

"LESBIANS AND THE HEALTH CARE SYSTEM, PERSONAL TESTIMONY BY N.Y. RADICAL LESBIANS," Violet Press, PO Box 398, New York, NY 10009, 13 pp.
. . .relates the experiences of eight lesbians in their dealings with general practitioners, gynecologists and analysts. The "straight" doctors assume that all the women's physical and psychological problems stem directly from their homosexuality, and try to force them into relationships with men (often sexual relationships with the doctor). This highly readable article ends with a list of demands: gynecologists fully acquainted with lesbianism; recognition of lesbian friends and lovers as true family members by hospitals and other institutions; more women doctors, particularly gynecologists; neighborhood women's clinics; and adequate preventive care.

A Gay Bibliography, Task Force On Gay Liberation, American Library Association, Box 2383, Philadelphia, PA 19103, 1974. Free
. . . thorough, up-to-date list of the best books, pamphlets, articles, and audio-visual resources available. It can be obtained by sending a stamped, self-addressed envelope.

Gay men...can show that they can do just fine, thank you, without the habits of this dying society. The more of this there is, the closer I think we'll be to bringing down the house of cards in which the Straight White Macho Male is living.

-- David Aiken

PERIODICALS

GAY ADVOCATE, Box 74695, Los Angeles, CA 90004. Biweekly, 13 issues /$4, men /women.

THE BODY POLITIC, 139 Seaton St., Toronto, Ont., Canada M5A 2T2. Bimonthly, 6 issues/$2.25 (USA), free to prisoners, men /women.

FAG RAG, Box 331, Kenmore Sta., Boston, MA 02215. Quarterly, 12 issues/$5, 50 cents ea., men.

GAY LIBERATOR, Box 631-A Detroit, MI 48232. Monthly, $3/ year, men /women.

GAY SUNSHINE, P.O. Box 40397, San Francisco, CA 94104, Bimonthly, 12 issues/$6; $10 1st class, sample copy 50 cents. Discount on bulk orders from gay and lesbian /feminist organizations. Men /women.

OUT, Box E, Old Chelsea Sta., New York, NY 10011. Monthly, $6 /year. Bulk prices available to gay and lesbian /feminist organizations, men /women.

LESBIAN TIDE, The Tide Collective, 373 N. Western, Room 202, Los Angeles, CA 90004. Monthly, $7.50 /year.

AIN'T I A WOMAN?, P.O. Box 1169, Iowa City, IA 52240. $5 /yr.

AMAZON QUARTERLY, A Lesbian Feminist Arts Journal, 554 Valle Vista, Oakland, CA 94610. $4 /year ($1 /issue).

FILMS AND TAPES

Feminist Women's Health Centers, 746 Crenshaw Blvd., Los Angeles, CA 90005

"Home Movie," 12 min. cl. $25/$18 (sale: $185/$150) An autobiographical film about lesbianism which combines current documentary footage of the lesbian community with actual old home movies of the filmmaker as a young child imitating her mother and as a high school cheerleader.

See also section on Women's Health.

RURAL RESOURCES

Forty percent of this country's poverty is in rural areas, although rural people constitute only 27% of the total population; this means that one person out of every four is poor in the rural USA. (Rural and Appalachian Health). This poverty is in sharp contrast to the wealth of the land. In agricultural areas, it is the big farmowners who get rich while small farmers lose their farms and farmworkers starve. In Appalachia coal operators make huge profits as they destroy the land through stripmining. Whole towns have been deserted when mechanization cuts out most of the jobs. It is no surprise that rural areas have been compared to colonies as resources are depleted while people get poorer.

There are some health problems common to all low income rural people. Substandard housing and poor diet are the major health hazards, with the pervasive poverty also reflected in impure water, inadequate sanitary facilities and insufficient clothing. Most people don't have the money to pay for medical care, and there is none available even when they do. Often facilities are far away and public transportation is nonexistent. One hundred thirty rural counties do not have a practicing physician, to say nothing of health care facilities. Doctors feel little desire to go to areas that lack the comforts and potential profits of cities. Social services are miles out of reach, and people who have a long history of self-reliance and independence may be unwilling to ask for help from welfare workers who can be racist or condescending toward country people.

Beyond these universal problems, each area has specific difficulties in getting health care. In the South,

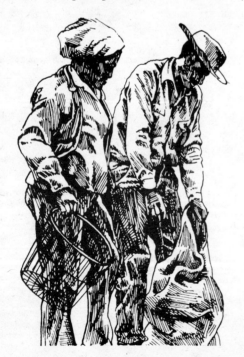

some groups such as the tenant farmers on the cotton fields of Mississippi and the sugar cane workers in Louisiana, are living in conditions virtually the same as those of their ancestors in the days of slavery.

In Appalachia there are health hazards for those who work in the coal mines and those who live around them. Acid run-off from the coal industry pollutes the water, low wages virtually guarantee inadequate diets, and in some areas the companies even control the local hospitals. Migrants are plagued by pesticides, low wages, long hours, and incredibly shabby living quarters on company property, far from the public eye. Residency requirements bar them from most public assistance programs. Special government programs help but are always tenuous; the Migrant Health Act, which provides the only source of health care for hundreds of thousands of people, is coming up for renewal or termination in June, 1974.

Black rural people have their own problems, compounded by the racism that also affects many migrants, Spanish speaking people in the southwest and Native Americans. For instance, the average Black Appalachian is two to three times poorer than the White Appalachian.

To talk with rural people is to be overwhelmed with their determination and pride. Many of the groups listed here are providing the only health care available in their area. It is frighteningly ironic that many of these projects are dependent on unreliable government demonstration project funding, while the government, through subsidies to coal operators, big farmowners, sugar growers in the South and others, perpetuates the system that destroys poor people's land and lives. With foundation funding equally tenuous, many clinics are trying to support themselves through sliding scale, Medicaid/care, and insurance payments. Although in the long run this is more stable than demonstration project funding and foundation grants, the lack of financial resources in the local community means that clinics face a constant scarcity of money.

If the cycle of rural poverty can ever begin to be broken, the massive profits that flow out of the land must go back to its people. Because rural health problems can not truly be eradicated without far-reaching economic restructuring, we are including general as well as health related projects and resources. For other rural groups, see the sections on Community Clinics, Third World, Occupational Safety and Health, and Health Personnel and Training.

ARKANSAS COMMUNITY ORGANIZATION FOR REFORM NOW (ACORN). . .a four year-old statewide organization of 4700 low-income and working class families who have organized in 42 local community groups to solve problems and build political power. Mostly, organizing has been multi-issued but programs have dealt with special groups like veterans and unemployed workers. Health work includes a small preventive dental clinic and an eye clinic. They also have a food buyers' club and handle welfare grievances, including foodstamp problems. The local social service agencies have learned that it is in their best interest to respond quickly to ACORN members' complaints. Contact ACORN, 523 W. 15th St., Little Rock, AR 72202, (501) 376-7151.

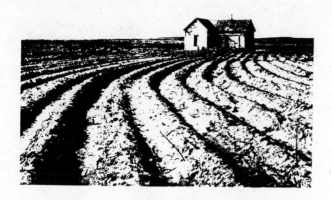

SOUTHERN MUTUAL HELP ASSOCIATION. . .is patiently and stubbornly building change among the sugar cane workers of southern Louisiana. Most of the workers live on plantations, in semi-feudal conditions of poverty and dependence. Work is seasonal; $1.80 or $1.90 is a high hourly wage and family incomes average $2,635 a year; housing is usually old and dilapidated. The diet of poverty contributes to obesity, hypertension, and other problems, besides direct results: malnutrition, stunted growth, retardation in extreme cases. Health care is hard to come by—and those who can't afford it may not be able to afford the bus fare and pay-loss involved in a trip to charity (state) hospitals in the cities. SMHA surveyed health needs, and after two years of trying got HEW funding to set up a health center. Now 2½ years old, the center has one full time doctor and three dentists (most people in the area had never seen a dentist). They provide services to all school children who qualify under HEW guidelines—preventive work is the goal, but they are still trying to catch up on treating already-existing problems. A fulltime volunteer nutritionist (a retired woman) helps patients with special diets, and carries education into the community. Three drivers transport people to the health center or, if necessary, to state-run hospitals. Outreach workers visit plantations to inform people of the center's services, give encouragement to those intimidated by the thought of dealing with doctors, and provide follow-up. The center is exploring third-party payments (medicare, medicaid, etc.) as a possible source of more secure funding than HEW's always-tenuous money. The Health Center is only one of SMHA's programs: they have initiated or aided self-help housing, adult education classes, a court case to win back wages for came workers, etc. In all cases, the goal is community development. Monthly community meetings on each plantation deal with questions like clinic hours and the small fees that go to support the health center—but they also provide a new sense of unity, a forum for communication, a first taste of self-determination. Whether working with housing or job training, SMHA does not look for the most "efficient" program, but for one that will build grassroots participation and community strength in an area where little organizing has been done since an attempt at farmworker unionization was crushed in the early '50's. Contact SMHA, P.O. Box 365, Abbeville, LA 70510 (318) 893-3912.

SOUTHERN REGIONAL COUNCIL. . .an excellent research and information agency which has been actively concerned with civil rights in the South for 20 years. They recently published Comprehensive Health Care: A Southern View, and also did a survey on outpatient utilization rates, hospitalization and other health statistics. Other health work includes testifying before congressional committees. Hunger and malnutrition have been a priority of SRC for the last five years. In 1972 they helped publish Hunger USA Revisited. Contact SOUTHERN REGIONAL COUNCIL, 52 Fairlie St., NW, Atlanta, GA 30303, (404) 522-8764.

NATIONAL SHARECROPPER'S FUND. . .has an impressive 30-year history of commitment to self-help and cooperative principles in rural organizing. They have provided technical assistance, paid organizers, and granted or helped find funding for a variety of projects: organic food-growing co-ops in Virginia and Georgia, health and housing work in Louisiana,

an organization for welfare rights in Arkansas and labor organizing among Black and White woodcutters. One thing leads to another—a farmer's marketing co-op may spark the formation of a sewing co-op to provide jobs, or a community campaign for improved health services. Supporting grassroots struggles in the grimmest of conditions, NSF sees the immediate goals as part of an effort to build whole communities based on a cooperative way of life. NSF lobbies in Washington, and their free newsletter, THE SHARECROPPER, keeps tabs on bills affecting migrants, tenant farmers, sharecroppers, and small farmers. Their literature exposes the exploitation of agribusiness corporations and tabs on bills affecting migrants, tenant farmers, sharecroppers, and small farmers. Their literature exposes the exploitation of agribusiness corporations and blasts government policies that cater to them; subsidies that go to the rich and ignore the poor; an administration that slashes rural allocations; research programs geared to the needs of big business rather than independent small farmers. NSF recently began a demonstration farm and training center in North Carolina to teach organic farming techniques, farm management, and organization of cooperatives. Contact NSF, 1145 19th St., NW, Suite 501, Washington, D.C. 20036 (202) 659-5620.

MISSOURI DELTA ECUMENICAL MINISTRY (MDEM) . . .operates in the six southeastern delta counties of Missouri with a credit union, co-op grocery store, a rural research depository, legal assistance program, and housing corporation. MDEM sends out community organizers to help neighborhoods fight for better social services. In one community devastated by spring floods in 1973, the local government concentrated on rebuilding only the wealthier sections of town, using government funds; however, with MDEM's help, the poor people successfully pressured the town to clear out the drainage ditches and put in sewage systems. A current MDEM-sponsored project is opening a dental clinic for low-income people. They have obtained donated equipment and strong community support, but are still looking for volunteer dentists. Contact MDEM, Box 524, Hayti, MO 63851 (314) 359-1718.

ORLEANS LEGAL AID BUREAU, INC (OLAB). . .is an OEO-funded legal services program for low income residents of Orleans, a small rural county in upstate New York. They pressure the Health Department to enforce safe housing laws when tenants complain about lead paint, inadequate sewage systems, and other problems; if necessary, they will bring suit against the landlord. They also pressure the health department to inspect and force correction of unhealthy migrant camps. OLAB's dealings with the welfare department center around foodstamp and Medicaid eligibility, making sure that no one is unlawfully excluded from these programs. They also do some referrals when faced with problems they can't solve, and direct people to local clinics, hospitals, and emergency food programs. Contact OLAB, 20 A. East Banks St., Albion, NY 14414, (716) 589-5628.

COUNCIL OF SOUTHERN MOUNTAINS . . . is an umbrella organization of Appalachian commissions working in the areas of welfare, employment, housing, education, mine health, safety, and compensations, youth advocacy, Black self-determination and more. They want to restore Appalachian identity and consciousness by promoting self-determination programs, Appalachian studies in local schools, and by preserving its beauty and culture. The Youth Commission published a directory of Appalachian groups and services. Contact COUNCIL OF SOUTHERN MOUNTAINS, Drawer "N", Clintwood, VA 24228 (703) 929-4489 or 95.

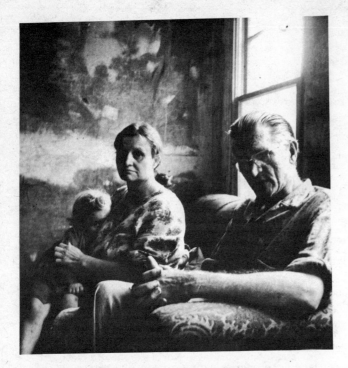

BLACK APPALACHIAN COMMISSION, INC...grew out of a reorganization of the Council of Southern Mountains in 1969. Its goal is to act as a tool to "assist the Black Appalachian community identify its problems, mobilize its resources, and deal more effectively with the institutional causes of the problems." Foundation-funded, BAC is run by an elected Board of Directors with representatives from eleven Appalachian states. The health component is very new, with emphasis on developing a coalition of poor and Black Appalachians to work for greater consumer control of health facilities, especially those funded by HEW and Appalachian Regional Commission (which has tended to ignore the existence of Blacks and other Appalachian minorities). The first program is a conference of Black professionals and community leaders to take place in the summer of 1974. Contact BAC, 52 Fairlie St., NW, Room 305, Atlanta, GA 30303 (404) 525-3416.

PEOPLE'S APPALACHIAN RESEARCH COLLECTIVE... is a research and writing collective working to develop an active analysis of the politics and economy of Appalachia. Their work helps local groups confront the region's colonizers. Their primary health-related work is in the area of occupational safety, although they also helped sponsor a Veteran medic's group. PARC publishes an excellent magazine, PEOPLE'S APPALACHIA and a resource book, Appalachian Reader, which is particularly helpful for Appalachian history classes. Contact PARC, Route 3, Box 355B, Morgantown, WV 26505, (304) 292-7663.

APPALACHIAN MOVEMENT PRESS...prints pamphlets telling the people's history of Appalachia, supports the Appalachian culture and provides information on the contemporary politics and economy of the region. Their aim is to aid the people fight for social, political and economic justice. For a list of their outstanding publications, contact APPALACHIAN MOVEMENT PRESS, P.O. Box 8074, Huntington, WV 25705 (304) 523-8587.

RURAL HOUSING ALLIANCE...is attacking one of the major causes of rural bad health—housing—by providing technical assistance and research to individuals and organizations combatting the rural housing crisis. Their technical assistance programs provide detailed advice on all phases of self-help housing, clarifying government regulations, information on federal programs, general background materials on house

plans, and methods of construction. The REPORTER tells about successful housing projects and exposes the faults and frailties of federal housing programs. RHA was instrumental in forming the National Rural Housing Coalition which lobbies for the interests of the rural poor. Contact RHA, 1346 Connecticut Ave., NW, Suite 500, Washington, D.C. 20036 (202) 659-1680.

DELMO HOUSING CORPORATION...is a longstanding organization made up of nine small rural communities in the Missouri bootheel. Delmo began in the 1940's when the government built houses for displaced sharecroppers in these nine communities with the intention of eventually selling the houses to the tenants at a low price. But with a change of administration, the government decided to back out and local landowners prepared to cash in on the deal. However, the people of the community organized themselves into Delmo, which acted as a financial intermediary, forcing the government to sell the houses to the sharecroppers at $800 a piece. Delmo still works with housing problems, but also sponsors several health projects. Their Migrant Health program serves a six-county area, operating under the Migrant Health Act, and provides financial assistance for medical care, drugs, hospitalization, dental work, and transportation to health facilities. They sponsor a pre-paid Family Health Center for migrants and seasonal farmworkers, and have an emergency loan fund. Delmo also works with the Regional Mental Retardation Center to find residential placement for retarded adults, and distributes sack lunches through the National School Lunch Program. Contact DELMO HOUSING CORPORATION, P.O. Box 354, Lilbourne, MO 63862 (314) 688-2565.

MIGRANT

ILLINOIS MIGRANT COUNCIL...staffs five clinics during peak season as well as pushing for the enforcement of laws to provide hospitalization and decent housing. IMC's governing

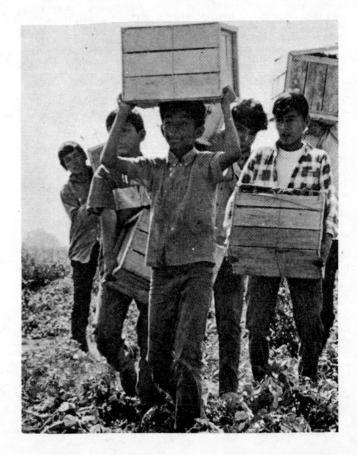

board is almost entirely elected by migrant councils, which are themselves elected by migrants in the state's seven regions. The clinics, open from March to October, provide general practitioner services, lab work, and can supply some drugs for free. Nurses and aides visit the camps for casefinding, follow-up, and health education. Illinois' Aid to the Medically Indigent law requires that townships pay hospital bills for those who can't afford to, but many townships are either unaware of the law or prefer to ignore it. The Council urges hospitals to provide care for migrants and collect from the township; where necessary, the Council has brought suit against townships. IMC is also pushing for enforcement of occupational safety and health laws covering housing and sanitation in migrant camps. Other IMC programs include adult education, and a legal program which has provided advocates for migrants in such areas as foodstamps, welfare, employment, and police relations. A spin-off of the local Catholic Archdiocese, IMC is funded by a combination of private, HEW, and Department of Labor grants. Contact ILLINOIS MIGRANT COUNCIL, 1307 S. Wabash, Chicago, IL 60605 (312) 663-1522.

RURAL MISSOURI, INC. . .provides a variety of services to migrant and seasonal farmworkers. Funded by the Department of Labor, they place people in non-migrant jobs and pay a training fee for a maximum 26-week period. So far they have been pleased with their success, although finding jobs is always a problem. They also operate an emergency aid fund to provide food, clothing and other necessities. This fund is from churches and other groups. Rural Missouri found that their government money was tied up in so much red tape that it was difficult to use in an emergency. However, they do plan to contract with United Migrants for Opportunity next year to operate an HEW emergency food and medical services project, while maintaining their separate fund. Rural Missouri is controlled by an elected Board of Directors, 61% of whom are migrants and seasonal farmworkers. Contact RURAL MISSOURI, INC., 418 Madison St., P.O. Box 204, Jefferson City, MO 65101 (314) 635-0136.

UNITED MIGRANTS FOR OPPORTUNITY. . .has a health services component to supplement inadequate federal, state and county projects in Michigan. Sometimes they reimburse local physicians for services to migrants; in other areas they have opened their own clinics. UMO has an HEW grant to operate an emergency food and medical services program in Michigan as well as contracts with seven other midwestern states to establish the program there. UMO helps people get on food stamps and gives them money to buy their food stamps if necessary. Those who are ineligible for foodstamps because of their transience can be reimbursed for money spent on food by UMO. Funded mainly by the Department of Labor, UMO also has a Migrant Scholarship program, a legal services program, a manpower training program, and provides housing and clothing through its emergency assistance program. Priority is given to farmworkers in hiring UMO staff. Contact UNITED MIGRANTS FOR OPPORTUNITY, 111 South Lansing St., Mt. Pleasant, MI 48858 (517) 772-2901.

VALLEY MIGRANT LEAGUE—HEALTH CARE SERVICES . . ."is providing comprehensive health care to migrant and seasonal farm-workers" in northwestern Oregon. The League, which is funded by HEW and the Department of Labor, opened its first clinic in January, 1973. At present they are operating one clinic, Centro De Salubridad, which provides year-round, full-time outpatient facilities, including a pharmacy, X-ray equipment and a clinical lab for analyzing urine and blood samples. Outreach work is done by community health aides and payment for services is on a sliding scale. Some patients are referred to the University of Oregon Medical School. In the summer, the Valley Migrant League plans satellite programs in three outlying areas. VML is controlled by a 24 member Board of Directors, all of whom are farmworkers or have been within the last two years. Other activities of VML include job training to help people leave the migrant stream, teaching English as a second language, and running a high school equivalency program. Oregon VML program allows the head of the family to go to school while continuing to support his/her family. Contact VML, 5103 Portland Rd., NE, Salem, OR 97303 (503) 585-9200, or Centro De Salubridad, 300 Young St., Woodburn, OR 97071 (503) 981-8888.

ASSOCIATED MIGRANT OPPORTUNITY SERVICES. . . offers three areas of service to Indiana migrants: legal, employment and health. In 1973 their health services consisted of a voucher system, whereby AMOS reimbursed physicians for fees resulting from treating migrants. Finding this system to be of questionable quality and providing little preventive care, they are now using HEW funds to establish two health centers in the major areas of migrant concentration in Indiana. To emphasize preventive care, they are training ex-migrants as health specialists; these specialists teach home health care, do follow-up visits and can "prescribe" food for hungry people with AMOS footing the bill. Health specialists will be operating throughout the state. Migrants who are too far from the two health centers can still use the voucher system which covers dental care, glasses, lab work, some hospitalization and more. AMOS also helps people get on welfare and foodstamps. They have forced the welfare department to accept more migrants through court cases challenging residency requirements. Contact AMOS, 806 E. 38th St., Indianapolis, IN 46205 (317) 925-9809.

EAST COAST MIGRANT HEALTH PROJECT. . .seeks to provide health care to migrants moving up the east coast. They do not try to establish their own clinics, since any one location is of limited value. Instead, they arrange to work with state or county clinics along the migrant stream. In the winter they have about 10 health workers in the field, mostly in Florida; in the summer the number rises to 25 or 30, including a few medical students and many religious sisters who work two to three months for subsistence pay, following the migrant stream through Georgia, N. Carolina, Virginia, and as far north as Delaware. Their central office in Washington DC keeps an eye on legislation that affects migrants, and lobbied for the emergency bill that forstalled the expiration of the Migrant Health Act in 1973. They organized a petition campaign among migrants, collecting thousands of signatures from Texas and the east coast, thus providing migrants a rare chance to speak for themselves in favor of the bill. ECMHP, like many other migrant projects, is currently dependent on Migrant Health Act funding, but they are exploring possible alternatives. Contact ECMHP, 1325 Mass. Ave., NW, Washington, D.C. 20005 (202) 347-7377.

California, Arizona, I make all your crops
Then it's north up to Oregon to gather your hops
Dig beets from your ground, cut the grapes from your vine
To set on your table your light sparkling wine.
—Woody Guthrie

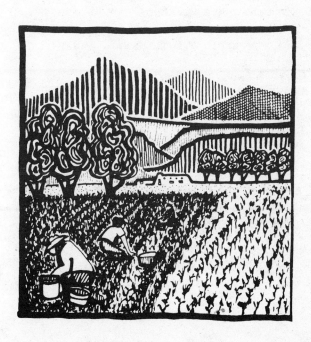

SOUTHWEST MIGRANT ASSOCIATION. . .operates a clinic serving about 50% of the 12,000 migrants in the San Antonio area. Their services, which are free to all migrants, include mostly curative and diagnostic work, although they also do routine pap smears, blood work and immunizations. Two dentists on their staff offer a full range of dental care, including plates. Funded by HEW, they operate a federal emergency food program and the Woman-Infant-Child Food Supplement Program. They are controlled by a community board, 2/3 or whom are migrants or seasonal farm-workers. Contact SOUTHWEST MIGRANT ASSOCIATION, 2327 Castroville Rd., San Antonio, TX 78237 (512) 434-0626.

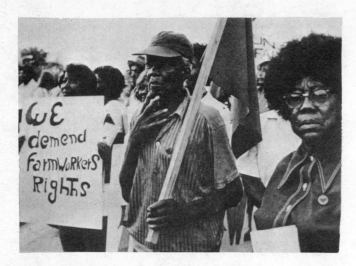

STRIP MINING GROUPS

SAVE OUR CUMBERLAND MOUNTAINS
General Delivery
Jacksboro, TN 37757
(615) 562-3371

CITIZENS LEAGUE TO PROTECT SURFACE RIGHTS
Joe Begley
Blackey, KY 41804
(606) 633-7660

COMMITTEE TO CONTROL STRIP MINING
Dr. Ted Voneida
3012 Lincoln Boulevard
Cleveland Heights, OH 44118
(216) 932-8708

ATHENS ECOLOGY GROUP
413 Baker Center
Athens, OH 45701
(614) 594-3161

FLOYD COUNTY SAVE OUR LAND
Irving Harris
Prestonsburg, KY 41653

APPALACHIAN GROUP TO SAVE THE LAND AND PEOPLE
Route 2, Box 340
Hazard, KY 41701

TOWN PLANNING COMMISSION
Mrs. Schuster
P.O. Box 337
Barnsville, OH 43713

CITIZENS TO ABOLISH STRIP MINING (CASM)
1703 Washington St. E., Room 205
Charleston, WV 25329

While the appetites of a growing industrial America have been met by the energy from these hills, and while some of her greatest fortunes have been founded here, the people who live here and who have so contributed to the development of their country, have as their reward poverty in isolation, slums, welfare, social security, unemployment, sickness, rock dust, black lung, soup beans, and food stamps.
—Our Land Too

RESOURCES

BOOKS

Rural And Appalachian Health, Robert Nolan and Jerome Schwartz, eds. Charles C. Thomas, 301-327 East Lawrence Ave., Springfield, IL 62703. 249 pp.
. . . is a collection of papers by a varied group of people, from a medical student to local organizers, on health problems in Appalachia. The range of the articles is wide. One discusses the declining number of doctors in a West Virginia area: in 1938 there were 80 per 100,000—today there are 28. Other chapters talk about specific health programs in Appalachia, or the role medical schools should take in rural areas. Some speakers touch on the roots of Appalachia's problems:"It would be wrong for us to encourage the belief that we can continue as an imperial power on a global scale, and, at the same time, make decent provision for our poor, because we are not about to do that."

Our Land, Too, Tony Dunbar. Vintage Books, 201 E. 50th St., New York, NY 10022, 1971. 231 pp. $1.95
. . . an important book documenting life in the cotton lands of the South and in the coal belt of the Appalachians. The first section relates Dunbar's experiences living with poor Black tenant farmers in the Mississippi Delta. The second section is written from tapes of conversations with a returned coal miner who discusses the people and problems of the Kentucky mountains. The book does not offer solutions, but warns against depending on institutional leadership to redress the crimes committed against poor rural people in the name of progress.

"The Health of West Virginia," Fred Rubin. Available from Louise Rice, 65 Chestnut St., Cambridge, MA 02139, 1971. 68 pp. $2.38
. . .a study of West Virginia: the present state of health delivery, why it's so poor and how it got that way. In addition to suffering from common rural problems such as lack of public services, West Virginians are controlled by the coal industry in every facet of their lives. The state has been exploited and left in poverty with enormous environmental destruction. Obviously this is not an area that will attract doctors; what few there are show little concern with preventive care and state health programs are pitifully inadequate. Rubin calls for radical change, citing Cuba as a good model of an impoverished region that significantly improved the general health of its people.

"Tied to the Sugar Lands," Peter Schuck, SATURDAY REVIEW OF THE SOCIETY, 488 Madison Ave., New York, NY 10022. May 6, 1972, pp. 36-42
. . . a hard-hitting, fast-moving expose of the Louisiana sugar cane business, centering on the US Department of Agriculture's role in the situation. The Sugar Cane Act of the 1930's, requires the USDA "to restrict the quantities of raw sugar marketed annually in the United States, reserving a specific quota for each domestic producer as well as import quotas for designated foreign nations." This cuts down foreign competition and keeps domestic sugar about three cents per pound above the world price. The act also provides for annual government subsidies to growers to limit production, totalling about $500 million each year. However growers are legally compelled to pay "fair and reasonable" wages to workers and the hourly wage must be determined by the USDA. In 1972, the USDA did a curious thing: the growers recommended a pay raise and USDA decided on a wage lower than the one suggested. The author feels that the USDA has consistently acted in the interests of the growers and has neglected to exercise its power to protect the worker.

"A Directory of Migrant Health Projects Supported Under the Migrant Health Act," HEW. Available from Bureau of Community Health Services, Program Services Branch, Room 12A, 33 Park Lawn Building, 5600 Fishers Lane, Rockville, MD 20852, May 1972. Free. Publication no. HSM 72-6601
. . . names 100 migrant health projects scattered throughout the US, including location, time of year when services are offered, peak migrant population, and number of patients

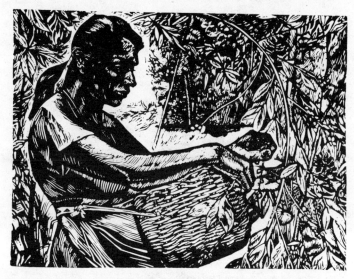

served per year. Most noteworthy is the ranking of each center according to services offered, from full-time comprehensive health services to mere consultation and coordination of "direct health care activities of the groups". Scary but not rare to see figures indicating migrant populations of 71, 000 of whom only 4,000 were served by clinics.

"1973-1974 BIBLIOGRAPHY ON THE APPALACHIAN SOUTH," Council of Southern Mountains Bookstore, CPO 2307, Berea, KY 40403. 31 pp. $.25
. . . outstanding collection of books, records, pamphlets and films including children's books, radical labor history, novels, and songbooks.

PERIODICALS

MOUNTAIN LIFE AND WORK: THE MAGAZINE OF THE APPALACHIAN SOUTH, Council of Southern Mountains Bookstore, COP 2307, Berea KY 40403. $4/year for students, members $5/others
. . . a monthly magazine with excellent articles on Appalachian heritage, unionization, Black Lung, mountain music, and much more.

PEOPLE'S APPALACHIA; A CRITICAL RESEARCH REPORT FROM THE PEOPLE'S APPALACHIAN RESEARCH COLLECTIVE, Rt. 3, Box 355B, Morgantown, W.VA 26505. $5 contribution/year
. . . high quality periodical with a radical analysis of Appalachian people's fight against poverty and "basic capitalist exploitation."

Delano, John Gregory Dunne, photos by Ted Streshinsky, The Noonday Press, 19 Union Square West, New York City, N.Y., 10003, 1971. 202 pp, $2.25
. . . a report on the United Farm Workers grape strike. In journalistic style Dunne tells the history of farm labor in California, and of the oppressive conditions of Chicano life in Delano. He describes the evolution of the strike, with the increasing tension between the migrant workers and the rest of the community and includes interviews with policemen, SNCC volunteers, Chavez, the mayor, the growers, farmworkers, and others connected with the strike.

FILMS AND TAPES

Appalacian Educational Media Project, Box 743, Whitesburg, KY 41858

"Buffalo Creek 1972: An Act of God?" 30 min. b&w $35 (sale: $250)
In 1972 a giant coal waste dam at the head of a hollow in Logan County, West Virginia, burst, sweeping 130 million gallons of water down the crowded valley of Buffalo. This film documents the people's fight against the coal company responsible for the disaster.

"Stripmining in Appalachia," 20 min. b&w $35 1973 (sale: $250)
Speaks with the voices of and for the powerless "little man" caught in the jaws of a cancerous industrial process.

Impact, 144 Bleecker St., New York, NY 10012

"Appalachia: Rich Land, Poor People," 59 min. b&w $55/$40 1969
The land is rich with coal, yet its people are denied adequate food, housing, or medical care. This film focuses upon Eastern Kentucky where mechanization of the mines has replaced people and jobs. Documents the first area in the US to be turned into an ecological wasteland.

"Migrant," 52 min. cl. $75/$60 1970
Focuses on the migrants of Belle Glade, Florida, a giant agricultural center. Shows the shame, frustration, hunger and despair that are part of the migrant's life.

"Hard Times In The Country," 58 min. cl. $65/$50 1970
The effects of consolidations in the food industry upon consumers and farmers are examined in this film. Also explores the influx of destructive outside corporations that farm for a loss as a tax write-off.

NBC Educational Enterprises, Room 1040, 30 Rockefeller Pl., New York. NY 10020.

"Valley of Darkness," 18 min. cl. 1970 $10
The only opportunity for employment in West Virginia is working in the mines. Dust causes Black Lung disease and there is the constant danger of explosion or cave-in, yet the economic and political pressures for business as usual go on.

APPALACHIAN NEWS SERVICE, P.O. Box 2921, Charleston, WV 25330, $12.50 annually for individuals, $25 for organizations. . .a monthly news service aimed at increasing regional awareness and solidarity. The articles are written by community people with a slant toward organizing, and cover such diverse topics as federal expenditures in Appalachia, coal miners'strike and interviews with local folksingers. Excellent resource for community papers and people involved in Appalachian politics.

CHICANO RESOURCES

As with other Third World people, the indignities suffered by Chicanos seeking health care are only one facet of the treatment of a racist society. Unemployment and school dropout rates are twice as high for Chicanos as for Anglos, and 80 per cent of the Chicano labor force is unskilled or semi-skilled. Thirty-six percent of the adult Spanish-speaking population is functionally illiterate.

There are currently 6.29 million Chicanos in the US, 85 per cent of whom live in Texas, California, New Mexico, Arizona, and Colorado. The gravity of Chicano health care problems is manifested by the fact that their TB frequency is 17 times the national average; that instances of parasitic worms in Chicanos is 35 times the national average; and that their life expectancy is 10 years lower than the Anglo life expectancy. "In 23 out of 25 reportable disease categories (mumps, TB, measles, hepatitis, food poisoning, etc.), East Los Angeles, which has the largest Chicano population in the US, ranked either first, second, or third when compared with other areas in Los Angeles."

Many Chicanos are migrants or live in rural areas, which makes health care doubly inaccessible. And, when health facilities do exist, there is little money to pay for care. For other Chicanos, the problem lies in the fact that they have entered this country illegally. Mandatory hospital insurance forms and doctors' questions carry with them the threat of eventual deportation. Language and cultural differences are also important barriers. After all, what is the point of paying for a visit to the doctor if you don't understand what s/he is saying or doing?

It is estimated that there are only 250 Chicano doctors trained and practicing in the US. In Los Angeles, 20 percent of the population is Chicano, yet only .005 percent of the doctors are Chicano (78 out of 14,203). New Mexico, with a 40 per cent Chicano population, has only 4 nursing students who are of Mexican descent (out of 140 students total). In 1971-72, there were only 247 Chicano medical students and 93 Chicano dental students in the US. This represents .005 percent of the total students studying in these two fields.

The following groups are working in a variety of change and health related areas. They should be able to put people in touch with local projects and serve as models for on-going programs.

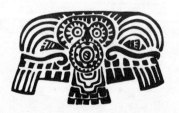

NATIONAL COUNCIL OF LA RAZA. . . serves as a research, resource and advocacy center for Chicano groups. The Council originated in 1968 in the Southwest with housing and economic development the main focuses; the national office opened in 1972 to provide back-up services to local projects and express the specific needs of Chicanos (as different from Puerto Ricans and Cuban) to federal policy makers. The National Council hopes to help local groups with funding. Chicanos por la Causa, the original project in the southwest, and several affiliate groups, offer programs in housing, economic development, health, drug abuse, etc. Recent projects of the National Council include an excellent study on nursing homes for the Spanish speaking and research into Chicano mental health and drug use problems. For information on their quar-

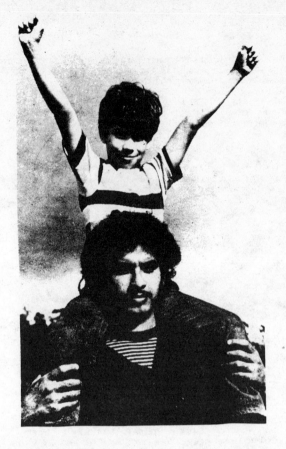

terly magazine AGENDA, nursing home study or general operation, contact NATIONAL COUNCIL OF LA RAZA, 1025 Fifteenth St. NW, Washington, D.C. 20005, (202) 659-1251.

RAZA UNIDA PARTY. . . is a Chicano political party with members in 21 states. The party grew out of a 1970 school boycott by 1700 Chicano students in Crystal City, Texas, a town whose population is 80% Chicano, but which was, prior to 1970, completely Anglo controlled. Following the student walk-out, Chicanos organized and gained control of all elected offices in the town. The pro-Chicano school board banned standarized IQ tests, non-union lettuce, dress codes, and army recruiters. For the first time in Crystal City, education was made truly bi-lingual and bi-cultural. Subsequently, the Raza Unida party has spread, with candidates running for state and local offices in Texas, California and Colorado. In 1972 the party's gubanatorial candidate in Texas received 7% of the vote and Raza Unida members were elected to half of the offices in the county near Crystal City. The national office publishes a newsletter and seeks to form coalitions with other Spanish speaking groups. Contact RAZA UNIDA PARTY, 519 E. Crockett St., Crystal City, TX 78839, (512) 374-2322.

CHICANOS POR LA CAUSA. . . exists to help bring about widerange change in the treatment and conditions of Chicanos. In 1968, when Chicanos por la Causa started after a high school boycott by Chicano students, the annual budget was $10,000; it has since grown to $500,000 with substantial funding from foundations and HEW. The three health projects sponsored are: development of a clinic in Jila Bend, Arizona, a town of 5000, located 60 miles from Phoenix; acquisition of an ambulance from the Public Health Department in Avandale; and education for school children and the general public around the availability of health facilities in Phoenix. They have also backed the successful election of Chicanos to the County Board of Directors and city and county health agencies. Chicanos por la Causa's commitment to economic development has led them to support the creation of two businesses and build 235 homes. The group is affiliated with the National Council of La Raza. Contact CHICANOS POR LA CAUSA, 903 E. Buckeye St., Phoenix, AR 85034, (602) 252-7191.

LA CASA LEGAL. . . offers legal services to a predominantly low income, Spanish speaking clientele. Chicano law students receiving both academic credit and a salary for their work, comprise most of the staff. La Casa states that it will not represent drug pushers or men who appear to have violently committed rape. Services are free for low-income people and on a sliding scale for the more affluent. Contact LA CASA LEGAL, 1660 East Santa Clara St., San Jose, CA 95116, (408) 926-2525.

SACRAMENTO CONCILIO. . . is an umbrella organization for 22 Chicano-oriented projects, serving a Spanish speaking population of 120,000. The overriding goal of the Concilio is to raise the self-image and economic level of Chicanos. Health related projects include: outreach workers who assist Spanish speaking people to use local medical services and sensitize the health establishment to the particular needs of the Chicano; Raza Drug effort, which educates, detoxes and generally works to prevent drug abuse; a hospital advocacy program, thorugh which Concilio workers accompany patients and speak in their behalf; and group and peer group counseling. With a budget of close to $1 million from the Federal Government and a staff of 55, the Concilio coordinates other such diverse programs as school and job placement, a legal center, production of radio and TV shows and a documentary film, and housing and general outreach for the elderly. The Board of Directors consists of representatives from the 22 member organizations. Contact SACRAMENTO CONCILIO, P.O. Box 896, Sacramento, CA 95814, (916) 444-6314.

INTERSTATE RESEARCH ASSOCIATES. . . provides technical and fund-raising assistance, program evaluation and back-up services to local projects. The staff and clientele are primarily Chicano with an interest in bilingual programs. Past work has centered in the areas of health, education, housing and personnel development. They are chiefly supported by consulting fees although they will occasionally work for free and have some skill in untangling the federal grant application bureaucracy. Contact IRA, 2001 Wisconsin, NW, Washington, D.C. 20007, (202) 333-0510.

MEXICAN-AMERICAN UNITY COUNCIL. . . conducts 3 health related programs: family health, which works with "high risk mothers"; adult mental health; and child mental health. The latter 2 projects involve outreach workers who deal with the entire family striving to relate mental stresses to societal factors. The family health project concentrates on identifying women whose physical condition or age results in high risk pregnancy, encouraging the use of birth control until the cause of the problem is cured. Six para-professional outreach workers visit the women while still in the hospital after delivery. They generally work with women diagnosed as having hypertension, diabetes, kidney problems, difficult delivery, or who are under 15 and single or over 37 with six or more children. The outreach workers (all of whom are women) encourage the mothers to take advantage of the hospital's free dispensal of contraceptives or to learn effective use of the rhythm method, since this is the only form of contraception acceptable to many women in the program. The staff, all of whom are Spanish speaking, do not view the use of birth control as permanent, but rather as an important measure until the women are physically stronger. A major problem has been maintaining contact with women in the program, although use of staff from the local community has minimized this. About 300 women are seen monthly. Contact MEXICAN-AMERICAN UNITY COUNCIL, 712 South Flores, San Antonio, TX 78204, (512) 225-4241.

RESOURCES

Pain and Promise: The Chicano Today, ed. by Edward Simmen, The New American Library, Inc., P.O. Box 999, Bergenfield, N.J., 07621, 1972. 348 pp, $1.25
. . . an anthology of essays and stories, from such varied writers as Cesar Chavez, Newsweek, and Jose Angel Gutierrez deal with the identity, source of discontent, and movement directions of the Chicano.

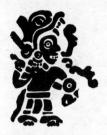

The Chicanos: Mexican-American Voices, ed. by Ed Ludwig and James Santibanez, Penguin Books, 7110 Ambassador Rd., Baltimore, MD 21207, 1971. 286 pp. $1.50
. . . a collection of stories, poems and essays on Mexican-American history, and Chicano life today. Sections focus on the Mexican migrant workers, life in a Chicano barrio, education efforts to improve conditions and the position of the Chicano caught between two cultures. Each section combines a description of group problems (i.e. the need for more bilingual education) with one of individual problems (i.e. a Chicano child who is forced by an Anglo school system to cut his hair). Cesar Chavez writes on how he began organizing; a barriology exam tests one on the meanings of such words as "capirotado", "pedichi" and "moocher"; the case of Los Siete is reviewed. This successful juxtaposition of varied literature is followed by a bibliography, and a list of related biographies.

"THE CHICANOS," North American Congress on Latin America, P.O. Box 57, Cathedral Station, New York, NY 10025, 1973. 32 pp. $.50
. . . full color history of the Chicano people in comic book form.

PERIODICALS

REGENERACION, PO Box 4157, Los Angeles, CA 90051. $5/5 issues.
. . . articles, analysis and poetry with an emphasis on Mexican-American women. Includes discussions of welfare and employment problems, latest coverage of political action and a wide range of poetry and short stories.

AGENDA, National Council of La Raza, 1025 15th St., NW, Washington, D.C. 20005. $10/year, quarterly
. . . exciting, well written articles covering such areas as mental health problems which Spanish people in the U.S. are faced with daily due to barriers of language and culture, the added oppression facing Spanish speaking women in the U.S. and the resultant lack of opportunity or incentive to change their position, and different approaches to solving drug problems with a strong emphasis on preventive education and establishing rehabilitation programs. An excellent resource for people working with issues affecting Mexican Americans and Spanish surnamed Americans.

EL GALLO, LA VOZ DE LA JUSTICIA, P.O. Box 18347, 1567 Downing St., Denver, CO 80218, $2.50/12 issues
. . . coverage of Chicano political action, with articles in Spanish and English. The focus is toward encouraging solidarity within the Chicano movement. Excellent photos and graphics.

FILMS AND TAPES

Ballis Associates, 5439 Carlton, Oakland, CA 94618

"I am Joaquin" 20 min. cl. $40
Epic Chicano film poem on La Raza experience from the Aztec Empire to the current farmworker movement. Produced by El Teatro Campesino, a Chicano theatre company which grew out of the Delano grape strike.

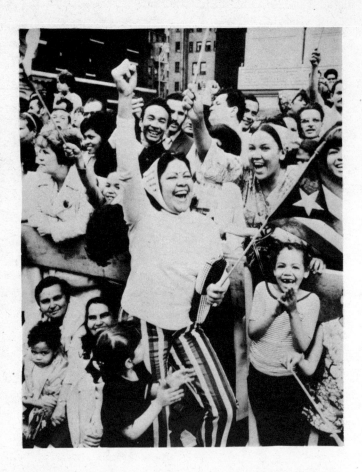

PUERTO RICAN RESOURCES

The 1970 census reports 1.55 million Puerto Ricans on the U.S. mainland, 58% of whom were born on the island and have immigrated. Many Puerto Ricans leave the island to escape the by-products of colonialism and underdevelopment, influding inflation, unemployment, and low-incomes. Yet for many Puerto Ricans, conditions in this country are not much better, and include the added factor of alienation.

Puerto Ricans in the U.S. live in urban ghettos—59% in New York City. As with other Third World people, unemployment rates are high, averaging 6.2% in 1970, well before unemployment became a widespread problem. For Puerto Ricans between 16 and 19 years old, the unemployment rate is 16%. High unemployment coupled with low average income (below $5000) and large families results in over-crowded housing, nutritionally poor diets and a high incidence of communicable diseases.

Even in New York, health care is not geared to the special needs of the Spanish-speaking. Often only a few, lower echelon hospital workers speak Spanish and the patient must wait until they are available to translate. Doctors become impatient and give only cursory exams. And, if Medicaid and Medicare forms are intimidating and confusing to the native English speaker, they are far worse for Puerto Ricans.

Transportation and availability of health services are also problems for the Puerto Rican, with only 37% of households owning cars. Given all the obstacles to seeking health care, many Puerto Ricans wait until illness reaches a crisis state. Thirty percent of New York City's drug addicts are Puerto Ricans. The City's lack of commitment to these people is manifested by the fact that there is only one bilingual comprehensive drug program in the metropolitan area.

Increasing the number of Puerto Ricans in the health professions is one way of improving the health services available to Puerto Ricans—a slow process at best. In 1971-72, Puerto Ricans comprised a mere .001% of the medical and dental students in the U.S. This is no surprise given the racist attitudes of U.S. educators and the fact that only 23% of the adult Puerto Ricans in the U.S. have graduated from high school.

The following groups represent both health related and general projects because the struggle for decent health care cannot be separated from the struggle to improve living conditions. Most are located in New York City, since the greatest concentration of Puerto Ricans on the mainland is located there.

PUERTO RICAN HEALTH SERVICES FEDERATION. . . works to generate change in the health care institutions serving New York's Lower East Side as well as providing multifaceted screening for the area. Workers, consumers, students and professionals all work together to pressure hospitals into providing better services for the local population of Puerto Ricans, Blacks, Jews, Chinese, Ukranians, etc. In addition, they operate the Batansas Unit, a 27-foot mobile unit equipped for screening of tuberculosis, sickle cell anemia, lead poisoning, hearing, vision, VD, urinary tract infections, Pap smears and hypertension. Sex, drug, and family education are also available for the approximately 400 people screened monthly. One full-time RN and several part-time MDs work with the Unit, making referrals to local hospitals when treatment is necessary. The Batansas Unit was originally operated as a drug program by a church, but when community people took it over in 1970 they changed the priority to screening and testing. Contact PUERTO RICAN HEALTH SERVICES FEDERATION, 35 Essex St., New York, NY 10002, (212) 982-2920.

UNIVERSIDAD BORICUA. . . offers bi-cultural, bi-lingual university education for Puerto Ricans on the mainland. Students take responsibility for planning their own curriculums, with Learning Centers set-up wherever there is a concentration of Puerto Ricans. Faculty members assist prospective students in obtaining Graduate Equivalency Degrees for those who have not completed high school. The word Boricua is derived from Boriquen, the name given by the Taino Indians to the island before its discovery by the Spaniards, reflecting the commitment of the Universidad to pride in Puerto Rican heritage. Contact UNIVERSIDAD BORICUA, 1766 Church St., NW, Washington, D.C. 20036, (202) 667-7940.

LA ALIANZA HISPANA. . . offers a wide variety of social services in the areas of education, literacy training, housing, economic development, employment, health and youth work. The only agency serving Boston's Spanish speaking population of 100,000, they provide vital bi-lingual, bi-cultural services. Their main health care work is doing referrals, although La Alianza has also pressured two hospitals into hiring bilingual staff. The program, with a staff of 25, has been funded by a Model Cities grant, however future support is needed. Despite the work of La Alianza, conditions for Boston's Spanish speaking population remain poor, with few bilingual health workers, and only limited attention from the local government. Contact LA ALIANZA HISPANA, 645 Dudley St., Dorchester, MA 02125, (617) 427-7175.

ASPIRA. . . . offers a wide range of services to New York's Puerto Rican community, although the emphasis is on youth and education. Programs, funded by foundations and the federal government, focus on drug education (addicts are referred to either Lincoln Detox or to SERA and other therapeutic communities), counseling and tutoring for high school students, college placement, scholarship, and loan assistance, college retention, and parent-student guidance. In an effort to increase the number of Puerto Rican health professionals, ASPIRA surveys medical schools and affiliated colleges to identify summer school programs for minority pre-med students and actively works to place Aspirantes in such programs. They also help students write medical school applications and prepare for the interview, and they arrange waivers for students unable to pay the Medical College Admissions Test (MCAT). In 1971-72, Aspira helped 14 students gain admittance to medical schools, representing a national increase of 38% in Puerto Rican admittance. The drug program does education in high schools and junior highs around the societal causes of addiction, including poverty, racism, and sexism. They oppose the use of methadone maintenance. Contact ASPIRA, 296 5th Ave., New York, NY 10001, (212) 924-8336.

ASSOCIATION OF COMMUNITY SERVICES . . . . is an ethnically mixed group writing a directory of health services in the Lower East Side of New York. The Association hopes to publish the book in Spanish and English, and it will be distributed free of charge. Other Association projects include daycare centers, housing specialists, education projects, parents' organizations, welfare advocacy and an employment office. Contact ASSOCIATION OF COMMU—NITY SERVICES, 152 Ave. D, New York NY 10009, (212) 533-2410.

RESOURCES

Puerto Rican and Community Service Organizations Throughout the United States, Migration Division, Department of Labor, Commonwealth of Puerto Rico, 322 W. 45th St., New York, NY 10036, 1973. Free
. . . extensive directory of organizations serving Puerto Ricans, ranging from activist groups to business associations. Each entry includes the address, phone number, director, type of organization and funding. Most groups listed are in New York, although 9 other northern states are included.

Puerto Rico, Showcase of Oppression, distributed by Latin American Publications Service, Box 12056 Mid City Station, Washington, DC 20005, 1970. 7 pamphlets, $2.50.
. . . collection of pamphlets on US imperialism in Puerto Rico. Covers the church, Operation Bootstrap, political development, cultural identity and more.

Palante Young Lords Party, Young Lords Party and Michael Abramson. McGraw-Hill, 330 W. 42nd St., New York, NY 10036, 1971. 160 pp. $3.95
. . . compelling story of the birth and growth of the Young Lords, a militant Puerto Rican revolutionary party. Through personal essays, political analysis and scores of photos, the sense of struggle and dedication of the Lords is forcefully conveyed. Discusses life in el barrio and prison, as well as the tactics and goals of the party. In a very beautiful way this book communicates Puerto Rican pride and strength.

Down These Mean Streets, Piri Thomas. Alfred A. Knopf, 201 E. 50th St., New York, NY 10022, 1967. 333 pp.
. . . moving presentation of life in Spanish Harlem, as lived by one Puerto Rican. This autobiographical novel follows the life of Piri Thomas from boyhood in Harlem, to a brief stay in suburbia, then back to Spanish Harlem, the South, and eventually to prison in New York State. Vividly portrays el barrio, life on the streets, heroin addiction and prison. Combining Spanish and English the style is compelling and driving.

"East 110th Street", Jose-Angel Figueroa, Broadside Press, 12651 Old Mill Place, Detroit, Michigan, 48238, 1973. 45 pp. $1.75
. . . a Puerto Rican poet writes of the lives of Latinos in New York City. Biting images reflecting anger at the political system are combined with songs of love for la Patria and the Puerto Rican way of life.

FILMS AND TAPES

Third World Newsreel, 26 W. 20th St., New York, NY 10011

"Don Pedro: La Vida de un Pueblo," 50 min. cl. $90, 1974 (sale: $600)
The story of one man who sees his children educated in Puerto Rican schools set up by gringo. They lose their cultural identity and become wanderers in Ponce, San Juan and New York where they serve the gringos in the most menial positions. Concludes with the old man teaching his grandchildren of a better way of life.

"El Pueblo Se Levanta ," 42 min. b&w $50, 1971 (sale: $350)
Traces the growth of the Puerto Rican Young Lords Party and their work in health, housing, education and nutrition. The film stresses the strength and power of the Puerto Rican people.

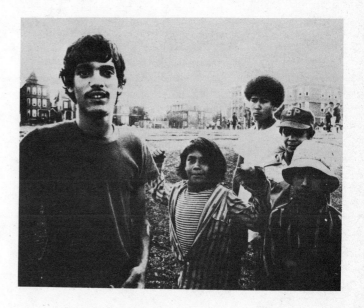

BLACK
RESOURCES

Being Black in the United States is a health hazard. It means running a much greater risk of: high blood pressure, infant and maternal mortality, sickle cell anemia, drug addiction, and low income. The average life span for Black people is 7-10 years lower than for Whites, and a 25 year old Black in the U.S. is four times as likely to die before reaching 40 as her/his White counterpart. Black infant mortality is nearly two times that of Whites and maternal mortality is four times the White rate. Researchers estimate that 35-40% of Blacks (twice the rate for Whites) suffer from high blood pressure, a disease directly related to stress and socio-economic status, as well as smoking and obesity. With the exception of sickle cell anemia, these higher incidences of poor health in Blacks can all be correlated to social and economic rather than physical causes.

The number one health problem for Blacks is high blood pressure, "the silent disease." Because it has no external symptoms, half of the people afflicted do not realize that they have high blood pressure until it manifests itself in kidney disease, a heart attack or a stroke. The danger of hypertension is increased for low-income people because they are not exposed to and cannot afford preventive care and screening.

Another serious health problem for Blacks is sickle cell anemia, a disease which causes the red blood cells to "sickle", resulting in poor physical development, weakness, enlargement of certain vital organs (heart, liver, spleen), paralysis of muscles, retarded growth patterns and a high susceptibility to infections. Victims commonly suffer from pneumonia, ulcerous sores, jaundice and infections.

Although one in five hundred Blacks has sickle cell anemia and nearly one out of ten carries sickle cell trait (genes which increase the probability of sickle anemia in the offspring), the disease has only recently become a "respectable" subject for study—and it still is grossly under-researched and over-publicized. Although publicizing a serious disease means greater public awareness, many Blacks believe sickle cell anemia publicity is geared to imply racial inferiority or to instill a false sense of progress in researching the disease. Government research priorities are blatantly demonstrated in the distribution of National Institute of Health grants. In 1968, NIH awarded 65 grants to cystic fibrosis research (which affects one in three thousand, with 98% of the victims White); 41 grants for phenylketonuria (an illness affecting one in ten thousand) and less than 24 grants for sickle cell anemia. In 1971 NIH gave more money to the University of Alabama than to all the Black schools combined.

The number of Black health professionals is another example of society's lack of concern for Third World health care. Although 10% of the population is Black, only 2% of the nation's doctors and dentists are. One in every 560 Whites will become a physician, while only one in every 3,800 Blacks will. The rate for RNs is somewhat higher (although far too low), with 4% Black. When one realizes that Federal tax monies support two-thirds of the cost of medical education, it becomes obvious that poor and Third World people are subsidizing the training of White students.

Only a small proportion of Black health groups have been included in this section, however Black groups are strongly represented throughout the rest of the catalogue. Also, many of the following groups are general resources rather than directly related to health, yet they nonetheless offer valuable assistance in organizing around health issues.

PEOPLE'S FREE HEALTH SERVICE. . . has tested over 5000 people for sickle cell anemia (SCA) and over 800 people for hypertension since 1972, on an outreach basis. Volunteers go door-to-door in Black communities, explaining the dangers and affects of SCA and hypertension and encouraging residents to receive a free test. Outreach workers are trained by the program and sales of the Black Panther Party newspaper cover tne cost of testing supplies. The service provided a free clinic, offering complete ambulatory care from 6-10 pm daily, although it was closed due to lack of funds; there are plans to re-open it in late-spring 1974. Through the clinic and outreach program the PFHS hopes to force existing institutions to be more responsive by soliciting free lab work and back-up services. Contact PEOPLE'S FREE HEALTH SERVICE, 418 H St., NW, Washington, D.C. 20002, (202) 544-9100.

MALCOLM X UNITED LIBERATION FRONT. . . is a cadre-type organization of 9 Blacks working for radical change. Their primary tactic is organizing, with significant work in the health field. Currently they operate a blood bank. Local people donate blood to the Malcolm X account and it is then given free to anyone needing it. This is an invaluable service since the going price for blood in the area is $45/pint. The Front has also pressured the local government into doing Sickle Cell Anemia screening as well as equiping and using a mobile unit to provide a range of testing and preventive services. Since the local Public Health Clinic is 6 miles out of town, the Front has convinced the health department to provide free transportation. Accessibility remains a problem and the Front sees the only immediate answer in free, local clinics —although they do not have the money to set up such clinics. Other work includes organizing around prisons, students and lack of community services. The all-volunteer staff makes decisions collectively. Contact MALCOLM X UNITED LIBERATION FRONT, 443 N. Macomb St., Tallahassee, FL 32301, (904) 224-0070.

TRIPLE JEOPARDY. . . works to make existing health facilities more responsive to the needs of Third World women and to raise women's consciousness about their bodies. The project is a response to the fact that Third World women are routinely used for experimentation and treated in dehumanizing and exploitive ways. Specific work includes familiarizing counselors with family planning, abortion, pre- and post-natal care and patient's rights. Plans include creation of a patient's advocacy program in area clinics. Contact TRIPLE JEOPARDY, 1633 W. Bristol, Philadelphia, PA 19140

SCARE. . . the first group to deal with sickle cell anemia in a serious fashion, has several chapters and a national office in San Francisco. Work involves: education in schools and communities about the dangers and implications of SCA; counseling for carriers of SC trait and people with the disease; distribution of information on SCA and hypertension and publication of a quarterly newsletter; free testing for SCA and SC trait; 24 hour emergency service, assistance with transportation, hospitalization and medical advice; free blood transfusions through maintenance of a blood bank at a local hospital; and research into causes and cures of SCA. The San Francisco office conducts screening programs at local factories and universities and is trying to purchase a mobile unit to facilitate screening for SCA and hypertension. They also conduct a summer camp for victims of SCA. Funding for the limited paid staff is from the United Crusade, federal, state and private grants. Contact SCARE, 2201 Stiener, San Francisco, CA 94115, (415) 563-6040.

NATIONAL ASSOCIATION FOR SICKLE CELL DISEASE, INC. . . . works on a national level to educate and advocate around sickle cell anemia. With 31 member organizations in 20 states, the Association carries on a wide range of programs: distribution of bibliographies and how-to manuals on setting up a local project; publication and distribution of pamphlets and position papers on sickle cell anemia for health professionals, legislators, grass-roots groups and employers; workshops on improving the quality of life for the child with sickle cell anemia; training in genetic counseling; and technical assistance for local groups. NASCD will assist in the formation of local projects, serve as a clearinghouse for sickle cell anemia information and provide referrals to testing and treatment centers. Contact NASCD, 945 S. Western Ave., Suite 206, Los Angeles, CA 90006, (213) 731-1166.

SICKLE CELL ANEMIA CENTER/HOWARD UNIVERSITY . . . offers a much needed service in researching the causes and cures of sickle cell anemia. The educational component teaches both professionals and lay people about SCA, how to test, etc. National scientific conferences have been sponsored by the Center and literature for the non-medical community has been widely distributed. On a local level, using a mobile van, the Center does screening, counseling and treatment. Patient care is done by health teams and involves the family of the individual. An NIH grant covers the cost of medical research into SCA. Located on the campus of predominantly Black Howard University, the Center offers technical and non-technical information on a crucially under-researched disease. Contact SICKLE CELL ANEMIA CENTER/HOWARD UNIVERSITY, 520 W St., NW, Washington, D.C. 20001, (202) 636-7884.

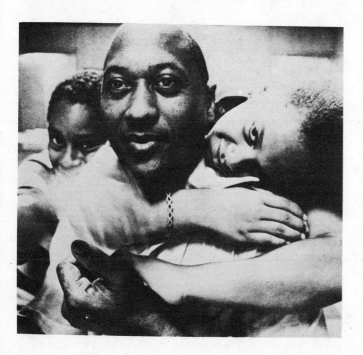

SICKLE CELL SOCIETY . . . assists people with sickle cell anemia and sickle cell trait as well as publicizing and researching the disease. The society was started in 1970 by a man suffering from SCA; he hoped to alert society to the fact that 1 of every 10 Blacks in the U.S. carries SC trait and 1 of every 500 succumb to the disease. Through outreach and testing programs, the Society has identified 200 SCA patients and 2000 carriers of the trait in Southwestern Pennsylvania. They provide genetic counseling, emotional support, medical referrals and emergency services. For patients with no other resources, the Society will help with medical bills, blood replacement, transportation to and from the hospital, education, job training and housing. In coordination with the Society, a large staff of doctors are researching SCA at the University of Pittsburgh medical school under a federal grant. Contact SCS, Medical Center East, Suite 742, 211 Whitfield St., Pittsburgh, PA 15206, (412) 441-6116.

BLACK PANTHER PARTY . . . is striving to achieve its goal of radical change through political education and service projects in Oakland as well as participation in electoral politics. The Oakland Community Learning Center, located in the East Oakland ghetto and operated by the Panthers, "is a complex of buildings with 35 rooms, a cafeteria, and a 300-seat auditorium, which has been used for art festivals and political meetings," as well as religious services. Programs include weekly bus transportation for families of inmates to area prisons; dance and music classes; women's self-defense classes; adult literacy; senior citizens' programs; a free clinic; and a community school for youth between 3 and 11. Based on the belief that providing good, free services makes people blatantly aware of the failings of the capitalist system, the Panthers are working to develop more local support. Such leaders as Elaine Brown and Bobby Seale have polled significant numbers of votes in recent elections in Oakland. Contact BPP, 8501 E. 14th St., Oakland, CA 94621, (415) 638-0195.

VIETNAM ERA VETERANS NATIONAL RESOURCE CENTER . . . was formed in reaction to the inadequate services provided by the Veterans Administration, particularly for Third World vets. The project works with 2700 vets projects around the country, many connected with campus veterans affairs offices; 90% of the local projects deal with Third World vets, for whom the Vietnam war was just one more devastating experience in their lives. The Center is currently compiling a national directory of vets projects, and doing a cross generational study of men affected by the Vietnam war— vets, POW's, resisters, evaders, deserters. In addition, it has begun to develop vets rap groups and works closely with a national group of Third World women veterans and women relating to male vets. The Center is working on a discharge upgrading project as well as advocating for individual counseling at the time of discharge. The Vets in Prison Project is trying to locate prisoners who are veterans and work for their release. Staffed 75% by Third World people, the Center strives to hook up skilled people with resources and projects, help with funding and promote information sharing, with major efforts geared to vets on the streets. Contact VEV-NRC, Room 767, 475 Riverside Dr., New York, NY 10027, (212) 870-2192.

SOUTHERN CHRISTIAN LEADERSHIP CONFERENCE... grew out of the Montgomery bus boycott in 1956 under the leadership of Martin Luther King, and has since maintained an important position in the civil rights movement. A large portion of the staff of 17 is engaged in voter registration and campaign activities in Alabama as well as education and advocacy around amnesty, prisons and civil rights. They publish a newspaper, SOUL FORCE, and a magazine, DRUM MAJOR. SCLC has 350 local chapters as well as 1200 affiliates in the U.S. and 2 abroad. Contact SCLC, 334 Auburn Ave. NE, Atlanta, GA 30303, (404)-522-1420.

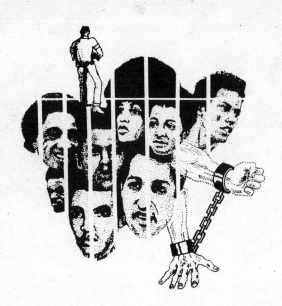

SOUTHERN POVERTY LAW CENTER... takes cases for Black and poor people in the south on a wide range of civil rights issues. Their services are free and the Center is supported by donations. Recent cases include: a suit against the federal government for the OEO funding of a family planning clinic accused of forced sterilization; defense of 3 Black men in North Carolina sentenced to the gas chamber for allegedly raping a White woman; and a suit against Governor Wallace of Alabama for obstructing the hiring of Black state troopers. SPLC, whose president is Julian Bond, offers a desperately needed service in a region crucially lacking in Black and progressive lawyers. Contact SPLC, Washington Building, Montgomery, AL 36101, (205) 264-1412.

RESOURCES

Sickle Cell Anemia—The Neglected Disease: Community Approaches to Combating Sickle Cell Anemia, ed. by Freya Olafson and Alberta Parker. University Extension, University of California, Berkeley, 2223 Fulton St., Berkeley, CA 94720, 1973. 109 pp. $3.00
. . . speeches from a California health center seminar program on sickle cell anemia and its treatment. The book discusses the causes, symptoms and genetic basis of SCA as well as how to set up a community program, the need to stress the difference between sickle cell anemia and trait, and the use of a coordinated approach (involving social workers, psychiatrists and physicians) to help victims. Throughout the book, the speakers discuss such issues as who should be tested (should testing be mandatory?), the need to proceed from "molecular research" about the disease, to designing screening, counseling and referral programs, and the effects of the recent campaign against sickle cell anemia (i.e. scaring people, who find they have a disease for which there is no cure). A bibliography gives information about other writing on sickle cell anemia.

Blood in My Eye. George J. Jackson, Bantam Books, 666 Fifth Avenue, New York, N.Y., 10019, 1972. 169 pp, $1.50
. . . a series of letters from the Black revolutionary prisoner, George Jackson. Heavily influenced by Marx, Lenin, and Mao, Jackson relates their writings to the situation of Black Americans today. He calls for an end to capitalism, and its replacement by "scientific revolutionary socialism". His own revolutionary commitment is witnessed by his active role as a political organizer, during his more than ten years in prison, despite the fact that he was frequently relegated to solitary confinement. "I've lived with repression every moment of my life", he writes, "a repression so formidable that any movement on my part can only bring relief, the respite of a small victory, or the release of death". George Jackson was shot in San Quentin, a few days after this book was completed.

No More Lies, Richard Claxton Gregory, ed. by James R. McGraw, Harper and Row, Publishers, Inc., 10 East 53rd St., New York, N.Y., 10022, 1972. 372 pp, $2.50
. . . a review of the myths of American history. Gregory stresses how "the continuing myth of American history dignifies the illicit acts of some and condemns the same acts when others do them". For example, George Washington "is revered. . .because he fought against oppression," while Black people seeking liberation are villified by White society. Similarly, Blacks called for law and order after the murder of Malcolm X, and of Martin Luther King, while Whites became interested in law and order only after the ghetto riots. Writing with insight and biting humor, Gregory expresses optimism backed with determination and conviction.

PAMPHLETS AND ARTICLES

"HEALTH, HEALTH CARE AND THE BLACK COMMUNITY," William M. King, Council of Planning Librarians, P.O. Box 229, Monticello, IL 61856, April, 1974, No. 555. 16 pp. $1.50
. . . bibliographical listing of scores of books and articles on health care for Blacks, covering material from the late 19th century to the present.

"Sickle Cell Anemia: An Interesting Pathology," Michael G. Michaelson, RAMPARTS, available in reprint from Louise Rice, 65 Chestnut St., Boston, MA 02139, 7 pp. $.31
. . . an excellent political and historical overview of sickle cell anemia (SCA), a genetic disease which kills one in every five hundred Blacks and poses a milder form of the disease to the two million Blacks who carry the sickle cell trait. The recent emphasis on SCA research is put in perspective with a brief history of the disease and the lack of interest in it by the White medical establishment. Condemns and documents the insincerity of the Defense Dep't, the AMA, NIH, and the general medical community in their approach to this "chic" topic. The current SCA research boom aims for quick results and high visibility, and its long-range consequences will not be medical so much as social and political. Points out that the significant work has been performed by community groups, such as the Black Panthers, who have consistently been the most motivated and productive in identifying and educating carriers of the trait and those affected by the anemia. "Current liberal enthusiasm about sickle cell anemia leaves deliberately unexamined the real roots of the Black community's chronic ill health." Articulate and convincing.

The federal government funds Sickle Cell Anemia prevention and education projects as well as some research. For names and addresses, contact DEPARTMENT OF HEALTH, EDUCATION AND WELFARE, Public Health Service, NIH, Building 31, Room 5A04, Bethesda, MD 20014.

PERIODICALS

THE BLACK PANTHER, Black Panther Party, 8501 E. 14th St., Oakland, CA 94621. $.25
. . . radical political coverage and analysis of Black news in the US and throughout the world. Articles include interviews with leaders of the Black Panther Party and news ignored by the established press. This paper has articles on Africa, China, Third World groups in the US and other anti-imperialist work.

TRIPLE JEOPARDY, Third World Women's Alliance, 346 W. 20th St., New York, NY 10011/P.O. Box 3065, Berkeley, CA 94703, $.25 in New York and $.30 outside the city
. . . covers the struggles of Third World women in the US in Spanish and English. Articles focus on Puerto Rico, forced sterilization, political prisoners, health and more. Excellent perspective on the triple oppression of Third World women: racism, imperialism and sexism.

NATIVE AMERICAN RESOURCES

With an average annual income of $1500, an unemployment rate of 45%, and 70% substandard housing, it is no wonder that Native Americans face serious health and nutritional problems. The statistics speak for themselves: average life expectancy for Native Americans is 46 years compared to 70 for the rest of the population; the Native American tuberculosis rate is 8 times the national average, with death from TB 4 times the average; Indian infant mortality is 2 times the average and the Native Alaskan infant death rate is 4 times higher than the national average.

Indians are considered "wards" of the government, lumped together with federal prisoners and drug addicts. Their health needs are supposedly met by the Indian Health Service (under HEW), although IHS only serves reservation dwellers, who currently comprise only 55% of the Native American population. IHS programs and facilities are extremely inadequate. Only 21 of 51 IHS hospitals have passed Joint Hospital Accreditation Committee standards, and a mere 15 meet Fire Protection Association and Uniform Building Code requirements. Many are now understaffed, and the situation will only deteriorate due to the end of the military draft, which gave doctors the option to serve with IHS instead of going into the Service. A not uncommon example is the Pine Ridge reservation hospital (South Dakota) which has 4 doctors for 13,000 people. In Navajo Nation, Arizona, IHS doctors are too busy to perform surgery on children with middle ear infections even though it can result in deafness and loss of equilibrium. The federal government shows no interest in improving conditions, as evidenced by Nixon's impounding of IHS funds for 4 of the past 5 years.

For non-reservation Indians, conditions are often worse. No special health facilities exist and, generally, doctors are unsympathetic to cultural and language differences. As with other minorities, there is a crucial shortage of health personnel. There are currently only 51 Native American physicians in the USA.

Underlying most health problems faced by Native Americans are the subtle and not so subtle actions of a racist government and society. Indian children are taken from their homes and sent to boarding schools where they are taught to emulate White culture. Adults must choose between refugee-camp reservations, under the authoritarian control of the Bureau of Indian (BIA), or move to urban areas, losing the scanty government assistance and cultural identity they have left. Reservation Indians are subject to regulation by the local, state, and federal government, including the BIA, the Department of Interior, and the House Committee on Interior and Insular Affairs.

As with other ethnic minorities in the US, Native Americans suffer a loss of culture identity, language, and self-respect in the process of adapting to a white society. One release from this forced adjustment is found in alcohol. AKWESASNE NOTES estimates that one in three adult Indians abuses the use of alcohol, with a correlatingly high number of arrests. According to Americans for Indian Opportunity, 33% of Native Americans are jailed at some time and many of these arrests are related to alcohol abuse. Every second Native American family has a relative who will die in jail. The Native American suicide rate is twice the national average, and cirrhosis of the liver (an alcohol related disease) is 4.7 times the national average.

Because health conditions for Native Americans can not be improved without drastically bettering housing, employment, nutritional standards, self-esteem, etc., the work fo the groups listed varies widely. All share a commitment to change and have at least a majority of Native Americans in decision-making positions.

AMERICAN INDIAN MOVEMENT. . . is the national political organization of radical Indians. Identifying three major destructive forces to Indians—Christianity, White-oriented education and the federal government—AIM works for "self-determination and the right to be and think Indian." Tactically, they have been involved in countless demonstrations and court cases, the most famous being the Trial of Broken Treaties and the occupation of Wounded Knee. AIM was formed in Minneapolis in 1968 to confront police harassment. Although Native Americans represented only 10% of the population in Minneapolis, they comprised 70% of city jail inmates. AIM organized a ghetto patrol, equipted with 2-way radios capable of picking up police radio calls. Whenever a call came through involving an Indian, AIM rushed to the area to defend the rights of the Indian involved. The Native American jail population was reduced by 60% as a result. AIM has 79 chapters in the US and Canada, and ties with native organizations in Australia and Micronesia. Contact AIM, 1337 E. Franklin Ave., Minneapolis, MN 55404, (612) 227-0651.

WHITE ROOTS OF PEACE. . . facilitates communication among Native American people through a traveling group, a newspaper (Akwesasne Notes), and the publication and distribution of books, posters, records, and calendars. The resident staff (about six) lives and works communally, writing and compiling books on the takeover of the Bureau of Indian Affairs building, the occupation of Wounded Knee and the subsequent trials, native poetry and more. They also distribute posters and over 65,000 copies (per issue) of Akwesasne Notes. The traveling group (6-20 members) does on the spot reporting of Native American news; meets with urban, reservation, prison and student groups to "promote Indian unity, strength in the Indian ways, and to give out information on Indian situations"; and speaks to college and church groups. Although not working directly in the health field, White Roots of Peace is an invaluable group for anyone involved in the Indian movement. Contact WHITE ROOTS OF PEACE, Mohawk Nation via Rooseveltown, NY 13683, (518) 358-4697.

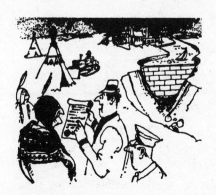

"It's quite explicit chief...only as
long as the sun shines & the rivers run.

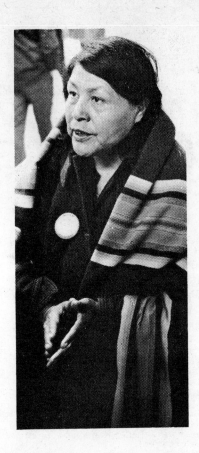

CALIFORNIA URBAN INDIAN HEALTH COUNCIL... is a coalition of 9 clinics serving low-income Native American communities. The Council, created in 1973, facilitates fund raising, data collection and information dissemination on federal health policy. CUIHC believes that the federal government is partially responsible for the migration of Native Americans from reservations to the cities (i.e. BIA relocation programs) and therefore should assume some responsibility for Native American health care in urban areas. The Council receives primary funding from HEW, which is then passed on to the local clinics. The goal is to help clinics move toward self-sufficiency through Medicaid, Medicare and insurance payments. Decisions are made by a Board of 9, with one representative from each of the clinics. Two people work as paid staff. For information on the individual clinics or the Council, contact CUIHC, 46 Shattuck Sq., Room 14, Berkeley, CA 94704, (415) 845-4491.

AMERICANS FOR INDIAN OPPORTUNITY... offers technical assistance to local Native American groups in an effort to increase economic power and cultural pride. They have formed legal defense and small business investment organizations and are currently working on a series of Indian movies. AIO is particularly active in the struggle to win Native Americans their legal rights in Court cases. Contact AIO, 1816 Jefferson Place, NW, Washington, D.C. 20036, (202) 466-8420.

WOUNDED KNEE LEGAL DEFENSE/OFFENSE COMMITTEE... is providing legal back-up for the 317 cases pending in federal, state and tribal courts resulting from the 1973 liberation of Wounded Knee. The 71 day occupation, which was supported by the American Indian Movement, dramatized both the federal government's continuous violation of the Fort Laramie Treaty of 1868 and it's support of an Authoritarian tribal government on the Sioux reservation. The Committee is currently representing people in Sioux Falls and Pierre, S.D.; St. Paul, Minn.; and Lincoln, Neb. The committee workers live and work collectively with support from donations. They write and distribute a monthly newsletter and an excellent background booklet, Remember Wounded Knee. Contact WKLD/OC, 333 Sibley Ave., Room 605, St. Paul, MN 55101, (612) 224-5631 or 2nd Floor, 100 North Phillips, Sioux Falls, SD 57101, (605) 339-9805.

AMERICAN INDIAN PRESS ASSOCIATION... writes and distributes weekly news packets on issues affecting Native Americans. With a slight bias toward federal and legislative actions, the packets cover issues often ignored by the straight press. Members of the Association (only Indians allowed) pay $40 for a year's subscription; non-members are charged $100. The Association also distributes the American Indian Media Directory (600 entries) and MEDIUM RARE, a monthly newsletter. Contact AIPA, Room 206, 1346 Connecticut Ave., N.W., Washington, D.C. 20036, (202) 293-9150.

AMERICAN INDIAN MOVEMENT/ST. PAUL... has set up a first aid clinic for people in St. Paul for the Wounded Knee trials. An RN permanently works out of the AIM office, with her salary paid by the county health department. Supplies and time for the first aid clinic are donated by area hospitals and health workers, enabling the clinic to provide free services. General check-ups are done, with referrals to more comprehensive clinics when necessary. AIM also screens the children attending their day care center. Contact AMERICAN INDIAN MOVEMENT, 553 Aurora Ave., St. Paul, MN 55103, (612) 224-4395.

NATIVE AMERICAN RIGHTS FUND... tries precedent-setting cases involving Native Americans. Their priorities include tribal existance, tribal resources and human rights, although they do some health related cases. Currently pending are cases on Native American access to state institutions for the retarded and the restraint of people in mental institutions. They have a growing Indian Law Library. Contact NARF, 1506 Broadway, Boulder, CO 80302, (303) 447-8760.

NAVAJO COMMUNITY COLLEGE... is the first institute of higher learning on an American Indian reservation. Having opened in 1970, it is completely owned and operated by the Navajo tribe and 90% of the students are Navajo. Historically, Indian students have done poorly in Anglo academic programs, largely because of problems of social adaptation. It was hoped that staying on the reservation for at least the first two years of college would ease this transition. The college has an open admissions policy to everyone with a high

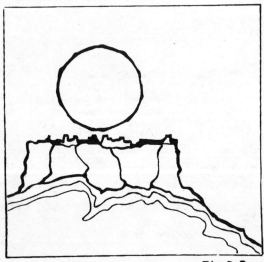

John De Puy

52

school diploma or its equivalent, and developmental studies are also offered. All expenses are covered by the government. Included in the offerings is a two year RN program, and massive nursing recruitment efforts throughout the 75,000 square mile reservation are just beginning. The curriculum stresses a cross-cultural approach, for example, a medicine man is on the nursing faculty. Although the majority of the administration are Indian, many of the academic faculty are White, because the college has had difficulty finding Indians with adequate training in these areas. Contact: Navajo Community College, Many Farms, RPO, Arizona 86503, (602) 724-3311.

NATIONAL CONGRESS OF AMERICAN INDIANS. . .
"gives the tribes a voice at the national level" through lobbying and education. A national congress is held annually, with representatives from approximately 90 tribes, where scores of resolutions are passed on Indian-related national and state issues. The 4-member staff in Washington, D.C. lobbies, offers technical assistance to local tribes, writes a monthly newsletter (THE SENTINEL), and keeps the tribes informed of changes in federal policy. The Congress first met in 1944. Contact NATIONAL CONGRESS OF AMERICAN INDIANS, 1346 Connecticut Ave., NW, Washington, D.C. 20036, (202) 223-4155.

UNITED SIOUX TRIBES OF SOUTH DAKOTA. . . recently conducted a survey on the adequacy of the Indian Health Service facilities in South Dakota. Results will be used to pressure the local power structure to improve. United Sioux Tribes provides more direct services in employment, housing and training. Contact UNITED SIOUX TRIBES OF SOUTH DAKOTA, P.O. Box 1193, Pierre, SD 57501, (605) 224-8862.

UNITED SOUTHEASTERN TRIBES. . . contracts with the BIA to provide health services for 6 tribes in the Southeast. They operate hospitals in North Carolina and Mississippi, as well as service units, mental health and alcohol programs in several other states. UST also focuses on the recruitment of Indians into health professions, the recognition of the skills of medicine men, environmental health, and water and sewage services. Non-health related work includes legal services, economic development, education and teacher training. UST is funded by the federal government, tribal dues, and private foundations. Contact UST, 1970 Main St., Sarasota, FL 33577, (813) 955-0281.

GREAT LAKES INTERTRIBAL COUNCIL, INC. . . . represents ten reservations and defines its priorities as: 1. economic development, 2. education, and 3. health. Health related work is diverse, including community health representatives on the reservations, working as advocates and trouble shooters; an elderly feeding program, bringing hot food to over 320 seniors daily; emergency food program to provide one week's commodities in a crisis; nursing recruitment program; and education and referrals around alcoholism. The Community health representatives oversee clinics on each of the reservations, provide transportation to clinics and hospitals, and work to lower the suicide and alcoholism rate. The Council believes that economic development is of prime importance in improving Native American conditions. Other programs include a Neighborhood Youth Corps, community organizing, and a pre-apprenticeship program. Funding is from several government agencies and the staff of 190 is 93% Native American. Contact GREAT LAKES INTERTRIBAL COUNCIL, P.O. Box 5, Lac du Flanbeau, WI 54538, (715) 588-3331.

NATIVE ALASKAN AND HAWAIAN

The Hawaians
16 J Market St.
Wailuku, Maui, Hawaii 96793

Mil-ka-ko
Box 786
Captain Cook, Kona, Hawaii 97604

Alaskan Native Brotherhood
1003 B St.
Juneau, Alaska 99801

Alaska Federation of Natives
1675 C St.
Anchorage, Alaska 99501

Indian-Eskimo Association of Canada
277 Victoria St.
Toronto, Ontario, Canada

RESOURCES
BOOKS

American Indian Medicine, Virgil J. Vogel, University of Oklahoma Press, 1005 Asp St., Oklahoma City, OK 584 pp. $12.50
. . . American Indian medical practices, and their influences on modern medicine. Native Americans used drugs to cure diabetes, syphilis, and many other diseases; an herbal concoction, which regulates the menstrual cycle, served as the precursor for today's birth control bill. Syringes, anesthetics, and antiseptics were used in Indian treatments yet, to date, little credit has been given by White society to the Indians for their contribution to modern medicine. A description of medicine man practices reveals the unmagical basis for some of their cures (i.e. removing pus through sucking; giving psychological support to a patient). The book includes an extended bibliography on Indian medicine, and categorizes therapies and drug use.

Custer Died for Your Sins, Vine Deloria, Jr., Avon Books, 959 Eighth Ave., New York, N.Y., 10019, 1969. 272 pp, $1.25
. . . a manifesto on the state of Indian life. Deloria describes the many mythes White society has created about Indians, the abundance of those who consider themselves "Indian experts", and how stereotypes and misconceptions have oppressed Indian people. He reviews laws and treaties with the U.S. government, government agencies involved in Indian affairs, the ways missionaries and anthropologists have plagued Indians, the relation between U.S. treatment of Blacks and of Indians, and the history of Indian leadership. He points to the urban Indians today as "the cutting edge of the new Indian nationalism", but stresses the need for co-ordination between urban and reservation Indians. Deloria applauds the efforts of Indians who have used such (political) tactics as demanding equal time, when ABC presented a "Custer" series.

Indian Health Service Recruitment Problems, Hearings before the Subcommittee on Indian Affairs of the Committee on Insular Affairs, United States Senate. U.S. Government Printing Office, 1974. 167 pp.
. . . 1973 hearings outlining the deplorable shortages of physicians and other health service personnel in the health facilities operated by the Indian Health Service. Special attention is given to the Doctor Draft Act (2 year IHS service in lieu of military service) and its effect on this shortage. Specific IHS facilities are examined with statistical data presented to bolster claims of insufficient staffing and funding. Good recommendations are made if only someone would act on them.

"A survey was taken, and only 15% of the Indians thought that the US should get out of Vietnam. Eighty-five percent thought they should get out of America."
—from Custer Died for Your Sins

PAMPHLETS AND ARTICLES

Remember Wounded Knee, Wounded Knee Legal Defense/
Offense Committee, 2nd Floor, 100 Phillips, Sioux Falls,
SD 57101, 1973. 32 pp. $1.00
. . . collection of articles and background information on the
occupation of Wounded Knee. Originally written as a press
kit, it includes statements by participants, the Fort Laramie
Treaty of 1868, the May 1973 agreement which ended the
occupation, a description of the cases and principle defendants, and information on AIM. Invaluable resource for anyone concerned with Native American rights and Wounded
Knee in particular.

**"GOVERNING BODIES OF FEDERALLY RECOGNIZED
INDIAN GROUPS",** U.S. Department of the Interior, Bureau of Indian Affairs, 1951 Constitution Ave., NW, Washington, D.C. 20001. May 1973. 33 pp. Free
. . . alphabetical and geographical listing of federally recognized tribes.

PERIODICALS

AKWESASNE NOTES, Mohawk Nation, via Rooseveltown,
NY 13683. 7 issues/year; minimum donation of $5 suggest-
ed, especially for institutions
. . . sensitive, proud and joyous coverage of the Native American struggle. The articles range from in-depth accounting of
Wounded Knee to original poetry; also covers Indian movements in other countries, particularly Central and South
America. Akwesasne Notes carries analytical essays, thoughtful book reviews and fine, fine graphics. Well worth the cost
(which helps support the work of White Roots of Peace).

FILMS AND TAPES

Impact Films, 144 Bleecker St., New York, NY 10012

"As Long As the Rivers Run," 60 min. cl. $125-$65 (sliding scale) 1971 (Sale: $600)
Documents the struggles of Indians fighting for fishing
rights on the Nisqually River in Washington. Indian songs
and narration are blended with village scenes, government
harassment and the take-over of Alcatraz.

Ballis Associates, 5439 Carlton, Oakland, CA 94618

"The Dispossessed" 33 min. cl. and sepia 1970 $50
A film on the Pit River Indians' struggle to regain their
lands and how this is related to farmworkers, ecology,
and foreign wars.

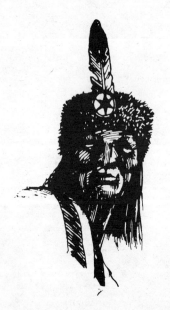

ASIAN RESOURCES

Asian Americans are an often ignored, yet important and growing minority in the US' They come primarily from Taiwan,
Formosa, Japan and the Philippines—all countries with long
histories of US involvement in economic and political affairs.
Asians come to the US in search of health and well-being--but
for many the dream soon turns into a nightmare of over-
crowded slums, long hours of work at low pay, and loss of
culture and family ties.

The principle Asian communities in the US are in Hawaii, San
Francisco, Los Angeles, New York, and Boston; most of the
Asians in these cities congregate in one section. Boston's
Chinatown, for example, has the lowest income of any neighborhood in the city, with 63% of the families having an income below $6300. Infant mortality and tuberculosis are
twice the city-wide levels. In 1968 immigration laws restricting the number of Chinese entering the US were removed, resulting in a five-fold increase in newcomers. Since social services and housing have not increased proportionately, problems of overcrowding and poverty among Asian American
populations have become accentuated in many areas of the
country.

The Asian American population can best be understood as
two distinct groups: first generation immigrants who speak
little English and live in inner city ghettos; and second and
third generation Asians, many of whom have been assimilated
into White society. Although both groups face problems, the
nature of their respective difficulties are quite different.

New immigrants experience serious language barriers, poverty,
high incidence of communicable diseases, lack of adequate
health care facilities, and stress. They work in the restaurants,
laundries and other small businesses common to Asian-American ghettos, living in conditions of urban poverty that most
tourists choose not to see. Many second and third generation
Asians have "made it", moving to White suburbs, sending
their children to college, etc. But in the process of "suc-
ceeding", many Asians have sacrificed their culture and family
ties only to meet persistent and continual racism from White
society.

Listed below are both health related and general groups. They
provide important services for Asians, as well as advocacy for
meaningful change.

I WOR KUEN. . . is a revolutionary organization of Asians.
In New York City they run a free clinic and book store, show
films, and are involved in Chinatown struggles. The San Francisco branch is setting up a committee to bring low-cost adequate housing into Chinatown. Made up mostly of poor and
working class people, and some students, they publish GET-
TING TOGETHER bi-weekly ($3.50/year), sponsor an alter-
native Chinese school, work with Asian Legal Services, and
with students organizing against U.S. imperialism in Southeast Asia. Contact: I WOR KUEN, 24 Market St., New York,
NY, 10002, (212) 267-5850 or 850 Kearney St., San Francisco, CA, 94108, (415) 398-2212, or GETTING TOGETHER,
P.O. Box 26229, San Francisco, CA 94126.

JAPANESE COMMUNITY SERVICES. . . operates a patient
advocate program for the San Francisco Japanese community.
The program offers information and referral services for patients, accompanies them to the hospital and explains and
translates medical terminology and procedures. Presently
JCS is involved in training a translator for the out-patient

clinic of a near-by hospital and in compiling a glossary of relevant Japanese health terms. The basic principles of JCS run throughout their program: 1. self-help—each individual gaining more control of her/his mind or body, 2. bettering the Japanese American community, 3. developing more of a sense of community, 4. ending discrimination by race, sex, and age. Contact: JCS, 2012 Pine St., San Francisco, CA 94115, (415) 929-7567.

YELLOW SEEDS CENTER... provides referral services for the Asian community, assisting anyone needing help with housing, immigration, social security, medicare, language problems, education, employment, draft counseling, income taxes, or recreation. Their newspaper, Yellow Seeds, informs Asian Americans and others of the issues confronting the Asian American Community. ($1.00 per year). Contact: YELLOW SEEDS CENTER, 1006 Winter St., Philadelphia, PA 19107, (215) 925-3723.

TWO BRIDGES NEIGHBORHOOD COUNCIL... works to improve the quality of housing, health, and recreation in the community and to create "human dialogue." As a subsidiary of the federal Homemakers program, the council offers workshops in nutrition, food preparation, and exercise. It also helps people enroll in federal food programs and fights for their implementation on local levels. Workshops have been conducted on child raising and child/parent relationships. In addition the Council has supported a local methadone clinic and the Chinatown Health Fair. It is presently fighting for a health clinic in a newly built community high school. Contact: Two Bridges Neighborhood Council, 179 Cherry St., New York, NY 10002, (212) 233-6457.

JAPANESE AMERICAN SERVICE COMMITTEE... was organized 27 years ago to help the Japanese Americans who were returning from relocation centers. Many of the Committees programs are now oriented toward the older Japanese or "issei," the first generation of Japanese-Americans. These programs include dental and medical clinics, a homemeal service, a homemaker service, a housing project, a "friendly visitors" service, a telephone-aid service, and, in the near future, a drop-in center. The Committee also runs a counseling service for family counseling, housing, employment, and health referrals. Although much of the Committee's funding is from government agencies, it also comes from community drives; the Board of Directors is chosen through a committee of community organizations. Contact: JASC, 4427 North Clark, Chicago, IL, 60640, (312) 275-7212.

ASIAN-AMERICAN ALLIANCE... works to increase the delivery of services to the Asian-American community. The Alliance has delivered workshops inside a variety of institutions from the Department of Social Services to the local community mental health center, VISTA to church groups. It has also worked to get more Asian-Americans on the directing boards of these institutions. Presently the Alliance is trying to get funding for a bilingual outreach program in the community to help the many non-English speaking people get more services. Contact: Asian-American Alliance, c/o Takoma Community House, 1311 South M St., Tacoma, Washington, 98405, (206) 383-3951.

RESOURCES

BOOKS

Roots: An Asian American Reader, Amy Tachiki, Eddie Wong, Franklin Odo, eds. UCLA Asian American Studies Center, Continental Graphics, 1971.
... covers a tremendous range of subjects with hundreds of references all in a radical perspective. Includes sections on identity, history, and communities. The book deserves careful reading.

Asian Women, available from Everybody's Bookstore, 840 Kearney St., San Francisco, CA 94108, 1971. 144 pp. $2.00
... excellent anthology of essays, poems, and photographs by women in the US and Asia. Intensely personal and political, the writings communicate strength, conflict, and the courage to fight and change. Topics covered include US military involvement in Southeast Aisa, sexism, and racism within the US, cultural changes confronting Asian immigrants and more. A joy and inspiration to read.

Longtime Californ', Victor G. & Brett D Bary Nee, Pantheon Books, 201 E. 50th St., New York, NY 10022, 1973. 410 pp. $10.
... personal accounts of Chinese immigrants to the U.S. Tells of the awful conditions that immigrants must endure on Angel Island before being allowed to enter the US; the constant effects of racism; the anger and frustration of the youth. This book offers an important insight into life in Chinatown.

Americans and Chinese, Francis L.K. Hsu, Natural History Press, American Museum of Natural History, Central Park West & 79th, New York, NY 10024, 1970. 493 pp.
... a tremendously sensitive, comparative study of American and Chinese cultures. Individualism is seen as the root of the competition that permeates all aspects of American life and is so different from the outlook of the Chinese. Out of Hsu's portrayal of Chinese culture come some radical alternatives for Americans. Important reading for White consciousness raising.

Outlines History of the Chinese in America, H. Mark Lai and Philip P. Choy. Distributed by Everybody's Bookstore, 840 Kearney St., San Francisco, CA 94108, 1972. 84 pp. $3.00
... comprehensive history of the Chinese in the US. The book covers Chinese-US relations, immigration, the role of Chinese laborers, racism and more. Although the use of outline form makes it a bit difficult to follow, the extensive detail make this book a very useful resource.

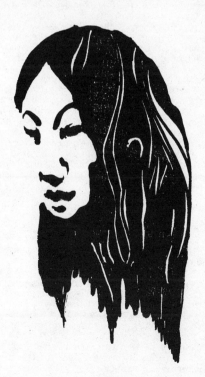

HOSPITALS

PROBLEM

In the past 100 years, the delivery of health care has evolved from a doctor-oriented, small artisan trade to one of the most profitable and swiftly-expanding industries in the country, grossing $83 billion per year. Hospitals have played an integral part in this transformation. What were once charitable, philanthropically supported institutions have become health care delivery factories focused on profits, research, education, prestige, and centralization of power. The three types of hospitals — voluntary ("non-profit"), proprietary (profit-making), and public (mainly federal, city and county) — are in a chaotic state of economic competition as each one seeks to protect and increase its own income and status. Businesspeople are recognizing proprietary hospitals and chains as prime, virtually recession-free investments, while medical schools are gobbling up voluntary and public hospitals to add to their increasingly powerful domains. The relationships between hospitals, medical businesses and schools are incestuous and manipulative, yet inevitable within the context of the health industry structure as it now stands.

At the heart of the health industry are medical centers, which have largely replaced individual hospitals as the bastions of medical power. Medical centers are usually built around a medical school or large teaching hospital. Other public or voluntary hospitals affiliate with the center to gain access to staff, facilities, funds, and status. Though the medical center may not have legal control over the affiliating hospitals, such connections as interlocking directorates tend to develop quickly. Medical centers' first loves are research, education, and prestige — all of which are pursued with great gusto. In order to win government, industry, and foundation research grants and to maintain its prestige, the modern medical center must attract top-flight researchers, scientists, and educators. These people must be lured with promises of large grants, interesting colleagues, a "good name" and plenty of research opportunities. This is where the voluntary and public hospitals come in. Their patients are material for researchers and teaching tools for educators. In addition, most voluntary hospitals have at least token community services. These services lend a facade of community responsibility to their sponsoring medical centers, besides filling their coffers with important government and foundation community development grants.

These feudal-type relationships raise ominous problems as powerful medical centers stake out their territory and consolidate the community's health resources under one or a few spheres of influence. In New York City, for example, three-fourths of the hospital beds are controlled by seven or eight medical centers. The influence of these centers is enormously disproportionate to the strength of the community and its people. As the directors of medical schools and their satellite hospitals gradually overlap, the power of each institution merges more and more with the others. These boards of directors are dominated by businesspeople, administrators, and physicians; there are few representatives of the consumers and workers who depend upon the health care delivery system for their health and livelihood. The people of a community end up with little control over its health resources and policy.

The medical centers and their affiliates did not reach their present status unaided — nor are they the only ones who profit. Medical centers are integrally linked to the leading financial and industrial concerns of their area. Banks are the prime beneficiaries of hospital expenditures. One New York City hospital spends $1.25 million a year in mortgages and interest — an average of $3 per day for each patient going directly into bank profits rather than improved care. Real estate is a major holding of some hospitals. In order to expand, an institution must have room to grow; so, in some cities, hospitals have become the largest and most negligent of absentee landlords. Living space is torn up and tenants displaced to make room for luxurious office buildings, concrete garages, and construction of hospitals, even where they are not needed. In Cleveland, two hospital projects were responsible for the displacement of 4,500 families, most of them Black. The only ones to gain from this frenetic expansion are leading area contractors and construction companies — often controlled by hospital trustees.

For the hapless consumer the problem does not stop here. There is still the myriad of hospital back-up industries (supply, lab, technological, insurance, etc.) which feed into and profit by the health care industry. In 1969, one sixth of the $62 billion expended for health care went to hospital supply companies which market everything from disposable catheter tubes to multi-thousand dollar kidney machines — as long as it is "anti-bacterial," clean, bright, and expensive. Much of the expense is wasted on needlessly exotic and duplicated equipment. In New York City, for example, fifteen separate hospitals developed open-

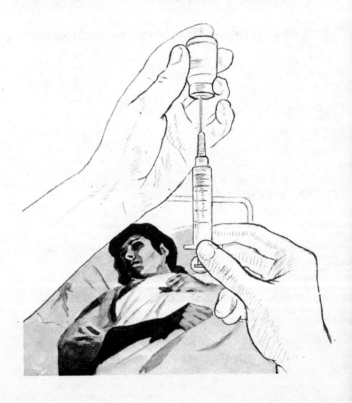

heart surgery units; but 83% of the open-heart surgery was performed by 7 hospitals (Health-PAC). The money that could be saved by sharing facilities could be used for preventive medicine, emergency care, or other services beneficial to the whole community. Consolidation is important to hospitals and medical centers only when it adds to their own profits, control, and prestige, not necessarily when it promotes lower costs and better patient care.

Irrational growth is reinforced further by hospital insurance programs. Most insurance payments (sometimes called third party payments) are made on a cost-plus basis. This means that all costs of a hospital are automatically assumed by the companies; there is no incentive for hospitals to keep costs down. But every time a hospital unnecessarily expands, builds, purchases, or wastes, the cost is passed on through the insurance industry to the consumer in the form of higher premiums, while those on medicaid/care must cover more of the cost out of their own pockets.

The consumer is, in fact, subsidizing the profits of hundreds of large and small industries at the expense of her/his own health and well-being. Nor can the consumer turn to a "higher authority" for redress of grievances; the government, rather than acting as a consumer advocate, is primarily concerned with further subsidizing health industries. Subsidies take the form of direct payments for care (medicaid/care), loans for hospital construction, research and education, grants, tax exemptions and deductions, etc. Most of this money enters the health care system with few and often unenforced controls.

Around sixty different federal programs funnel money into health services, yet there is only minimal planning and direction of how and where government resources should be spent. Government money is funnelled heavily into research, usually emphasizing exotic diseases that affect Whites, and drug research that benefits the military and the drug industry more than consumers. Community health services and preventive care take low priority. Research on drugs and rare diseases has its importance, but the money spent on it far outweighs the number of people it benefits. For example, it is more profitable for a medical center to contract for obscure research than to contract for outpatient care. So, while research develops more and more refined cures for complex diseases, the poor continue to suffer from diseases whose cures have long been known.

Other government funding programs have similar drawbacks. Many hospitals would not be in existence without the help of the Hill-Burton Construction Act, yet often they are permitted to ignore the law's requirement that they serve a significant portion of the indigent community. Medicare and medicaid do nothing to slow the rise of hospital costs; and when the amount medicare or medicaid will pay for a particular service falls too far below what hospitals are charging, these patients are refused beds in favor of private patients whose insurance can reimburse costs fully.

Government complicity in skyrocketing profits and inadequate care takes subtler forms, too. Many voluntary hospitals enjoy a tax-exempt status, yet use their tax-exempt money for further expansion rather than their stated purpose of improved "charitable" community service. This, combined with lack of planning, has allowed the existence of hundreds of empty beds in one section of a city or county, while in another section people have to wait weeks to be admitted. Hospitals will maintain many empty beds,

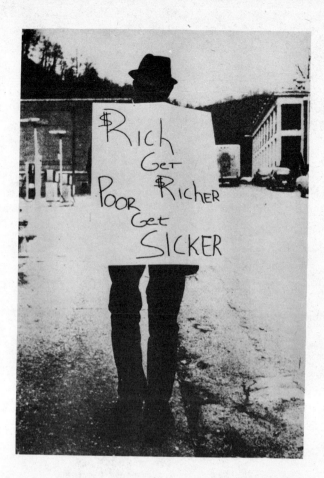

knowing they bring in an average of $84 per day when they are filled; this is still more profitable than providing good outpatient and indigent care. All in all, the result of government involvement in the health care industry is chaos for the consumer and easy money for the provider. The amount of money we pay into the system is little indication of the quality or quantity of the care we receive. It is, instead, an indicator of the economic well-being of the hospital and hospital-related industries.

We, as patients and as hospital workers, are up against a situation in which our health and well-being take second place to the needs of an expanding industry. It is a situation, too, in which those who control the industry use all the divisive stereotypes that plague our culture to keep us from working together, and perpetuate the centralized control of the medical establishment. Thus, racial, male-female, and professional-worker splits are reinforced by the hospital business.

Institutional racist and sexist attitudes are reflected in a variety of ways. Less time and money is spent on training Third World people and women in the society as a whole and within the medical training structure in particular. Thus, women, Blacks, Spanish-speaking peoples, Native Americans, and Asian Americans usually occupy the bottom strata of the hospital hierarchy. White male doctors learn their trade on Third World and poor patients but build their actual practice around White middle-class patients. These factors affect the way minority groups and women are often treated in the hospitals — more like research subject matter than people.

Reinforcing this dehumanization is the fact that most medical centers use poorly equipped and understaffed public hospitals as dumping grounds for poor, often Third World people who are deemed "uninteresting cases." Yet such a patient who displays unusual symptoms or has a rare disease may be given the most comprehensive treatment in the best-equipped of hospitals; it's a good learning experience for the young, White male students.

Adding insult to injury, hospitals spend millions of dollars each year for gimmicky publicity that covers up their racist and sexist attitudes. That money could improve patient care and upgrade workers' training rather than being used to maintain a cheap facade of humanitarianism.

Other ploys used by hospitals to undermine any kind of popular move against their institutional control are union-busting and dividing the community from the workers. Hospitals use classic red-baiting scare techniques to squash worker organizing and community support. They try to pacify workers with small favors and promises that are never kept. To cut community support, hospitals blame the high costs of hospital care on higher wages for workers, when in fact it is largely waste, high administrative salaries and the profit-margins of related industries which send costs spiralling up. Inadequate patient care is also blamed on workers, when in fact the responsibility usually rests with inadequate staffing and inefficient planning.

Hospital workers are pushing firmly for the decent livelihood and regard for their rights that have been denied for years. Meanwhile a growing patients' rights force is exerting itself in the form of in-hospital and citywide advocacy. At the same time, poor, middle-income and working class families are organizing and forming coalitions to define and meet their communities' long term health needs. The fight is difficult and sometimes the needs of community, workers and patients conflict painfully. Solving these conflicts is all the more important because all segments of the health movement are working towards one goal: to take profit out of the health care system and put the people back in.

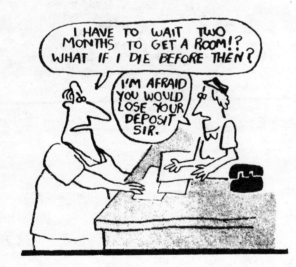

PLATFORM

First and foremost, of course, is our right to good health, resulting from effective preventive health care programs in our communities. In addition, hospitals must accept and abide by a minimum bill of patients', workers' and community rights. Some of these rights, though often ignored, are written into the law; but a legal precedent for many of them is yet to be established . . .

I. THE PATIENT'S RIGHT TO TREATMENT MUST COME FIRST . . . including the right to be treated comprehensively by well-trained health personnel in any hospital when life is in danger . . . to have transportation provided to and from the hospital . . . to free daycare while keeping doctor's appointments and visiting in-patients . . . to have help in finding a place to stay when leaving the hospital, in getting financial aid, in contacting relatives, and in getting other support services to help resolve emotional problems resulting from illness . . . to receive further treatment at a convenient time and place.

II. THE RIGHT TO DIGNITY, COURTESY, AND PRIVACY MUST BE RESPECTED...including the right to be addressed courteously and respectfully...to be in an enclosed area during examinations or treatment — with people not directly involved in care requiring the patient's permission to be there... the right to have access to our own medical records, which must remain confidential unless otherwise released by court order...the right to know who wants to see our records, why, and how this will benefit us, and the right to refuse them permission...the right to refuse to be filmed, photographed or publicized...and to leave the hospital when we choose unless a contagious disease is involved.

III. THE RIGHT TO INFORMATION MUST BE RECOGNIZED...including the right to automatically receive a patients' rights handbook upon entering the hospital...to know the regulations of the hospital...to have explanations in a comprehensible language of our condition, treatment, and prospects for recovery...the right to know the names of the medical people specifically responsible for us...to be completely informed of all letters or conferences about us...to know of any affiliations between the hospital we're in and other health care institutions (teaching or research hospitals, for example)...the right to be told the reasons for transfer to another hospital and the other options that are open...to have help in applying for medicaid/care...and to have a full explanation of all bills...and the general right of the community to full access to information concerning the functioning of the hospital.

IV. THE RIGHT TO INFORMED CONSENT MUST BE STRICTLY OBSERVED...including the right to delete any section of any form before signing it...to refuse to be used as a teaching object...to know, before receiving treatment, all possible side effects, what exactly will happen, how much it will hurt and for how long, the cost, the length of hospitalization required, and what alternatives are available...the right to change our minds after consenting to treatment...to be treated by a doctor other than the one originally assigned... to know, before consenting to being used in an experiment, what risks are involved, possible side effects, whether the experiment has been done successfully before, whether it will benefit us personally or only medical science, what other options there are...and the right to refuse permission for any experiment or treatment.

V. PATIENTS, WORKERS, AND THE COMMUNITY MUST BE FREE TO ORGANIZE TO PROTECT THEIR INTERESTS...workers in particular must be guaranteed the right to unionize...to go on strike...to collective bargaining...to a decent wage, job security and respect...to compensation and/or retraining if disabled on the job...to free daycare facilities, health benefits, maternity/paternity leave, paid vacations and other fringe benefits available to many workers...to career advancement opportunities through on-and off-the-job training...the right to non-discriminatory treatment for Third

World people, women and older workers...to have job expectations set out clearly in a comprehensible language...the right to self-determination within the workplace and the union structure, including the right to meet, to have some control over working conditions, to advocate for patients without fear of reprisal, and to distribute information.

VI. HEALTH CONSUMERS, ORGANIZERS AND WORKERS MUST HAVE EFFECTIVE GRIEVANCE PROCEDURES...

including the right to easy access to an independent advocate not responsible to the hospital...the right to procedures through which an advocate can present our grievances to the people responsible and, if no action is taken, to a community board...most importantly, the right to form community boards, composed of workers and community people, democratically elected, and having significant power in the formulation of hospital policy — in hiring, firing, and fiscal decisions.

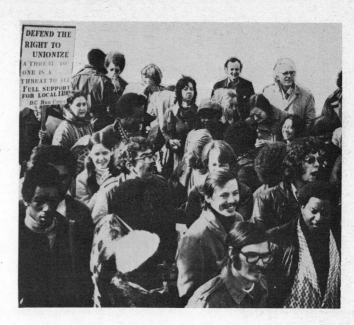

PROGRAM

RESEARCH YOUR COMMUNITY OR WORKPLACE THOROUGHLY

1. Know your rights. Learn which of those listed in the Platform have strong legal precedent in your state; however, lack of such precedent should not stop you from asserting rights that should be yours as patients and workers. If you are a patient, question everything that is done to you, and insist on clear, comprehensive answers.
2. Dig into the local, municipal, and state health power structures. Find out who's really in control, who caters to their interests, where the money comes from and where it goes. Explore the backgrounds, weak spots and conflicting interests of administrators, board members, city officials, etc. Familiarize yourself with conditions in the community and existing laws. Analyze what you've learned, try to figure out the trends, what the area administrators are planning and how to counteract them.
3. Hospital workers aren't covered by the National Labor Relations Board, meaning that their right to organize is not protected by federal law; only twelve states offer this protection. It is important to take this into account when planning tactics, since administrators won't hesitate to use the most drastic measures, including job termination, to halt organizing activities. Plans must be made accordingly, including perhaps feeling out other workers and the community for support and researching union possibilities.

ORGANIZE AS A STRONG VIABLE FORCE

1. To bring your community or workplace together, focus on the most widely felt and pressing problems. Formulate a basic set of demands and decide how you will present it to the administrators.
2. Develop communications with other community groups — recognize your common interests, trade information and tactics, form coalitions.
3. If possible, get out your own publication (ranging from a leaflet to a regular newspaper) to inform people and draw their support. Seek friendly publicity from local community or radical publications.
4. Community coalitions should actively support worker demands and struggles for organization as workers in turn should recognize the value in presenting a united front to the administration. Such coalitions can generate powerful energy for redirecting the priorities of the health system to benefit patients, community and workers.

EMPLOY MULTI-LEVEL PRESSURE TACTICS, choosing those that are appropriate to your community and your own group's level of strength.

1. Play on the hospital's fear of publicity by using the local media to expose violations of patients' and workers' rights and misuse of government funds or tax-exempt status. Draw on your research to expose conflicts of interest — those who influence health policy in their own behalf and against the community's interests.
2. Rally the community by spotlighting one particularly flagrant violation of a patient's rights, or the discriminatory firing of a worker, etc. Bring mass malpractice and class action suits against doctors and local medical societies. Picket the hospital (officials often find this very embarrassing), stage peaceful sit-ins.
3. Decide whether to challenge an institution's Joint Commission on the Accreditation of Hospitals accreditation by pointing out overcrowded conditions, etc. (the threat is that marginally operating hospitals may close rather than improving conditions). Call public assemblies, hold hearings, lobby before legislatures, attend hospital board meetings to bring issues before the community and the medical elite. Educate yourselves and the entire community about the health system as a whole.
4. Protest unnecessary construction of new hospitals by publicizing existing empty hospital beds. Form tenant unions to stop hospital expansion and subsequent dislocation of a community it doesn't serve.
5. Appeal to the hospital's often over-worked house staff (nurses, interns, doctors, etc.) for an active show of support. Sympathetic house staff have at times supplied community organizers with valuable information about the hospital's inner workings; they have assisted workers in "sickouts" (by signing medical excuses for mass absences from work) and "heal-ins" (admitting masses of people to the hospital to emphasize the inadequacy of staff, facilities, and efficiency). They have also occasionally participated in efforts to gain a greater say in policy for workers.
6. Strikes are often the most effective (if sometimes the most costly) tactics in the workers' struggle. Less drastic actions such as refusing to perform certain tasks or abide by certain regulations can also result in significant gains. New York workers, for example, staged a "billing action" — they withheld $750,000 worth of the patients' billing sheets which the city needs to redeem funds from the government.

DEVELOP EFFECTIVE GRIEVANCE PROCEDURES

1. Courts, though sometimes useful, are biased, costly, extremely time-consuming, and generally no place to be — which makes it essential to build strong non-judicial enforcement structures. Insist on an explicit code of patient's rights, made available to each patient upon admission. Demand a patient advocacy system within the hospital, responsible to the community, to represent patients and negotiate their problems with professionals and administrators.
2. Negotiate for community boards composed of community and worker representatives, to which the administration must answer. These boards should have a powerful voice in hiring, firing, fiscal decisions, and hospital policy. They should also handle any problems the advocates are unable to resolve, and carry on continuing education of the community and hospital personnel regarding patients' rights

and workers' rights.

3. Workers should have community support in fighting for their own strong grievance mechanisms when negotiating a union contract.

REMEMBER

Demystification is the key. Refuse to be intimidated by hospital jargon, dress and professionalism — doctors and administrators exist as technical consultants to serve you, not as gods to do with you what they will. The medical establishment will only be responsive to our needs when we force it to be. Know your rights and expect to fight for them.

Organize and negotiate creatively and resourcefully. Give up minor demands for major victories; be willing to pad your demands with a few you can afford to sacrifice. Keep a constant awareness of the totality of your struggle. Don't remain a crisis-oriented or single-issue organization. Continue to grow and keep the pressure coming — it takes years to effect significant change. Meanwhile the power structure will do all it can to divide us and turn us against ourselves — be on the lookout for co-opting tactics. Once the patients/workers/community realize the power they have collectively, the most important battle is won.

PATIENTS' RIGHTS

People's anger at the health care system, and determination to change it, are often sparked by experiences as a patient. Patients are frequently subjected to impersonal and inadequate care, indignity, and intimidation. They are showered with complex forms, x-rayed, photographed, and talked about (not to) in pretentious medi-code. In addition, test results are often significantly delayed and even incomplete. They are experimented on, operated on, and used as "teaching material" -- frequently without their informed and educated consent and almost always without full information in their own language about their condition, options, and possible side effects. The underlying assumption is clear: the patient is expected to surrender all control over her/his body to the professional, who, after all, has the resources and know-how to make an educated decision. This attitude is especially prevalent in the treatment of the most powerless -- the poor, Third World people, old people, and women. However, in a system dominated by research and profit, it is unsafe for anyone to passively accept the treatment offered them. The patient must take active responsibility for her/his own recovery.

Many health activists consider patient advocacy the first step in pushing health care institutions to be responsive to people's needs. In various ways, the following groups are working toward a strong patient representation system responsible to a community/worker-controlled hospital board. Some groups have instituted in-hospital patients' assistance programs; some run legal aid projects; and some have formed city-wide advocacy programs. But the problems are many. The legal rights of patients are largely undefined, untested, or non-existent. Getting out information about these rights is difficult and frustrating; hospitals often block even the most minimal educational projects such as waiting room "complaint tables", leaflet and handbook distribution, etc. When an advocate is able to enter a hospital, s/he often has little power to redress grievances. The same holds true for many community/worker boards at this time. Nevertheless, both are vital vehicles for consciousness-raising and together can form a foundation for effective community involvement. A vigorous patients' rights program can secure immediate benefits to individual patients; such benefits

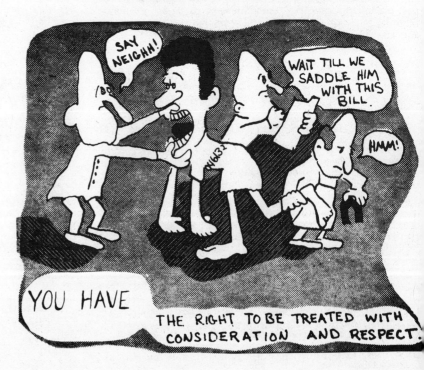

SAY NEIGHH!

WAIT TILL WE SADDLE HIM WITH THIS BILL.

HMM!

YOU HAVE THE RIGHT TO BE TREATED WITH CONSIDERATION AND RESPECT.

can generate the energy for the longer task of restructuring the health care system.

A strong patients' rights program must center around a patient advocate who is hired by a community group and is responsible to the entire community. Upon entering the institution, patients should receive material advising us of our rights; these rights should also be publicly posted throughout the hospital. In addition, it is essential that the advocate have a private office space and be easily accessible to all patients daily. Above all, any advocacy program must have the power behind it to effectively follow through on legitimate patient complaints.

(See sub-section on Research, in Health Personnel and Training.)

MEDICAL COMMITTEE FOR HUMAN RIGHTS PATIENTS RIGHTS CLEARING HOUSE. . .is being set up by the national office of MCHR to establish and spread communication in the area of patients rights. They plan to gather written material from people with patients rights organizing experience all over the country. They forsee a newsletter, speakers' bureau, and possible development of a patients advocacy training program. Conferences and workshops to educate community groups and workers about patients rights are another possibility. Contact MCHR, P.O. Box 7155, Pittsburgh, PA 15213, (412) 682-1200.

LUTHERAN HOSPITAL GRIENVANCE COMMITTEE. . . was founded in 1972 by organizers from the Cleveland Legal Aid Society and low-income families of the West Side. They surveyed 300 homes to define the needs of the community and researched the power structure of Lutheran Hospital. Lutheran had no pediatrician on call, though the hospital is situated across from a housing development; there were no translators, no follow-up in the emergency room, no transportation, no drug dispensary in the evenings, etc. The Committees first meetings explored abuses suffered by community people in the hospital and the commonality of the problems that Whites, Puerto Ricans and Blacks were having. A public meeting with the Chief Administrator and a few trustees, good publicity from the local newspaper and TV, and further pressure from the Committee brought concrete results: the hospital hired a pediatrician and set up a clinic in the housing project. The administration offered to make the Grievance Committee the official Hospital Community Advisory Board, but the people saw this as a token, co-opting ploy and refused. The committee feels its strength lies in its community origins and support. A VISTA slot has allowed a community woman to work fulltime on the project. Contact LUTHERAN HOSPITAL GRIEVANCE COMMITTEE, c/o Raheema Basherruddin, 2320 Bridge, No.186 and 187, Cleveland, OH, 44113, (216) 861-3399.

YALE-NEW HAVEN PATIENTS ADVOCACY PROGRAM
. . . grew out of a 1968 community survey examining patient treatment in the hospital, especially the emergency room and clinics. Stories of waiting in line for hours, and of patients (particularly the Spanish speaking) being ignored and rudely treated by the staff, led the community to decide that a patient advocate was needed. A central office was established in 1969 with an advocate to explain bills and terminology, to represent patients in the emergency room, in clinics and in disputes with attending doctors. Each patient admitted receives a bilingual patients' rights handbook and a flyer explaining how to contact the patients' assistant. The patient advocate is responsbile to an outside agency and not to the hospital itself. Most complaints are handled on a one-to-one basis with the offending professional or staff person. Few have been taken to higher-ups. The emphasis now is on bilingual services, explaining insurance, and billing. Contact: PATIENT ADVOCATE, Yale-New Haven Hospital, New Haven, CT (203) 436-8480.

PEOPLE'S LAW SCHOOL/BAY AREA MEDICAL COMMITTEE FOR HUMAN RIGHTS. . . are collaborating on a patients' rights manual. A class on patients' rights has been initiated at the People's Law School. Believing that teaching must provide specific tools and tactics for real change, the school is structured around students taking on research projects and pulling together actual cases. The health law field is still very undefined, and it's important that lawyers know how to test the laws in both traditional and creative ways. Besides specific ways to litigate for patients' rights, the course covers the rights of advocates and health workers who advise and care for patients. Students will be asked to contribute to the manual that is being prepared. Contact MCHR, P.O. Box 7677, San Francisco, CA 94119, (415) 842-5888.

MARTIN LUTHER KING HEALTH CENTER. . . was formed to provide comprehensive family medicine and support services such as training, employment, and advocacy to the Bronx. Their in-house patients advocacy program, one of the first in the country, began in 1970. After consulting with patients, community members and staff to learn what problems most concerned them, and possible solutions, a patients rights book was composed, an advocate assigned, and a grievance procedure instituted. The booklet, geared to the local community, was distributed to each employee of and family using the health center; distribution and discussion tables were set up in hospitals, community organizations, and housing projects (on rent day). An update of the manual is now in process. In addition to an in-house organizer, MLKHC does community advocacy around housing, welfare, and social services. Originally, advocacy was done by an independent department within MLKHC, but funding constraints have resulted in a switch to family health workers. As MLKHC is forced to change from OEO to HMO funding, financial and bureaucratic restrictions will result in a reduction of services. Contact MLKHC, 3674 3rd Avenue, Bronx, NY 10456, (212) 992-9100.

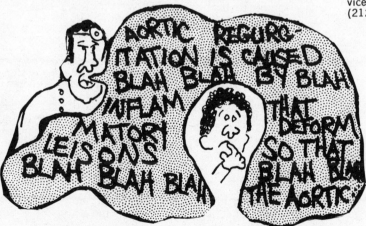

THE RIGHT TO BE TOLD WHAT'S WRONG WITH YOU IN LANGUAGE YOU CAN UNDERSTAND.

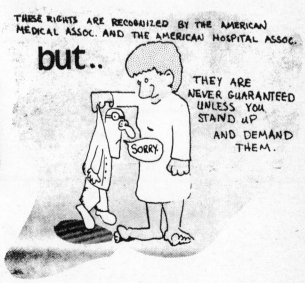

SOURCES OF PATIENTS' RIGHTS

1. United States Constitution

2. Federal laws and regulations (e.g., Medi-caid, Medicare)

3. State laws and regulations (e.g., the Public Health Law and State Hospital Code, the Ghetto Medicine Law, the Health and Hospitals Corporation Act)

4. Common Law

5. Professional ethics, including the Hippo-cratic Oath

6. Other promulgations of professional bodies (e.g., the American Hospital Association's Statement on a Patient's Bill of Rights, the Preamble to the Accreditation Standards for Hospitals of the Joint Commission on Accreditation of Hospitals)

7. Rules and regulations of individual hospi-tals and other health facilities

8. The moral sense of the community

(Health-PAC)

PITTSBURGH FREE CLINIC PATIENTS ADVOCACY PROGRAM . . . takes a city-wide rather than one-insti-tution approach to advocacy. The program grew out of the free clinics' observation that many of its patients need help in dealing with the hospital they are referred to. Three training sessions were set up to start the pro-gram. The first featured Health Law Project people dis-cussing legal rights of patients, how they differ from eth-ical rights, and the functions of various advocacy programs. The next sessions included administrators and workers talking about hospital procedures, the development of an advocate job description, review of referral information, and interviewing techniques. Advocates operate a desk at the free clinic for immediate problems and medical referral, collect and disseminate information about differ-ent facilities in the area, set up feedback systems to see if patients are satisfied with the clinic and with referrals, and accompany patients needing hospitalization or other care to the institution. Advocates will also speak to commu-nity groups, urging them to being their own advocacy program, and will share information to help such prog-rams get going. The clinic hopes to have enough resour-ces and strength to handle complaints from all over the city within six months. They plan to open a storefront office in the heart of the Pittsburgh Hospital empire area. Contact PFC, East End Christian Church, S. High-land and Alder, Pittsburgh, PA 15206, 412-661-5424.

NATIONAL HEALTH LAW PROGRAM . . . is an OEO-funded legal back-up service working on a comprehensive patients' rights manual. The book will focus on the specific legal rights -- as opposed to the human and moral rights —— of patients. It will outline what can be expected from health law and attempt to educate lawyers about the health care system; an appendix will cover specific precedent-setting cases. NHLP sees its work in patients' rights as a useful tool, not as an end in itself -- people must go on to organize around specific issues such as emergency care and outpatient services. Contact NATIONAL HEALTH LAW PROGRAM, 10995 Le Conte Ave., Rm. 640 Los Angeles, CA 90024, (213) 825-7601.

BRENTWOOD HOUSING PROJECT/CHILD-PARENT AD-VOCACY PROJECT . . .is producing a patients' rights hand-book with Jacksonville Legal Services. In an effort to in-volve community people in the book's preparation, outreach workers from the advocacy project provided transportation and day-care for people to come to community meetings and discuss their problems as health care consumers. The group hopes the book will be a catalyst for further organizing ef-forts. It deals with general patients' rights and the specifics of getting decent care in Jacksonville. It offers such practi-cal suggestions as how to make clinic appointments, what to bring to appointments, how to get transportation to medical facilities, what special services are available to the communi-ty, and what local free clinics offer. With the support of a University Hospital of Jacksonville pediatrition, the Brent-wood group is talking about instituting patient-staff commit-tees to deal with specific problems and pressuring the hospi-tal into using the booklet for an in-service training require-ment for hospital staff. Contact BRENTWOOD HOUSING PROJECT, CHILD ADVOCACY, Jacksonville, FL 33206 (904) 353-1933.

HEALTH LAW PROJECT . . . does research, teaching and advocacy around health law problems, encompassing such issues as accessibility, availability, accountability, quality of care, and the financing of institutions and care. Com-posed of lawyers, health workers, students, a community organizer and researcher, the group provides consumers with the information and technical resources to "develop their capacity to make health systems and institutions publicly accountable." HLP has used informed consumer pressure and litigation to force changes in and fully im-plement the medicaid children'sprogram. The project has supported community patients' rights committees and has done fine work with old people and prisons. Publications include information on national health in-surance, Blue Cross/Shield, medicare/aid, and prisons, guides for health consumers and workers, a patients' rights handbook and many more. Funded by OEO, HLP oper-ates under the auspices of the University of Pennsylvania Law School. Contact HEALTH LAW PROJECT, Univer-sity of Pennsylvania Law School, 133 S. 36 St., Phila-delphia, PA 19174 (215) 594-6951.

CITY-WIDE HEALTH COMMITTEE. . . is a coalition of neighborhood-based health groups and the local Medical Com-mittee for Human Rights working for comprehensive and re-sponsible care for the people (especially the poor) of New Or-leans. The group started by assessing "abuses of basic patients' rights" at Charity Hospital and exposing "just how unrepre-sentative. . . of the patient population" the hospital board is. With this information, the Committee (representing 10 low-income neighborhoods) negotiated its own appointment as the patient advisory committee to the Director of the hospi-tal, with a patient advocate selected by and responsible to the Committee. The group has since written a brief, excellent analysis of the program; its strengths, weaknesses, and impli-cations for the future of the patients' rights movement. The basic lesson is that, if a patients' rights organization is to be an effective force in changing hospital policy and ocrrecting underlying problems, it must become a "viable community-worker controlled institution with an integrated system of in-take, counselling, referral and follow-up, and an adequate staff to carry out its demanding functions. . . Otherwise, it is no more than a complaint department of sorts, and most like-ly serving the hospital more favorably as a PR gimmick than it does the patients' needs." The Committee feels that it had laid the basis for such a strong organization by winning input into hospital policy. Yet, because they lacked adequate staff to work as patient advocates and also research needed institutional changes, little further progress has been made. City-Wide representatives also sit on an all-consumer board for three Model Cities out-patient clinics—comprehensive clinics with scaled prices, receiving back-up services from area hospitals. Contact MCHR, P.O. Box 30362, New Orleans, LA 70130, (504) 861-7926.

RESOURCES

"PATIENTS RIGHTS AND ADVOCACY," Medical Committee for Human Rights, P.O. Box 7155, Pittsburgh, PA 15213. 15pp. Free
. . . a collection of model manuals on patients' rights used by such groups as the National Health and Environmental New Haven Hospital in Connecticut. Some materials are both in Spanish and English. Each manual includes clear explanations of patients' rights, how to obtain them, how to express dissatisfaction (frequently and forcibly) and descriptions of standard hospital practices. Prototype guides for groups organizing around patients' rights.

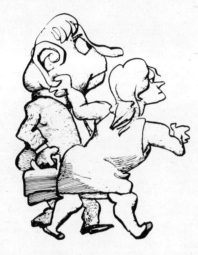

"BOSTON MCHR PATIENTS RIGHTS HANDBOOK," P.O. Box 382, Prudential Station, Boston, MA 02199. In production as we go to press, price undecided.
. . .excellent, comprehensive and sensitive resource on the needs and rights of patients from the time they enter the hospital until they leave. Specific sections deal with the emergency room, admissions, and the going home process, besides the usual listing of in-hospital rights. Criteria for effective patient advocacy are included, as well as a more complete discussion of the politics of patients' rights than is normally found in such handbooks.

"Patients Rights Book", New York City Patients Rights Group, c/o Harf, 256 City Island Ave., Bronx, NY 10464, 1974. 25 pp. Free
. . . another good model patients rights manual. The book is especially good in that it ties in the commonality of patients and workers in fighting for better health care. Tells what both can do to improve care and how they can help each other in their respective struggles. The book ends with a concise, easy-to-understand statement of the politics of the health industry.

"YOUR RIGHTS AS A PATIENT," St. Louis Chapter of Medical Committee for Human Rights, 6010 Kingsbury, St. Louis, MO 63112. 31pp. Free
. . . discusses patients' rights in public or private general hospitals as provided for in the Preamble to Hospital Accreditation Standards and in a Statement of the American Hospital Association. Comprehensive, written in a straightforward, concise style, the pamphlet presents a brief analysis of why the health care system is inadequate and what workers and patients can do about it.

"Your Rights as a Patient," Health Law Project, 133 S. 36th St., Philadelphia, PA 19104, Free
. . .presents the rights of patients and their legal and administrative sources. These include lawsuit decisions, statutes, medical or hospital ethics, federal medicaid/medicare requirements, and JCAH standards. Good resource for lawyers and patients, though it may be a bit dated.

"PEOPLE'S GUIDE TO HEALTH CARE: HOW TO ORGANIZE A HOSPITAL GRIEVANCE COMMITTEE," Alice Schottenstein, Legal Aid Society, 2108 Payne Ave., Rm. 707, Cleveland, OH 44114. 10 pp. Free
. . . the story of the Lutheran Hospital Grievance Committee on Cleveland's West Side. It provides an excellent model for groups challenging the power structure of medical institutions such as hospitals, beginning with the initial community survey to collect specific grievances and leading up to the group's first confrontations with the chief administrator. One important omission: the pamphlet makes no mention of any attempts to establish communications with workers at the institutions involved.

FILMS AND TAPES

AFL/CIO, 815 Sixteenth St., NW, Washington, D.C. 20006

"Where It Hurts," 28 min. cl. 1971 $3.00
Produced by HEW, this film depicts the helplessness of the patient when s/he becomes ill and has to find a way through the complex maze of medical specialities, hospitals, and other health institutions.

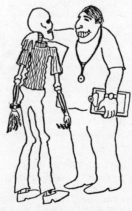

"THERE, THERE YOU DIDN'T HAVE TO WAIT THAT LONG"

COMMUNITY COALITIONS

Community coalitions are one of the most effective ways to build support for the re-direction of one hospital's priorities or of a community's health care delivery system as a whole. Issues that coalitions form around include hospital expansion, monopoly control of health services, the absence of clinics or emergency services, transportation, mal-practice, hospital closure, and lack of community control. Approaches vary from holding public meetings to operating speakers' bureaus or testifying in city councils. Researching the financial and official power structure of a community and defining its needs are necessarily first steps for many groups. With well-documented information and a basic analysis of the problems, a coalition can expect to attract good people and work up considerable clout in effecting change. Carefully planned and creative legal approaches are an important tool at this time. Demanding public representation on boards and challenging tax-exemptions, federal funding, and city supervisory agencies can open up whole vistas of control. The following groups present an exciting variety of approaches in organizing to change the medical priorities of whole cities.

SEATTLE PUBLIC HEALTH CARE COALITION. . .formed almost three years ago to fight the Nixon administration's proposed closure of the Public Health Service hospital in Seattle, the main public hospital in the area. The group is exceptionally broad-based and effective, encompassing all those who stand to lose by the closing: Native Americans, merchant sailors, military retirees, hospital workers, free clinic people for whom the hospital provided back-up services. The well-organized and informed group has embarked on a five-point program: 1. keep the hospital open under federal funds; 2. expand and modernize the hospital (coalition architects worked out plans); 3. expand services to include extended care facilities, drug rehabilitation, and day care for patients and workers; 4. study the health care needs for the region; 5. work for eventual community/worker control. Organizing tactics included a petition drive to familiarize the people with the issues (they netted 50,000 signatures in support of the hospital); demonstrations; and testimony in Congressional hearings. The group received good publicity from local TV stations, due at least in part to its unusual composition. Their first success was obtaining an injunction against closure. Their demonstrations and lobbying efforts helped push through a federal law setting up conditions HEW had to meet before it could close Public Health Service hospitals. By Feb. 1973, the HEW plan failed to meet the specifications; for example, all people served by the hospital were not covered by the new plans. Only one-third were partially covered; Native American health service alone would have suffered a 50% decrease. The coverage that was planned entailed channelling HEW funds into contracts with private providers, thus ensuring that some one would get another slice of profit from money allocated to health care for the poor. In spite of Nixon's displeasure, Congress has finally passed an amendment stating that none of the remaining eight Public Health Service hospitals can be shut down without specific Congressional approval. With this in itspocket, the SPHC Coalition is now able to take on the task of rehabilitating the hospital to its status as of 1970 before funds started gradually decreasing. It is sending out questionnaires to relevant people, pressuring for a consumer board, and trying to obtain the cut-off back-up services for area free clinics. The strength of this amazing group lies in its sensitivity to the community, its ability to bring together such diverse elements in a common fight. Contact SPHCC, 402 15th Ave., East, Seattle, Washington 98112, (206) EA 2-6698

PEOPLE'S HEALTH MOVEMENT. . . is a three-year mass organization of workers in health and industry, community members, and students in health and sciences. Their main principles are that "decent health care is the right of all people regardless of class or social status" and that "good health care is not possible because there are huge profits to be made from selling health care." PHM's original eight demands, submitted to the City Council and the Board of Health in 1971, included eight comprehensive health centers with satellite services, a working relationship between the Cincinnati College of Medicine and neighborhood clinics, a network of regular and emergency transportation for patients, much stronger environmental programs, and inspection of stores and factories for health and safety hazards. Supporting community efforts to get local health centers, and helping to develop a lead poisoning detection program were among the group's first focuses. PHM also proposed and won a charter amendment expanding the Board of Health and shortening terms from ten years to three; a PHM caucus now sits on the Board. Through them, PHM's major demand for community controlled health centers has been realized: "Communities can now contract with the city to run their own health services, and we are now preparing community health committees to assume control of their clinics." In January, 1972, PHM decided to take on Cincinnati General Hospital. Demands for immediate changes in the emergency room were ignored, but after considerable struggle, the City Council agreed to hold hearing. Testimony from hundreds of individuals and groups brought drastic conditions into the open, but again nothing happened. PHM concluded that the city and university had no intention of changing things because the Medical School ran General for its benefit—to teach, to do research, and to make money. PHM proposed taking General from the university and putting it under a new, independent board, responsible to patients and workers at General, with the majority of members elected by the people. To get the proposal onto the ballot, about 12,000 signatures were needed; PHM collected nearly 23,000 in 14 months, speaking to hundreds of groups in the process. The city fought dirty and long, finally going to court to keep the issue off the ballot. The city lost once, and appealed to a higher court. As things stand now, the appeals court has ruled against PHM and the community. But the fight for better health care goes on. Contact PHM, P.O. Box 19284, Cincinnati, OH 45219.

NEW YORK COALITION FOR COMMUNITY HEALTH. . . exists as a resource group for community advisory boards and others who usually have little power and must rely on community pressure to back up their proposals. The Coalition includes people from planning agencies, neighborhood health councils, and hospital community boards. Committees are studying such areas as hospitals, legislations, the Comprehensive Health Planning Board, and mental health programs. Coalition members are available to speak at workshops and groups. The organization's main concern now is the control of area health resources by CHPB and the Health and Hospitals Corporation. So far the CHPB has devised elaborate work programs for setting up community boards, but not acted on them. The Coalition is questioning the way CHPB wants to set up the boards, the fact that they have made up their own guidelines and violated them, and their nearly total lack of community input. A suit has been brought challenging the fact that the same person heads both CHPB and HHC. Added to their interlocking directorates, this situation means that the same complex of powerful people make health plans, reviews those plans, distributes funds, etc. The Coalition is searching for a community member to be the new president of the HHC. Contact NYCCCH, c/o Wessler, 214 E. 2nd St., 4th Fl., New York, N.Y. 10009.

CITY-WIDE HEALTH CONSUMERS COALITION. . . organized to obtain free, comprehensive, and preventive medical care for the people of Milwaukee. Traditionally there has been little, if any, work done to prevent diseases in the poor communities, and emergency care has been costly and inaccessible. The major medical facility in Milwaukee, Downtown Medical Services, was closed three years ago, but re-opened after lobbying by the 27th Street People's Free Health Clinic. After this victory, the 27th St. Clinic and the People's Committee for Survival organized the city-wide coalition to demand more responsive care from DMS. The coalition now draws the support of many community groups, including Eastside Community Organization, Indian Consumers Coalition, and Welfare Rights Organization. The present county board which controls DMS is not representative of, nor responsive to, the downtown community. A community board, which will include workers from DMS, is the first goal of the coalition. Then the following programs are sought: free screening and education for sickel cell, TB, lead poisoning, and high blood pressure; an outreach program employing community residents; hiring of more Third World staff to reflect the make-up of the community; and a citizen-controlled grievance procedure.

As the coalition wins community control at DMS, it would like to see similar struggles waged around other health facilities in Milwaukee. Contact PEOPLE'S COMMITTEE FOR SURVIVAL, 2456 North 3rd Street, Milwaukee, WI 53212, (414) 263-5251.

HEALTH TASK FORCE/OKLAHOMA CONSUMER PROTECTION AGENCY...

in connection with the Medical Committee for Human Rights has intensively researched the Oklahoma City hospital and economic power structure. Studies show that the health care system is in the hands of a few leading businesspeople who use their position to benefit themselves and selected colleagues. The task force educates the public about health issues and uses the law creatively to make hospitals responsive to patients, rather than profits. Suits are being brought against one hospital's plans to use $3,000,000 in federal Hill-Burton money for a maximum security parking facility; at issue is the violation of public trust by a supposedly public body. Other suits have been brought against hospitals for charging as much as $325 in pre-admission fees. One of the task force's most striking findings is that Oklahoma City has 1200 excess hospital beds. The building and maintenance of these beds (based on fantasy "boom" projections of area businesspeople), and the hospitals' stockpiles of

self-perpetuating hospital board. Yet they made little headway and were constantly thwarted by the businesspeople who controlled the board. Although the citizen's group effectively used the county hospital to educate people about health resources in Durham, who controls them and who should, they failed to win community representation on the board. Demoralized and losing members, Citizens Concerned went through a self-evaluation in the summer of 1973, and analyzed what they had done wrong (focusing too much on a single issue, failed to develop a long-term strategy). In the fall the group re-emerged better organized and more ready to take on the Durham medical and business establishment. Four ommittees concentrate on organizing petitions, working with the media, sending out speakers, and fund-raising—and one of the group was finally nominated to the hospital board. Members of Citizens Concerned were instrumental in preparing a report by the Health Planning Council of North Carolina defining the needs of that region, and have incorporated many of its suggestions into their over-all strategy. The group also puts out a newsletter and good, locally-oriented pamphlets dealing with community control of hospitals and health care in general. Contact CITIZENS CONCERNED ABOUT DURHAM HEALTH CARE, P.O. Box 1225, Durham, NC 27702, (919) 286-3512.

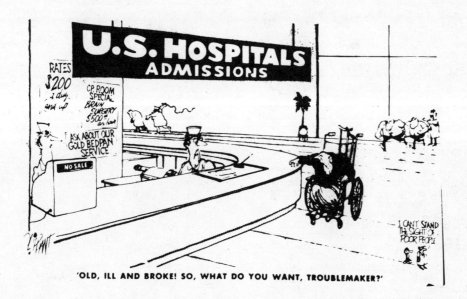

'OLD, ILL AND BROKE! SO, WHAT DO YOU WANT, TROUBLEMAKER?'

exotic equipment, have diverted money from needed outpatient clinics and emergency services and into the hands of contractors, supply companies, and banks. The Task Force has brought suit to force the hospitals to close these beds and quit shifting their excess maintenance costs to patients (third party insurance cannot, because of the price control laws, raise their payments to absorb the extra consumer burden). Action is also being taken to revoke local hospitals' tax-exempt status or force them to use their estimated $22.5 million in tax-exempt money for community services. In the past two years, Task Force members have noticed a definite, if subtle, change of attitude in this conservative city. People are less likely to argue that "we need all the hospitals we can get;" they have begun to ask how much the hospitals cost, and who benefits. Contact: OKLAHOMA CITY CONSUMER PROTECTION AGENCY, P.O. Box 60060, Oklahoma City, OK 73106, (405) 521-0245

CITIZENS CONCERNED ABOUT DURHAM HEALTH CARE...

organized in 1971 around the issue of a $20 million hospital being planned and built with community property taxes but with virtually no poor or working class input into its construction and services. Concern centered around location and transportation problems, lack of adequate clinic and emergency room space, the fact that the hospital board represented only the upper class of Durham, and the fact that there was no coherent planning for the overall health needs of the people of Durham. For over a year, the group's main goal was getting community representation on the

VIETNAM VETERANS AGAINST THE WAR...

has locally and nationally opposed the conditions and policies of Veterans Administration Hospitals. VVAW issues include the fact that many Vietnam vets are discriminated against in treatment and benefits, that Post-Vietnam Syndrome (a psychological reaction to the horrors of the war) is not recognized as a war-related tragedy by the VA, and that most VA hospitals have inadequate drug units—a major problem as many Vietnam vets come back addicted to the heroin so prevalent in SE Asia. Because less-than-honorable discharges (often given because the soldier became an addict while in the service) are discriminated against, VVAW calls for a universal discharge. VVAW is is doing agitational—as opposed to alternative-building—work since they feel the VA has a responsibility to deal with whatever happens to people in the military. Political action (including demonstrations at VA hospitals) and community education are prime focuses. Reports on VA hospitals are published in VVAW's affiliate newspaper, WINTER SOLDIER. The conditions of the hospitals ranges from fair to intolerable (rats roaming the floor and patients shooting heroin in the elevators). VVAW has publicized the fact that the VA's doctor-patient ratio is lower than in regular hospitals, and that, although claiming to have no money to improve services to vets, the head of the VA wants to cut back on appropriations. Contact VVAW National Office, 827 W. Newport, Chicago, IL 60657, (312) 935-2129.

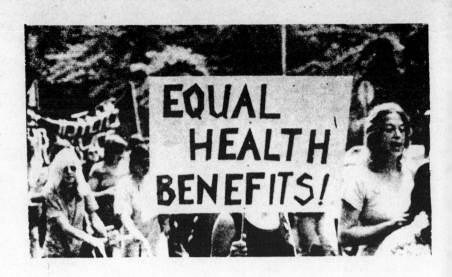

NEIGHBORHOOD SAVE OUR HOMES COMMITTEE...
is an excellently organized tenants' group that has been fighting hospital expansion for years. Columbus hospital (a voluntary, yet publicly subsidized institution) decided to tear down two tenements in order to build a parking area and luxury apartment building. After buying the tenements in 1969, Columbus induced over half the tenants to move by allowing the buildings to physically deteriorate—a classic landlord tactic. But the tenants organized, forcing the hospital to answer 23 housing code violations in criminal court. The tenants also filed a suit blocking a $39 million state mortgage for the hospital expansion. A compromise was worked out: the hospital got its mortgage money in return for a contract guaranteeing that the tenements would not be demolished, that the tenants could stay, that repairs would be made and that the tenants would not be bribed to move by relocation fees. But as the hospital reneged on its agreement and allowed deterioration to continue, community pressure built up again. In November, 1972, more than two hundred local residents marched on the hospital, charging it with "medical imperialism. . .victimizing the poor, rather than serving them." The tenants' committee obtained a restraining order on the hospital and filed a half-million dollar damage suit alleging breach of contract. The hospital counter-filed, claiming interference with hospital management. . .and the fight is still going on. The Save Our Homes Committee hopes to force the hospital to sign a permanent ban against eviction. This group is a model of strong community organizing around specific issues. It has used publicity effectively, obtaining good press coverage in community and city papers, and gaining the support of progressive city council people, mayoralty candidates and state assembly people. The Neighborhood Save Our Homes Committee is affiliated with other tenants' groups fighting institutional expansion under the name City-Wide Save Our Homes Committee. Contact **CITY-WIDE SAVE OUR HOMES COMMITTEE**, P.O. Box 651, Madison Square Station, New York, NY 10010, (212) 777-6346.

When striking Lincoln hospital workers were threatened with dispersal by the police in the spring of 1969, one worker commented wryly, 'They (the administration) don't know their own power— they just have to threaten us with violence. If we thought we were going to be injured this close to Lincoln, and be taken there, we'd all throw up our hands.'

—The American Health Empire

409 HOUSE. . .has been organizing against hospital expansion in the Haight-Ashbury district of San Francisco for four years. One effort centered around the U. of California's plan to build a 14 story dental building. After acquiring much property by direct purchase and gaining equal "right of eminent domain" status with the state to buy the rest, the university publicly announced plans to tear down the monstrous building and eat up another block of housing. 409, with other community people, challenged the plans as being overly destructive of the neighborhood. They called, instead, for satellite clinics to train and give service to community people. The fight ended in compromise, with the state legislature appropriating funds for a structure half the original size and the university building two 40-chair satellite clinics. A current struggle centers around a Catholic voluntary hospital's plans to tear down 48 housing units and displace 150 people in order to build a plush new doctors' office building. Again, the hospital was granted the right to eminent domain and issued a "conditional use" zoning permit allowing them to violate the zoning standards for the area. The tenants plan to file a suit claiming that granting "eminent domain" is unconstitutional and that the housing code states that only property owners can obtain conditional use permits. Feeling the group has been too defensively oriented, 409, in conjunction with the health committee of a local Community Development group, also plans to set up a People's Health Resource and Advocacy center. Over the past few years, this tenants group has established good relationships with hospital workers and medical students at the U. of California hospital; they have supported each other's work against expansion, and for day-care, better working conditions, and better care in the hospital. Contact 409 HOUSE, 409 Clayton, San Francisco, CA 94117, (415) 863-5498.

EAST HARLEM HEALTH COUNCIL. . .started in 1968 and lists as members both health providers and consumers, representing the area's Puerto Rican, Black and White population; the by-laws guarantee a consumer majority on the Board of Directors and a consumer chairperson. The Council maintains an overview of all health related activity in East Harlem including community health fairs, cancer, TB and hypertension screening, hospital policy and expansion. Particular attention is paid to the quality of ambulatory care, enactment of medicaid and Social Security programs, and the elderly. The Council works to increase the availability of care, decrease impersonalization of services, and get more bilinguals working in local facilities. Although the effectiveness of the Council varies with the composition and enthusiasm of the Board of Directors, it is a definite force in East Harlem health politics and can effectively cut through hospital red-tape in obtaining services for its constituency. Rapport with area hospitals has improved, although relations with the city government continue to present problems. In addition to its advocacy role the Council, with city funding, conducts a walk-in drug program. The 80 participants participate in a de-toxification program before entering; the main thrust is on education and vocational training. Contact EAST HARLEM HEALTH COUNCIL, 217 E. 106 St., New York, NY 10029, (212) 831-2800.

PUERTO RICAN ASSOCIATION FOR HEALTH AFFAIRS
. . . has two chapters serving as watchdogs for the Puerto Rican community. They define the major health related problems of Puerto Ricans as lack of bilingual services, poor diet, lack of health facilities for low-income neighborhoods, and inadequate follow-through for care. The city-wide chapter, primarily composed of health professionals, keeps abreast of developments in city health policy and lobbies for the Spanish speaking community. The second chapter, El Barrio Chapter, is located in East Harlem and pressures local hospitals to provide better services. They call for a restructuring of priorities, and bilingual, bi-cultural personnel on all levels. Tactics involve meeting with leaders of the health institution, infiltration into positions of power and possible use of class action suits. Most of their dealings have been with New York Medical Center and Mt. Sinai Hospital. Both chapters are staffed by volunteers with no substantial funding. Contact PUERTO RICAN ASSOCIATION FOR HEALTH AFFAIRS, City-wide chapter, 197 Haver Meyer St., Brooklyn, NY 11211, (212) 384-1507; or El Barrio Chapter, c/o Improved Services to Puerto Ricans, 80 5th Ave., Rm. 1204, New York, NY (212) 924-4845.

EAST HARLEM TENANTS COUNCIL. . .serves as a health advocate for the local community. They have surveyed the general and emergency care services of Mt. Sinai, Metropolitan, and New York Medical Hospital, meeting with hospital administrators in an effort to obtain implementation of their suggestions: increased bilingual services and community people on hospital boards. Tactics are non-confrontational, generally involving meetings and negotiations. In addition, the EHTC sponsors a project to educate the parents of mentally retarded children on the special needs of the retarded. Contact EAST HARLEM TENANTS COUNCIL, 2193 3rd Ave., New York, NY 10035, (212) 427-7100.

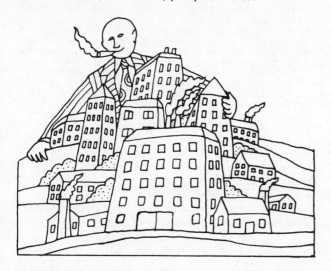

CONSUMER COMMISSION ON THE ACCREDITATION OF HEALTH SERVICES, INC.. . . .is trying to close the information gap about health care services by providing consumers with "heretofore buried, unpublicized" facts on the quality and high costs of health services. Besides publishing a wealth of investigative materials on New York City area hospitals, they have been helping community groups get involved in hospital accreditation procedures. Helped along by extensive New York Times coverage, this has so far resulted in consumers winning the right to accompany the Joint Commission on Accreditation on its rounds, to have their complaints against the hospital heard by the Joint Commission, and to have the findings of the Joint Commission made public. A group in Nassau County not only succeeded in getting more women and Blacks on the hospital board, but brought enough publicity and pressure to bear to force the administrator to resign. CCAHS itself is run by a board of 2/3 consumers and 1/3 providers. Only

a year and a half old, it eventually hopes to rate area hospital services and to identify the deficiencies and superiorities of each institution. Overall, the commission is a good model for beginning to make institutions accountable. Contact CONSUMER COMMISSION ON THE ACCREDITATION OF HEALTH SERVICES, INC., 4 West 58th St., New York, NY 10019 (212) 752-0888.

WEST SIDE CITIZENS FOR BETTER HEALTH SERVICES, INC. . . . grew out of a confrontation between a local hospital and the low-income White/Latino/Appalachian community of Cleveland's west side. As a result of that struggle, the city of Cleveland began building a health center for the West Side, but with no plans for a board representing the community. Community people involved in the original confrontation banded together to fight for community control of the health center; within a few months they became incorporated as the West Side Citizens for Better Health Services and elected their first community board of directors. With funds from a local foundation and help from medical students in the Student Health Organization, WSCBHS created a $7 million proposal for a comprehensive community controlled health care system for Cleveland. The plan was turned down by the city because they lacked money; and also, the citizens' group felt, because the city was not interested in finding the funds for a plan involving worker/community control. As an alternative to the planned city health center, WSCBHS set up the Near West Side People's Free Clinic with a grant from the Metropolitan Health Planning Corp. WSCBHS still hoped to install their clinic in the yet unopened city health facility. This didn't come through, but when the city facility opened in 1972 WSCBHS began working to make the administration of the center responsive to the community. Today, although the city health center still has no community board, a community/staff committee has been formed as a result of meetings between WSCBHS and the city health administration. WSCBHS is now the political arm of three free clinics: NWSPFC, the Tremont Free Clinic, and the newly opened Riverside Free Clinic. They are also working on a program called "New Concepts in Nursing" which is trying to install nurse practitioner training local nursing schools, establishing a system of pocket medical cards (carrying information on allergies, medication being taken, chronic conditions such as heart trouble, etc), and studying the air pollution from local steel mills. They are building ties with workers in the city's West Side health center in hopes that with the community and workers pushing together, they will be able to achieve community/worker control. Contact WSCBHS, Inc., 1965 West 44th St., Cleveland, OH 44113, (216) 281-4242.

RESOURCES
PAMPHLETS AND ARTICLES

"PEOPLE'S GUIDE TO HEALTH CARE—THE POLITICS OF HEALTH CARE," Terry Demchak, Barbara Ehrenreich and Cleveland Women's Liberation, Health Task Force, Legal Aid Society, 2108 Payne Ave., Cleveland, OH 44114, 1972. 15 pp.
. . . a succinct political analysis of Cleveland hospitals in their non-medical roles: "as employers of thousands of people, as repositories for large amounts of investment capital, and as centers of real estate empires." The pamphlet identifies the health power structure in Cleveland (Money Oligarchy, Old Aristocracy, Front Men and Professional Promoters), then demonstrates who profits and who suffers from institutional expansion.

The issue is not the old and almost comfortable issue of archaic plant or antiquated apparatus. The issue is Black people. The issue is white medicine. The issue is colonial health care in its most blatant and most devastating form, the issue is two-class medicine in a racist and divided social order. Yet these are the words nobody wants to use.
—Jonathan Kozol, Ramparts

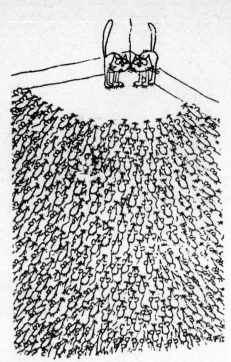

"Well, don't just stand there—negotiate!"

"Hospitals for Sale (and Other Ways to Kill a Public Health System)," Elinor Blake and Tom Bodenheimer, RAMPARTS, 2054 University Ave., Berkeley, CA 94704, Feb., 1974. pp. 27-33
. . .the story of the impending collapse of public health care. County hospitals are closing down or going private, leaving 20 million Americans who are ineligible for Medicaid or unable to buy health insurance with no place to go. "As long as a small underfinanced public system coexists with a large wealthy private one, there will be competition for paying patients, doctors, money and power. And the private system will win." This is a factual, well-documented report of a grim development in the US health delivery fiasco.

HEALTH/PAC BULLETIN, 17 Murray St., New York, NY 10007, Oct., 1973, pp. 1-24 $.60
. . .in an editorial entitled "Public Hospitals: Going, Going, Private," and in two articles about Bellevue and Boston City Hospital, this issue documents control of private institutions (i.e., medical centers) over public hospitals because of their dependence on the medical centers for medical resources. The public system has become "an adjunct of the private system, partly performing functions the private sector prefers not to perform in its own facilities, partly providing a setting in which the private sector may carry out its own pet projects at public expense.

"OKLAHOMA CRUDE: EVERYTHING'S COMING UP HOSPITALS", Health/Pac Bulletin, No. 157, 17 Murray St., New York, NY 10007, April 1974, pp. 1-9
. . .an excellent indicative summary of the waste and profiteering resulting from the manipulation of the hospital industry by leading financiers in Oklahoma City. This report by the Oklahoma Consumer Protection Agency documents how purchase and maintenance of excess beds means higher prices and less service for consumers and greater profits for the hospital and construction industry, corporate lawyers, architects, surveyors, appraisers, management consultants, and money lenders. While expensive beds are lying idle, the 17 voluntary hospitals and one public-supported hospital are cutting down on indigent care (violating tax-exemption policy) and charging pre-admission rates.

"THE ACCREDITATION OF HOSPITALS: A GUIDE FOR HEALTH CONSUMERS AND WORKERS," Health Law Project, Univ. of Pennsylvania School of Law, 133 South 36th St., Philadelphia, PA 19104, 1971. 29 pp. Free
. . . an excellent how-to article for groups challenging Join Commission on Accreditation of Hospitals (JCAH) approval of a hospital. Without accreditation by JCAH hospitals cannot receive Medicare funds or have interns and residents; JCAH approval is based on the hospital's answers to a questionnaire and an inspection. JCAH works hand-in-hand with the hospitals. The once-yearly inspection is announced in advance, so the hospital can be at its best; and there is often no chance for citizens to express their dissatisfactions. After explaining how JCAH functions, the article outlines a strategy for challenging accreditation, and explains the risks involved (the hospital may choose to close rather than improve standards). Appendices cover JCAH standards and the Association's basic position on hospital responsibility (a vague statement in favor of patients' rights). A clear, practical guide for local organizers.

"The Hospital Business," Ronald Kessler, THE WASHINGTON POST, available from Health-PAC, 17 Murray St., New York, N.Y., October-November, 1972, 11 pp.
. . .an impressive expose of conflicts of interest and other financial abuses in such area hospitals as the Washington Hospital Center. Kessler offers an astounding array of facts in this series of six articles, revealing the lack of public accountability of hospitals that has been a major factor in increasing costs. Hospital costs rose 110% between 1965 and 1972, accompanied by a mere 27% increase in services. Kessler found hospitals taking a great deal of government money, yet operating as private institutions "run by trustees who generally elect themselves." At Washington Hospital Center, "10 of the 38 trustees of the hospital, and four former trustees, have been involved in conflicts of interest when they or their companies did business with the hospital. . ." The importance of this investigation in demonstrating the decadence of hospital administrations cannot be overestimated.

HEALTH/PAC BULLETIN, 17 Murray St., New York, NY 10007, May, 1972, pp. 1-14 $.60
. . .the first article in this issue, "How to Build a Hospital," tells how Blue Cross, Medicare, and Medicaid have provided hospitals with a steady, guaranteed income and construction allowances totally at the hospitals' disposal, resulting in great cost to the public as patients and as taxpayers. "Save Our Homes" discusses a coalition of New York tenant groups fighting hospital expansion. "Off With Their Beds" reveals NY City's Health Service Administration's efforts to turn over to private institutions the public responsibility for providing health services in municipal hospitals.

"THE CLOSING OF ST. FRANCIS HOSPITAL: A CASE STUDY OF THE POLITICS OF HEALTH PLANNING," Peter Rothstein, prepared for Health/PAC, available from Medical Committee for Human Rights, available from Louise Rice, 65 Chestnut St., Cambridge, MA 02139, 1967. 28 pp. $1.15
. . . offers a detailed report on the decision-making involved in closing St. Francis, a voluntary hospital in South Bronx, New York. South Bronx is characterized by great poverty, poor housing, high unemployment, and inadequate emergency and in-patient facilities. By tracing the decision to close St. Francis, the author shows the Archdiocese of New York's lack of regard for community needs (residents and hospital workers continuously protested the decision). Although somewhat ponderous and technical in style, this article issues a powerful call for "1. basic revision. . .of public policy-making procedures for all hospitals and health services in New York City; 2. A public body with the power to carry out total health planning for all people and areas of the city; and 3. all deliberations, meetings, reports and decisions must be open to all citizens. This agency must be accountable to all people of the city."

"ON THE MATTER OF COMMUNITY RELATIONS: THE CONSUMER MOVEMENT IN HEALTH CARE AND THE ALBERT EINSTEIN MEDICAL CENTER," Edward V. Sparer, available from Health Law Project, University of Pennsylvania School of Law, 1335 S. 30th St., Philadelphia, PA 19104, 1971. 49 pp. Free
...a good overview of the health movement, covering community voice in hospital decisions, patients' rights and professional accountability. Sparer ends his paper with suggestions on how Albert Einstein Medical Center should incorporate greater consumer rights, health practices, and policies, and creation of a structure to allow for "consumer scrutiny and criticism of those practices and policies."

PERIODICALS

PEOPLE'S HEALTH, P.O. Box 12577, Seattle, WA 98111
...is truly "A Voice of Seattle's Health Movement," jampacked with all the happenings in Seattle and major health movement events nationwide. Hospital worker coverage is emphasized—the need to unionize, the limitations of the union, the rank-and-file's role in organizing and fighting for union democracy, the need to work with the community to improve care, etc. It also deals with Nixon's health cuts and their political significance ("...social welfare programs were never designed to attack the root causes of poverty: the fact that our society's economy is operated for corporate profits, not to satisfy human needs.") Though not connected with The People's Health Care Coalition, the paper gives ample coverage and support to its work. Articles on general news events (Wounded Knee, Vietnam) and features on other health care systems (like Cuba) supplement regular features like a special women's page, book reviews, and Indian health news.

NEW YORK COALITION FOR COMMUNITY HEALTH NEWSLETTER, c/o Wessler, 214 E. 2nd St., 4th Floor, New York, NY 10009. Free
... supplies solid, up-to-date information on health happenings in New York City. Detailed information on federal, state, and local agencies and programs is presented, including step-by-step information on how to deal with governmental red-tape in moving toward consumer control over delivery and financing.

HEALTH PERSPECTIVES, Consumer Commission on the Accreditation of Health Services, Inc., 101 W. 31st St., New York, NY 10001, $25/year
... a valuable periodical on hospital accreditation, with information on the make-up of hospital boards of trustees, whose interests they serve, the role of the consumer in hospital accreditation, and hospital reimbursement rates from Blue Cross, Medicaid, and Workpeople's compensation. HEALTH PERSPECTIVES advocates greater hospital accountability to consumers; the information it provides will help people move towards this end.

HOSPITAL WORKERS

If patients suffer periodically from the health care system, hospital workers are abused daily by the institutional inhumanity of the hospitals. Yet too often workers' fights are slighted or even ignored by other health and community activists. Workers' welfare and livelihood is integrally related to the hospitals and other health institutions that activists are trying to change. Such struggles can be very threatening for aides, technicians, food service and maintenance people who sometimes barely manage to eek out a living from their hospital workplace. Community people may take out their frustrations with the hospital on the workers; the hospital, after all, is only one of many alienating institutions community members encounter every day. But if the radical re-direction of the health care system is to be fully realized, workers must be insured their rightful place in the restructuring; the rest of the health movement must be sensitive to their needs and support their demands for a decent income, dignity, a voice in policy matters, and control over their workplace and lives. Further, hospital workers are a central element in efforts to implement patients' rights or other community control programs. Workers many times represent the community around the hospital and are the most effective day-to-day force in protecting that community's interests. Only by attacking the institutions from the outside and the inside can real change be achieved.

Hospital workers have been among the most exploited members of the workforce for decades. Working conditions were — and still are — terrible: long hours (mostly spent standing up), irregular shifts, many hours of overtime with no extra pay, and often no compensation, paid leave or health insurance. Job security, many times, simply does not exist.

There have been improvements in recent decades. Unionization drives have hit many metropolitan areas and workers are gradually winning a decent livelihood. (For instance, wages have tripled in New York in the past 10 years.) Yet with the whole economic and political order against them, hospital workers have not won gains easily. Most hospital jobs are low-skilled and dead-end; they often attract the powerless and those with no marketable skills. — especially foreign and Third World people, women, and those who have recently migrated from rural areas. These conditions make the workforce on the most transitory in the country. Nor is the law on the side of hospital labor.

Neither federal minimum eage guidelines, nor the National Labor Relations Board cover hospital workers. Voluntary hospital workers have no federally protected rights to organize and hold union elections, and only 12 states have instituted such protection on their own. Most hospitals oppose worker organizing with a vindictive passion. Some administrators actually make their living jumping from one hospital job to another for the sole purpose of busting unions. The American Hospital Association publishes a 78-page handbook with step-by-step descriptions of how to break organizational drives. Hospital tactics include deliberate misrepresentation of facts and outright lying — everything from saying union dues and initiation fees will offset any wage gains made by the union to announcing cancellation of key worker strategy meetings. More severe divide-and-conquer measures include supervisors taking various workers aside for "personal chats" about the evils of the

At New York City's Columbia Presbyterian Hospital a worker was fired in 1967 for her organizing efforts. Thirty years earlier, her father was fired at the same hospital for the same reason.

union, red-baiting, and buy-off techniques (promising immediate token wage or benefit gains to dissipate union appeal). In Detroit, a hospital director deliberately leaked a fake inter-office administrative memo stating that a key union organizer had successfully been bought off and needed only $5,000 more to throw the election entirely. The union lost the election, of course, but they are suing the hospital administration for "unfair labor practices." Such tactics are not isolated incidents; they are the norm. Cutbacks are also used as a divisive weapon. Workers are told that increased wages drain hospital resources, with the implied threat that the hospital would have to cut back on positions open, lay off workers, or even close down completely. This is a frightening prospect for a worker trying to support a family. Many hospitals do in fact exploit union organizing as an excuse to lay off workers and save money. They also use the attrition approach — they simply fail to hire new employees to fill vacant positions. This of course causes division, anger, and resentment of the union among those left with more work. In reality, it is things like needless equipment, over-construction and general inefficiency that force hospitals into financial disasters.

In spite of overwhelming odds, the fight for unionization has gained momentum. Unions have been successful in giving workers solid bread-and-butter gains in the past 10 years. These include substantial wage increases, leave and vacation, health insurance, pension plans, and workpeople's compen-

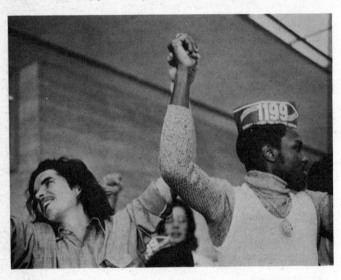

sation. For the first time, workers are protected against re-assignment, firing, and arbitrary disciplinary actions. The major unions have begun upgrading programs and are making headway in establishing daycare and walk-in clinics for workers and their families. Although there are several unions organizing hospital workers, two of the largest are Local 1199 (Drug and Hospital Workers of the American Federation of Retail and Wholesale Clerks) and the American Federation of State, County and Municipal Employees (AFSCME). Local 1199 began as a small local of drug store employees in the mid-50's and began to expand rapidly in the early sixties. Mainly Black and female, the union has been a focus of the Black, labor and Civil Rights movements. Now the only national union that is organizing health and hospital workers exclusively, 1199 organizes mainly in voluntary hospitals. AFSCME organizes workers in state, county, and municipal hospitals and nursing homes. Because wages are controlled by the state, AFSCME mostly bargains for benefits and job security. The union has begun a series of health institutes to educate stewards in dealing with the health system — trying to project and deal with changes in the system before they occur. They also have training programs to upgrade workers, and have helped hospital worker-community coalitions, many of which deal with the dismantling of state hospitals and homes for the retarded

Although unions are an important vehicle for securing workingpeople's rights, they are far from perfect. Many are more democratic in theory than in practice. Rank and file participation and divergence from the union line may be stifled in a number of ways. Union hierarchies are of-

ten well-entrenched and the leaders insure their position through meeting procedures and election rules that are stacked against those who lack the hierarchy's support. Control of the unions is usually centralized in the national office, thus alienating workers even more. Dissent is isolated, and union higher-ups will often put a higher priority on negotiations with management than on listening to the voice of the workers. Hospital workers unions, in general, lack the ability or will to deal with non-bread-and-butter issues. Many hospital workers feel it is up to the rank-and-file to insure workers' rights through a two-pronged struggle, pushing for more democracy and responsiveness in the union even while fighting management.

Because of the nature of this subsection, we feel it is necessary to diverge from the regular catalog format. Most of the problems encountered in hospital worker organizing are universal — as are the methods employed to overcome them. So group descriptions on our regular model would be repetitive rather than informative. And most hospital workers are being organized by only a few major unions. More importantly, some of the groups and individuals we contacted, for obvious reasons, do not want to be specifically named. So we are presenting descriptions of worker actions within and without the context of the union, and of the rank-and-file push for union democracy, without cataloging them into specific groups.

In the movement for workers' rights, a few particular conflicts stand out. Hospital worker organizing began with Local 1199 in New York City. The union there is now a strong force in the health system. In fact, members of 1199 went out on the largest strike against hospitals ever reported in the fall of '73. At issue was the refusal of Nixon's Cost of Living Council (CLC) to allow wage increases promised two years earlier. The Council justified this refusal under the banner of upholding Phase III wage controls — but hospital workers were one of the few groups to be so strictly held to Nixon's dictates, as wages of those higher on the economic ladder continued to soar. The strike marked the first time any union struck over CLC's anti-union policies. Yet, beneath the surface struggle against management was the quieter, equally important fight of the rank and file to control their union. For months, workers pressured the union hierarchy to strike. The union repeatedly stalled in the process of arranging a strike vote, with admonitions of "patience," and "the time is not right." Even when the union finally gave in, it seemed at times more concerned with its image in the eyes of management than with its responsibility to the workers. Only part of the workforce was called out, thus dissipating strength. The union head issued assurances that other workers would be called out "if needed," but never got around to seeing the need. The leadership of other hospital unions issued directives that their workers should not leave work in support of 1199's strike. Some workers from other unions joined 1199's picket lines anyway, as an expression of the need for unity. Workers felt that, had the leadership followed their needs more closely, the strike would have been significantly more successful. As it was, hospital workers gained only half the wage increase originally promised them — a gain largely dissipated by inflation.

Union hierarchies' inattentiveness to the rank and file, or actual efforts to stifle dissent, have been a problem in various other cities as well. In one New England industrial city, the firing of a hospital worker for union organizing sparked a two-year fight for union recognition. At one time, two-thirds of the hospital unit being organized had signed recognition cards, indicating that they wanted the union to represent them. But by the time the election was called, only one-third voted yes for union recognition. It is true that the administration waged a particularly vicious, underhanded campaign, including reams of red-baiting anti-union literature balanced by token concessions. Yet, many workers in that city place heavy blame for the loss on the union. They claim that the rank and file was not consulted on important issues, that the union organizer ran the campaign with an iron hand and in fact reneged on decisions reached democratically in union meetings. Many of the leaflets distributed and tactics used by the workers actually came out of the national office rather than from their own local. The workers, therefore, felt alienated from their own drive for unionization. Many came to look upon the union as an "outside force," reinforcing management's attitude. Though discouraged, the workers at this medical center are slowly beginning to regroup, with the knowledge that their own initiative is their most powerful tool.

Things do not always happen this way. Many organizing campaigns are encouraging examples of solidarity among workers and between the workers and their community. A striking example is the struggle in Pikeville, Kentucky, still going on as the catalog reaches completion. More than 200 of the 237 workers (5 out of 6 of whom are women) have been on strike since June 10, 1973. It is a classic business vs. working class confrontation. The 30-person hospital board is dominated by eastern Kentucky mining interests; it refused to negotiate or "even speak one civil word with the strikers." "Workers have been subjected to threats, intimidation, court injunction and contempt citations, and physical violence from the hospital management and the people working with them." (SOUTHERN PATRIOT) The business community is solidly behind the management — as are most public officials. Guns have been pulled on pickets, rocks have been thrown at them, and a car owned by the mayor's cousin entered the hospital grounds at 60 mph, dislocating a strike leader's shoulder. But working people in the area support the strike solidly. Miners and other workers join the picket lines, and the Black Lung Association supports a boycott of Pikeville business places. A "Concerned Citizens" committee has put out support leaflets in the community, while truck drivers refuse to cross picket lines to deliver supplies. When the union put up roadblocks on the highway to ask passing motorists for contributions to their strike fund, they collected over $1000 each day. As one striker says: "The businessmen know that when we win this strike, the whole city is going to go union. That's why they're fighting us so hard."

Charleston, South Carolina, is another outstanding name in hospital labor and community organizing history. Unionized in the late sixties, the strikers (mostly Black women) gained the support of the entire civil rights movement as well as union leadership. The strikers risked everything at a time when hospital workers' organizing efforts had barely begun, but won the support of the community in their 110 day ordeal. The community boycott of White businesses and a famous march led by Ralph Abernathy played an important part in the workers' final gains: the rehiring of laid-off employees, union recognition, and a new level of respect.

In Chicago, medical and nursing students rallied behind worker demands and participated in leafletting and general support actions. The union opened its membership to the students, some of whom were later expelled from school for

their activities.

An interesting experiment in worker-staff control comes out of San Francisco. There a hospital-affiliated clinic is controlled by worker-staff teams who meet daily to discuss everything from general clinic policy to the cases of particular patients. Most important, decisions are made collectively. Although many issues concerning class, racial, and ethnic differences remain, the participants feel the program is trying successfully to establish open, honest cooperation between all health workers. A positive side-effect has been the discovery that patients generally prefer the non-hierarchical structure of the clinic to regular top-down situations. (See also Health Personnel and Training).

Washington, D.C. is one of the major cities in which community support for hospital workers is being actively sought. In the winter of '73-74, fifteen workers were suspended and 25 fired for participating in a two-hour lunch-time peaceful sit-in in the hospital lobby. At issue is the administration's total refusal to even listen to workers' demands for union representation. Since that time, union organizers and workers have actively solicited the support of the Black and White DC community. Meetings of union and community people have been held regularly and committees set up to educate the public and recruit its help in fighting a particularly reactionary medical center, whose affiliate university is the largest private employer in the District.

A major attempt at worker control by mental health workers was staged at four state-run mental hospitals in Topeka, Kansas, in June 1968. Kansas Health Workers Local 1271 presented a list of demands to the administration, including the following: community control of the hospitals, recognition of their right as public employees to negotiate with the state, comprehensive in-service educational and career development programs, union approval of all hiring and firing, a forty-hour work week, and a panel of workers to develop a "platform of hospital reform." When the deadline for meeting the demands had passed unacknowledged, the workers declared the hospital administration illegitimate and indifferent to people's suffering. Taking care not to disturb clinical relations, they took control of the wards in an effort to demonstrate what ideal health care could actually be. The only authority they recognized was that of the union stewards. In addition, an in-service training program was organized for workers, staffed by sympathetic psychiatrists, doctors and social workers. Although the hospital superintendent had seven workers arrested, (including the union chairperson), suspended sixty workers, and fired the doctor/advisor, they managed

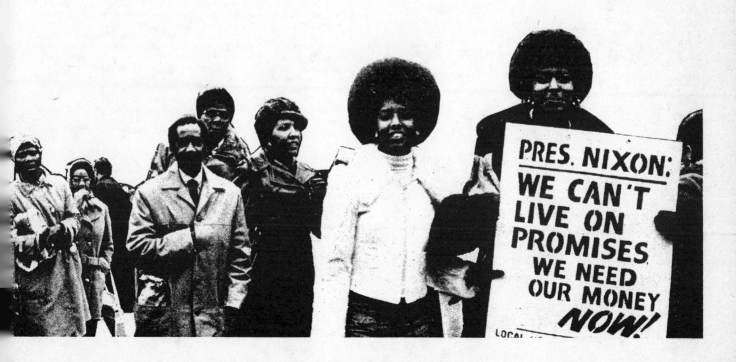

PRES. NIXON:
WE CAN'T
LIVE ON
PROMISES
WE NEED
OUR MONEY
NOW!

to hold control of the wards until a court injunciton and re-straining order was issued. However, further confrontations, meetings and the training program continued. Labeling their action a "work-in" rather than a strike, the workers empha-sized their desire to link up the patients' interests with their own through the slogan "We Care".

Perhaps the clearest embodiment of the issues involved in community-worker control is the series of actions that have taken place at Lincoln Hospital since 1969. While many workers' struggles have centered around the pressing needs of the workers themselves, Lincoln is a dramatic example of workers pushing for changes to benefit the entire com-munity. Lincoln is a physically deteriorating city hospital in New York's South Bronx, affiliated with the liberal Al-bert Einstein School of Medicine. In 1969, Black and Puer-to Rican mental health workers, with professional support, took over the community mental health center; four work-ers had been fired and promises of para-professional career upgrading and worker participation in administration had not been acted upon. During the take-over, workers con-tinued to provide patient care despite arrests, suspensions, and closure of the clinic. Community people were called in to help make decisions and form policy, although work-ers at Lincoln feel the action was weakened because there had not been time to build a broad enough base of com-munity support. In the end the take-over succeeded only in winning conventional gains (job security and pay), but the take-over definitely set the stage for further change. Lincoln was relatively quiet on the surface for a year, but during this time the Health Revolutionary Unity Movement (HRUM) came into being, bringing together Puerto Rican and Black workers and community people. Then, in the spring of '70, "Think Lincoln" evolved. It was a coalition sparked by HRUM, including workers, community people and street gangs. A complaint table was set up and seven demands emerged which were presented to the administra-tion. These included door-to-door preventive health ser-

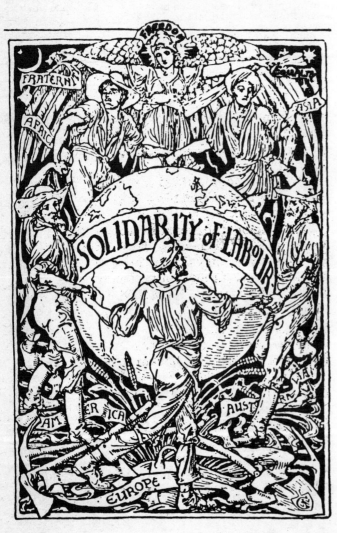

vices, day care for workers and patients, total community-worker control of all services, and construction of a new building. Think Lincoln arranged an intensive screening and education program to educate community residents about communicable diseases and to "place responsibility for health problems at Lincoln's door." The administration was unresponsive; to express the seriousness of their demands, 100 members of Think Lincoln, the Young Lords Party and HRUM occupied for one day part of the Nurses Resi-dence building (which contains administrative offices). As a result, a day care center was begun, and ground was bro-ken for the new building that has been promised for years. But not long after the take-over, an abortion performed at Lincoln killed a young Puerto Rican woman. The death was seen as a symptom of neglect and low-quality care. Community pressure forced the resignation of the head of the obstetrics department. Meanwhile, the hospital had ob-tained an injunction preventing community groups from en-tering the hospital and workers from meeting in the hospi-tal. The injunction, which stifled organizing and provided grounds for harrassment of workers by guards and adminis-trators, specifically named such groups as HRUM, Young Lords and Think Lincoln, along with any other community person or worker. Several months, later, however, there was a take-over of one floor of the administration depart-ment around the issue of starting a detoxification program. Despite harrassment, the de-tox program has grown and thrives; it is entirely staffed and run by community resi-dents.

The Pediatrics Collective, made up of both workers and pro-fessionals, was a focal point of support for Think Lincoln. The collective demanded the resignation of the department head because of his inability to administer and his resistance to community and worker control. He left, taking with him most of those staff people who had supported him. The new department head, a Puerto Rican woman, re-established de-partment meetings in which workers participated with staff in making departmental decisions. Workers and staff gained a say in recruitment and a diverse group of attending phy-sicians were hired to fill the vacancies. Recruitment of Puerto Rican doctors was begun. Later, clerks at Lincoln protested city budget cuts by holding up medicaid forms, thus preventing the city from receiving reimbursement. Al-though the tactic was imaginative and potentially forceful, the action failed because no strategy was worked out to gain support from other departments in the hospital and other hospitals in the city.

Organizers at Lincoln have confronted many of the basic problems in moving toward community and worker control. "The issue of worker/community control has developed at Lincoln with more emphasis on worker than community." Yet the workers at Lincoln are themselves part of the com-munity. The first worker take-over, during which patient care was carefully maintained, pointed out the connection between worker demands and community needs. Yet there remain tensions between users and providers of health ser-vices. Workers, for instance, often feel threatened by com-munity demands for more services coupled with administra-tive refusal to hire more workers and increase pay. Worker organizing has become the dominant issue at Lincoln, based on the conviction that those related to the institution daily have a greater chance of changing it. But the need to work out relations with the community continues. As one worker organizer says: "We lay out what the problems are ...(and)...point out the division around worker and commun-ity is not their fault. We try to show them why this hap-pens."

The administration reinforces community-worker divisions through such ploys as blaming workers for the poor quality of care. The administration also perpetuates divisions between Blacks and Puerto Ricans. For instance, after the program to recruit Puerto Rican doctors began, the hospital virtually stopped hiring Blacks. Such tactics have been used over and over to set minority people fighting with each other to pro-tect minor gains. At Lincoln, unity between Puerto Ricans and Blacks has been striven for consciously all along. The fact that such groups as HRUM and Think Lincoln could bring Blacks and Puerto Ricans together has been a major factor in building their strength.

Over the past couple of years, activity at Lincoln has chan-ged in emphasis. Workers, many of them once active in the dramatic take-overs of the past, now see the need for "ground-floor organizing" as the key to building a strong class-conscious base for change. They are mainly involved in day-to-day political education through such tools as their newsletter. Many workers feel that the hospital unions are hopelessly bogged down in bureaucracy, are not the democratic organizations they claim to be, and are unresponsive to the needs of the rank and file. Therefore, an important part of radical caucus activity is directed toward pointing out the limitations of the unions. They attend union meetings, pushing for more democratic structures and pressuring stewards to act on worker grievances rather than just talking. Radical workers at Lincoln feel it is their role to push beyond bread and butter issues to deal with questions of social change.

Unions Organizing Hospital Workers

Drug, Hospital, and Nursing Home Employees Union (Local 1199) 310 W. 43rd St., New York, NY 10036, (212) 582-1890.

American Federation of State, County, and Municipal Employees 1155 15th St., NW 20005, Washington, D.C. (202) 223-4460.

Service Employees International, 900 17th St., NW, Washington, D.C. 20006, (202) 296-5940.

RESOURCES

PAMPHLETS AND ARTICLES

R118
HEALTH/PAC BULLETIN, 17 Murray St., New York, NY 10007, July-August, 1970, pp. 1-20. $.60
. . .despite its age, this issue offers an excellent analysis of unskilled and semi-skilled hospital workers in their struggle for unionization and their common grounds for aligning with consumers. Includes a history of the fight for hospital unions and a critique of Local 1199, the March 1970 worker strike at San Francisco General Hospital, and worker actions around the country that go beyond bread and butter issues.

"Tremors at San Francisco General," HEALTH/PAC BULLETIN, 17 Murray St., New York, NY 10007, February, 1972, pp. 1-15 $.60
. . .documents workers' battles between 1970 and '72 to improve conditions and patient care at San Francisco General Hospital, where administrative responsibility is "divided between an inflexible, penny-pinching city bureaucracy and an academically oriented affiliate institution, the University of California Medical School."

"A Matter of Life and Death: The Scandalous Conditions at Boston City Hospital," Jonathan Kozol, RAMPARTS, 2054 University Ave., Berkeley, CA 94704, April 1973, pp. 21-25
. . .a scathing denunciation of institutional racism as manifested in medical care. Kozol focuses on Boston City Hospital, which serves mainly low income Black and Spanish speaking people. Temporary loss of its accreditation in 1970 precipitated the forming of a coalition of interns, residents, and nurses, who began bombarding the press with horror statistics and stories. The extreme cases of understaffing and medical negligence are less enraging than the stories of exploitation of patients for teaching purposes through unnecessary procedures, including surgery. Read this to renew your sense of outrage.

HEALTH/PAC BULLETIN, 17 Murray St., New York, NY 10007, January, 1972, pp. 1-16
. . .classic stance on the necessity for hospital workers to take the lead in institutional organizing, as exemplified by "the emancipation of Lincoln" hospital. See HEALTH PERSONNEL AND TRAINING for a complete review.

"PEOPLE'S GUIDE TO HEALTH CARE: FOR HEALTH WORKERS", Legal Aid Society, 2108 Payne Ave., Cleveland, OH 44114, 1972. 7 pp. $.25
. . . separating the hospital heirarchy into 1. management and doctors and 2. everybody else, this booklet notes that an immediate source of workers' alienation—management—"is hard to spot and even harder to reach or to change. So, one's frustration is turned on other workers. . . and on patients." Lists steps for organizing to obtain more rights and benefits, as well as better patient care.

PERIODICALS

TRANSFUSION, c/o New England Free Press, 60 Union Square, Somerville, MA 02143. Free.
. . . a monthly paper by and about workers who "want to provide health services in an atmosphere in which health is given in response to need, not social conditions, where health services are controlled by the workers and patients . . ." Articles cover Boston area hospital worker organizing, poor work conditions, problems with unions. Features have included such things as health care in other countries women's clinics, and more. Generally of high quality with good analysis, the paper is written in Spanish and English.

STETHOTRUTH, P.O. Box 156 Hamtramek, MI 48212. $2/year
. . . aimed at North Detroit Health workers, the paper promotes a 5-point program including the right to free complete and preventive health care. Articles are mainly concerned with union struggles although some reprints from other periodicals cover everything from health care in China to drug industry rip-offs.

"HOSPITAL WORKERS' NEWSLETTER," Lincoln Hospital Workers, P.O. Box 677, Bronx, NY 10451. monthly/Free
. . . Spanish/English paper dealing with issues important to Lincoln Hospital workers (announcements, how to fill out grievance forms, how to use the union machinery), as well as more general political questions affecting all hospital workers. Past issues have discussed big business' role in causing inflation, and racism—what it is and how it is used to divide Black and Puerto Rican health workers. Much space has been devoted to talking about the limitations of the unions (1199 and 420), and what actions the rank-and-file have taken to secure their own demands. An underlying goal of the paper is to unify workers and build a strong class consciousness.

EMPLOYEES ORGANIZE—EMPLEADOS ORGANIZEN, United Stanford Employees, Local 680, Service Employees International Union, AFL-CIO, PO Box 7152, Stanford, CA 94305.
. . . packed with a wide range of articles, relating to Stanford workers from ongoing accounts of their specific struggles to monopolistic practices of US oil companies, sex discrimination suits won by women and shows of support for workers in other fights. A "Serving the People" column appears regularly, devoted to health concerns of the workers; written by sympathetic Stanford house staff, it includes information on the value of various health plans, how to save money on prescription drugs, and more.

FILMS AND TAPES

Newsreel, 26 W. 20th St., New York, NY 10011
   "Lincoln Hospital," 15 min. b&w $20
   Workers and community people attempt to take control of a community mental health center in a New York City public hospital. The film exposes the contradiction between the corporate/university controlled medical facilities and the health needs of the people.

Audio-Visual Center, Indiana University, Bloomington, IN 47401
   "Like a Beautiful Child," 24 min. b&w $5.75
   Narrates the story of Local 1199 of the Drug and Hospital Employees Union, and tells how and why it began and developed.

HEALTH PERSONNEL AND TRAINING

PROBLEM

Since the 19th century, when formal, standardized training began pushing out folkhealers and midwives, the US health system has been dominated by White middle-class male doctors who have attained a status that keeps them "beyond criticism, beyond regulation, and very nearly beyond competition."

A military-styled hierarchy has evolved in the health field, complete with uniforms, pins, ranks, titles and chains of command—and the physician sits at the top of the hierarchy to call the battle plans. The doctor is a major force behind the policies that determine the sex, race and size of the health workforce, the quality and type of medicine practiced, the geographical area the workforce will serve, and the cost to the consumer for the health care. Physicians are in a position to command the highest wages paid to any professional. They have created an aura of mystery and awe around themselves so successfully as to be seen as virtual miracle workers. Thus, we are led to believe that the most basic knowledge of how to care for our bodies can only be obtained by years of highly technical training and mastery of a complicated language. We also make the mistake of assuming that the scarcity of health personnel is somehow due to the degree of difficulty in learning the skills and length of training time, rather than the result of limitations placed on the number of people trained in health careers.

The breakdown of health careers reflects the racial, sexual, and class prejudices of the society at large. At the top are White male doctors; only 2-3% of all doctors are Third World, and eight percent are women. Doctors are followed closely by dentists, pharmacists, social workers, and administrators; in the middle are largely White women nurses and technicians; and at the bottom, Third World aides, dietary workers, and housekeeping staff.

This type of occupational hierarchy inevitably induces conflicts among the personnel at each job level and helps maintain the dominance of doctors. These conflicts prevent innovative changes in occupational rules that would contribute to an equitable distribution of power, recognition, and meaningful work for all. This would mean better health care for everyone.

There are many forces that keep patients and workers from challenging the doctors' dominance. Through the images presented by media writers on TV shows like "Marcus Welby, MD", and through direct experience with the health system, the public has learned to internalize the mystique of professionalism. All health personnel have developed their own form of professionalism; the doctor's version is the most pervasive. While professionalism could mean competence in a skilled trade, it has come to mean doctors' use of secrecy and "medi-code" to create such an air of mystery that most people can't understand what they are talking about and are afriad to ask. For instance, physician-caused deaths, of which there are estimated 200,000 annually, are called "iatrogenic" rather than mistakes. Professionalism means that doctors will not criticize a colleague in front of non-doctors and often do not disclose mistakes to a patient for fear of threatening the image of infallibility. The overall result of professionalism is almost total control for the doctor.

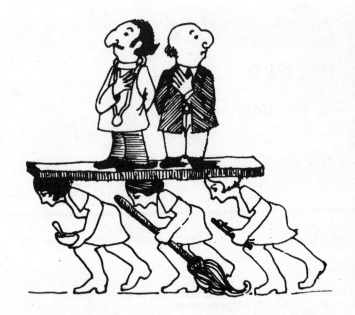

The physician's authority is heightened by intentionally limiting the supply of doctors and other health personnel. The outcome of this professional birth control is that every part of our country is experiencing personnel shortage. Currently there are 2000 patients for each family care physican and 2/3 of those practitioners serve the richest half of the US population. Rural areas suffer the most from the shortage since they have only 1/3 the practitioners of urban areas on a per capita basis.

Partially because of the US personnel shortage, there has been an influx of foreign-trained workers, mainly from Indian, Korea, Philippines, and South American countries. Besides providing a cheap source of labor, foreign physicians, nurses and technicians readily submit to professional authority due to threats of losing certification and licensure, and even deportation. Importation of foreign health personnel allows this country to avoid dealing with its shortages of health workers while it drains the resources of countries who have health problems much greater than our own.

The American Medical Association, which is the largest and most powerful body of organized physicians, is also the most affluent and powerful professional group in the US. Historically the AMA has opposed all progressive health legislation by a variety of red-baiting tactics: Old age and unemployment insurance was described by the AMA as a "definite step toward communism or totalitarianism." State health agencies to reduce the death rate of mothers and children were fought because they "tended to promote communism." And free diagnostic service for handicapped children were denounced as a "socialist regulation."

Other public-interest health measures the AMA has opposed (in the past) influde free innoculation against diptheria, polio, and smallpox, federal grants for medical school construction and low interest health student loans, and of course, Medicare. They are also well-known for collusion with the drug and tobacco industry. Nationally, the AMA wheels and deals on a budget of over $35 million, more than a third of which comes directly from drug companies in the form of advertising in the AMA Journal. Nearly all of this budget goes to support lobbying and through its political arm, American Medical Political Action Committee, to contribute to the campaign of conservative candidates who oppose public-interest health legislation and support such conservative stances as the continuation of the war in IndoChina.

The AMA's influence is most directly felt in their monopolistic policies on health personnel. By limiting medical student enrollment through opposition to new schools and student financial aid, the AMA has ensured that a majority of traditionally oriented middle-class applicants gain admission, thus preserving the political conservatism of the profession. The AMA control extends to all health workers since it is one of the major accrediting agencies of health science schools, and also of personnel, through state licensing boards. The AMA also does its best to limit hospital admissions privileges to patients of AMA members. Resisting the transfer of medical skills to non-physicians is another of their tactics.

MEDICAL EDUCATION

Being selected for medical school is seen as a privilege and an honor to the applicant. The faculty embrace first year students with "Welcome colleague, you're one of us now." But neophytes in this most exclusive fraternity endure a "hell-week" four years long. From the beginning students find themselves barraged with more information than they can possibly assimilate. The overwhelming amount of studying leaves them with little time to analyze the underlying values or question the professional approach. The pressure to learn is tremendous, for it is implied that any neglected information could result in a wrong decision at a crucial time. In some schools the pressure is so overwhelming that 20% of the students use tranquilizing drugs regularly and an even greater number seek psychiatric counseling.

Women's credentials must be of higher quality than men's to get into medical school, and the interviews they are forced to crawl through are filled with implications that they surely will quit after a few years to assume wife and motherly functions. School itself is a constant, isolating, uphill battle against intimidating instructors, sexist learning materials, and highly threatened, competitive male students. Once out of school, women have a much harder time earning recognition and positions of greater responsibility.

Many students begin their training committed to the delivery of patient-oriented primary care. Yet in most cases by the time they graduate, they have become much less community oriented, and often have chosen careers of specialty practice or medical research. This change has several causes. Nearly all the physicians with whom the student comes in contact are researchers or specialists, so involved with their tiny niche in medicine that they offer no support or encouragement to students concerned with primary care. A school which offers courses on medical economics, community health problems, social organization, and human ethics beyond a superficial level is unusual. And it is rare that a student leaves medical school with the interpersonal skills and cross-cultural understanding necessary to serve the community.

UNDERUTILIZATION OF PROFESSIONALS

Focus on the MD as the sole provider of medical care usually results in gross underutilization of other health workers with highly specialized training and skills. Aside from nurses, three examples of these are dentists, pharmacists and social workers.

Pharmacists are just now beginning to be educated towards healing rather than retailing, but they are drastically underused. Adverse drug reactions constitute over 1,500,000 hospital admissions a year; drug education by pharmacists for doctors and patients, complete drug histories and monitering of patients' drug-taking could substantially reduce this figure. Dentists are also overtrained and could be offering more total preventive care.

Although trained in counseling skills, social workers end up spending their time dealing with rigid hospital procedures—pushing papers to try to get services for those in need. Any individual client advocacy they manage to do merely scratches the surface of the patient's problems, which the hospital perpetuates and occasionally causes.

NURSES

Nurses are next in line in the occupational pyramid. It is their job to play patient's advocate while supporting the doctor's ego; this means passing along quick, accurate judgments to the physician as unobtrusively as possible, being supportive yet submissive. In such ways these victims of "the handmaiden syndrome" earn the distinction of being "a damn good nurse." Nursing suffers from decades of discriminatory sexual stereotyping. It has traditionally trained women into passivity because this is the famale ideal our society reinforces. This supporting role meshes neatly with physician/male superiority and is perpetuated by those in control. Many women have had to conform to this role because nursing has provided their most accessible route into semi-responsible positions in the health field. The government has traditionally funded nurisng education at 1/5 the level of medical training, though the total number of nursing students triples that of those in medical schools.

The men who join the nursing profession (2% of all nurses) consistently receive higher salaries, are promoted faster and assume many leadership positions. When women advance they usually lack decision-making powers and budget control over their own departments in the hospital; in universities they have little voice in general nursing education policy, and sometimes receive lower salaries than professors of other colleges within the same institution. This is hardly surprising; many nursing schools do not train women to be leaders or to stand up for themselves. Nursing education tends to be extremely rigid and concerned with the right way of doing things. Creativity is discouraged to the extent that nurses have little faith in their own judgments or perceptions by the time their training is over.

Internal division is a pervasive problem of nursing. Presently the field spans everyone from the relatively untrained nurses's aides to the nine years of post-secondary training towards a Ph.D. usually required of supervisors and directors. For example, nurse practitioner programs can require anything from prior Registered Nurse (RN) experience and a few months special training to a master's degree. White middle-class women are mainly recruited into baccalaureate degree programs, and Third World women are often channeled in as aides and Licensed Practical (or Vocational) Nurses (LPN, LVN). Even the universities that do token recruitment of Third World students rarely have adequate retention programs which are committed to keeping students in school. Thus, the percentage of Third World women in policy-making nursing positions is negligible. Hospitals rarely cover the education and training costs necessary for advancement, and educational programs give no credit for past uncredentialled training or experience. Few outside the middle class have time or money to quit work and go back to school full-time.

Such barriers to advancement are reinforced by the professionalist attitudes of the elite in the nursing world—those with degrees. In their fight for responsibility and respect from the physicians and administrators, they often vent their frustrations by exerting control over those lower on the ladder. As long as nurses keep fighting against each other, they leave the MDs on top.

With such status bickerings compounding the problems of mediocre pay, long hours, alienating tasks, and little job fulfillment, or autonomy, it is small wonder that the field has had a turnover rate of 60% each year and that approximately 1/3 of the RNs in this country are not actively practicing. Often those who don't quit move on to teaching and administration.

The nurse's role is confusing and undefined; traditional nurses' duties have been taken over by a variety of new occupations from medical social workers to registered medical record librarians, inhalation therapists, dieticians and more. Each new specialist in the health field is a potential threat. Further confusion stems from the emergence of the nurse practitioner (clinician) programs which train nurses extensively in specialities from gynecology to geriatrics to family practice. They have proven especially valuable in rural counties and ghetto areas where doctors are scarce. Gradually these practitioners are gaining the legal right to practice independently without any doctor. But expansion into more skilled areas just compounds the identity dilemma: is the nurse to assume the more primary care services that were once only the doctor's domain: is s/he to remain as a technical assistant; or is s/he to assume a nurturing function distinctly separate from but complementary to the doctor's role?

One nursing student "tells of being severely disciplined for failing to wake a patient in order to change his bed linen. Her explanation that the patient had not slept for several nights and that he needed undisturbed sleep more than clean linen was judged irrelevant."
—Health/PAC

The nursing field is currently barren of leadership—the American Nursing Association (ANA) represents only about ¼ of the RN's and mainly involves itself in self-interest struggles to preserve professionalism. However there is evidence of some slight stirrings among the Student Nursing Association to become more issue-oriented. The likelihood of their setting up a nationwide hypertension screening program hints of a desire to become more community oriented and to depart from the ANA line.

Beset by their own division, it is easy to understand why nurses have failed to organize to any great degree. Some ANA chapters have been doing collective bargaining since 1964; other nurses consider it "unprofessional" to organize. A growing number of RNs concerned with issues such as understaffing and the resulting low quality patient care are already putting aside past attitudes and joining hospital workers' unions. Whether this trend towards worker unity will take the form of fighting for change in the entire health care system remains to be seen.

PHYSICIAN'S ASSISTANTS

The position of Physician's Assistant (PA) was purportedly designed to extend health care to more people by employing former military medics as doctor's aides, giving more primary care than nurses, but less than physicians themselves. However, many people see these programs as the AMA's answer to nurse practitioner programs—a stop-gap measure against nursing—and female—expansion into the doctor's realm.

For the health establishment, the PA represents token concessions to the personnel shortage without paying the money necessary to train more doctors.

Many state Medicare programs reinforce PA dependence on the doctor by only providing reimbursement for services rendered when the physician is supervising. This same dependence prevents PAs from providing more family practice-type care to the general population. In most states, they are so closely tied legally to the physician that they must instead follow him/her down the road to his/her particular specialization. Another problem with the PA program in general is that many of those with PA training are unable to find physicans to employ them.

There are many similarities between the training involved in some PA and nurse practitioner programs since they both are being taught more specialized medical skills. The basic difference seems to be that the NP is taught to provide more of a nurturing function. This involves trying to meet the patient's total physical and emotional needs rather than just treating medical symptoms, and providing preventive counseling and support about how to deal with the causes and effects of the illness. Combining the NP & PA into one job classification seems natural; it would help fight expanding occupational fragmentation, sexual stereotyping in jobs, and extend more skilled personnel into the public domain by releasing the PA's from the physician's control.

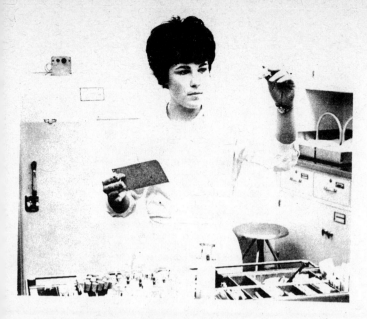

(from a nurse): Whenever I told a doctor I was going back to school, the response was invariably, 'why?'
--MS., Aug. '73

OTHER ALLIED HEALTH WORKERS

Just above the base of the pyramid are the myriad of workers in the allied health occupations struggling for professional status. Fitting into over 375 specialized job categories in all, these allied health workers include all personnel providing "professional" and "technical" support to doctors, dentists, RN's, pharmacists and social workers. For every sophisticated piece of machinery, complicated new lab technique or intricate new operating system, dozens of new occupations abound. These range from inhalation therapists to X-ray equipment repair technicians, occupational therapy associates to medical record keepers. Under each of these titles are subgroups of technologists, technicians, assistants and aides, as well as divisions of these. Each title is indicative of a different length and type of training program.

Since the paraprofessional concept mushroomed in the early 60's, most of these workers have gained little more than new titles. Earnings are still meager, hours bad and responsibility minimal. Some of these people see the patients 10-15 times as often as doctors do, yet are rarely consulted on any kind of decision-making about the patient's welfare.

As with nurses, the fight intensifies to hold onto one's turf with the advent of each new occupation. Going back to school for more training and higher job status is prohibitively expensive for many. Government funding is a mere trickle when it comes to such training, and the hospital is not about to dip into its profits to train people they have a vested interest in keeping in their places. For the hospitals, "stuffing more in at the bottom" is by far preferable to the costly upgrading of those with years of experience.

Under the all-encompassing banner of allied health personnel is a hazy division between those 25 or so categories of licensed (at least in some states) technicians who consider themselves the "legitimate" professionals, and those who are not formally licensed, often referred to as the "new professioinals." The former group has in a sense "made it"—their training has become somewhat standardized, their wages higher, and their job security and mobility improved. Yet they have now become formally locked into tasks often as boring and routine as those performed by unlicensed workers. To secure their status, many of them must ally themselves with doctors and the "ideology of professionalism."

Besides the patients, those to suffer most directly from licensed personnels' emulation of physicans' behavior are the unlicensed, who are often equally skilled but lack the official credentials to prove it. This group covers a huge gamut of job categories from nutrition aide to family planning counselor. Whereas many have high school diplomas, additional training is usually received on the job, in community centers or in universities; it is in no way coordinated, standardized or accredited, making mobility to other jobs requiring credentials impossible.

The training programs for all these occupations are largely in a state of refined chaos: there are different standards and curriculum for the same job, uncoordinated training for different levels of the same job, and unrelated training for related occupations. Community training programs for jobs in local clinics often end up taking pressure for such training off the institutions themselves. However, these jobs rarely fit into the existing institutional structure and the community then must assume responsibility for employing everyone it trains in more jobs that lead nowhere. Vertical coordination of these training programs is virtually nonexistent—a health worker with years of experience and any amount of related education must still start from the bottom if s/he wants to become a doctor.

Trying to link up people with personally rewarding positions that also fulfill health wo/manpower needs is one of the most complex problems facing health activists and planners. Whereas growing numbers of allied health workers are represented by unions, so far the unions have been more involved with bread and butter issues than as agents of significant change. The process of deciphering the health occupational hierarchy is a bewildering one; what appear to be deep-seated irrationalities are rational in the context of a profit-making system. Any real change must involve sweeping innovation in the entire structure of the health care delivery system. So far the paraprofessionals concept has been little more than a further pacification of the community in order to perpetuate the existing order. Professionals have refused to allow the concepts of new careers to do much towards constructively reorganizing health services.

LICENSING, CERTIFICATION AND ACCREDITATION

Licensing, certification and accreditation procedures for regulating personnel reflect the chaotic duplicity in health occupations and training programs. The prcess begins when an occupation gains enough strength and power to formally "professionalize" itself—it forms an association, sets rigid education and training entrance requirements, certifies members and pushes to be recognized by licensing boards. Each connecting operation is dependent on the others—generally, workers must train at accredited institutions to be certified by their future professional association to be licensed by their state board, to be hired by the health institution. To compound this confusion, there are multitudes of agencies to perform each function.

The certification or registration procedure itself is a voluntary mechanism governing qualifications for the profession in an attempt to standardize the workforce. Commonly determined by each professional association, these entry requirements usually consist of a set score on a written exam based on education, a degree or diploma of some sort, and a fixed amount of clinical experience. These often indirectly serve to establish a profession as the domain of a particular race, sex or class. And as a profession fights for status, it inevitably raises these requirements (particularly educational ones), shutting out workers who have plenty of experience but lack the extra academic preparation.

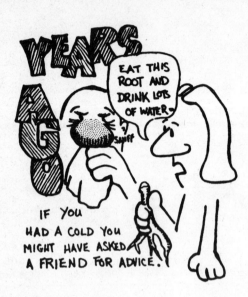

IF YOU HAD A COLD YOU MIGHT HAVE ASKED A FRIEND FOR ADVICE.

The next step, licensure, grants a profession a legal monopoly over a specified set of skills, approves the educational program, and officially establishes a profession's entrance requirements, though these are usually a reflection of the certification qualifications. The licensure board which sets these requirements is composed of professionals from one's guild, or from the guild above it. For example, LPN's are not licensed by other LPN's, but by RN's. In approving education programs, the licensing boards of many states actually only rubber stamp the accrediting done by a plethora of private accrediting agencies which often establish variable standards for the same or related occupational programs. In addition, one institution sometimes has to meet the standards of several such agencies. The AMA's Council on Medical Education is one of the most active of these accrediting groups, and does not hesitate to pass over programs allowing workers mobility or other advantages threatening to the doctor's autonomy.

Other problems abound. Professions which are licensed in some states are not in others. Moreover, within an institution, "scope of practice" laws as governed by licensing may have little meaning, since workers are often asked to perform tasks they're unlicensed to do, if it saves the institution money. Yet if they tried to perform such skills outside the institution, they could be prosecuted. And if they overstep "professional" bonds—by possibly going on strike, or exhibiting other insubordinate behavior, they risk decertification. Thus health workers learn to stay in their place. Indeed, the last line of the medical technologists' pledge is: "I do not want to encroach upon anyone else's premises."

Recently there has been a move afoot to take licensing power from the states and give it to the institutions themselves. Supposedly this would help insure public accountability, increase the number of health workers and provide for more updating of skills. However, this would give the hospitals final responsibility for arbitrarily dividing labor and tasks of all but doctors and dentists. State boards would have some input, but job security would be totally dependent on the whims of administrators and doctors, and worker mobility would be greatly decreased since a position in one institution might not trans-

fer to another. And the hospital could still pay workers low wages, yet "license" them to do more complex responsible tasks. Strongly supported by the AMA and the American Hospital Association, the idea is just as vehemently opposed by the other professional associations. No substantial action has been taken as yet; still, the possibility of these institutions gaining the even greater measures of control that licensure power would bring is a grim one.

Licensing has done little in the way of protecting the public from professional ineptness and exploitation—there is no formal mechanism for periodic review of health workers to insure they are keeping up their skills and to keep them publicly accountable. Though licensure is legally bound to provide "a system of continuous control over the licensed," in practice, licenses are essentially granted for a life-time.

In a token attempt to make doctors more accountable, the federal government is currently in the process of setting up a new quality control system of professional standards review organizations (PSRO). These will purportedly review doctors' payment requests under Medicare/caid, insuring that valid reasons exist for ordering patients into hospitals, performing operations or prescribing drugs. Established under HEW's new Bureau of Quality Assurance under the Office of Professional Standards Review, the PSRO office itself is headed by a physician (surprise, surprise!); a national council supervises and evaluates operations. The yearly report they are to submit covering PSRO activities is regarded as the concession to public accountability.

Boards are also being set up on state and local levels. Local membership is open to all area practicing doctors, and AMA-controlled medical societies are presently pushing to be recognized as official PSRO units. With rotating panels of doctors reviewing one another's work, it is highly unlikely they will often deny one anothr payment or impose fines for violations. Consumer representation is prvided for only on the state coordinating councils, which will occupy four of eleven

WHAT WAS KNOWN ABOUT HEALTH CARE WAS PRETTY MUCH SHARED THROUGHOUT THE POPULATION. BUT CAPITALISM AND MODERN MEDICINE MADE IT POSSIBLE FOR RICH MEN TO HOARD KNOWLEDGE. THEY ARE RESPECTFULLY CALLED "DOCTORS." DIPLOMA $$$$ TAKE 2 ASPIRIN AND DRINK LOTS OF WATER $5 PLEASE

seats (two nominated by the state governors and two chosen by HEW); all other seats are held by physicians. As one doctor put it, "Professional standards are an inherently professional responsibility." These boards will have access to valuable information on comparative costs and quality of care by doctors throughout the state, but there is little reason to believe it will be used to significantly control quality of care, considering board composition. The AMA, initially violently opposed to the idea of being "strait-jacked" by such a machanism, has adroitly reversed strategies and is now usurping control of the operation. Meanwhile, other powerful professional groups such as the American Association of Physicians and Surgeons continue to battle against any public regulation of doctors.

RESEARCH

The shove that keeps the US medical system rolling comes from research. To maximize the profits of the health industry, its market must continuously expand, essentially through the efforts of research and its associated technology. Research is the most common way of bringing federal money into the health industry in a process that lacks consumer input or control, since it is channelled through universities and health institutions. Over half of the operating budgets of the nation's medical schools have come from federal research grants. However, Nixon's recent federal cutbacks in health spending threatened to reduce medical school budgets by at least 25%.

The road to prestige for doctors and health institutions is paved with research grants. That prestige is not measured by the number of people who will benefit from the new information, but by the amount of research money controlled. Clearly the public's image of the virtuous medical researcher is somewhat distorted. "What you hear and see about progress in medicine is often staged by PR men, press agents, and medical journalists. The information. . . tends to be selective, overstated, generally long on form and short on substance." (Medical Economics) With federal research money diminishing, PR people find they have a tougher job; researchers have even faked successful results to increase their chances of renewed funding.

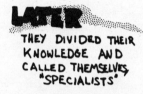

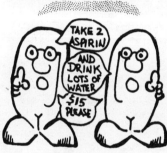

Medical centers often divert money from patient service to seductive recruitment campaigns offering scientists high salaries, carpeted offices, and even private swimming pools. A healthy return on their investment comes to the center when the researchers arrive with their equipment and staff resources. The center then has access to goods that would otherwise be out of its financial reach, its name on any publications that come from the research, and an additional source of income obtained from charging for overhead expenses, such as office space and equipment which may amount to 60-70% of the grant. (Health/PAC)

Usually implicit in the agreements between researchers and medical centers is that the former will spend part of their time teaching in the medical school. Medical education tends to suffer because professors are picked on their research ability, not on teaching skills.

Much research today is theoretical, redundant, irrelevant, and inapplicable. Urgent needs where groundwork has already been laid are ignored: pre-natal care, nutrition, sanitation, and diseases such as TB. Experiments tend to be overly repeated. All too often the thrust of original research tends to be towards relatively rare diseases that are concerns of the middle and upper-classes, such as muscular dystrophy and cystic fibrosis, rather than diseases that affect Black and poor people, like sickle cell anemia and hypertension. And when new successful treatments are discovered, often they are not implemented because of the expense involved and personnel shortages.

Medicine and the military join hands in the area of research. The late sixties and early seventies produced a flurry of documents revealing the extent of the US's involvement in chemical and biological warfare. Both gas and infectious dis-

ease weaponry research projects were uncovered and were either "justified", disposed of, or moved to a new secret location. Presently, very little is known about the state of medicine's current complicity with the military. It is known, however, that at least 46 medical schools and hospitals have Defense Department contracts, indicating a continuing high degree of involvement.

One of the most disgusting aspects of research is the sheer disregard for the lives of those who are experimented upon. The people usually exploited in the experimentation process are the disabled, the retarded, the incarcerated, and women, many of whom are Third World people. The institutionalized patients in the wards of big city hospitals or in the charity wards of teaching hospitals are often unknowingly involved or coerced into experimental treatments and drug screening. One famous example is the US Public Health Service's Tuskegee Syphillis Study from 1939 to 1972 in which 400 Black men with syphillis were observed and left untreated well after penicillin was discovered as a cure for the disease. In the Congo, live virus polio vaccines have been tested on people by US corporations. An example is the work of Dr. Sol Krugman who conducted studies on the elimination of hepatitis at Willowbrook State School on retarded children. Because of the unsanitary conditions at Willowbrook, virtually every resident contracted hepatitus and usually dysentery within six to twelve months of entering. Instead of working to improve the terrible conditions of the school, Dr. Krugman performed "controlled" experiments on cures for hepatitis. As a militant group of medical school activists put it, "The problem wasn't hepatitis—it was Willowbrook!"

The issue of "informed" volunteers taking part in experiments is a crucial one. Even when an experiment is explained to the participants, facts and risks can easily be distorted by the researcher. After the explanation, volunteers must "consent" to their participation through a process which requires the volunteer's signature on a consent form. Many of these forms "release and forever discharge" the researchers and anyone else involved "from liability for injury which may result directly or indirectly from the performance of these investigations." While permissible in the strict legal sense, for private industry this type of wholesale consent has been banned from use in HEW funded research. However HEW has yet to enforce these regulations; they neither require that the wording of consent forms be cleared with them nor that copies of the form be submitted.

Medical and health-related research is a necessary component of any health system. Potentially, it can bring about new, low-cost treatments available to those with the greatest need, discover health hazards in work-places before injuries, and establish the most efficient uses of health personnel and resources. To serve the best interests of all people, research must be conducted by an enlightened and accountable breed of researchers who will not forget their community responsibility.

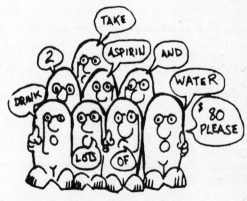

WHERE WILL IT END?

PLATFORM

The divisive hierarchical structure of our health system corresponds to the structure and design of our society. The roots of the problem are far too deep for a few reformist measures to eradicate. Until the entire system is shaken and reordered along more equitable lines, however, we see organizing for the following changes as a beginning.

I. HEALTH TRAINING SCHOOLS MUST INSTITUTE PROGRAMS THAT MEET COMMUNITY PERSONNEL NEEDS. THEY MUST ENACT:

1. large-scale recruitment programs that introduce all the health occupations to men and women of all races, ages and classes, with emphasis on breaking down traditional stereotypes of who performs what skill.

2. admissions policies to redress the dominance of White middle-class males. Enrollment should reflect the population of the country with preference to those experienced in the health field. Admissions decisions should be made by boards consisting of students, faculty, workers, and community people. Importation of personnel from other countries should be discouraged. Tuition should be on a sliding scale, and eventually all health training programs must be open to everyone and financed with the profits of the health industry.

3. comprehensive retention programs for those with poor academic preparation or from different socio-cultural backgrounds, including tutoring programs, personal counseling and flexibility in course load.

4. a core curriculum of preparatory work for all those entering health occupations which emphasizes preventive aspects of health care, stressing community health needs and a political and economic understanding of the entire health system. This curriculum will encourage general skills over specialization and will emphasize all opportunities in health fields. It will also include an introduction to all areas of health care and the fundamental concepts of health and disease as related to people of all races, sexes and ages, encouraging self-help techniques. All students will spend significant training time in rural and/or urban areas.

5. health career ladders for everyone in the health field, extending from the core curriculum and providing multiple points of entry into a variety of skill levels. Workers-students will receive credit for past experience, and performance will be stressed as well as education. Such programs must be coordinated and standardized nationwide to allow for greater worker mobility. Training must be tied in to accredited educational institutions and trainees will receive credential every step of the way.

II. HEALTH DELIVERY INSTITUTIONS MUST DEMYSTIFY THE PROFESSIONAL'S ROLE AND GIVE BETTER QUALITY CARE BY:

1. promoting patient education about our own bodies.

2. instituting a nationwide system of interdisciplinary health teams. Workers of various skill levels will each provide different services for the patient but will all work together to deal with the patient as a whole person, including the effect of illness on the family, curative and preventive measures, counseling, etc. All team members will move towards equalizing input on decision-making. The functions of each team member must be periodically re-evaluated by the entire team on the basis of serving community needs rather than conforming to traditional job stereotypes.

3. insuring job equality and job attractiveness for every member. Easy access to child care facilities will be provided as well as complete health benefits for workers and their families from the institution. In-service continuous training must be available part-time or full-time, paid for with institution funds. Part-time jobs must be open for those wishing to continue education or devote extra time to families. Also, institutions must force government and insurance companies to provide medicare/caid reimbursement for services provided by health teams.

4. looking to models offered by other countries, to see what systems have been most effective in best serving the greatest number of people.

III. LICENSURE, CERTIFICATION AND ACCREDITATION PROCEDURES MUST WORK FOR PUBLIC/WORKER PROTECTION:

1. Health occupational categories must be consolidated into a basic few, leaving fewer titles and less specialization, so that each job category will cover a broader range of skills.

2. Every health occupation will be licensed on a standardized national scale to allow for worker mobility; licensing and certification must be quickly attainable, with consideration given to clinical experience and present performance as well as education. In addition, licensed health personnel and their patients must be given hospital admittance services at all times, regardless of the professional organization they belong to.

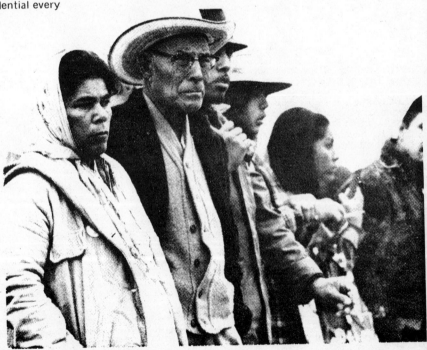

3. All health workers must periodically come before consumer/worker boards for licensing review to insure that they've maintained their skills and kept up with advances in their field.

4. Accreditation of health-related institutions must be controlled by community boards, with worker representation, on the basis of general national standards which insure quality but not rigidity.

IV. HEALTH WORKERS MUST BE DISTRIBUTED WHERE THE NEED IS GREATEST

1. All health workers should spend a significant time period working in shortage areas. One method of doing this is the British model, whereby a national board decides how many doctors can practice in a given region.

2. Special efforts must be made to train health workers from rural and inner-city communities and encourage them to return to these areas to serve.

V. HEALTH-RELATED RESEARCH MUST BE MADE ACCOUNTABLE TO THE PUBLIC BY:

1. ending the exploitation of Third World people, women, the poor and the incarcerated as research subjects (and) by assuring that everyone who does participate in research experiments has complete knowledge of all aspects of the project and its possible side effects.

2. establishing mechanisms for research proposals and grant monies involving possible risk to people or the environment to be administered by consumer-controlled review boards.

3. researching alternative methods of practicing medicine (acupuncture, homeopathy) and publishing the results of all research, including failures.

4. insuring that all research personnel serve significant time in clinical health work before beginning straight research; (and) that throughout their careers they maintain contact with the community through continual part-time or periodic full-time direct service.

5. spending the most resources dealing with the most pressing needs of all the people. More funds should also go into responsibly funding a variety of innovative model health care delivery demonstration projects, although if people in an area depend on a demonstration project's services, something must take its place when its funds run out.

The Constitution of this Republic should make special provision for Medical Freedom as well as Religious Freedom. . . . To restrict the art of healing to one class of men and deny equal privileges to others will constitute the Bastille of medical science. All such laws are un-American and despotic. They are fragments of monarchy and have no place in a Republic.

—Benjamin Rush, M.D.
Surgeon General of the Continental
Army of the United States

In the struggle to deprofessionalize the health care system and humanize services, it is imperative that communities, workers, sympathetic professionals and health science students unite in a common front. Many of the following points are directed at such coalitions, while others are designated for specific groups.

ACT IMMEDIATELY ON THE HEALTH PERSONNEL CRISIS

1. Health science students: form stronger ties with students outside your specific field; begin meeting to discuss curriculum relevancy, professionalism, faculty attitudes towards women and Third World students.

2. Patients' rights and advocacy groups: work with sympathetic professionals to demystify the medical profession and develop community-based self-help programs.

3. Community coalitions should build around such issues as institutional expansion, the absence of public clinics, malpractices, and lack of community control; chip away at the artificial divisions between consumers, workers, and professionals.

START CHALLENGING EXISTING HEALTH PROGRAMS

1. Health science students: use examples from foreign health systems and your own ideas to develop alternative courses and demand that they be integrated into the curriculum. Boycott classes irrelevant and divisive to health science students; agitate for preceptorships in rural and inner-city areas, and for practicums in different health careers.

2. Health science students: research your school; expose statistics on women and Third World admissions and retention rates; expose sexist and racist faculty and administrators, unearth vested interests between the health industry and school authorities. Working with community groups, protest the presence of drug company salespeople pushing their overpriced and often dangerous wares through gifts to students and professionals. Create leaflets and newspapers to disseminate indictive information or leak it to community and worker groups.

3. Hospital workers: unionize your workplace and, after a bargaining unit is established, push for an open-ended training and upgrading program to allow workers to further their education.

4. Find out what public health programs there are in the state; discover how much and in what form government money is coming in for local health services. Survey neighborhoods to learn how many and what type of health personnel are in that area working; find out office locations, rates, and who they serve. Investigate health science recruitment practices on the high school and college level; publicize abuses of federal programs and spotlight these programs' specific weaknesses; make it known how much tax money is subsidizing publically unaccountable health schools, institutions and professionals. Pressure local, state and federal health authorities to increase financial aid to low-income students; demonstrate at high schools and colleges that employ career counselors who advise women and Third World students to become nurses and aides while advising White males to study medicine.

5. Fight to change HEW policies and funding priorities. One place to begin is nominating responsible communities' members to state and federal Professionals Standards Reviews Organizations, since PSRO council members will have access to potentially indictive information on the variations of cost and quality of services in different regions of the state and country. This includes information on which doctors and hospitals are overcharging, overoperating, etc. Consumer council members will be able to spot which local PSROs are not doing their jobs.

6. Work with sympathetic lawyers to bring anti-discrimination suits against institutions' and federal agencies' practices in hiring, entrance into training programs, etc.

7. Watch-dog the local medical society and the state and national AMA; obtain copies of their financial statements and expose any questionable sources of money; reveal their stands not only on health care but on all social issues; monitor their involvement with all levels of PSROs.

WORK TOWARDS CONTROL OF THE HEALTH IN YOUR COMMUNITY AS A LONG-RANGE GOAL

1. Professionals: make your services available to low-income citizens; expose incompetent personnel who embarrass, abuse, and overcharge their patients; build solidarity with other health workers and the community by offering them technical assistance and by sharing skills and responsibilities, establishing non-hierarchical structures through health teams; get copies of proposals for current and future research otherwise unavailable to laypeople; expose research results that have been covered up.

2. prepare, on a community basis, your own health school admissions and core curriculum plans (send a copy to us); develop a model team-oriented health delivery program using salaried workers whose emphasis will be on primary and preventive health care, paid for on a sliding scale.

3. Formulate and propose city and state legislation to gain control over school admissions, professional licensure, accreditation, and research priorities. Use referendums to bring community issues to the whole community.

RESEARCH

Getting through most medical research publications requires a technical scientific background and a cup of strong coffee to figure out such basic questions as what was being studied, relevance of the work, how it was carried out and whether the work succeeded in its intent. People concerned with the procedures and direction of research but lacking science experience face the initial problem of obtaining medical journals (14,000 to chose from) and articles. Some can be found in local libraries, but local colleges and universities will probably have the most complete collection of publications.

Those planning action around objectionable research can find information on most of the past and current research in local institutions from the Public Relations or Public Information officers there. Ask for a description of all research projects currently underway, who is paying for it, and how much money is involved. A lot of institutions like to brag about this sort of thing, so if you conceal your real motivations, this information might be easier to get. If anyone tries to dissuade you from seeking this information, don't back down! If the research is federally funded, and if it does not carry some security classification, say the magic words "Freedom of Information Act" your open sesame to government information.

If the project is not covered by the Freedom of Information Act, or if it has a security classification, publicize this refusal or classification. This might raise the curiosity of others and might be enough publicity to open the door to what you want to know. Also work to build ties with sympathetic workers who may have access to "inside" information that researchers have "neglected" to mention in their results.

While none of the groups listed below are solely involved with watchdogging medical research, most have a liberal or radical perspective on science in general and may be helpful in providing information about questionable research.

SCIENTISTS AND ENGINEERS FOR SOCIAL AND POLITICAL ACTION (SESPA), 9 Walden St., Jamaica Plain, MA 02130, (617) 472-0642.

NATIONAL ACTION RESEARCH ON THE MILITARY-INDUSTRIAL COMPLEX (NARMIC), 112 S. 16th St., No. 1, Philadelphia, PA 19102, (215) 563-9372.

SANE, 318 Massachusetts Ave., NE, Washington, D.C. 20002, (202) 546-4868.

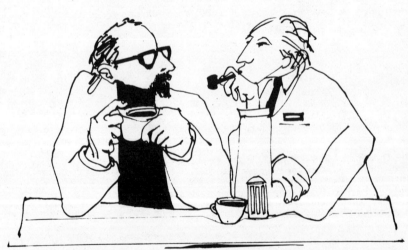

It's perfect really, it kills every living thing within 200 miles, without otherwise altering the ecological balance.

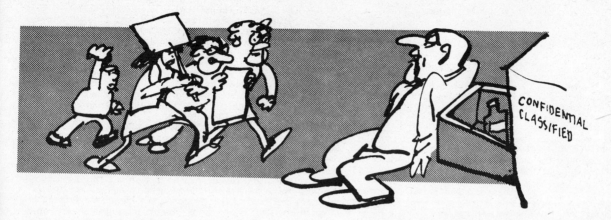

HASTINGS CENTER INSTITUTE OF SOCIETY, ETHICS, AND LIFE SCIENCE, 623 Warburton Ave., Hastings-on-Hudson, NY 10706, (914) 478-9764.

RESEARCH GROUP ON HUMAN EXPERIMENTATION, c/o Dr. Bernard Barber, Dept. of Sociology, Barnard College, New York, NY 10027, (212) 280-4359.

RESOURCES

BOOKS

<u>The University-Military-Police Complex,</u> North American Congress on Latin America, P.O. Box 226, Berkeley, CA 94701, 1970. 89 pp. $1.50
. . . is a well-documented, although somewhat outdated book which includes a directory of military research organizations, a survey of institutions working specifically in the area of chemical and biological warfare, and a review of the Law Enforcement Assistance Administration's 1969 research contracts, plus much more.

<u>The D.M.S. Marketing Intelligence Guide,</u> available by specific request from NARMIC, 160 W. 15th St., Philadelphia, PA 19102, 1974. (215) 563-9372
. . . is a very expensive, rarely available set of Defense Department listings of yearly civilian contracts on weapons research and military procurement. The set is divided into four sections: contracts by institutions, description of weapons systems, contracts in each county of the US, and electronics contracts.

PAMPHLETS AND ARTICLES

"CRITICAL LOOK AT HUMAN EXPERIMENTATION," Concerned Rush Medical Students, c/o Gordon Schiff, Box 106, 1743 W. Harrison, Chicago, IL 60612, March, 1974. 4 pp. Free
. . . a furious expose of the work of Dr. Sol Drugman who researched hepatitis cures by infecting retarded children at Willowbrook State School with the disease. Analyzes Krugman's actions in the perspective of "the modern medical school/teaching-research hospital complex" whose research priorities distort the health care system.

"Death, Doctors, and Defense," Howard Levy, <u>HEALTH/PAC BULLETIN</u>, 17 Murray St., New York, NY 10007, March 1972, pp. 10-14
. . . discusses the more than 10 year radiation study at the University of Cincinnati Medical Center, funded by the Department of Defense (DOD). The research, which aimed to "understand better the influence of radiation on the combat effectiveness of troops," was done primarily on poor Black people, all of whom were suffering from supposedly inoperable cancer. But DOD reports show that many of them were in relatively good health when the experimentation began and may not have been aware of the dangers involved in radiation exposure. "Of the total of 87 patients for whom complete reports are available, 21 (24%) died within 38 days."

"PREPARED STATEMENT FOR THE HOUSE SUB-COMMITTEE ON HEALTH HEARINGS, PROTECTION OF HUMAN SUBJECTS ACT", Bernard Barber. Available from author, c/o Department of Sociology, Barnard College, Columbia University, September 28, 1973. 6 pp. Free
. . .written from Barber's findings during two studies of biomedical research institutions using human subjects. He pleads strongly for government regulation of medical research since he has found that patients are often abused in research experiments, particularly "the ignorant, the poor and the ethnically despised."

"SOME 'NEW MEN OF POWER: THE CASE OF BIOMEDICAL RESEARCH SCIENTISTS," Bernard Barber, Dept. Sociology, Barnard College, Columbia University, New York, NY, January, 1970. 4 pp. Free
. . . points out that biomedical researchers involved in human experimentation are monitored by review committees that are ingrown, particularistic, and narrow in viewpoint. Barber calls for biomedical researchers from other institutions and sociological-legal-ethical experts on review committees, as well as better legislation.

PERIODICALS

<u>SCIENCE FOR THE PEOPLE,</u> SESPA, 9 Jamaica Plain, MA 02130. $10/year, includes membership to SESPA
. . . is a radical publication which analyses the role of science and technology in national and international politics. The magazine also serves to keep local SESPA chapters in touch, presents examples of activities useful to local groups, brings issues and information to the attention of the readers, and offers a forum for discussion.

<u>RECON,</u> P.O. Box 14602, Philadelphia, PA 19134. $3/year
. . . is a monthly newsletter on the US military machine. Radical in its perspective, Recon serves as a "people's moniter" of the Pentagon. Good for keeping abreast of the US progression in chemical-biological warfare.

PROFESSIONAL ORGANIZATIONS

In reaction to the racism of the health care system and how it affects both Third World workers and patients, a variety of organizations of Third World health personnel have formed. These tend to be more progressive than their White counterparts such as the AMA. They are concerned with things outside their professional self-interest like the social and political problems of obtaining health care for Third World people. They also work to unite Third World health personnel to destroy the economic and attitudinal barriers which have traditionally been used to keep minorities out of health careers.

Another kind of organization exists whose membership consists of liberal and radical health activists who are working both from the inside and the outside to create major political and economic change in health institutions and in society as a whole.

MEDICAL COMMITTEE FOR HUMAN RIGHTS . . . is a nationwide organization of professionals, students, community people, and activist health workers concerned with radical social change, especially in health related fields. Work is currently being done on industrial and prison health issues, mental health, patients' rights, and a national health plan. Chapters can be found in most major cities. (See also section on Health Planning and Financing). Contact National MCHR, PO Box 7155, Pittsburgh, PA 15213, (412) 682-1200.

WOMEN'S COALITION FOR POSITIVE ACTION (WCPA) . . . is composed of women employees—from housekeeping staff to those in top level positions—at New York City's Harlem Hospital, and "is in the process of toppling the hospital's (male) administrative echelon. . . in order to restructure and redirect the hospital's activities and services" to better serve the community which finances it. Supported by the National Black Feminist Organization and Manhattan Women's Political Caucus, the Coalition was recently formed in protest of the complete omission of women from the promotion list circulated by the hospital's director. At their insistence, the administration agreed that the screening committee for job applicants include 50% women, and that women be appointed to three top-level positions formerly held by men. Although they fulfilled the first demand and also hired a woman (from WCPA) as associate director, they have failed to act on the other two promised appointments, and WPCA is working with the Equal Employment Opportunities Commission to force them to follow through. Composed mostly of employees from the lower level of the health hierarchy, the Coalition is set on fighting elitism (both internal and external). Currently they are giving input into an affirmative action program to upgrade women and minority people, and are establishing a women-staffed rape crisis center at the hospital; they are also concerned with revamping the nursing school, instituting meaningful career ladders, setting up daycare centers, establishing a community preventive health care center, and basically reviewing "the men who have been in power for years." Contact: Women's Coalition for Positive Action, c/o Cecile Boatright, 354 West 123rd St., New York, NY 10027, (212) 865-6400.

STANFORD HEALTH WORKERS SUPPORT GROUP. . . is a significant example of professionals coordinating support among other staff for hospital workers' organizing efforts. Intentionally keeping a low-key, non-initiating profile, they are working with the United Stanford Employees to help them win bargaining power from the administration. This involves writing articles for the USE newspaper to share their technical knowledge on everything from HMO's to health insurance; supporting arbitration and other grievance procedures by providing assistance from their health collective to the union; and using their skills and status to give general support to workers' actions, such as providing them with medical certification for "sick-outs." Members of the group are also involved in individual research projects on the Chilean health system under Allende, a follow-up study on community organization resisting hospital expansion in Boston, and a study of private foundations in the health system. The latter focuses on how "such foundations provide continued financial support—in the form of investments and deposits—in financial institutions and corporations which are responsible for repressive actions in IndoChina, Latin America, and other parts of the Third World." Contact STANFORD HEALTH WORKERS SUPPORT GROUPS, c/o Howard Waitzkin, Department of Medicine, Stanford University Medical Center, Stanford, CA 94305, (415) 497-5906.

NATIONAL MEDICAL ASSOCIATION (NMA). . . is a predominantly Black organization of over 6,000 physicians which formed in 1895 in reaction to the racism of the AMA. While its structure of composite medical societies parallels that of the AMA, the NMA certainly takes a more progressive stand in health issues, especially those that affect low-income people. The Association's projects include a sickle cell anemia program, a recruitment program which aims to reach a minimum goal of 12% minority representation in medical schools, and the distribution of publications related to Black diseases. The JOURNAL is the official medical publication of the NMA. Contact: NATIONAL MEDICAL ASSOCIATION, 1717 Massachusetts Ave., N.W., Suite 602, Washington, D.C. 20036, (202) 462-4200.

CONCERNED CHICANO NURSES. . . active since 1969, is an angry group determined to make the LA community respond to Chicano health needs. Though they say it is like pulling teeth, they have effectively brought pressure to bear on university chancellors to admit more Chicanos and have demanded representation on minority advisory committees. In the county hospital, they have also managed to institute Spanish classes for staff, bilingual telephone operators and Spanish signs for patients. Major effort is directed a recruiting Spanish-speaking high school students into the health care professions. In addition, they hold workshops with other Third World groups on common issues, and publish a newsletter which acts as a clearinghouse for job opportunities. They are also working for curricular change in health schools which will gear itself to meeting Chicano's particular health needs and more public health needs in general. Highly frustrated with the present health care system, they hope to eventually organize their own Chicano nursing school. Contact: CONCERNED CHICANO NURSES, 2016 E. First St., P.O. Box 33407, Los Angeles, CA 90022, (213) 223-4021 (Pauline Dorsey).

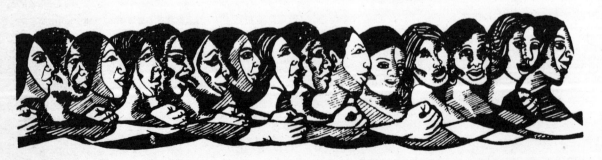

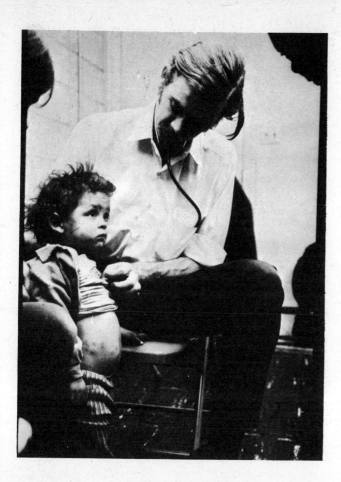

AMERICAN PUBLIC HEALTH ASSOCIATION. . . issued a national health care program which incorporates "consumer-majority policy-making boards at every level of administration" and provides for recruitment and support of racial/sexual/economic minorities who are largely excluded from many health careers. Recently APHA has been working around the issues of involuntary sterilization, eliminating lead-based paint poisoning, health conditions in prisons, biomedical experimentation on the institutionalized, community health education, breaking the monopolistic practices of Blue Cross/Shield, and getting recognition for "new professionals." Black, Chicano and Women's caucuses have all developed within APHA; at the 1973 convention the Black and Chicano caucuses took over the governing council, demanding representation on the policy-making committee. The organization publishes a monthly newspaper, THE NATION'S HEALTH, and an informative monthly magazine. Contact: AMERICAN PUBLIC HEALTH ASSOCIATION, 1015 18th St., NW, Washington, D.C. 20036, (202) 462-4200.

CREATIVE HEALTH SERVICES, Inc. . . . is a brand new independent corporation of nurses providing a whole range of health care for the middle class community. Services are prevention-oriented, from birth control and abortion counseling, to care of the chronically ill, hypnosis and gay counseling, and establishing occupational health and safety programs. Currently they are offering two courses, one of which deals with concepts of self-actualization; the other, "Our Bodies Ourselves," teaches women self-help and how to use the health system. Though a fee-for-service organization and presided over by a man (the other 15 are women), CHS offers an interesting example of non-physician-provided healing, counseling, and preventive care at moderate to low cost on a group practice model. Contact CREATIVE HEALTH SERVICES, INC., 4645 E. Colfax Ave., Denver, CO 80220, (303) 321-0567.

CALIFORNIA INDIAN NURSES ASSOCIATION. . . are working to bring more Indians into all nursing programs to help provide better health care to the Indian community. In contact with nursing schools around the state, they nominate students for scholarships, advertise available staff positions to the 200 Indian nurses they are in touch with, advise schools on recruitment of Indian students, and answer general requests. They hope to do high school recruiting, and help older nurses go back for more education. They encourage students to work on Indian summer projects and try to funnel nurses into the 23 Indian Health Programs in California. Contact: CALIFORNIA INDIAN NURSES ASSOCIATION, c/o Indian Health Unit, State Department of Health, 714 "P" St., Sacramento, CA 95814, (916) 322-2950.

ASSOCIATION OF SPANISH WORKERS IN HEALTH AND HOSPITALS IN NEW YORK CITY, INC. . . . has a membership of 2000 Spanish speaking health workers ranging from social workers and hospital administrators to orderlies and hospital housecleaners. Energy is currently devoted to publicizing the needs of Spanish speaking employees in 8 hospitals and encouraging on the job training and advancement. The Association strives to work closely with the hospital unions, while acting as an advocate for the needs of Spanish speaking workers. Contact: ASSOCIATION OF SPANISH WORKERS IN HEALTH AND HOSPITALS IN NEW YORK CITY, c/o Jose Maldonado, Gouverneur Hospital, Room 660, New York, NY 10002, (212) 374-4200.

COUNCIL OF BLACK NURSES. . . is a professional group of Black RN's working towards increasing the number of Black nurses, especially in policy-making positions, and towards improving health care to the LA Black community. Their major efforts are directed at recruitment and retention which involves sponsoring workshops and career days in high schools, giving tutorial help to individual students, helping nursing students prepare for the state board exams, providing limited scholarships, and helping to match up qualified Black people with education and job opportunities. Contact: COUNCIL OF BLACK NURSES, c/o Betty Williams, 5544 Summerholl Road, Los Angeles, CA 90043, (213) 825-0816.

NURSES NOW. . . is a national taskforce of the National Organization for Women; it helps nurses and women gain their rightful share of decision-making power in health care delivery. "Women in health care are under-represented (they comprise 75% of the health workforce) not because of a lack of qualified people but rather because those in power do not think it necessary to consult us." NN is rallying nurses to assert themselves. On a local level, NN has become a contact group for nurses who were harassed or fired for challenging poor hospital practices; they also lobbied at the state legislature and have been developing a short curriculum on "Trends in Nursing" to "carry the feminist message to young women who need alternatives to sexist teaching in schools of nursing." One of their members went as a delegate to the ANA convention to pressure that organization towards more forceful actions. Other work revolves around speaking and educating at nursing schools, conventions, and civic groups, spreading their ideas and fighting tremendous opposition from hospitals and administrators; they also aim to work with other feminists in solving health care problems. For $.50 they offer a fine consciousness-raising packet on nursing and feminism, including a bibliography of helpful articles and instructions for starting an NN group. Contact NURSES NOW, P.O. Box 5156, Pittsburgh, PA 15206, (412) 683-2670.

NORMAN BETHUNE COLLECTIVE.... formed out of the old Student Health Organization in 1971, and is named after one of the heroes of the Chinese revolution. The collective consists of politically active nurses and doctors in the Detroit area who are trying to develop within themselves a racism- and sexism-free consciousness while organizing for radical change in the availability of health care. Their work has centered around the Detroit General Hospital because it is there that they find the sharpest contradiction between the technical possibilities and the actual quality of care. Collective members spend much of their time in discussions with medical students at Wayne State University where they hold Community Medicine seminars which cover such things as collective lifestyles, health care in the US, the drug industry, the role of the physician, the profit motive, and the students' career future. A bi-weekly speakers program has also begun which deals with similarly important topics. The collective's newsletter is distributed to students and hospital workers. They are also trying to set up weekly meetings among all the workers in each ward to discuss how service can be improved. Contact NORMAN BETHUNE COLLECTIVE', 206 Salem, Highland, MI 48203, (313) 883-3684.

ASSOCIATION OF AMERICAN INDIAN PHYSICIANS... aids in the recruitment, counseling, placement and financing of Native Americans for health careers. The AAIP's work is similar to National Chicano Health Organization. Contact AAIP, 721 NE 14th St., Oklahoma City, OK 73104, (405) 235-5862.

BAY AREA BLACK NURSES ASSOCIATION... organized in 1969 because they felt the official nursing organizations weren't addressing themselves to the problems of Black nurses and patients—career mobility, recuitment and training of more Black nurses, and sensitivity to Black community interests and lifestyles. With the Council of Black Nurses in Los Angeles, they sponsored a conference and to make Black nurses in the state aware that they were all grappling with the same problem. Since then this activist BNA chapter has been involved in community projects such as health fairs, recruiting in health schools to get minority students into health careers, pressuring for increased Black enrollment in nursing schools and acting as patient advocates for community people. Recently they received a grant to establish a minority student counseling center which will formalize much of the work they've been doing all along—helping student challenge the racist faculty, giving them emotional support, and tutoring them with academic work. They realize that overall they have been doing a lot of what the nursing schools themselves should be doing, and they are working with Black doctors to pressure these administrators to be more accountable. Contact BAY AREA BLACK NURSES ASSOCIATION, c/o Margaret Jordan, 2122 Junciton, El Cerrito, CA 94530; or write BNA clearinghouse for local chapters, c/o Lauranne Sans, Dean, Tuskegee Institute, Tuskegee, AL 36088, (205) 727-8011.

COUNCIL OF HEALTH ORGANIZATIONS (COHO)... is a loose connection of activist organizations representing health professionals, workers and other groups interested in health issues. Its main purpose is to facilitate the exchange of information on individual projects. COHO has also worked to bring suit against the National Institutes of Health for their shoddy safeguards on psychosurgery, and representatives have been sent to testify before several congressional hearings. Public statements, for example, denouncing the Indochina War, are also issued upon concensus of all groups. A current project has been to locate jobs for Chilean health workers who have fled their country or who must have jobs guaranteed before they can leave. Contact COUNCIL OF HEALTH ORGANIZATIONS. c/o Physician's Forum, 510 Madison Ave., New York, NY 10022, (212) 688-3290. PHYSICIAN'S FORUM has an orientation similar to COHO's, as does PHYSICIANS FOR SOCIAL REPSPONSIBILITY, P.O. Box 8804, Boston, MA 02144.

NEW HUMAN SERVICES INSTITUTE... acts as a resource on new careers programs throughout the country, offers over 150 publications, including bibliography, and a funding guide. Contact: NEW HUMAN SERVICES INSTITUTE, 184 Fifth Ave., New York, NY 10010, (212) 924-4777.

RESOURCES

BOOKS

<u>One Life, One Physician: An Inquiry into the Medical Profession's Performance in Self-Regulation,</u> Robert S. McCleery, MD, and others. Public Affairs Press, 419 New Jersey Ave., S.E., Washington, D.C. 20003. 1971. 167 pp. $5.00
... a Ralph Nader Project report on the affect of self-regulatory controls on the quality of health care, concluding that the medical profession does not merit the trust of society and that a patient cannot be reasonably sure s/he is receiving quality care. Recommends the establishment of a National Board of Medicine.

<u>THE MEDICAL OFFENDERS,</u> Howard and Martha Lewis, Simon and Schuster, 630 5th Ave., New York, NY 10020, 1970. 377 pp. $7.95
...documents the vulnerability of patients in the hands of their doctors, many of whom are prone to performing unnecessary surgery, fee splitting and profiteering. The book is a good one for destroying the myth of the infallible, ethical physician, but is limited in its reformist views. Suggests opening licensing boards to public review, barring physicians from owning pharmacies and drug companies, and overhauling emergency care system.

<u>Women in White,</u> Geoffrey Marks and William K. Beatty. Charles Scribner's Sons, 597 5th Ave., New York, NY 10017, 1972. 240 pp. $6.95
... a collection of brief histories of important women in medicine. Good for background information.

PAMPHLETS AND ARTICLES

"THE HEALTH PROFESSIONALS: CURE OR CAUSE OF THE HEALTH CARE CRISIS," David Hapgood, available from Louise Rice, 65 Chestnut St., Cambridge, MA 02139, June 1969. 7 pp. $.30
...points out the dangerous absurdity of permitting the health industry to regulate itself and the crisis situation which has resulted. In every state, licensing boards are controlled by doctors. As Hapgood points out, "No industrial lobbyist in Washington, even in his most fevered dreams would dare imagine such bliss. Very good introductory material.

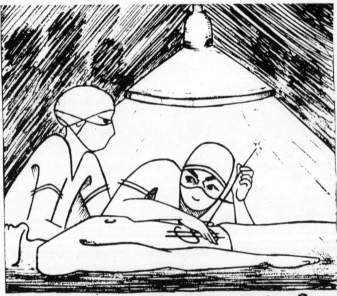

interesting operation doctor? no just a routine sendachectomy.

"Getting By With A Little Help From Our Friends," Barbara and Al Haber, available from Louise Rice, 65 Chestnut St., Cambridge, MA 02139, 1967. 11 pp. $.44.
. . . asserts the value of radical political work in the professions. The Habers advocate organizing to fight the power structure of institutions where radical professionals work, and fighting to challenge the way the profession is practiced, through alternative models such as free clinics.

"The Patient Auction Block," Roger Rapoport, NEW TIMES, 1 Park Ave., New York, NY 10007, January 11, 1974. pp. 19-22.
. . . a sickening account of doctors who sell patients to southern California corporate or doctor-owned hospitals. As a result of overbuilding by profit-oriented medical entrepreneurs, one-third of Los Angeles County's 32,230 hospital beds are empty. "The biggest suppliers own or operate private emergency rooms from which they divert patients to hospitals for cash."

PACKET ON ANTI-AMA PROTESTS, Quentin Young et al, available from Louise Rice, 65 Chestnut St., Cambridge, MA 02139, 1969-1971. 11 pp. $.44
. . . includes "Welcome to Chicago," by Quentin Young, 1970; "American Murder Association," by Richard Kunnes, 1969; statements by Oliver Fein and others to the AMA conference, 1969; and "chapter Takes on AMA," from HEALTH RIGHTS NEWS, 1971. For the most part, the articles are good. Oliver Fein's statement is valuable for its listing of six major ways the AMA has contributed to the current crisis in health delivery.

"The Nursing Profession: Condition Critical," Trucia D. Kushner, MS., 370 Lexington Ave., New York, NY 10017, August 1973. pp. 72-77, 99-102
. . . describes the lowly position of nurses in the medical field. "The hospital system has exploited the nursing profession, used its cheap productivity, and ignored its craving for dignity and respect. And because of insecurity, lack of money and lack of political power, the profession has cooperated." The article includes some disgusting quotes from doctors talking about nurses and provides a good general overview of problems in nursing.

"Sex Discrimination: Nursing's Most Pervasive Problem," Virginia Cleland, AMERICAN JOURNAL OF NURSING, 10 Columbus Circle, New York, NY 10019, August 1971. pp. 1542-1547
. . . an excellent article, exposing the myth of nursing autonomy and documenting numerous examples of sexism in medicine. Leadership in nursing is "weak and unimaginative" since "administrative positions. . .are available only with the approval of the male systems in medicine, hospital administration, and high education." Dr. Cleland calls for courageous and outspoken leaders who will improve the lot of nurses and demand a greater part in making decisions that affect the profession.

"WOMEN IN HOSPITALS: WORKING FOR THE MAN," Amy Brodkey and Gale Grumbles, available from Louise Rice, 65 Chestnut St., Cambridge, MA 02139, March, 1972. 4 pp. $.20
. . . discusses the worker hierarchy in hospitals, and the lack of advancement opportunity. Often the patients suffer when powerless women workers have no outlet for their hostilities towards arrogant male doctors. The article points out that union organizing may be only a partial solutuion for women since the unions themselves tend towards male domination.

. . . Another social worker described one of her most important tasks as the education of doctors to enlighten them about the conditions of extended care facilities. She took residents on field trips to the state hospital's geriatric wards to which many patients were discharged. The medical supervision tried to st stop the trips because they objected to 'upsetting' young doctor doctors by exposing them to the horrible conditions to which they would be sending patients . . .
—Health/PAC Bulletin, Sept. '70

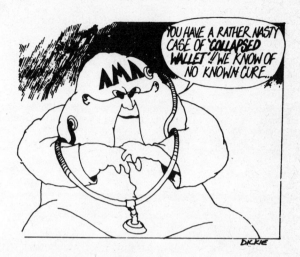

YOU HAVE A RATHER NASTY CASE OF 'COLLAPSED WALLET'! WE KNOW OF NO KNOWN CURE...

HEALTH/PAC BULLETIN, 17 Murray St., New York, NY 10007, January, 1972. $.60. pp. 1-16
. . . expounds the theory that non-professional hospital workers must take the lead in institutional organizing. This crucial issue explores the relationship between professionals and non-rofessionals in the context of efforts to improve patient care and work conditions at Lincoln Hospital. These efforts have come from a number of sources between 1969 and 1972. Three groups, the Young Lords Party, the Health Revolutionary Movement, and Think Lincoln (a coalition of professional and nonprofessional hospital workers) occupied the Administration building over the firing of mental health workers. The Young Lords and HRUM also set up a heroin de-tox program in the Administration building. And the Lincoln Collective of doctors from Pediatrics, Medicine and Psychiatry, has worked to break down job hierarchies, give support to workers, and provide more continuous care to the community. Although the Collective has gone through many changes since this article, the analysis of its problems and accomplishments is invaluable to radical professionals. Perhaps the hardest and most essential concept for the Collective to accept was the attitude of Third World workers and community people towards professionals: "Their role is to serve the people with their technical skills in human ways. We know what class they're coming from. They must understand that they are the weakest link." An important resource.

"Hospital Workers: A Case Study In The 'New Working Class'", Barbara and John Ehrenreich, NEW REPUBLIC, 1244 19th St., NW, Washington, D.C. 20036. January, 1973, pp. 13-26
. . . analyzes the structure of job classifications in hospitals with a clarity and shrewdness typical of the Ehrenreichs' fine work. The hospital benefits from the "class and caste antagonisms that are bound to arise between the allied professionals and the workers."

"Health: Women's Work", Susan Reverby, HEALTH/PAC BULLETIN, 17 Murray St., New York, NY 10007, April 1972. pp. 15-20
. . . discusses the place of women in the health field, specifically the role of nurses. Concludes that "to achieve job control, status, decent wages and some measure of job fulfillment professional workers must join with health workers at all levels in a struggle which would make these goals possible for all."

"WITCHES, MIDWIVES, and NURSES: A HISTORY OF WOMEN HEALERS," Barbara Ehrenreich and Deirdre English, Glass Mountain Pamphlets, P.O. Box 238, Oyster Bay, NY 11771. 45 pp. $.75
. . . explores women's role in medicine from witch-craft to the nursing profession. Especially revealing is the description of the US medical scene in the early 19th century. Folk-healers, midwives, and other lay practitioners, who in most cases knew as much or more than any formally trained "regular" doctors, were legally prohibited from practicing. Ironically, there "was no body of medicine to be trained in," but the "regular" doctors soon completely dominated the medical field. The authors stress the need for women health workers and consumers of today to combat the privilege and sexism of the medical profession. A fresh and revolutionary perspective on medical history.

The interview of a Boston University School of Medicine Student for an internship at a Boston University teaching hospital last year included detailed questions about her method of contraception, rather than her plans for a career and her goals as a physician; this hospital has not had a woman intern for years.
—"Women Interns and Residents,"
Leah M. Lowenstein, MD

"THE DOCTOR-NURSE GAME," Leonard I. Stein, available from Louise Rice, 65 Chestnut St., Cambridge, MA 02139. January 1968. 5 pp. $.15
. . . is a fascinating, yet disturbing article exposing the demeaning and repressive games that preserve male dominance in the medical field. For example, it would be a direct threat to the doctor's authority if the nurse were to make a direct recommendation. So instead of saying, "Doctor, I recommend a retention enema for Mr. Brown," she must say, "A retention enema has proven effective in the past," or something equally non-committal.

"Social Workers: Keeping the Pieces Together," Michael Smuler and Connie Epstein, HEALTH/PAC BULLETIN, 17 Murray St., New York, NY 10007, September, 1970, pp. 11-12
. . . "The human needs which cannot be disregarded, suppressed, channeled, and controlled by the routine procedure for compartmentalizing people's health needs are turned over to the social work staff."

PSRO: DOCTOR ACCOUNTABILITY OR CONSUMER DISASTER, Robert E. McGarrah, Jr., Patricia Kenney, Leda R. Judd, Health Research Group, 2000 P St. NW, Washington, D.C. 20036, 1973. 14 pp. Free
. . .factual information on the Professional Standards Review Organization (PSRO), set up "to review doctor's payment requests under Medicare and Medicaid." The purpose of this article is to give the public the information necessary to "demand full implementation of the legislation's limited public accountability requirements."

PERIODICALS

CONSUMER CLEARINGHOUSE FOR PSRO ACTION, Health Research Group, 2000 "P" St., NW, Washington, D.C. 20036. $1/year
. . . is a quarterly newsletter which details developments in the government's PSRO (Professional Standards Review Organizations) policies and gives accounts of what communities and consumers are doing to gain some control in the PSROs. The Clearinghouse also describes efforts of the AMA and other monopolistic groups to amend and repeal sections of PSRO legislation.

Today one finally has the right and even the duty to be, above all things, a revolutionary doctor . . . But now the old questions reappear: How does one actually carry out a work of social welfare? How does one unite individual endeavor with the needs of society? We must review again each of our lives, what we did and thought as doctors, or in any function of public health, before the revolution. We must do this with profound critical zeal and arrive finally at the conclusion that almost everything we thought and felt in that past period ought to be deposited in an archive, and a new type of human being created . . .
—Che Guevara

STUDENT ORGANIZATIONS

Organizing has not reached major proportions among health science students; radicals don't usually get admitted in the first place and the few students that are concerned with real change must maintain a hectic, high-pressure classroom and study schedule which barely allows for any type of non-academic activity. Many professional groups have student counterparts with varying degrees of commitment to change.

The late sixties and early seventies saw the student health movement blossom with the Student Health Organization (SHO), which was dedicated to political change. Nationally, SHO attempted to initiate community-controlled summer education and service projects, like patient advocacy programs and screening programs in poor urban and rural areas. But SHO students gradually realized that these projects let health institutions off the hook, by fulfilling what should be the institutions' responsibilities while improving poor people's images of the health professions and medical schools. Their response to this predicament was to turn to direct political action in the institutions themselves: preventing medical school expansion at the expense of neighborhood housing (Mission Hill near Harvard), demanding increased minority admissions and financial aid (Philadelphia), and forcing teaching hospitals to be more responsive to patient needs (Columbia). While only a few organizations still use the SHO title, a number of student groups continue with a similar spirit.

In contrast to the SHO, the Student American Medical Association (SAMA) presents a credo of "Concern, Commitment, and Action," while actually limiting itself to obtaining discounts on insurance, accommodations at the local Hilton and Ramada Inn, and Chrysler automobiles. SAMA offers preceptorships in Appalachian areas, but participants are assigned only to areas lacking community organizing and seldom return to practice in this part of the country after completing training. From its traditional stand on professional roles to the drug company ads in its magazine, "The New Physician," SAMA is little more than an adolescent AMA.

Most of the following groups are currently working in three general areas: reforming admissions and curriculum, exposing vested interests as well as sexist and racist policies in health institutions, and educating themselves and their communities in social and political factors affecting health. Some student groups do community service and free clinic work on the side, while other groups make this type of activity their main focus.

CONCERNED RUSH HEALTH STUDENTS. . . have been battling the dual standard of health care for "public" patients and "private" patients at Rush Presbyterian St. Luke's Medical Center. The predominantly Black "public" patients receive rushed care, segregated into older buildings, and are used for the teaching of medical students and house staff. CRHS focused on the treatment inadequacies in the OB-GYN department by initiating a weekly lunchtime series of speakers and discussions, called "The People's Grand Rounds." They dealt with institutional racism, sexism, and alternatives to institutional care for OB-GYN patients; this brought a strong positive response from the hospital's workers. Two public forums were also organized for people to publicly vent their frustration and anger about the center's practices. Other CRHS projects include organizing resistance to drug industries, setting up an information and literature table in

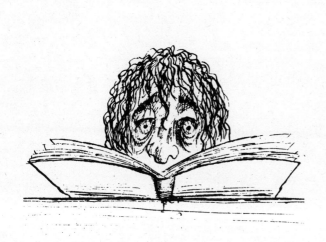

and administration, the collective members have not been successful in generating the support required to force the administration to act on their demands, but the administration may tokenly concede to some of the collective's demands through minor student representation on the admissions committee. Their model curriculum, "THE PROGRAM IN BIOSOCIAL MEDICINE," is aimed at primary care and community medicine; it has been published and is available for $.75 (55 pp.). Contact HARVARD BIO-SOCIAL CURRICULUM COLLECTIVE, 12 Parker Hill Ave., No. 1, Roxbury, MA 02120, (617) 566-4971.

STUDENT HEALTH COALITION at Vanderbilt University . . . was created in 1968 to work with rural and urban communities and help them meet their health care needs. This has involved responding to invitations to sponsor 26 summer health fairs in Tennessee, Kentucky and Virginia, which reached 17,000 people. Afterwards two students remain in each community to give support on follow-up projects, steering clear of a decision-making role. The Coalition tries to maintain contact with the communities and makes resources available, while imposing a policy of non-reliance between students and community. Emphasis is also placed on non-medical problems which affect health, such as helping people get Medicaid/care cards, cleaning up impure streams, working with anti-strip mining coalitions, and other local community groups. Students from the humanities (including law) as well as from the sciences form the coalition, which is student directed, planned, and implemented. So far, it has offered a different kind of educational experience to over 400 students. According to a student survey, this experience strongly influenced the career plans of many of its participants. Other concrete results of coalition activities include the addition of 3 courses to the university curriculum related to the needs and objectives of the coalition and the transference of skills, such as grant-writing, to local community groups necessary for the preservation of their autonomy. In addition, 15 of the 18 communities they've worked with have started their own health councils, and 12 of the councils are operating health clinics. In 1970, the Coalition helped create the Center for Health Services, which acts as a funding umbrella for the Coalition's and other student/community projects. Administered by a student/faculty/community board, the center establishes guidelines which must be met by all projects to preserve the integrity of the community and foster community involvement. Contact: STUDENT HEALTH COALITION, c/o Center for Health Services, Station 17, Vanderbilt Medical Center, Nashville, TN 37232, (615) 322-4773.

OTHER END OF THE SPECULUM . . . brings together women medical students to talk about feminism and to deal with the problems women face in obtaining and providing health care. With a focus on general feminist politics, they have also initiated discussions with doctors and hospital staff about the sexist treatment of women patients and employees, particularly in the OB-GYN Department. The group published a women's issue of the student newspaper, SYNAPSE, that covered both women in medical careers, and specific female health problems. They feel they've made male med students aware of feminist issues, but have yet to make them sensitive. Contact OTHER END OF THE SPECULUM, 858 Clayton St., San Francisco, CA 94117, (415) 661-8042.

the hospital, fighting racism and sexism in medical education, and exposing callous practices in research and human experimentation. Contact CONCERNED RUSH HEALTH STUDENTS, c/o Gordon Shiff, Box 106, 1743 W. Harrison, Chicago, IL 60612, (312) 733-5151, ext. 157.

A 36 year old Black Portuguese female was admitted for sterilization. According to the medical student, there was a discussion on teaching rounds with a senior resident as to "whether they could 'get' a vaginal hysterectomy 'out' of this case. . . ."
Student: Why is tubal ligation the last choice?
Resident: We want the teaching experience. . . She's 36 and doesn't need her uterus.

Quoted by Jonathan Kozol, Ramparts

SHOT IN THE ARM. . . is an organization of politically active medical students at the University of California, San Francisco, that works to unify the students while exposing some of the myths of medicine through rap sessions with new students, and a booklet on the detrimental consequences of professionalism. Their ability to force the faculty to adopt a pass-fail grading system by organizing the students to leave their names off exam answer sheets seems to indicate a wide student support for them. In another project, Shot in the Arm people have been working with the Prison Law Collective in collecting evidence for a class action suit against San Quentin Prison. Some members have also been working with the United Farm Workers in providing clinical aid. Future activities may include organizing a brigade to health workers to visit Cuba. Contact SHOT IN THE ARM, 850 Clayton St. San Francisco, CA 94117, (415) 661-8042.

HARVARD BIO-SOCIAL CURRICULUM COLLECTIVE. . . is a group of Third World medical students at Harvard Medical School who came together for the purpose of challenging the school's administration and organized students around the social-political aspects of medicine. The Collective recognized that students who appear to be a threat to the traditional role of the physician are usually screened out of medical school in the admissions process. Thus, they demanded changes at Harvard that centered around student control of admissions and curriculum, as a means of establishing a broad power base from which admissions could be opened up. Pressured to maintain their studies, and harassed by the faculty

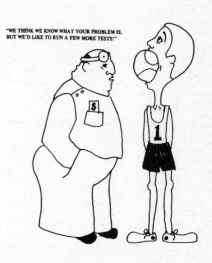

"WE THINK WE KNOW WHAT YOUR PROBLEM IS, BUT WE'D LIKE TO RUN A FEW MORE TESTS!"

CONCERNED NURSES CAUCUS... of the Student Nurses Association of California (SNAC) was organized two years ago by students who felt SNAC wasn't meeting their needs. They now have several members on the SNAC board to make it more responsive, and have active chapters in Los Angeles, San Francisco and San Diego. They have fought against nursing schools who are trying to decrease enrollment, and who are discriminating against radical students, those of racial minorities, and others who don't conform. They marched 500 strong in Sacramento to protest the California Nursing Association's bill which made individual nurses pay for mandatory continuing education; in addition, they received a great deal of publicity for their march in Los Angeles to alert the public to cutbacks in nursing programs and understaffing in hospitals, which they feel directly affects patient care. At a recent SNAC convention they sponsored a range of resolutions which were passed; that SNAC defend students' rights by pushing for joint grievance committees of students and faculty; that nursing school populations proportionally reflect the state racial population; that curriculums cover the health care of all people, not just the White middle class; that the employer be responsible for release time and cost for their continuing education; that SNAC support minimum staffing standards in hospitals; and that when workers strike, SNAC support the students' refusal to take over their jobs. Contact CONCERNED NURSES CAUCUS, c/o Barbara Hertz, 1908 Charnwood, Alhambra, CA 91803, (213) 223-5236.

. . . And I've had my fill of putting it to blacks. I learned to draw blood on old black ladies. I learned to do pelvics on young black women. I learned to do histories and physicals on black bodies and on a few wrinkled and run down white ones. . . Medical barbarism. . . it permeates hospital life. Needless tests, justified on educational and experimental bases. Poorly supervised procedures, repetitive examinations. . . Endless technical discussions at the bedside, the patient excluded except for necessary information, a piece of meat to be thumped and prodded and exposed. . . all in the name of high quality, scientific care. It's a farce. And a drag, and it's brutal. That's why I'm leaving. . . .

—from an open letter to the Deans of the University of Pennsylvania School of Medicine, by a 3rd year med student

STUDENT HEALTH PROGRAM FOR MIGRANT FARM WORKERS AND RURAL POOR... brings together over 45 multidisciplinary health students to live and work from October to May in rural Colorado communities which have a high influx of migrant workers. Medical, nursing, dental, nutrition, nurse practitioner, and physician's assistant students provide free screening and testing services to the children of migratory and rural families in morning clinics; evenings and weekends are devoted to clinics for adults. The program follows up these services with educational and self-help workshops, and teaches the students community health skills in the administration of medical needs and in analyzing health systems within rural communities. Contact STUDENT HEALTH PROJECT FOR MIGRANT FARM WORKERS AND RURAL POOR c/o Dr. Stephen Barnet, University of Colorado Medical Center, Container 2582, Denver, CO 80220, (303) 394-8740.

STUDENT NATIONAL MEDICAL ASSOCIATION... is an "association of minority students in pursuit of medical education. . . which will equip them with knowledge and skills to provide quality care to minority and disadvantaged people." Through its organization of 97 chapters at medical schools across the country, SNMA distributes information relative to minority problems and education. Special SNMA programs include a preceptorship program which gives its members experience in both ghetto and rural health delivery, a sickle cell anemia program, and a national study on minority women in medicine. Contact STUDENT NATIONAL MEDICAL ASSOCIATION, 2109 E St., NW, Washington, D.C. 20037, (202) 337-4550.

BLACK STUDENT ORGANIZATION... brings together Black students at Tufts University Medical and Dental Schools in an advisory and support organization. Committees have been established to work on a variety of projects ranging from talking with Black undergrad pre-medical students at Tufts to getting medical students to live with and help the residents in a housing development for the elderly. The organization has also arranged a special orientation for new Black students and have set up a program of rotations in community clinics in Black neighborhoods. Contact Black Student Organization, Tufts Medical and Dental Schools, 136 Harrison Ave., Boston, MA 02111

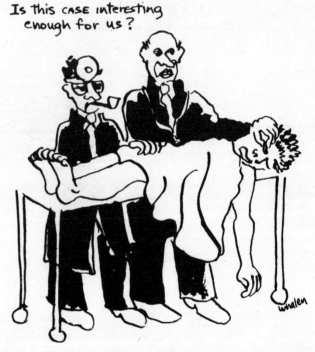

Is this case interesting enough for us?

COUNCIL FOR HEALTH INTERDISCIPLINARY PARTICIPATION/UNIVERSITY OF MINNESOTA... is one of the most active CHIP chapters in the country. Their main activity is in community projects, two of the most successful being drug and VD education projects in the state high schools. CHIP's multi-media shows and rap sessions in these two areas have been well-received, and the students are constantly invited back. They also initiated a recruitment program for Black and Native American high school students which the University has since adopted on a city-wide basis. A CHIP experimental course on health teams training was so successful that the University agreed to institute it as part of the curriculum. The University is also giving credit for a CHIP-initiated course on counseling in birth control and family planning clinics. Students have been involved in a wide number of additional projects, from working in free clinics, to providing health care at Wounded Knee trials in St. Paul, and publishing a monthly newsletter. Their campus/community credibility is high, and they serve on university policy-making committees with full voting privileges. Contact COUNCIL FOR HEALTH INTERDISCIPLINARY PARTICIPATION, University of Minnesota Health Sciences Center, Minneapolis, MN 55455, (612) 373-8969.

BLACK MEDICAL STUDENTS' ASSOCIATION... was organized to give academic and emotional support to Third World medical students at St. Louis University. Through its pressure, Black student enrollment has increased from two students in the school to the present total of 40. BMSA has two representatives on the admissions committee and hopes to raise the Black population of the school to 20%. To prepare incoming Black students for the culture shock of medical school and to expose them to successful and politically aware Black medical students, BMSA has initiated a summer orientation program. There is a tutorial program to aid these students once they begin classes, and upperclass members donate old books to lower level students to cut down on costs. BMSA has gone into St. Louis Black and other Third World communities to do sickle-cell and hypertension counseling and screening, and to discuss public health issues. Contact BLACK MEDICAL STUDENTS' ASSOCIATION, 1402 S. Grant, St. Louis, MO 63104, (314) 534-5206.

STUDENT NATIONAL DENTAL ASSOCIATION... is dedicated to increasing minority representation in dentistry; membership is open to anyone willing to work for this goal. Presently 12 of the 56 dental schools in this country have no minority students—and whereas the ratio of White dentists to the White population is 1:3,000, the corresponding minority ratio is 1:12,500. Though less than two years old, SNDA has 24 chapters around the country and national recognition has already given them some power to effect curricular change and improve recruitment/retention on their respective campuses. Contact STUDENT NATIONAL DENTAL ASSOCIATION, c/o Howard University College of Dentistry, Washington, D.C. 20001, (202) 636-6400.

RESOURCES

PAMPHLETS AND ARTICLES

"The Enterprising Medical Middle: Student AMA," Robert Richter, HEALTH/PAC BULLETIN, 17 Murray St., New York, NY, 10007, Sept., 1970. 5 pp.
... this article, prefaced by an excellent editorial on professionalism, gives a history of SAMA, "the world's largest and richest student professional organizations," and analyzes the reasons behind SAMA's tendency to provide superficial answers to complex problems.

"THIS IS YOUR LIFE, A PREVIEW OF MED SCHOOL," Shot in the Arm, 858 Clayton St., San Francisco 94117. 15 pp. free
... honest and personalized perspective on med schools, a kind of warning for the newly enrolled student with radical views. The pamphlet also includes the account of a third year med student who has found strength and support in a collective of other political conscious medical students.

"ALTERNATIVES FACING THE RADICAL IN MEDICINE," Ollie and Charlotte Fein, available from Louise Rice, 65 Chestnut St. Cambridge, MA 02139, 1964. 2 pp. $.08
... good but limited perspective on the political value of organizing a neighborhood clinic. Written when the authors were interns, the article raises some important issues on radical opportunities for doctors.

"LOOKING INTO HEALTH CARE," Candy Alt Crowley, Student American Pharmaceutical Association, 2215 Constitution Ave., NW, Washington, D.C. 20037, 1974. 21 pp. Free
... discusses the National Student Conference of Health Manpower held in March, 1972, focusing on interprofessional cooperation and minority health care problems, "especially the recruitment and retention of minorities in the health sciences." The report discusses how health teams can improve patient care. The Third World section is extremely worthwhile, concentrating on Chicanos and Native Americans.

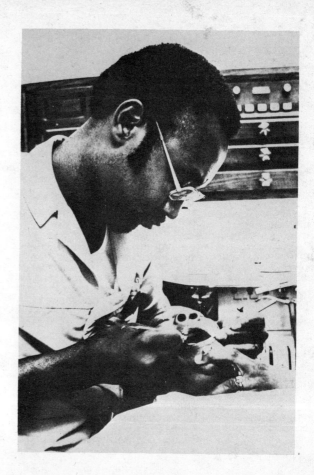

"THE AMERICAN STUDENT DENTAL ASSOCIATION (ASDA) COMMUNITY HEALTH MANUAL, A GUIDE FOR ESTABLISHING DENTAL HEALTH FACILITIES," ASDA, 211 East Chicago Ave., Chicago, IL 60611, 1972. 40 pp. Free
... a how-to guide covering many basic aspects of planning, implementing and running community dental health clinics. Though written for dental students, it has general application for any groups establishing community projects, emphasizing meeting a community's cultural needs, and insuring that the project will be continued once the students are gone. Covers potential funding sources, how to write grant proposals, and guidelines for delivering care. The list of resources (available separately from ASDA) includes helpful material for those working in urban and rural communities.

Twenty-five million American people are presently without a tooth in their heads... Twenty-four out of twenty-five young children suffer some form of dental disease by the time they reach school age... Nine out of ten people reaching the age of sixty today will not have any teeth of their own.

—The Tooth Trip

"CATALOG OF DENTAL HEALTH PROJECTS," Jack Tenenbaum, Committee on Community Health, American Student Dental Association, 211 East Chicago Ave., Chicago, IL 60611, 1972-3. 40 pp. Free
... provides information on over 80 community projects initiated and run by dental students in conjunction with communities around the country. These include working with migrants, Native Americans, prisoners, mental patients, the deaf, and communes; services range from sponsoring career days in high schools to mobile screening and teaching preventive dentistry, in addition to providing direct dental services.

**"ALTERNATIVES TO STANDARD PHARMACY PRAC-
TICE,"** Student American Pharmaceutical Association,
2215 Constitution Ave., NW, Washington, D.C. 20037,
1973. 30 pp. $1.00
. . .lists opportunities available in non-standard forms of pharmacy practice. Includes a nationwide list of free clinics and
drug information centers, and a list of excellent periodicals
which describe alternative health care positions. This report
represents an unusual direction for student professional organizations, although it sticks to service-oriented programs
and neglects to mention cooperative pharmacies, or suggestions for the student to create his/her own pharmacist's role.

"Doctors Dilemma: Doctors' Organizations," Fitzhugh Mullan,
HEALTH RIGHTS NEWS, 542 S. Dearborn St., Chicago, IL
60605, March 1972. pp. 4
. . .brief but important analysis of the two prevalent trends
in medical student organizations: interns and residents committees seeking better pay and fringe benefits, and groups focusing on progressive forms of health delivery, such as free
clinics and community medicine residencies. The author believes that both trends fail to promote true, radical change.
Concludes that the Lincoln Collective and house staff association at Cook County Hospital are examples of the small
groups of house staff collectives that are challenging "the notion of a pristine health service education," working for basic
changes in the health care system.

PERIODICALS

SYNAPSE, Synapse Publication Board, University of California, San Francisco, CA 94143. $3.00/year
. . . is one of the best health science school newspapers. Written by students, Synapse covers an incredibly wide range of
topics, from a rebuttal against racist genetic theories, to the
dreadful health conditions at a California prison, the ominous
plans for a psychosurgery center in the state, and student support of a faculty member denied tenure. Special issues are
also published, including ones on Women's Health and Chicano Health.

TRAINING

In a field which includes over 125 recognized occupations
and 250 specializations of these, the corresponding training
programs are "suffering profusely from lack of coordination."
They not only overlap, but are usually too long, expensive
and theoretically rather than practically oriented. General
trends are moving towards even greater specialization, further reinforcing the segmentation of health care delivery.
Many workers have been forced to be so preoccupied with
credentials and pretensions of professionalism, that they're
becoming over-trained. Efforts to implement new training
concepts that will radically change this situation rather than
reinforce it are difficult because of the control of the AMA
over licensure of workers and accreditation of training. The
long educational routes presently necessary to gain job credentials are in large part responsible for the personnel shortages. This is infuriating not only to consumers, who suffer
from the resulting low quality care, but especially to those
who want to enter the health field but lack access to the
training. Neither is the government of much assistance—
afraid of "oversupply", Nixon just cut the '75 health wo/
manpower training budget by nearly $200 million, which
has all but erased most federally funded training programs.
Though some token efforts have been made, such as "shortening" programs from four years to three, (this just means
going to school all year round), admissions are still tightly
controlled; generally curriculums are dry, intimidating and
highly pressurized.

Nursing is an especially fragmented field, including nearly 20
different types of programs. Many of the nursing diploma
schools are now closing because of their inability to compete
with degree-granting programs of community colleges. In
many cases, however, the training in diploma schools has been
far more clinically useful than the college nursing courses,
which are geared more towards administrative skills.

One of the worst aspects of nursing training in general is the
molding process. Some schools go so far as to discriminate
admittance policies against those who are overweight or otherwise fail to conform to the "attractive female" image. Activist and Third World students particularly are the victims of
the "flunk-out policy" of many schools, which intentionally
admit more students than they can handle. Those lacking the
proper attitude, who try to challenge the system, are often
told they are not 'cut out' for nursing, or should consider
LPN rather than RN or baccalaureate training. Meanwhile,
supposedly progressive medical anthropology courses continue to reinforce ethnic and racial stereotypes: Blacks don't
trust doctors; Chicanos use sickness as an excuse to get out
of work; Jews and Italians complain too much. However, isolated pockets of resistance do exist in which students are exposing racist and elitist practices and insisting such changes
as bilingual courses in Spanish-speaking areas.

It is difficult to generalize about programs training other
health personnel. There are "career ladders" of various types,
but in the words of one workers, they "start at the bottom
and work down"—that is, you can advance to a certain level
through work experience, but if you want to go farther still,
you must quit, go back to school and virtually begin again.

Community clinics often have training for their own personnel which are usually more flexible and practical than college programs, but other institutions will rarely accept these
workers' qualifications because training varies so much from
clinic to clinic. Such community training programs reflect
the irresponsibility of those who design and fund them. They
are intended to crank out large numbers of people as quickly
as possible, with no thought of providing more than direct
services to a few more people for a temporary period of time,
as specified by the grant money. In many cases, trainees are
merely being prepared to fill positions already held by other
poor community people, not to actually ascend the career
ladder.

To avoid this type of careless planning that benefits neither
workers nor patients, changes must be made in the whole concept behind health science training. Training programs for all
health workers should be inter-disciplinary, starting with a
"core" curriculum that all workers would go through together
on an equal basis. (see Platform). Integrated with this concept is that of the career ladder. After a year or so of the
common core curriculum, some students would funnel into
the institution, working full-time (or part-time, while continuing training part-time). They would have the option of
coming back for more training anytime to a level on the ladder commensurate with the experience they'd gained. Others
would remain in training for longer periods of time, and then
branch off, again with options open for returning. In this
way, anyone with ability and desire could work at their own
rate of speed up to the most skilled positions, whether neurosurgery or hospital administration. Such open channels between multiple entry and departure points are an effective
way of eliminating occupational barriers as well as class, sex,
and racial ones.

Most present training programs are designed to work within
the system, yet they can also be seen as intermediate steps
towards more far-reaching change. These include coordinating college academic programs with hospital training, giving
graduates first priority for jobs in that hospital; doing task

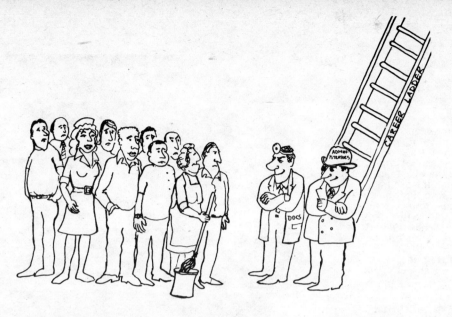

analysis of jobs by defining people by what skills they have rather than their job title, and credentialing them accordingly; doing more in-hospital training and upgrading of all present employees; pulling motivated students from minority communities and intensively preparing them to succeed in professional schooling. Non-exploitative experimentation must be encouraged to determine what systems work best for patients and workers and why, with the overall goals of combining quality care with meaningful and equal employment opportunities.

DR. MARTIN LUTHER KING JR. HEALTH CENTER...
once offered an excellent career ladder program for employees from the community, whereby they could work up to professional or administrative status, if desired, and receive a $50/week stipend from the Center for expenses, while taking time off to attend classes. They received credentials for their training, giving them mobility in the traditional health hierarchy. Theoretically, the complete ladder is still functional; however, OEO cut the stipend funds and now workers must finance their own education, which is impossible for many. The Center also trained community residents for entry-level jobs in the community health field, such as medical assistants and family health workers. While attending the initial eight-week training program, participants received a $50 weekly stipend. They then participated in further specialized training ranging from three months (medical assistant) to two years (X-ray technician). If MLK had no openings, they could work in other neighborhood health centers. Before funds were cut, MLK had made an arrangement with other health institutions to train workers in their certified labs while the Center paid her/him a stipend; at the end of training the person would be hired by the institution. Now, however, hospitals are unable to hire in spite of staff needs because they too have had personnel budget cuts. The Center has had poor luck in trying to obtain foundation funding for more training, and banks have generally refused to give students educational loans. Since the training program started in 1966, 509 people have been trained, 429 of whom are still working in the health field. Many of those presently in leadership roles worked up from the bottom ranks. 75% of the Center is staffed by community people; all non-community residents accept jobs at the Center with the understanding that they leave when a community resident is trained to take their place. Contact DR. MARTIN LUTHER KING, JR. HEALTH CENTER, Training Department, 400 East 169th St., Bronx, New York 10456, (212) 992-9100.

URBAN PRECEPTORSHIP PROGRAM... is an excellent eleven-week course for health science students, college students, and community organizers, covering medicine in communities and using the Chicago metropolitan area as a model. Seminars are led by community health organizers, health professionals and academic authorities, with topics ranging from the distribution of health personnel to the relationship between health care institutions and the community. There are also research projects involving field work in urban health problems. Contact URBAN PRECEPTORSHIP PROGRAM, Department of Preventive Medicine and Community Health, University of Illinois at the Medical Center, 835 South Wolcott, Chicago, IL 60012, (312) 966-6646.

THEME HOUSE IN COMMUNITY MEDICINE... is an undergraduate credit program at University of California at Berkeley studying the economic, political, and social—including racial, sexual, and cultural—aspects of the nation's health system. Students work with a faculty member in a topic-oriented small group, integrating readings, lectures, and seminars on the health system with projects or field work in health institutions. Some of the small group topics: "Organizing for Community Health," "Women as Providers" and "Consumers of Health Care," "Aging and Health in America," and "Asian American Communities and Health." Theme House also presents open colloquiums, for example, on "The Health of the Farm Workers," and "Women's Health Care: Self-help, Childbirth, and Delivery," and movies such as "Away with All Pests, and "Salt of the Earth." This is one of the most progressive, pre-health programs in the US Contact THEME HOUSE IN COMMUNITY MEDICINE, University of California, Berkeley, CA 94720, (415) 642-3205.

HOSPITAL LEAGUE-LOCAL 1199 TRAINING AND UPGRADING FUND... provides union members an opportunity to get out of dead-end jobs. The Fund operates a school for those seeking to finish high school or wishing to brush up on courses required for further education. If a member wants to be trained in a new field and has the necessary qualifications, the Fund will assist her or him in getting into the desired program through the union's contacts with training schools. To make it possible for the members to stay in school, the students have tuition and books paid for by the fund and are maintained at 80% of their former wages. In two years, 250 members have graduated into new technical and professional jobs and another 700 are in full or part time classes. Contact TRAINING AND UPGRADING FUND, 310 West 43rd St., New York, NY 10036, (212) 582-1890.

COMMUNITY HEALTH MAJOR... is an undergraduate major at the University of Kentucky, "the father of community health." The unique program, which leads to a B.S. in health sciences, was designed because it was felt that communities needed workers that were other than technically trained in the health sciences. Participants in the program learn to determine the extent and priorities of health problems, to promote specific community action, and to secure financial, moral and wo/manpower support for the plans. The faculty stress the necessity for graduates to challenge the present health system and to get outside of the White, middle class culture. Contact DEPARTMENT OF COMMUNITY HEALTH, HEALTH, College of Allied Health Professions, Albert B. Chandler Medical Center, University of Kentucky, Lexington, KY 40506, (606) 233-6361.

HOWARD UNIVERSITY COLLEGE ALLIED HEALTH SCIENCES... is designed to train Third World people in allied health skills: for instance, physicians' assistants, medical technicians, and occupational and physical therapy. The fact that a bachelor's degree is granted makes the college stand out from the many allied health training programs wh which lock the students into associate degrees. The BS degree provides the graduates with a base to work their way into top health planning and administration positions in the country so that the needs of Third World communities may be better met. Contact HOWARD UNIVERSITY COLLEGE OF ALLIED HEALTH SCIENCES, Howard University, Washington, D.C. 20001, (202) 636-7565.

SEATTLE CENTRAL COMMUNITY COLLEGE... offers an associate degree RN program geared to students who are on public assistance, are in public housing, are heads of households, have poor academic records (though they must have high school diplomas), or who have no "saleable skills". Eighty-seven percent of the students in the college are on financial aid; 60% are Third World; and most have at least two children. The retention rate in the RN program is over 75% (as compared to an average of 50% in many minority recruitment programs) because it is aimed at preventing failure by helping students learn to help each other work out their problems and gain self-confidence. Course loads are adjustable, and if students are having particularly difficult family or personal problems they are encouraged to drop out briefly and come back when things are okay. If students fail courses they can retake them immediately, and special tutoring and counseling is available for those having academic problems. The nursing program itself has a strong community emphasis—each quarter students do their own projects in the community; many graduates are hired by the community clinics they do projects with. The program focuses strongly on cultural differences and there is much honest encountering and communication between students and staff. This program has an unusually high commitment to personalizing and humanizing education. Contact SEATTLE CENTRAL COMMUNITY COLLEGE, Division of Allied Health Curriculums, 1718 Broadway, Seattle, WA 98122, (206) 587-4161.

HEALTH SERVICES SCHOOL... opened in 1973 at Johns Hopkins University to train middle-level health professionals. Students are admitted to the two-year baccalaureate program after two years of studies elsewhere, or if they have had previous experience enabling them to pass an equivalency exam. This is meant to attract graduate nurses, military medics, and medical technicians to the school. Efforts are being made to attract students from local community colleges and hospital training programs. There are also plans to create "work-linkages" with other student programs at the Hopkins medical complex to implement team concepts in clinical experience with nursing and medical students participating. Contact HEALTH SERVICES SCHOOL, Office of Student Development, Johns Hopkins University, 624 N. Broadway, Baltimore, MD 21205, (301) 955-5897.

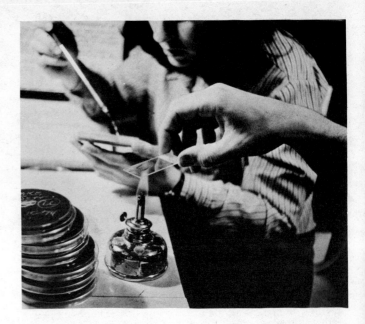

CASA LOMA INSTITUTE OF TECHNOLOGY... was begun in 1966 on OEO funds to train community people in paramedical careers in efforts to help pull them out of poverty and serve community health needs as well. Casa Loma offers associate degree programs in licensed vocational nursing, dental technology, physicians' assistantships, respiration therapy, and legal assistantships. By federal guidelines, the student body is 1/3 Black, 1/3 Chicano and 1/3 White, and many are veterans and/or unemployed. Most have families. Only the dental technology program requires a high school diploma, and the school helps interested students get this equivalency; it also hustles grants and scholarships for those not on the GI bill, and no student has been denied yet for lack of funds. The program successfully places over 90% of its graduates, most in the local community. In most programs, 80 credit hours of classroom and on-the-job training are crammed into a year's time because "that's the absolute longest time a poor person can survive without working during the day." The staff is largely Third World, and double as counselors. The school has successfully gone to court several times to challenge a licensing board's refusal to license qualified students with criminal records. Contact CASA LOMA INSTITUTE OF TECHNOLOGY, Pacoima, CA 91331 (213) 899-2622

HIGH SCHOOL FOR THE HEALTH PROFESSIONS... is a program where high school students elect to attend a special school to learn about different health careers. Located at the Baylor Medical Center since its beginning in 1972, the school offers the usual array of high school courses, except that phys. ed. and health classes have been replaced with pre-med courses, supplemented by lectures and demonstrations from health workers from a variety of professions. Women make up one half of the 200 people enrolled, and ethnic and racial minorities are represented in a proportion equivalent to that in the Houston area population. Other communities have shown a strong interest in this program, and its success will largely determine whether similar programs will be established. Contact HIGH SCHOOL FOR THE HEALTH PROFESSIONS, 1649 Braeswoods, Houston, TX 77025, (713)795-4629. For information on a similar program, contact CLARA BARTON HIGH SCHOOL FOR HEALTH PROFESSIONS, 901 Classen Ave., Brooklyn, NY 11225, (212) 636-4900.

INDIANA UNIVERSITY SCHOOL OF MEDICINE... has set up seven community-based satellite medical schools throughout the state. Students are taught basic medical sciences their freshman year and go to the main medical center in Indianapolis for their clinical experience. They may elect to stay in Indianapolis or return to one of the satellite schools for the final two years and internship. Contact INDIANA UNIVERSITY SCHOOL OF MEDICINE, 110 W. Michigan, Indianapolis, IN 46202, (317) 264-8416.

ALBERT EINSTEIN COLLEGE OF MEDICINE. . . received an OEO grant in 1969 to train a "new maternity care-centered health professional" or "health extern." This was to experiment with a new way of delivering maternal/family services while making health care more accessible to the medically needy Bronx Community. A Community Health Advisory Council was recruited to help select community trainees and to give direction to the program. Applicants were required and to give direction to the program. Applicants were required to have a high school diploma, and went through 13 months of intensive training in clinic, classroom and field. Their technical training was similar to the gynecology instruction given to Einstein medical students, and they received a small stipend for living expenses. They staffed two community clinics and a mobile unit. The health externs provided sex education, nutritional counseling, prenatal care, health education, and referral. Great emphasis was placed on outreach and follow-up work. But in 1973 training funds were cut off and the clinics are being forced to close down as well. The highly skilled health externs who received no formal transfer credentials for their training can now only qualify for positions on a nurses' aide level. This is because Einstein lacked an undergraduate college program to provide them with the credit they earned. This program is an outstanding example of the irresponsibility of program planners and funders who refused to deal with making permanent improvements in wo/manpower development and in the health hierarchy. For more information on the training program, contact Irwin Kaiser, Bronx Municipal Hospital Center, Pelham Parkway and Eastchester Rd., Rm. 709, Bronx, NY 10461, (212) 430-5214.

VETERAN MEDIC GROUP. . . was formed by former Vietnam medics to seek ways of using their medical skills to serve mining communities and other medically lacking areas. With the help of the United Mine Workers, community leaders, nurses and doctors, the 50 member VMG established the Black Lung Home Respiratory Care Service where veteran medics work under a physician's supervision; the group has also developed an upgrading and recruitment program of veteran medics for a one year physician's assistant preceptorship. The VMG was successful in gaining academic credit for veterans with military experience and training. Emergency care and rescue classes have been held by VMG members in several communities. Contact NORTH WEST VIRGINIA VETERAN MEDIC GROUP, 463 Wilson Ave., Morgantown, W.VA 26505, (304) 292-7763, or SOUTHWEST VIRGINIA VMG, c/o Will Cantrell, Emergency Room, Appalachia Regional Hospital, Beckly, W.VA 25801.

THE GALVESTON PLAN. . . utilizes a multi-health occupation program of instruction based on a common core curriculum and specialized clinical education. This innovative project at Galveston College encompasses "career ladder" and baccalaureate goals in training students in occupations such as electroencephalography, and radiological technology. The core curriculum is structured so that the students first take the required courses for graduation at the same time they investigate the fields of health care available in the program. Students can withhold their decisions on a career until they've been exposed to a number of different fields. The major drawbacks seem to be that the program fails to include the more entrenched professions such as nursing and medicine. Contact THE GALVESTON PLAN, Registrar, Galveston College, 4015 Avenue Q, Galveston, TX 77550, (713) 763-1275.

EAST BALTIMORE COMMUNITY CORPORATION AND THE JOHNS HOPKINS MEDICAL INSTITUTIONS. . . have developed and are training "non-physician family health teams" to provide continuous care on a family basis and to break down the doctor/nurse dichotomy. Aiming to operate at a lower cost than doctor and nurse "teams," they function through HMOs and are trained to give 80% of the primary care required for a given population. Each team is composed of a health advocate, health assistant and health associate; ideally eight to ten teams, backed up by three to five doctors and a few other health specialists, will serve 25,000 people. This innovative training program is presently being tried in Baltimore's inner city and is designed for community people from all socio-economic levels, to give horizontal and vertical career mobility. The advocate is the catalyst for helping patient and family utilize helpful community services. The assistant does check ups, manages chronic illnesses, and helps families and groups with health related problems. The associate is responsible for day-to-day team operation, treating mild to moderate health problems and referring serious problems to doctors. Working with one or two assistants and two to four advocates, the associate is either selected from assistant ranks or has been trained as an RN or military medic. (This is an effort to get nurses and corpsmen working together.) The basic course for each level worker involves six months or 860 hours, emphasizing family and community health, teamwork, and developing communications skills. Presently the first two levels are tied in to community college programs, and third to Johns Hoskins School of Health Sciences, allowing for horizontal input from other health careers and non-health areas, and facilitating worker mobility from the family health tract to other health fields. A similar approach to this innovative model is being adapted to a middle class community in Columbia, Maryland. Contact Archie Golden, c/o Johns Hopkins University School of Health Sciences, 624 N. Broadway, Baltimore, MD 21205, (301) 955-6426.

PHILADELPHIA CENTER FOR HEALTH CAREERS, INC. . . . provides a free, complete informational service, responding to all inquiries with appropriate literature on various health careers opportunities. The Center also offers individual counseling to minority and disadvantaged people seeking training in health skills. The counseling is followed up by assistance with the application process to the desired training program. Contact PHILADELPHIA CENTER FOR HEALTH CAREERS, INC., 311 S. Juniper St., Philadelphia, PA 19107, (215) 735-4332.

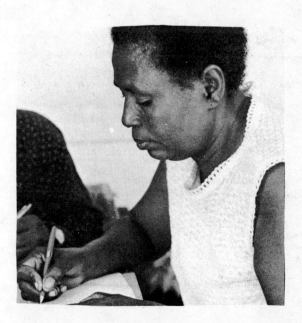

PRE-HEALTH SCIENCE PROGRAM. . . is a proposed project of Antioch College West. The program seeks to take a group of twenty low-income Third World people and women experienced in health care and help them enter careers in the medical professions. The students, after being recommended by community health centers and clinics, would be given credit from Antioch for their academic and/or vocational training. Students could then begin the program at an advanced level with the hope that they will complete the Pre-Health program and receive their baccalaureate degree in two years. They will participate in an intensive investigation of health science and health care delivery from a multi-disciplinary approach, with topics ranging from its political and economic aspects to discussions with other health workers of the frustrations and rewards of their jobs. Classes will also be given in chemistry and biology to satisfy medical school requirements. Finally, this academic experience would be followed up with individual counseling to get each student into the school in which s/he has the best chance of gaining admissions. Contact PRE-HEALTH SCIENCES PROGRAM, Antioch College/West, 3663 Sacramento St., San Francisco, CA 94118, (415) 931-6170.

RESOURCES

BOOKS

Health Professions Education Master Plan, A Part of Phase III of the New Jersey Master Plan for Higher Education, Office of Health Professions Education, New Jersey Dept. of Higher Education, 225 W. State St., Trenton, NJ 08625, 1973. 360 pp. $5.00
. . . establishes a framework for assuring an adequate supply of qualified college-trained wo/manpower to insure quality health services in the state. The plan provides an interesting model for what all states should be thinking about—training programs which meet societal needs and provide students with a total view of the human condition as well as give them technical competence. Emphasizes the team approach, career ladders, recruitment/retention programs, and consumer representation on state licensing boards.

PAMPHLETS AND ARTICLES

"HUMAN VALUES AND MEDICAL EDUCATION FROM THE PERSPECTIVES OF HEALTH CARE DELIVERY," Leslie A. Falk, Benjamin Page and Walter Vesper, Dept, of Family and Community Health, Meharry Medical College, Nashville, TN 37208, 1971. 14 pp. Free
. . . discusses the role that medical schools can play in training physicians who "know the etiology of social illness" through familiarity with such areas as inner city and rural conditions, health care beliefs and delivery among minorities and the poor. The authors cite Meharry Medical school's approach to community health, and the school's neighborhood health center.

"The Woman as Medical Student," CENTERSCOPE, Boston University Medical Center, Boston, MA, July/August 1971, pp. 6-8
. . . two medical students write of experiences women commonly face while in school: domineering males, condescending teachers, absence of females on the faculty and refusal to be taken seriously. "There are as many daily oppressive moments: . . . the doctor who comes in and begins his lecture, 'My, we have some lovely young ladies here. . .' or even worse, the doctor who will only address the class as 'Men. . .'" Well documented with statistical findings.

"Medical School Sweepstakes," Oliver Fein, A. Sandra Abramson, Michael Gordon, HEALTH/PAC BULLETIN, 17 Murray St., New York, NY 10007, Oct., 1972, pp. 2-14
. . . discusses the possibilities for a new medical school in New York City: the politics involved, the different proposals for medical schools, and an analysis of each in terms of who would control it, Third World orientation, and its municipal hospital relationship.

"Health Systems and New Careers," Alan Gartner, HEALTH SERVICE REPORTS, c/o New Human Services Institute, 184 Fifth Ave., New York, NY 10010, February, 1973. pp. 124-130
. . . a good analysis of the new health careers and their affect on the present health care system. Describes some new training programs and what a successful program should entail; concludes that the new paraprofessions should fight for career ladders, joining with consumers to increase efficiency in health care delivery.

HEALTH/PAC BULLETIN, 17 Murray St., New York, NY 10007, Nov. 1972. 16 pp. $.60
. . . attacks the fragmentation of health workers. Articles focus on licensure, and a new category of health worker, the physician's assistant. The licensing article is a broad analysis of job definitions within the health field. With typical force and accuracy, HEALTH/PAC writers point out the problems in fighting for licensing of more health personnel.

"PHARMACY EDUCATION RESPONDS TO CHANGING HEALTH CARE NEEDS," American Association of Colleges of Pharmacy, 8121 Georgia Ave., Silver Springs, MD 20910, 1974. 12 pp. Free
. . . good overview of innovative training programs in pharmacy. It does not pretend to be a comprehensive listing, but shows the move towards training patient-oriented pharmacists through programs emphasizing the special health needs of rural people, Native Americans, nursing home patients and many others.

"NURSING EDUCATION: TEACH THE WOMAN TO KNOW HER PLACE," Vicki Cooper, Paula Balber and Judy Ackerhalt, available from Louise Rice, 65 Chestnut St., Cambridge, MA 02139, September 1970. 4 pp. $.17
. . .describes the way nursing education teaches students to conform to their position as "minor cogs in the health system wheel." Women enter the profession with a desire to serve and often end up serving the hospital's needs instead of the patient's.

As for the relationship between the doctor and the nurse, it provides a leavening of the day. It's nice to have someone smile at you. I find it a change of pace. I like the difference—it's a pleasant release. I could never have a male secretary for these reasons.

—a male physician

PERIODICALS

HEALTH POLITICS: A QUARTERLY BULLETIN, Committee on Health Politics, New York University, 547 La Guardia Place, New York, NY 10003, April 1972. 11 pp. Free
. . . centers on health manpower, calling for a more rational, regionalized system of health care and spelling out the major issues in wo/manpower, licensure and certification, etc. A very extensive bibliography adds to the usefulness of the issue.

HEALTH MANPOWER REPORT, Capitol Publications, Inc., Suite G-12, 2430 Pennsylvania Ave. NW, Washington, D.C. 20034. $55/yr or $50 w/check in order
. . . an excellent bi-weekly report packed with information on legislative, judicial and administrative developments affecting health personnel. It gives detailed accounts of new university and government wo/manpower training programs and is an important resource for anyone desiring a comprehensive view of all that's going on in this area.

ALLIED HEALTH TRENDS, Association of Schools of Allied Health Professions, One DuPont Circle, Suite 300, Washington, D.C. 20036. Free
. . . published monthly, helpful in its occasional brief descriptions of new or innovative training programs as well as its notifications of area workshops and conferences.

MINORITY RECRUITMENT

Until all education training in this country is free and open to everyone, it is imperative that health training institutions commit themselves to actively recruiting and admitting Third World people, women, the poor and the over-25. Efforts must begin when public education does, and teachers and counselors should strive to make all children equally aware of opportunities in all the health occupations.

Presently, few schools are doing more than token recruitment of minorities. When the California Nurses Association surveyed its state nursing schools, of those that bothered to respond, only about 1/5 even "indicated they were actively and specifically recruiting minority students." And admissions decisions made with significant input from the underrepresented students themselves are virtually unheard of. Some schools are even seriously considering cutting out what recruitment and admissions programs they do have, on the basis that the students recruited "just haven't worked out." Blame is obviously placed on the student rather than on the program itself.

For women applying to medical schools, the picture is improving with intolerable slowness—presently 8% of doctors are women, a little over 10% of present medical students are female. Only a couple of schools have begun to talk about setting quotas for women at 50%, and scarcely a program exists which judges women's credentials equally with men's, and which encourages women to go into all types of practice, particularly gynecology.

For Third World students, specific problems center around admissions criteria and lack of adequate retention programs. The results of tests geared to the White middle class culture and educational background are usually the prime standards for admittance, rather than evidences of past and present motivation, commitment, along with more accurate measures of ability. Retention programs are criticized for taking the burden off educational institutions to give adequate education in the first place, but until they improve, it is essential for all committed recruitment programs to follow through with affective retention programs to help Third World students succeed, through remedial and tutoring programs as well as supportive personal counseling. Institutional responsibility to the student should not end until s/he has passed any applicable state board exams.

NATIONAL CHICANO HEALTH ORGANIZATION... has undertaken a nationwide effort to recruit Chicanos into the health professions. NCHO helps Chicanos to get into health science school, attempts to keep them there until they graduate, and, after graduation, steers them back to the barrio. NCHO's membership includes all types of community health workers, health science students and health professionals. Recruitment and counseling starts at the junior and senior high school and continues through the professional schools. This involves encouragement, tutorial assistance, career information, and a centralized financial aid information center. NCHO can also provide the latest information on institutions where Chicanos stand the best chance for admissions. For the future, NCHO is developing health career information kits, summer jobs for students and a recruitment film. Further plans are to bring suits against institutions who adhere to unrealistic and discriminatory admissions policies and who have only a token number of Chicano students. Contact NATIONAL CHICANO HEALTH ORGANIZATION, 1709 W. 8th St., Suite 517, Los Angeles, CA 90014, (213) 483-7167.

MINORITY ADVANCEMENT PROJECT... of the Massachusetts College of Pharmacy, accepts students with marginal academic records from Boston's inner city, with the intent of giving them a good undergraduate education, after which they will hopefully continue with pharmacy studies. Full tuition is paid the first two years of study, after which the school helps them get loans and scholarships. Supportive services of counseling, tutoring and remedial courses are available and the retention rate is about 80%. The pharmacy program itself includes a year of clinical emphasis and stresses the team approach. Contact MINORITY ADVANCEMENT PROJECT' Massachusetts College of Pharmacy, 179 Longwood Ave., Boston, MA 02115, (617) 734-6700.

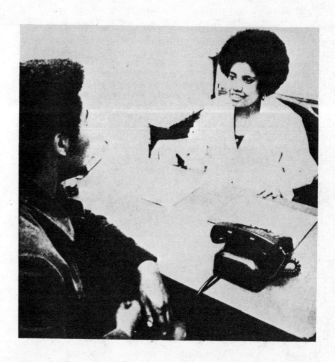

OPEN THE DOORS WIDER IN NURSING (ODWIN)— HEALTH CAREERS... helps minority people in the Boston area prepare for a health career suited to their interests and abilities. Presently they are working with about 300 students of various ethnic backgrounds and ages, 90% of them Black. The training is provided free. Upon coming to the center, students are tested on their English, math, and science skills, and an individual plan is made out to deal with their deficiencies. Less than 15% drop out of the program and they often achieve four-six years academic growth in two years. The staff, which is 50% Third World, helps them apply to health career programs for admission and academic aid, often meeting with school officials themselves. Great emphasis is placed on building student's self-images. A major problem has been schools accepting these students when they weren't ready. The student often flunks out and blames the failure on her/himself. ODWIN also gives workshops to faculty from Boston area schools to help them understand the needs and feelings of these students. There are also discussions on making admissions decisions, ODWIN tries to make faculty aware that they often do not expect these students to succeed and that attitude is internalized by the students. Examples of institutional racism in textbooks and elsewhere are also demonstrated. Contact ODWIN—Health Careers, 55 Dimock St., Roxbury, MA 02119, (617) 445-1290.

CENTRAL RECRUITMENT COUNCIL... originated in 1969 at Harvard Medical School by Third World physicians to recruit minority house staff for the Boston teaching hospitals. Three symposiums on health care in the ghetto brought support from 104 Boston organizations. CRC was then able to work out a plan to finance its work through an agreement with the teaching hospitals whereby each institution would contribute $100 per internship position. Recently CRC researched and exposed statistical evidence indicating racial bias in current intern placement systems all over the country. The Council works in three main areas: they bring in non-Bostonian Third World students to work in clerkships in urban Third World communities; they recruit minority house staff for Boston hospitals; and they counsel Third World health science students anywhere in the country. Contact CENTRAL RECRUITMENT COUNCIL, P.O. Box 463, Prudential Center Building, Boston, MA 02199.

EAST LOS ANGELES HEALTH MANPOWER CONSORTIUM, INC.... is a group of Chicano and Indian community activists with professional backgrounds in health and manpower who are working to get a greater percentage of their people into area educational training programs in universities and hospitals. This involves exposing high school students to health careers, counseling and tutoring them; a major focus has been dealing with high school counselors who had been guiding minority students to vocational/technical careers rather than ones requiring greater skill. The consortium has compiled a health career directory listing information on 82 different health careers to aid counselors in making students aware of all the possibilities. They are also working closely with other health-oriented Chicano groups and HMO's in the area. Generally they are trying to break the subtle patterns of discrimination in hospitals and schools by pressuring for: better upgrading programs; bi-lingual professionals; courses training professionals how to deal with health needs of cultural groups; Third World representation on accreditation and certification boards as well as on admissions committees; federal monies earmarked for minorities actually going to this purpose; and other educational institutions to accept local community college credits. Contact EAST LA HEALTH MANPOWER CONSORTIUM, INC., 1251 South Atlantic Blvd., Los Angeles, CA 90022, (213) 263-9313.

BAY AREA RAZA COALITION FOR HEALTH... places interested Chicano college students in its five area clinics which serve predominantly Spanish speaking and low-income patients. Students are paid a stipend for 20 hours of work per week and receive course credit. Graduate students in the health professions offer them counseling and supervision. Started in 1972, the Coalition encourages Chicanos to return to el barrio after health training is obtained; this is a fine example of clinics coming together to better serve the community. BARCH also has an outreach program in local high schools, encouraging students to consider a health career. In the summer they send a mobile dental clinic to migrant camps. Contact BARCH, 1477 Fruitvale Ave., Oakland, CA 94601, (415) 261-9502.

MEDICAL COLLEGE OF GEORGIA... has an Educational Assistance Program for Special Students in the Baccalaureate Nursing Curriculum, funded by HEW. Geared to students with a combined score below 800 on the SAT's, as long as they have a GPA of 2.0, the program recruits students through high school guidance counselors. They spend the summer taking special preparatory courses and start regular college in the fall. Supportive services throughout the year include group and individual rap sessions, as well as tutorial assistance. The latter have been so successful that these services are to be extended to the entire campus. Course loads can be flexible, and students are allowed considerable time leeway in completing the RN program. In addition, the school continues to work with students if they fail the national exam the first time around. Contact MEDICAL COLLEGE OF GEORGIA, School of Nursing, Augusta, GA 30902, (404) 724-7111.

PROJECT IODINE... is a demonstration RN project in three schools—North Carolina A & T University, traditionally Black, and two White schools, Polk Community College in Florida, and the University of Southern Mississippi—to recruit and graduate students "from different cultures and educational backgrounds." Approximately 130 students are in the program so far, recruited mainly from the institutions' backlog of those once rejected. Most participated in summer courses to become oriented to the schools and develop proficiencies in basic skills. Supportive services include group and individual counseling, tutorial sessions in academic problem areas and labs, learning labs with visual aids, and smaller learning groups. Such activities, which were initiated for this project, are now being made available to the rest of the student body at each school as well. The project has financed campus coordinators at each school to try to implement methods of meeting students' needs. Campus and regional workshops are being held to help faculty better understand these needs and how to adjust their courses, curriculum and teaching methods accordingly. Through comprehensive evaluations, the project hopes to determine how educationally disadvantaged students can succeed in nursing, and then share this information with other nursing schools in the region. Contact PROJECT IODINE, c/o Southern Regional Educational Board, 130 Sixth St., NW, Atlanta, GA 30313, (404) 875-7611.

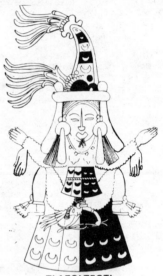

TLAZOLTEOTL
goddess of medicine and maternity

CHICANOS IN HEALTH EDUCATION... was formed in 1969 by the first group of Chicanos to come to the University of California/San Francisco's health school. CHE's efforts center on the recruitment, admission and retention of Chicanos throughout the state of California and the South West into health professional schools. On the community level, CHE's work has been co-ordinated with the Bay Area Raza Coalition For Health, and on the regional and national level with the National Chicano Health Organization. CHE has also been devoted to raising funds for Chicano clinics, and sharing their culture and heritage with the rest of the school. Contact CHE, Rm. 250, Millberry Union, 900 Parnassus, San Francisco, CA 94122.

MEXICAN-AMERICAN HEALTH PROFESSION SCHOLARSHIP FUND... provides scholarships during undergraduate study, counseling, and tutoring. Many Mexican-American students must hold one or more jobs to support themselves while in college, detracting from the time they have to study and prepare for the Medical College Admissions Test. To qualify for a scholarship ($1000/year for three years is the proposed amount) the student must be unable to obtain funding from traditional sources; show promise to succeed in medical school; express a social consciousness and desire to work with Chicanos; and be Mexican-American. The Fund would like to work with similar projects in other states. Contact MEXICAN-AMERICAN HEALTH PROFESSION SCHOLARSHIP FUND, 201 North Marie St., Suite 606, San Antonio, TX 78205, (512) 224-2842.

RESOURCES

PAMPHLETS AND ARTICLES

Minorities in Nursing, Minority Group Task Force. California Nurses' Association, 185 Post St., San Francisco, CA 94108, 1973. 80 pp. $3.00
. . . a thoroughly documented report demonstrating that Third World nurses are typically lower-paid than Whites, and underrepresented in schools of nursing and in positions of authority. Also discusses attitudes of White nurses who in some cases felt they were victims of reverse racism, indicating a real lack of awareness of institutional racism. The report is unusual in its content, having come out of the conservative ANA, but the organization has yet to act on this report's recommendations for combatting institutional racism.

" 'CHARET:' STATUS OF DENTAL HEALTH IN THE BLACK COMMUNITY," National Dental Association, 1130 Mondawmin Concourse, Baltimore, MD 21215, 1972. 86 pp Free
. . . includes outlines of problems and recommendations that came out of "Charet," a conference sponsored by the National Dental Association to discuss such problems as the lack of Black or minority input on dental health policies, and the inadequate economic base in Third World communities to purchase dental services.

"CRC TIME TABLE," Wilbert C. Jordan, MD, and the Central Recruitment Council, P.O. Box 463, Prudential Center, Boston, MA 02199, March, 1973. 1 pp. Free
. . . written by Third World professionals to help Third World medical students plan out their four years of school.

"EARLY AFRO-AMERICAN MEDICAL EDUCATION IN THE US: THE ORIGINS OF MEHARRY MEDICAL COLLEGE IN THE 19th CENTURY," Leslie A. Falk, Meharry Medical College, Nashville, TN 37208, 1972. 17 pp. Free
. . . traces the origins of Black medicine in the US as it relates to the opening of Meharry Medical College, one of two predominantly Black US med schools. The article begins with the days of slavery, when Blacks were legally prohibited from practicing medicine because "such doctors might foment insurrection," and gives an intriguing overview of the events that led up to the establishment of Meharry.

PERIODICALS

SALUD Y REVOLUCION SOCIAL, National Chicano Health Organization, 1709 W. 8th St. Suite 517, Los Angeles, CA 90017. Free to NCHO members
. . . aims to inform and motivate Chicano students into the health professions. One section reviews different health careers, and information on financing the training. Other sections offer health news covering such areas as nutrition and VD, and information about programs available for minority students in various universities. Stresses the need for Chicano professionals to return to Chicano communities to practice.

HEALTH TEAMS

One of the most effective methods of breaking the medical hierarchy and delivering one class of quality care for everyone is through the use of health teams. These are groups of health workers—not only doctors, but social workers, dieticians, aides, and others—making full use of their combined skills to deal with each patient individually as a total entity, rather than as an arm, tooth, or file folder. Ideally, each member's skills are valued equally, since all are integral to the patients' well-being. Major decisions on treatment and care are made collectively, with input from the patient, the keynotes being cooperation and coordination of services.

To build a national network of such teams, the ground-work must be laid in health training schools, where students can begin to cross traditional occupational boundaries. These teams must then be incorporated in all types of health delivery systems, concentrating on preventive, nurturing care, and working with other community services to help families improve health-related conditions such as inadequate housing. The teams could operate on various levels, with some providing more direct primary care and others giving more specialized care to larger regions.

Various concepts of health teams are being used more and more in rural areas. In many cases, the doctor stops in only periodically while the rest of the team does most of the care. Predictably, the biggest problems are in relationships between professionals and non-professionals, which often more closely resemble that of horse to rider than of real teamwork.

Though HMOs and group practices may purport to be teams of sorts, these are hardly operated on a concept of worker equality. Such concepts are threatening to many professionals, particularly doctors, who are used to controlling fellow workers as well as patients. Yet teams provide a sharing of the responsibility the doctor has had to shoulder alone in the past. And the patient certainly benefits from the chance to relate to a group working with, not on, her/him.

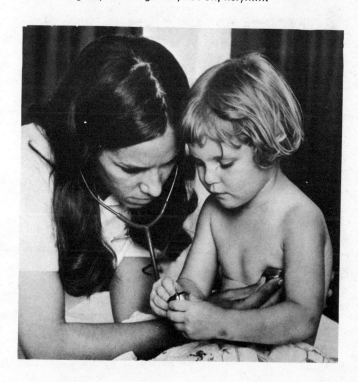

FAMILY HEALTH CENTER... is an outpatient clinic in San Francisco General Hospital, aimed at providing total preventive health care. This includes present medical problems, teaching people how to prevent future ones, and discussing problems related to employment, housing, emotional needs family conflicts, etc. Any city resident can receive care there, and people are billed according to their ability to pay. The clinic operates in two teams, each of which works half the time; about sixty patients are seen daily. A clerk, family health workers, nurses, nurse practitioners, social workers, family doctors (including four women interns and a nutritionist) make up each team. Before each work session starts, the entire team meets to discuss any problems regarding patients or clinic operation. A steering committee, composed of representatives of each category of worker does most of the policy-making. When staff grievances occur between two people which can't be solved in meetings, each person selects a spokesperson and the entire group chooses a third, to work it out together. The clinic is funded through OEO and city funds, and an OEO board of community people retains final hiring/firing control. Though the clinic is dedicated to providing real team-delivered care, it is undergoing a long uphill struggle to overcome worker divisions of class, race, sex and job category, and to define new roles for themselves. Through weekend retreats, direct encounters, meetings and consciousness-raising, they have tried to effectively deal with the conflicts inherent in any such attempts to bring about major changes. Contact FAMILY HEALTH CENTER, 995 Potrero Ave., Ward 81, San Francisco, CA 94110, (415) 648-4323.

UNITED HEALTH SERVICES (UHS)... is the result of the coalition of four clinics in rural Kentucky and Tennessee which joined forces in 1972 to get government funding. UHS is governed completely by a community board composed of members from each clinic. Community control is a very important concept at UHS; there are farmers, miners, coal truck drivers, and housewives on the board making the decisions that affect their health care. Professional staff advise the boards, but have no vote. The clinics each handle about 20 people daily and are all staffed by locally trained people from the community who do lab work, advocacy, outreach work, and a variety of other services from finding transportation to helping people get on food stamps. They operate as teams, centering mainly around the nurse practitioner who handles 80% of the cases. A team of a family physician, a clinical pharmacists, and a pharmacists aide spend one day a week at each clinic. The pharmacist and aide take drug histories and confer with the nurse practitioner about continuing medication. UHS is starting a dental program soon and recently got revenue-sharing money from the county and state. Currently they generate half their income through reimbursement by third party payments, Medicare/caid and United Mine Workers; though they still receive 50% government funding, they hope to soon become self-sufficient. Patients pay on a sliding scale. Contact UNITED HEALTH SERVICES, Clairfield, TN 37715 (615) 424-8492

KENTUCKY JANUARY... is a three week mandatory credit program in January for students in the College of Allied Health at the University of Kentucky. The school contracts with private health facilities to accept the students. Teams of six-seven students are sent to rural and inner city areas around the state to learn about community needs and the impact of community systems on health care within the community, spending time in the courts, schools, mines, industries, etc. They also rotate through acute services facilities, from laundry room to surgery, and then observe community health services. Other students work in clinical teams, geared to learning by doing. During this period, students are forced to work and live closely together. Contact KENTUCKY JANUARY, Medical Center Annex 3, University of Kentucky Medical Center, Lexington, KY 40506, (606) 233-6361.

DISTRIBUTION

INSTITUTE FOR HEALTH TEAM DEVELOPMENT... is an action research group dedicated to developing curriculum for health science centers in primary care using interdisciplinary teams. Feeling that team training experiences ought to be integrated into the schools in a legitimate way, the Institute has recently written a model course to help faculty teach team concepts; faculty have a tremendous effect on socializing students into their professional roles, and their behavior often contradicts the whole concept of teamwork. Starting in the fall of '74, intensive workshops will be held for interested faculty members from all over the country to teach them how to teach team concepts, family dynamics, and worker-patient relationships. Institute workers will follow up the workshops by helping participants implement these courses in their home settings. The Institute also publishes a monthly newsletter with information on relevant programs at universities, ongoing work in the field, listings of conferences and reviews of helpful literature. Contact: INSTITUTE FOR HEALTH TEAM DEVELOPMENT, 10500 Summit Avenue, Kensington, Maryland 20795, (301) 933-7060.

RESOURCES

Health Care Teams, An Annotated Bibliography, Vol. I., Monique K. Tichy. Institute for Health Team Development, Montefiore Hospital, 3329 Rochambeau Ave., Bronx, NY 10467, 1974. 250 pp. approximately $3.00.
... reviews books, articles and pamphlets about health teams describing the particular team's goals, functions, decision-making, patient involvement, how the team relates to the community or institution, student/faculty involvement, and teaching method used. A variety of different types of teams are described—family doctor health teams, nurse-centered teams, dental teams, mental health teams and pediatric teams, to name a few—located in the U.S. as well as in other countries. The evaluations of what has or hasn't worked and why is especially helpful.

"Appropriate Utilization of Health Professionals," Virginia Cleland and Dawn Zagonik, JOURNAL OF NURSING ADMINISTRATION, 12 Lakeside Park, 607 North Ave., Wakefield, MA 01880, November/December, 1971. pp. 37-40
...shows how the nurse clinician can make health care more efficient by performing tasks that doctors now do. This fits in with the idea of a health team that takes away the omnipotence of the doctor's position and provides better total care for the patient.

"THE PHARMACIST'S CLINICAL ROLE," Gordon R. Baldeschwiler, available from Alan J. Brands, Chief Pharmacy Officer, Public Health Service, HEW, 5600 Fishers Lane, Rockville, MD 20852, 1972. 8 pp. Free
... describes the author's work at Neah Bay Indian Health Center in Washington. Part of a health team with a doctor and a nurse, his duties consisted of performing laboratory and X-ray work. His story is a good example of how pharmacists' skills can be put to better use.

"CLINICAL PHARMACY SERVICES IN THE HOSPITAL," Allen J. Brands, Chief Pharmacy Officer, Public Health Service, HEW, 5600 Fisher Lane, Rockville, MD, 20852, Sept., 1973. 24 pp. Free
... an exciting view of the possibilities for pharmacists to improve hospital patient care: taking drug histories, evaluating drug therapy during hospitalization, counseling patients on drug use, and supervising drug therapy for patients with chronic diseases. Points out the fallacy in creating new health professions while nurses and pharmacists are not permitted to put much of their extensive training to use.

Several efforts are underway to begin to correct the under-representation of health personnel in rural and inner-city areas. One approach is for schools to offer, limited clinical and preceptorship opportunities (lasting up to 10 weeks) while retaining their traditional curriculum, in hopes that medical school graduates will settle close to the area with which they have had contact. A preceptorship is basically a program through which a student studies a specific type or area of medicine, such as gynecology or community medicine, under the supervision of a physician. In a second type of program, the medical education is decentralized; Students spend from several months to a year at satellite training centers scattered throughout a region. A third type recruits rural and inner-city inhabitants to enter training programs at all levels of the health field.

The first type of program seems to be the weakest; thus far, the rate at which the personnel return to the community after graduation has been insignificant. Because of their brevity and slant towards service rather than patient education, these programs often leave the community no better able to deal with its health difficulties than before As expressed by one radical educator, the real value lies in the exposure they give middle-class students to lifesyles vastly different from their own. At the least, this can help people see the health system's failings more clearly and begin to question their conditioning.

The most valid approaches appear to be the second and third options described above. Decentralizing the training process exposes the health student to a variety of health delivery settings and their particular health problems while guaranteeing a supply of health workers to the communities. Programs recruiting people from scarcity areas often achieve the highest return to community rate because the recruitees tend to have a high sense of appreciation for the problems caused by the lack of adequate health care. It is disheartening to note that these two approaches seem to be used least.

FRONTIER NURSING SERVICE. . . owns and operates a small hospital and five nursing outposts in eastern Kentucky, covering 1,000 square miles. Formed in 1925 to better meet rural people's health needs, the service originally did outreach work via horseback. Nurses and social workers still work with people in their homes when necessary; stress is placed on preventive care, and a physician is available for referral. In a population of 18,000 the service annually helps 12,000 people. It also sponsors the Frontier School of Midwifery and Family Nursing which gives graduate nurses a 16 month course in midwifery and rural primary care techniques. The family nurse who graduates is the equivalent of a nurse practitioner and may also continue in the course to be certified as a midwife. Contact FRONTIER NURSING SERVICE, Wendover, KY 41775, (606) 672-2317.

HEALTH MANPOWER DISTRIBUTION PROJECT OF THE NATIONAL HEALTH COUNCIL, INC. . . . acts as a clearinghouse for information on rural and inner city wo/manpower shortage areas. More specifically, through a survey of health schools around the country, they are developing an incredibly comprehensive file of incentive programs used to encourage students to practice in these areas. They hope to find out what's worked and what hasn't, and then make this information available. Recently, they funded three demonstration projects in New Orleans, Maine and Appalachia to test different methods of influencing health students to practice in needy areas after graduation. Guidelines for such projects emphasized the importance of the team approach in health care delivery as well as the necessity of community and provider input into the development of each project. HMPD puts out an "ANNOTATED BIBLIOGRAPHY ON HEALTH MANPOWER DISTRIBUTION," and "INCENTIVE PROGRAMS AIMED AT CORRECTING HEALTH SCARCITY PROBLEMS." Contact HEALTH MANPOWER DISTRIBUTION PROJECT, NATIONAL HEALTH COUNCIL, INC., 1740 Broadway, New York, NY 10019, (212) 582-6040.

PROJECT PORVENIR. . . places teams of senior health science students (medical, nursing, and pharmacy) into two New Mexico communities that have not had physicians. While each student spends only eight weeks in the project, there are still many opportunities for insight into the meaning of health as it relates to social, political and economical factors. In addition to clinic work, students carry out health education programs, home outreach projects, and special projects such as integration of folk and modern medicine. Contact PROJECT PORVENIR, University of New Mexico Health Science Center, North Campus, Albuquerque, NM 87131, (505) 277-3532.

MAYO CLINIC PROGRAM. . . was started by the University of Florida Medical School to give community-oriented comprehensive health care service in physician-less Lafayette County, 60 miles away. Community medicine residents, nursing and allied health students staff the clinic, providing care to people in the area and receiving a valuable learning experience as well. Students have become involved in community education, writing a health column for the local weekly paper, and giving talks in the schools on health-related topics. Contact MAYO CLINIC PROGRAM, Department of Community Medicine, College of Medicine, University of Florida, Gainesville, FL 32610, (904) 392-2994.

RESOURCES

"Boycott Health Corps," Irwin Redlener, HEALTH RIGHTS NEWS, 542 S. Dearborn, Chicago, IL 60605, June 1972. pp. 12-13
. . .calls for a boycott of the National Health Service "until the bureaucrats and legislators restore its potency." Redlener argues that the act has been rendered powerless by a major budget slashing and the fact that local government professional societies can keep the corps out of their area.

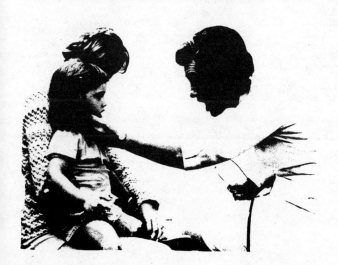

When health care is free, too many people come to doctors with nothing wrong . . . Let's face it, after three generations of welfare, there are people who have forgotten how to work.
—Dr. Charles Hoffman
former AMA President

MENTAL HEALTH

Psychiatric patients occupy approximately 50% of all hospital beds in this country; one in ten Americans is hospitalized for "mental illness" at some point in their lives. Often those who are hospitalized are the people society deems least productive economically and most offensive socially. Sixty percent are women; the rate of admission for Third World people to state and county hospitals is 1½ times that of Whites. There is also a large proportion of "rebellious youth" committed by their parents for any reason from smoking marijuana on up. And it is no surprise to find old people in mental institutions, many of whom are alone and poor with no place else to go. For many, mental hospitals are revolving doors—once committed, their rate of return is high.

Whereas an illness implies an organic disease, the term "mental illness" used in its popular sense has no medical significance at all. Its value lies in its ability to classify people who go outside the bounds of nonconformity that society is willing to tolerate. Most of those sensitive to the issues of mental health prefer the term "problems in living," feeling this is a more accurate description of what troubled people are going through.

The mental health industry rests on the omniscient and authoritarian image of the mental health professional. Psychiatrists have assumed powers equal to those of law enforcement officers, but without the safeguards the legal system is supposed to provide. They are able to label deviants and sentence them to an indeterminate stay in an institution that leaves them with a permanent stigma. Yet the supposed infallibility of psychiatrists rests on shaky ground. Their arbitrary judgements can mean living death for masses of confused, troubled, angry people. An example of professional fallibility is the Rosenhans study in which nine "sane" people lied their way into being committed. Once in the hospital, they reverted back to their natural personalities yet were unable to prove their "sanity" to those in power.

In a mental institution psychiatric records replace criminal records; hypodermics and chemicals replace guns and bars; hospital administrators replace wardens and aides replace the guards. Just as the term "rehabilitation" has been perverted to give prison officials free rein to perpetuate any number of indignities and atrocities on inmates, the term "treatment" has been similarly redefined in regard to mental patients. Powerful drugs used indiscriminantly have dangerous side effects, including everything from paralysis to loss of judgement and mental coherency. Electro-shock treatments, a process by which brain cells are electrically stimulated, can produce loss of memory in a short time and can turn people into vegetables if used extensively. Yet their long-term therapeutic value, like that of psychoactive drugs, is doubtful. The most dramatic example of unlimited power of the therapist is found in the recent upsurge of psychosurgery: the cutting away of portions of the brain to drastically alter behavior.

COMMITMENT

Two thirds of the mentally incarcerated are committed to institutions involuntarily and denied their legal and human rights in the process. The commitment procedure in this country is generally shockingly brief, vague and easy to carry out, although the particulars vary from state to state. It is vital to understand that involuntary commitment to an institution against one's will is an act of power, in direct violation of an individual's liberty and dignity. Most groups organizing in mental hospitals agree that those who have committed violent crimes should be separated from other people, but they must be insured procedural safeguards, fair trials, the right to prove their innocence, and the recognition that they can be physically isolated but not mentally controlled.

There are three basic types of commitment: involuntary emergency, involuntary non-emergency, and voluntary. In many state hospitals, most of the patients originally enter under emergency commitment statutes. Such commitment is supposedly based on the patient's potential danger and need for treatment, both of which are vaguely defined by nearly all the states. By most estimates, fewer than 5% of those in institutions are truly dangerous to themselves or others (Prisoners of Psychiatry). Seldom is anyone committed for a proven "act of danger" to someone else. More often it is the eccentric old person in the park, the bothersome neighbor, the suspicious-looking stranger, or the family member who fails to abide by clan or societal mores. The undefined statutory working of commitment laws paves the way for friends, relatives, psychiatrists, and judges to polish their own social biases into "sincere concern," "medical opinions," and "court findings" that often end up in commitment.

Emergency commitment is roughly equivalent to "arrest," or "preventive detention," in criminal law. In most cases, an individual can be committed if there are "reasonable grounds" to believe s/he may be "mentally unsound." The guidelines for determining such illness are not only arbitrary, but are often imposed with sexist, classist and racist biases. Once committed, a person loses all rights for the length of commitment, which can range from one day to more than 30 years. After initial confinement, one usually is entitled to a perfunctory court hearing. However, the hospital can prevent a patient from attending her/his own hearing. If the patient is allowed to be present—after being heavily drugged, deprived of any emotional support and legal help—s/he is unlikely to present a very convincing picture of competence to an intimidating judge. In contrast to criminal law, the system deposits the burden of proof on the patient to prove her/his sanity. The procedure for commitment on an involuntary, non-emergency statute, is similar to the process above.

Conditions inside mental hospitals are often filthy and destructive. The life of an incarcerated mental patient is one of unbearable tedium, structure, and depersonalization. Most are drugged to the point of not feeling and some go for weeks and months at a time without seeing a physician. These brutal institutions are run authoritarianly, by the psychiatrists and administrators. In addition, many doctors in state institutions are foreign (the AMA prevents them from being licensed for private practice) and can hardly communicate effectively with patients.

Often nurses, aides, social workers and other staff spend more time with the patients and understand their situations better than the doctors in charge. But because of the institutional hierarchy they must accept the doctors' recommendations for what may be harmful or unnecessary treatment. Overworked and underpaid, they feel helpless to make real changes and are taught only one way to deal with patients' needs. Thus, many workers gradually harden themselves and become part of the conditions that once appalled them.

MENTAL PATIENTS' RIGHTS

Although the abolition of mental warehouses is an ultimate goal of most mental patients liberation groups, the immediate necessity of knowing the moral and legal standards which state and private institutions can be made to live up to is also of great importance. This knowledge can mark the difference between an indeterminate institutional stay and the road back to dignity and self-determination. The rights listed below represent a cross-section. Some have been legally won and some are those which mental patients around the country are using as organizing points. Remember that laws existing in one state are often ignored in practice. Even the most "progres-ive" laws have built-in clauses permitting denial of statutory rights if it is in the patient's "best interest."

People incarcerated in mental hospitals have the right to free legal counsel and effective, safe treatment. They have the right to refuse any therapy, medication, or treatment, mechanical restraints or experimentation. They have the right to keep their possessions, not to be locked out of their room, and to communicate privately with anyone they choose. Any patient has the right to periodic review of status and access to all hospital records concerning her/him. Mental patients should be fully informed of their moral and legal rights and must be allowed to organize within the hospital. They should have the right to effective grievance procedures and input into institutional policies through patients' councils, and outside support mechanisms. They have the right to live in the least restrictive environment possible, the right to evaluation by other than medical personnel, and the right to be present at their own hearings. They should be protected from self-incrimination and should receive a fair wage for any voluntary work. Upon leaving the hospital, patients should be helped to find housing and employment. The state has the duty to prevent discrimination in all forms including insurance, owning property and other civil matters. The most basic right a person has is the right to live in dignity and pride, without fear of reprisal for nonconformity to arbitrary social constraints.

The mental patient's right to treatment has been the center of much legal action lately, highlighted in the Alabama case of Wyatt vs. Stickney. As in this case, the basic reason for bringing suits against institutions for not treating patients is that new treatment standards set by the court (such as increased staffing) are often too high for the institutions to afford; this forces them to release large numbers of patients. However, the problems of the "right to treatment" approach are that the state has no obligation to provide any aftercare for released patients, and the treatment given to remaining patients is of questionable value. Also, this approach does not really challenge the idea of involuntary commitment.

THERAPY

Dealing with the mental health profession in the hospital or through private therapy can be very destructive for a person already overstimulated by the complexities of our society. Therapy can be purchased at an average of $40 an hour for a psychiatrist, and about half that for a psychologist. Methods of therapy range from the drawn-out, expensive, analytical visit to the "walk in, talk to the doctor for five minutes, and get your weekly supply of drugs" approach. A typical therapeutic relationship is a vertical power structure, with the professional on top and the patient on the bottom. The therapist's role is to be objective and all-knowing, while the therapee's role is to be appreciative, passive, and unquestioning. Most psychiatrists will not even see a patient until s/he admits to being "sick," and consequently to being completely dependent on the professional to make her/him well.

Many of the problems in living people face are direct results of a society which usurps an individual's power and ability to function as an autonomous free-thinking entity. Yet it is a rare psychiatrist who will deal with underlying social condi-

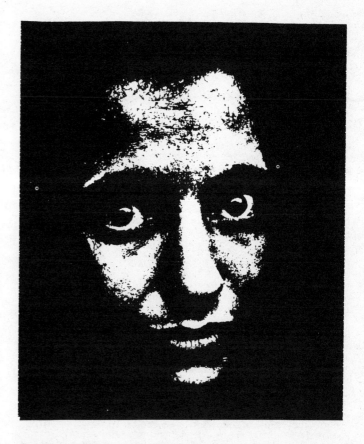

To be taken without consent from my home and friends; to lose my liberty; to undergo all those assaults on my personality which modern psychotherapy knows how to deliver; to be re-made after some pattern of 'normality' hatched in a Viennese laboratory to which I never professed allegiance; to know that this process will never end until either my captors have succeeded or I have grown wise enough to cheat them with apparent success—who cares whether this is called Punishment or not: That it includes most of the elements for which any punishment is feared—shame, exile, bondage, and years eaten by the locust—is obvious. . . . Even if the treatment is painful, even if it is life-long, even if it is fatal, that will be only a regrettable accident; the intention was purely therapeutic. . . . But because it is 'treatment,' not punishment, it can be criticized only by fellow experts and on technical grounds, never by men as men and on the grounds of justice.

—C.S. Lewis, "The People Helpers"

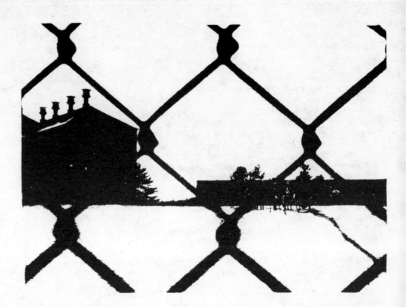

tions that spawn people's problems. Equally unusual is the doctor who will help patients develop the skills to take control of their lives and change such an environment. The whole nature of psychiatry works towards reinforcing a person's dependence on outside forces.

Half of a psychiatrists' training is medical and all the criticisms of the medical profession are applicable to them. Rather than seeing patients as total entities, psychiatrists are trained to separate out certain parts of a person's behavior and slap on labels such as schizophrenic or paranoid. Dealing primarily with the symptoms of troubles, they rely heavily on drugs and other artificial behavior-changers, like shock therapy, to relieve a patient's anxiety or depression. As an instructor at one of the country's leading medical institutions told his students: "Medicate to the point of toxicity and reduce the dosage one level." This is cheaper and less time-consuming than dealing with the root causes of a person's problems; it is also extremely dangerous. New mood and mind-altering drugs are placed on the market each year, seldom adequately tested and controlled. No one government agency has complete overview on the preliminary human experiments necessary to market them, and often patients are not even informed of possible side effects.

ALTERNATIVES TO INSTITUTIONALIZATION

The direct result of mental incarceration is to leave patients with the stigma of treatment and an uncertain future. Developing viable alternatives to institutionalization is and must continue to be a prime focus of those concerned with humanizing care for people with problems in living.

In 1963 under Kennedy's administration, Congress authorized the National Institute of Mental Health to set up a network of community mental health centers throughout the country. This act, sometimes referred to as "a keystone of managerial liberalism," intended for the centers to provide emergency care for community as well as "rehabilitation" for those who "chronically act in aberrant ways." A deeper purpose was for them to supposedly deal with the "social problems" of many inner-city communities as a whole. Many activists have legitimate fears about such government-funded social action programs pacifying community members by teaching them to accept their situations and diverting community leaders from more militant challenges against repressive conditions. Yet few if any of these community mental health centers have initiated programs effective enough to warrant such concern.

A major problem has been lack of community input in the centers from their original planning and design through their current operation and policysetting. Ideally, participation in community-based facilities could help take the fear out of "mental illness" Yet whereas all centers must have some form of community advisory boards, usually these boards were set up sometime after the center was already in opera-

tion, to meet Federal guidelines instead of to truly involve community members. The people on the boards are rarely representatives of the grass roots community; rather they are from service agencies and businesses. Often they work in the system themselves and don't question the medical model of most psychiatric treatment or have any knowledge of alternative care. Even if such were not the case, it would not make much difference, since the boards are only advisory and have little real power over the operation of the center. The professionals who run the center spend most of their time in management, severely limiting the amount of time that can be spent in delivering direct services. Therefore, pill-pushing is often nearly as common here as in the state hospitals. In other centers professionals have used funds for their own ends, experimenting on isolated cases with their pet "cures", rather than using the money in the community's interest.

The centers have done little to try to coordinate mental health services in the community and even less to publicize to community members the services they do offer. This is reflected in the minimal degree of walk-in services, advocacy, and comprehensive follow-up, as well as the absence of complaint procedures. Though their basic intent was to do mainly out-patient care, they often provide a similar or even greater percentage of in-patient services. It is no wonder that community people see such centers not as serviceable community-oriented and run clinics, but merely as extensions of the city and state institutions they fear and despise.

Whereas some centers do attempt to involve more community members by training and hiring them as paraprofessionals, such jobs are often dead end. That is, the training is usually not connected with any accredited educational institution. The mainly poor Black women who end up in these jobs as family outreach workers often provide more effective service than do the licensed professionals, but they have no standardized credentials to show for their skill when they try to get a similar or more advanced job in another institution. One center in Chicago has tried employing ex-patients themselves along with its academically-credentialed professional employees, hoping they could teach each other skills. However, class differences, professionalism and intimidation have been major stumbling blocks to their working together as effective teams.

The concept of local centers is a valid one. But it is imperative that they be planned, controlled and staffed by the community and linked with community struggles for self-improvement, through drug programs, better housing, schools, etc. Emphasis should be placed on outreach and direct services, both preventive and crisis intervention. Ideally, these centers should be an active force in helping people become aware of society's oppression and how to fight it.

The concept of halfway houses to help people who have been incarcerated get back into the day-to-day struggle of living has been around for quite a while. Ideally such places can help ex-patients regain the strength and self-confidence to deal with the outside world again in a positive way. If mental health involves being in control of our lives, then this can be an opportunity to regain that control in an affirming atmosphere. Such environments must encourage people to make decisions, to accept responsibility for determinging their own lives once again. This means that house residents, along with staff, must have full control over house policies, house rules, who may come and who should leave (including staff). However, after long months and even years of institutionally-conditioned helplessness, the struggle back can be a slow and painstaking process. Having others around who can relate to these feelings and be supportive rather than paternalistic is vital.

Unfortunately such houses are rare. In many cities "halfway houses" are actually shelter care facilities—dingy hotels—for those released from institutions who have absolutely no place else to go. They are over-crowded and usually profit-making: in many cases, residents never see their welfare checks as these go straight to the owners. Ex-patients' dependency on the mental institution is merely transferred to the halfway house, and residents are still treated as if they are being hospitalized. Only "trouble-makers" receive any type of individual attention.

Such services as community mental health centers and halfway houses are most often used after problems have surfaced. As with medical health problems, however, it is necessary to penetrate further and deal with the sources of difficulties rather than with symptoms. Such primary prevention concepts are growing rapidly and finding expression in a variety of experimental programs around the country. This entails helping people get in touch with all the factors that produce tensions—families, jobs, etc.—and learning to deal with these effectively. It means assisting people in learning how to respond to stress, how to make better choices. Present prevention programs are concentrating on working in schools, home, offices, and other areas to set up models, laws, and curriculums to help people learn to be more human. Self-help is an integral concept here: learning to do our own problem-solving with the support of others.

ORGANIZING FOR CHANGE

Former mental patients, and community people who have become aware of their plight have already started combining forces in this move for change. As one ex-patient activist put it: "You must first change your view of yourself, get it together, know where you're at, where you're going and how to keep from being messed over getting there." To do this, they're forming support/affirmation groups, communes and other alternatives. At this point, consciousness-raising and education are cornerstones of the movement. This includes everything from spreading awareness of the issues through the media to performing street theatre, to picketing offending institutions and professional meetings. While some people are putting their energy towards in-hospital organizing, this approach is studded with inherent difficulties. Outsiders have a tremendously hard time getting into the hospital; once in, they often find patients thoroughly de-energized, intimidated, suspicious of more outsiders looking out for their interests, and doped almost to the point of immobilization.

Most state laws relating to mental patients need redefining in the patient's actual best interests. Mental patients, ex-patients, radical professionals, public interest lawyers and other concerned people are lobbying and testifying to have these laws changed. Some legal services groups and schools are setting up classes for lawyers and students interested in mental health law, while others are initiating advocacy systems, including trying to contract with hospitals to represent patients. Several legal resource and back-up centers are collecting relevant data on mental health law and litigation. In addition, several precedent-setting cases have been won over the last few years, including a Michigan case outlawing experimental psychosurgery as an invasion of privacy.

There is a tremendous need for more people to become acquainted with mental health law, how to change it, and how to use it advantageously. For example, it is difficult to get psychiatrists on the witness stand, but once in court, lawyers have had notable success in exposing the fallibility of their opinions, often resulting favorably for the patient involved. However, the legal approach alone is a limited one—it is often predicated on the assumption that large-scale mental incarceration is valid if patients are generally treated humanely and fairly, given all their rights. Even people legally challenging involuntary commitment don't necessarily accept responsibility for the deeper problems of how to prevent commitment in the first place, how to support those who have problems in living once they're out of the institutions, or of how to humanize society's attitude towards mental illness in general.

Far more energy is required, to bring substantial changes in attitudes and ultimately in practice: research area institutions and publicize inhumane conditions and practices; go to court and lobby, publish and distribute patients' rights handbooks, demonstrate against psychosurgery. Encourage the development of mental health teams—radical psychiatrists, lawyers, social workers and other community people to visit patients in institutions, give them support and work to get them out. Write examples of "model" legislation to present to Congresspeople, teach community classes about self-help vs. professional infallibility, promote patient-run halfway houses, instigate primary prevention programs, aid patients released from institutions in finding housing, jobs and friendship. Help bring test cases which challenge present statutes and would contribute toward significantly changing conditions—on a massive scale such cases could have a huge impact because, as one legal activist put it, "the system rests on a rotten foundation"

Set up community resource centers which can turn people on to various community alternatives to traditional therapy, from those oriented toward humanistic psychology and family therapy, to rap groups, bio-energetics, women's/men's groups, radical therapy, transactional analysis, yoga, or anything that will help people understand their experiences. Along with this, encourage people to work with community coalitions to push for community-worker control of state and private mental hospital boards, and community mental health centers. For above all, it is essential that the struggle not end with meeting the individual's needs of the moment or with a specific legal fight—rather, we must all work to help each other relate our personal problems in living to the oppressive social forces of our society and commit ourselves to changing them. (See also Community Health, Hospitals, Health Personnel and Training.)

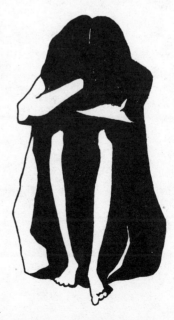

If a system is making its people sick should we attempt to cure the people and place them back into the system, or should we change the system?

—Ernest Mann

RADICAL PSYCHIATRY CENTER. . . is a political working collective of 15 people doing personal problem-solving in groups. They believe that "personal problems" are inseparable from political factors, and that a major focus of problem-solving is to identify and confront oppressive forces. Intentionally anti-professional, the Center's workers are White, middle- and working-class men and women, over half of whom are gay. Their work includes offering action-rap drop-in groups, for women; and for men/women together, which do on-the-spot problem-solving and generally introduce people to their way of working. In addition, there are small, on-going problem-solving groups which meet regularly with two facilitators from the Center; these are for people who want to change their lives, many of whom want to gain a political analysis as well. The Center also recently offered a nine-month training program for 30 people from the community and from the country at large, to share political perspectives and skills with them so they could set up similar projects and lead problem-solving groups; they plan a second training program beginning this fall. Basic priorities of the Center have centered around sexism. They are starting to deal with classist conflicts, and are working to understand how these ideologies at the same time support the capitalist state and generate "personal problems." They publish a bi-monthly newsletter. Contact RADICAL PSYCHIATRY CENTER, 2333 Webster St., Berkeley, CA 94705, (415) 548-2782.

ASSOCIATION OF PSYCHOLOGISTS FOR LA RAZA. . . is a splinter group of the American Psychological Association with approximately 100 Spanish-speaking members. The loosely structured group works to improve psychological care for the Spanish speaking. Contact ASSOCIATION OF PSYCHOLOGISTS FOR LA RAZA, c/o Floyd Martinez, 1414 N. Gate Sq., Reston, VA 22070, (703) 471-4631.

CITIZEN'S COMMISSION ON HUMAN RIGHTS. . . was formed in mid-1969 as a result of the involuntary incarceration of a Polish immigrant who was given intensive electroshock treatment. Since he spoke no English, he had no way of showing his mental competence, but he finally managed to communicate with a hospital aide. This resulted in getting the man legal counsel and a hearing, for which an independent psychiatrist was brought in to examine him. The psychiatrist was Thomas Szasz, who spoke Polish and helped obtain the man's release. Condemning the control tactics of psychiatry on unwilling citizens, this action-oriented group has been instrumental in securing the release of a number of mental patients hospitalized against their will, has taken testimony from ex-patients about psychiatric abuses, and has conducted a vigorous campaign for the adoption by hospitals of a bill of rights for mental patients. They also exposed the existence of a large psychiatric computer program which made available to virtually anyone the complete psychiatric history of mental patients. With chapters in 11 major cities and on 10 college campuses, CCHR is presently devoting much of its energy to lobotomy and psychosurgery projects. This involves a major lobbying project in Washington and intensive research documenting and exposing instances of lobotomy and psychosurgery all over. They are also engaged in personally inspecting and rating state mental hospitals around the country, even possibly writing them all up in a consumer's guide format. Despite the fact that the Commission is sponsored by the Church of Scientology, they have worked closely in the past with such groups as MCHR and ACLU, and are dedicated to insuring the rights of mental patients. Contact CITIZEN'S COMMISSION ON HUMAN RIGHTS, c/o Stephanie Hamilton, 5930 Franklin Ave., Los Angeles, CA 90028, (213) 464-5192, ext. 76, or (213) 464-4055.

TWICE BORN MEN PROJECT. . . came together in 1971 to try to deal with Bay Area veterans' post-Vietnam syndrome. 7.8% of California's over-16 male population are veterans; the project mainly works with those "high-risk" vets who have been turned down for jobs and/or have often been in prison, and spend most of their time on the streets. They report that presently 11% of federal prisoners are veterans, 80% of whom were never "in trouble" before. More US veterans of the Vietnam War have died since their release from active duty, many from suicide or drug overdoses, than died in the war itself. TBM exists to help the vets work through feelings of anger and frustration, turn them on to the skills they have and open them up to alternatives (job, school, etc.) Outreach is done in local bars, and the project (composed of vets, with help from sympathetic psychologists) works with the vets in both 1-to-1 and group sessions, all free. Feeling that it is important that the men not become too isolated, after time is spent in all-male vets groups they are encouraged to become part of TBM's mixed groups which may include wives, other ex-cons or juvenile delinquents. Special family therapy sessions are held to help the women the vets are relating to understand the inability of the vet to feel. Seeing PVS as a microcosm of what's happening in American society, the project also gives workshops and speeches around the country, encouraging people to work in their own communities and accept responsibility for PVS until it disappears. Contact: TWICE BORN MEN PROJECT, c/o Jack McCloskey, 4171 26th St., San Francisco, CA 94131, (415) 282-5414.

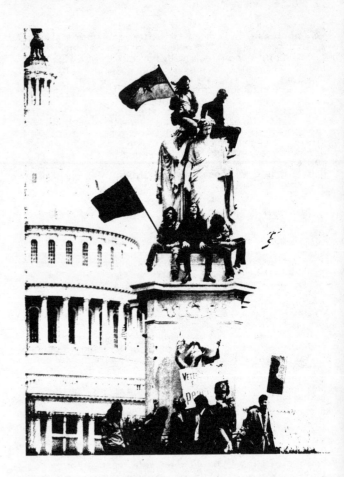

NATIONAL CLEARINGHOUSE ON POST-VIETNAM SYNDROME. . . is a referral/information service on Post-Vietnam Syndrome (PVS). Currently it is compiling a comprehensive research library on PVS (see review) and can put people in touch with PVS rap groups around the country. Contact VIETNAM VETERANS AGAINST THE WAR/ WINTER SOLDIER ORGANIZATION, NATIONAL CLEARINGHOUSE ON PVS, 2532 N. Holton, Milwaukee, WI 53212, (414) 562-9371.

PSYCHOLOGISTS FOR SOCIAL ACTION. . . "is part of the struggle to eradicate racism, sexism, militarism and poverty" and has active chapters in New York, Boston and Washington, D.C. Current projects are centered around the following major concerns: "exposing the bankruptcy of the hypothesis that intelligence, even IQ, is predominantly inherited"; eliminating sexism/racism/elitism from psychology teaching materials; opposing psychosurgery; examining the social/ethical consequences of forms of behavioral control; advocating for victims of the Vietnam war; supporting victims of the Chilean coup; and working for free, human and humane psychological and medical health care." They also offer an excellent monthly newsletter, "Social Action" with detailed articles about their projects and concerns. Contact PSYCHOLOGISTS FOR SOCIAL ACTION, Box 463, Planetarium Station, New York, NY 10024 or call Rosalind Gianutsos (516) 294-8700, Ext. 7484.

EMERGENCY CONFERENCE TO SAVE MENTAL HEALTH IN ILLINOIS. . . is a statewide coalition of over 20 on-going groups—from unions to social service agencies to ex-patients groups to professional associations—which organized because they were upset about the direction of mental health care in the state. Specifically, the State Department of Mental Health has been cutting back 10% a year on funding for state-provided mental health care (by closing hospitals and day centers for example) without implementing new ways to staff and fund community facilities to help people who want some continuing form of assistance. The Conference feels the state is moving too quickly without making adequate preparations for the displaced people involved, thus forcing communities to impose local taxes to pay for new facilities. In March of '73 the emergency conference of over 1,000 people was called to plan a strategy for fighting this irresponsible policy. The result of their labors was the proposal of a bill, now in the state legislature, which would basically subject all department actions to reviewal by community boards located in each of the 7 regions of the state and composed of community-selected consumers and non-profit-making providers groups. These would hold public hearings and review all cutbacks and reductions of services and grants, having veto power to stop the closings if they felt the department hadn't made provisions for valid alternatives to be established. Already, the precedent-setting proposal has been a cohesive force in pulling people together all over the state and giving them a new sense of self-determination. Supportive actions are building, ranging from lawyer's considering bringing right-to-treatment suits, to local communities pressuring their representatives to sponsor the bill. Though not a permanent group, the conference is a good example of community groups uniting to pressure for public accountability. Contact EMERGENCY CONFERENCE TO SAVE MENTAL HEALTH IN ILLINOIS' 3435 Dearborne, Rm. 706, Chicago, IL 60616, (312) 939-4987.

PATIENT'S ADVOCATE OFFICE. . . in Fergus Falls Minnesota State Hospital, has been fighting great odds to demand the rights of the mostly poor people involuntarily incarcerated there. The advocacy office was recently set up as a result of a recent Minnesota welfare policy stating that there must be an advocate salaried by every state hospital; unfortunately, general enforcement so far has been lax. All patients are contacted upon entering the hospital and are given a pamphlet describing the advocate's functions and how to contact her/him. Most time is spent in attempting to get people released from the institution. They are also trying to get money to fund a legal aid group in the town, since without such back-up assistance their powers are limited. Future plans of the advocate's office include organizing a course to teach advocacy from the patient's point of view, to social workers. Contact Bill Johnson, OFFICE OF THE ADVOCATE, Box 157, Fergus Falls, Minnesota 56537, (218) 739-2233 Ext. 263.

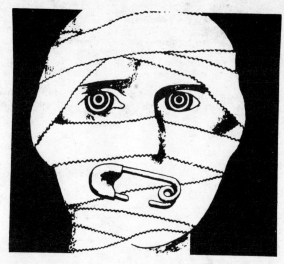

AMERICAN ASSOCIATION FOR THE ABOLITION OF INVOLUNTARY MENTAL HOSPITALIZATION, INC.
. . . acts mainly as a national educational clearinghouse, information center and referral service. Its membership directory includes listings of professionals sympathetic to the cause, whom people can contact for help. They lack the funds to fight cases in court and hope instead to spur people to take action themselves. Thomas Szasz, a well-known civil libertarian in the field, chairs the board; the Association also publishes "The Abolitionist", a compendium of pertinent legal opinions, book reviews and articles. Contact AMERICAN ASSOCIATION FOR THE ABOLITION OF INVOLUNTARY MENTAL HOSPITALIZATION, INC., 301 Sedgwick Dr., Syracuse, NY 13203, (315) 474-0131.

POLITICAL PSYCHOLOGY COLLECTIVE. . . is a socialist-oriented study group of 10-25 graduate students, social workers, and community organizers. With MCHR they have co-sponsored two forums—one at a New York hospital on "Medicine and Social Control," for workers allied with health services, which historically traced strains of racism, sexism and individualism in psychology. The other forum, "Race and Intelligence," discussed why the theory of a genetic relationship between race and intelligence is taught, and how to fight it. They participated in a contingent which unsuccessfully tried to pass a resolution against racist rulings about IQ and race at a meeting of the American Psychiatric Association. Presently they are writing a political critique of Thomas Szasz's work on involuntary committment. Contact POLITICAL PSYCHOLOGY COLLECTIVE, c/o Jules Kerman, 3411 Wayne Ave., Apt. 10-A, Bronx, NY 10467, (212) 798-4224.

METROPOLITAN CENTER FOR PROBLEMS IN LIVING
. . . serves subscribers to the prepaid group practice medical care plan, which is available to United Auto Workers as well as other employee groups. Though physically part of Detroit's Metropolitian Hospital, the clinic is relatively autonomous. The staff is composed of psychologists and social workers, as well as psychiatrists, and great emphasis is put on staff equality and personal autonomy. This means that when people call for an appointment, they are automatically assigned to the next staff person in line; another priority is that patients be seen with within 3-10 days after they call. The staff will only work with clients who come to the clinic voluntarily, rarely do psychological testing and abstain from recording information in the outpatient chart (although there is an administrative record that a person has been to the clinic.) Clients are charged $2 per visit. Most staff reject the concept of "mental illness" and refuse to prescribe medication; they stress the importance of people taking responsibility for decisions. Though initially they participated in an NIMH nationwide study of the users of psychological services under prepaid plans (consisting of patients answering a few questions), MCPL has since ceased to cooperate, feeling this was dehumanizing, deceiving and indirectly coercive since the end results of the study could conceivably work against the patients' best interests. Contact METROPOLITAN CENTER FOR PROBLEMS IN LIVING, Metropolitan Hospital, 1800 Tuxedo, Detroit, MI 48206, (313) 869-3600.

ASIAN AMERICAN MENTAL HEALTH FEDERATION...
was begun in September '73 with the immediate goals of set-
ting-up mechanisms for communication between groups, providing a vehicle through which the Asian-American community can advocate for its needs, and make people more aware of
the demands of the Asian community. Funded by NIMH,
they have been in contact with groups all over the country,
have established preliminary communications through a newsletter, and have held conferences in a variety of geographical
regions. Contact ASIAN AMERICAN MENTAL HEALTH
FEDERATION, 150 Eighth St., San Francisco, CA, (415)
626-2737.

CHANGES... is a loosely-knit group of 50-100 people, mostly students, who meet regularly and work with each other
in therapeutic self-help settings. A common technique used
is Carl Rogers' method of reflective listening. They also staff
a crisis hotline and a general rap line for the Chicago area.
Contact CHANGES, 5655 University, Chicago IL 60637,
(312) 955-0700.

RESOURCES

BOOKS

Radical Psychiatry, ed. Phil Brown, Harper, 10 E. 53rd St.,
New York, 10022, 1973. $2.95
. . . a 28-article anthology explaining the origins of radical
psychology, expounding the belief that problems in life can
only be understood in a social framework. The section on
the sociological approach disclaims the concept of mental
illness and analyzes the use of mental hospitals to further the
"pathological" medical base. "The Marxist Foundation"
analyzes the powerlessness, repression, and alienation we
confront daily. "Fighting Back" is a loose collection of tactics used to fight institutional psychology, including a mental
patients bill of rights. This anthology provides a nice overview of where we've been, where we are, and inspiration for
where we must go.

Myth of Mental Illness. Thomas Szasz, Anchor/Doubleday,
245 E. 47th St., New York, NY 10017, 1961. $2.25
. . . the classic refutation of the medical model of "mental
illness", comparing this to the medieval concept that a person is possessed by demons. Indispensable reading for those
committed to helping clear away the cobwebs of discrimination and oppression of those with problems in living.

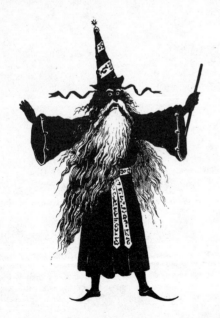

The Madness Network News Reader, Madness Network News
Collective, Glide Publications, 330 Ellis St., San Francisco,
CA 94102, 1974. 192 pp. $5.95
. . . a provocative collection of articles, poems, graphics and
personal statements pulled mainly from past issues of the
MADNESS NETWORK NEWS paper. Providing a "forum
for people who know madness well", it covers everything
from drugs and psychosurgery to the role of the law, and
how to effect radical change in psychiatric institutions;
also featured are selections from Ken Kesey, R. D. Laing,
Jessica Mitford and Thomas Szasz.

**The Manufacture of Madness: A Comparative Study of the
Inquisition and the Mental Health Movement**, Thomas Szasz.
Dell, 245 E. 47th St., New York, NY 10017, 1970. $2.95
. . . "A comparison of the medieval Inquisition and contem-
porary control through psychiatric authority. . ."

Radical Therapist. Radical Therapist Collective. Ballantine
Books, 120 E. 50th, New York, NY 10022, 1971. 292 pp.
$1.25
. . . a collection of the old RADICAL THERAPIST (now
ROUGH TIMES). Selections cover working towards a theory
of radical therapy, a look into Laing's Kingsley Hall, and a
statement by the Insane Liberation Front. Also discusses
rampant sexism in psychology and the need for communities
to have control over community services. Other essays are
concerned with the rights of children, a gay manifesto, and
a radical psychiatry manifesto.

The Age of Madness, ed. Thomas Szasz, Doubleday/Anchor,
Garden City, N.Y. 11530, 1973. $2.95
. . . a frightening account of the history of psychiatry presented through documentary and literary sources. Szasz
backs up his theory that psychiatry has been labelling people
as mentally ill when they were confronting action problems
in living or came into conflict with authorities. In 1851, the
Americal Journal of Psychiatry gave medical 'proof' of the
correlation between being Black and being mentally ill; in
1860, Elizabeth Packard was committed for opposing slavery
and Calvinist authoritarianism; the discoverer of lobotomy
won a Nobel price in 1935. Literary references are interwo-
ven with the factual material to provide a more complete
account of the role between psychology and social oppression,
with excerpts from Sylvia Plath, Jack London, and Anton
Chekhov. Although Szasz is considered a civil libertarian,
the essence of his book has a radical perspective on the politics of psychiatry.

*When you see a psychiatrist, you can say there is going to be a pa-
tient. Because psychiatrists cannot exist without creating or turning people into patients.*

—R.D. Laing

Repression or Revolution, Michael Glen and Richard Kunnes,
Harper Colophon Books, 49 E. 33rd St., New York, NY 10016,
1973. 189 pp. $2.95
. . . provocative analysis of therapy as a tool of capitalist society to maintain the status quo. "Implicit in therapy is the
assumption that the socio-political system is adequate. . .and
that it is the patients who are inadequate and must more than
reform their ways." The authors, who have a strong Marxist
analysis, see therapy as inherently reactionary and blunting
of the political impulse. "The treatment, unfortunately, has
become part of the illness." They see organizing by lower
status health workers and mental patients themselves as the
key to effective change in the mental health field and call
for new community-based training programs. An insightful
book for understanding the class base of psychiatry.

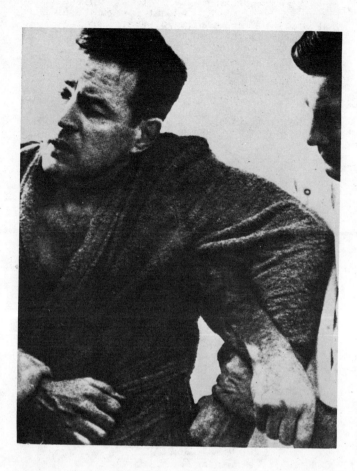

Asylums, Irving Goffman. Aldine Publishing Co., 529 S. Wabash, Chicago, IL 60665, 1961. 386 pp. $12.95
. . . the classic sociological analysis of the oppression of total institutions, especially mental hospitals. <u>Asylums</u> first examines total institutions in general, then focuses on public mental hospitals. It shows how inmates are introduced into the institution, how they are stripped of their identity and roles, and the ways the inmates and staff adapt to the environment. Excellent resource.

Rough Times, The RT Staff, produced by Jerome Agel, Ballantine Books, 201 East 50th St., New York, NY 10022, 1973. 238 pp. $1.65
. . . the second invaluable anthology of articles pulled from the RT magazine, dealing with mental hospitals, professionalism and oppression as mental health. Includes selections on China, Mental Patients Liberation Project, a debate on the myth of professional skills, union organizing, how to face down the man, people's psychiatry sheets on handling drug emergencies/suicides, and lobotomies and prison revolts. "Psychological oppression is a pervasive aspect of modern capitalism. The choices of bourgeois existence are madness, total apathy and conformity."

Ideology and Insanity, Thomas S. Szasz, Doubleday/Anchor, Garden City, New York, NY 11530, 1970. 263 pp. $1.95
. . . Szasz warns of political tyranny disguised as psychiatric therapy: "under the guise of a health ethic, psychiatry may easily become an all-powerful social force for regulating human behavior." His book covers the "psychiatric dehumanization of people" through mental health services in school and university, courts, community health centers and psychiatric hospitals. Szasz argues convincingly that "conflicting human needs cause problems in living—not insanity."

The Politics of Experience, R. D. Laing. Ballantine Books, Inc. 101 Fifth Ave., New York, NY 10003, 1967. $.95
. . . radical analysis of psychiatry; one of the best.

The Divided Self, R. D. Laing. Pelican Publishing House, 433 Gravier, New Orleans, LA 70130, 1970. $1.45
. . . existential study in sanity and madness.

To be a revolutionary, you must be a little loco—and you must never be afraid.

—Che Guevara

Going Crazy: The Radical Therapy of R. D. Laing and Others, ed. by Hendrik M. Ruitenbeek, Bantam Books, 666 Fifth Ave., N.Y., N.Y. 10019, 1972. 308 pp. $1.65
. . . is a collection of 21 articles reflecting many different facets and schools of radical therapy. Basically all are united in rejecting the application of psychiatric structure and theories to mental illness. Includes writings on R. D. Laing's community for psychotics, Kingsley Hall; the role of women in radical therapy, clinical experiences with therapeutic communes in the US, and psychiatry's oppression of homosexuals (unfortunately the discussion centers on men.)

Racism and Psychiatry, Alexander Thomas and Samuel Sillen. Brunner and Mazel, 64 University Place, New York, NY 10003, 1970. 176 pp. $7.50
. . . two mental health professionals trace racism in psychiatry in this country and call for more mental health facilities for Blacks as well as an end to racist attitudes among mental health professionals. Unfortunately, the authors are still bound to the medical model of "mental illness".

The Death of Psychiatry, E. Fuller Torrey, M.D., Chilton Book Company, Dept. PW 12874, Radnor, PA 19089, 1974. 234 pp. $8.95
. . . shows how psychiatry got where it is, why it is destructive in its present form, and therefore, why it should die. Recognizing mental illness as a misleading label, he calls for a system of social supports to help people deal with their problems in living. In place of psychiatry, Torrey advocates more fully integrating the study of human behavior into education so we can learn to cultivate better interpersonal relationships and conserve human resources.

PAMPHLETS AND ARTICLES

"CITIZEN PARTICIPATION IN MENTAL HEALTH: A BIBLIOGRAPHY", No. 559, William R. Meyers and Robert A. Sorwart, Council of Planning Librarians, P.O. Box 229, Monticello, IL, 1974, 15 pp., $1.50
. . . good reference tool of both conventional and radically-oriented resources.

"HUMAN EXPERIMENTATION", A Submission to the House Subcommittee on Public Health and the Environment, Citizen's Commission on Human Rights, 5930 Franklin Ave., Los Angeles, CA 90028, 1973. 14 pp.
. . . a clear readable report based on hundreds of pages of research and letters (mainly between drug companies and experimenters) which were removed from the Missouri Institute of Psychiatry. The report has resulted in a statewide moratorium in Missouri on psychiatric drug experimentation on state mental patients. It documents the various drug experiments and immediate effects on patients (no long-term follow-up studies of effects were even done); the lack of informed consent (doctors even lied to relatives about possible side effects); and the conflicts of interest (using state funds to test for private industry.) It also discusses general human experimentation in prisons, psychosurgery abuse around the country, the failure of the FDA to adequately protect the public, the 5 bills introduced in the 93rd Congress that deal with human experimentation, and a declaration of human rights for mental patients. Concludes that legislation must bring an immediate halt to experimentation on prisoners and mental patients, that Congressional investigations be launched into the FDA's role in drug experimentation in all its forms, and that legislation be introduced to protect all people's rights and safety from such abuse.

The public has to recognize that they cannot trust scientists and doctors and health administrators to tell them the truth about what they need for their own health and what's really going on about human experimentation.
—Paul Lowinger, M.D.
Professor of Psychiatry and Bio-Ethics

VVAW/WSO National Clearinghouse on Post Vietnam Syndrome Research Library, put together by Milwaukee chapter of Vietnam Veterans Against the War/Winter Soldier Organization, 2532 N. Holton , Milwaukee, WI 53212, 1974, about 170 pages and growing, price ranges from $6/vets to $50/ federal government
. . . contains over 100 different articles relating to PVS and the emotional needs and problems of Vietnam Vets. Written by vets, news reporters, and sympathetic mental health professionals. The library covers indictments of the Veteran's Administration, descriptions of PVS rap groups, information on vets drug and employment problems, military psychiatry and struggles of Third World vets. The hardest impact by far is felt from the personal letters and poems from vets in prison and out, the stories of vets' postwar suicides, the descriptions of their shame, guilt, rage, alienation, terror, disorientation, and "psychic numbing". "You get chewed up in the Vietnam war machine and get spit out unfeeling. Then you are just the fingers that pull the trigger." There are many examples like Don Kemp, still full of fear after his war experiences, in prison for life for killing his wife during a Vietnam flashback nightmare. It's painful reading and terribly important for those of us who haven't yet come to grips with how our society has totally shut the war and its results out of our minds, neglecting to deal with its victims in our own country in a humane, sensitive supportive way.

"Crisis in Child Mental Health: A Critical Assessment," Group for the Advancement of Psychiatry, 419 Park Ave. South, New York, NY 10016, 1972. $1.00, 138 pp.
. . . criticizes the government's Report of the Joint Commission on Mental Health of Children, claiming that it doesn't really attempt to understand the underlying factors in the anti-child attitudes abounding in our culture. GAP makes its own recommendations on improving child mental health services (including doing follow-up studies of the effectiveness of present programs.) Most valuable is the appendix of the mental health grid, which outlines in some detail particular services needed by all ages of children, such as home visiting programs to support families with troubled children, drug education, and halfway houses for adolescents.

"A BIBLIOGRAPHY OF MATERIALS USEFUL FOR CHANGE IN MENTAL HOSPITALS", No. 533 and 534. Council of Planning Librarians, Post Office Box 229, Monticello, IL 61856, Feb. 1974. 80 pp. $80.00
. . . an academic, library-oriented bibliography of hundreds of books and articles on mental hospitals.

"Psychologists: High Priests of the Middle Class," Dorothea D. Braginsky and Benjamin M. Braginsky, Psychology Today, December 1973, or order from Mental Patients Resistance, P.O. Box 185, Croton, NY 10520. Free
. . . decries the bond between psychology and "mainstream values", the "handholding between psychologists and the managers of society". "Psychologists translate the suspicions that we all share into research hypotheses. Then they 'scientifically' correct the misfits' behavior". The authors give as an example a study of the diagnosing of mental health problems of patients expressing "new left political philosophies": "The results show that the more politically deviant the patient was, the more the diagnosticians said he was mentally disturbed." They feel that in order to really communicate with and help people, psychologists and psychiatrists must become humble, meet their clients as equals, and face "the human condition without trying to classify it by the lights of prevailing ideology."

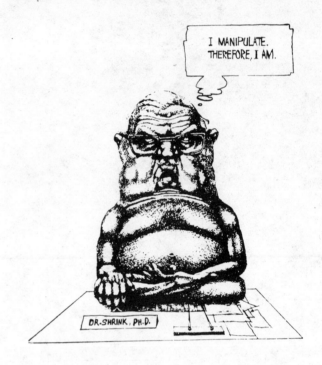

"Ethnicity and Mental Health, Research and Recommendations," Joseph Giordano, National Project on Ethnic America of the American Jewish Committee, Institute of Human Relations, 165 East 56th St., New York, NY 10022, $1.00, 1973. 50 pp.
. . . discusses the importance of understanding the different cultural values and special situations of lower middle class White ethnic people in America today—their feelings of powerlessness and alienation which have definite tie-ins with their emotional well-being—and the necessity of community mental health services (and professionals) in particular to better meet their needs.

"The Performance of Paraprofessionals in the Mental Health Field", Alan Gartner and Frank Riessman, New Careers Development Center, 184 Fifth Ave., New York, NY 10010, 1971. 20 pp.
. . . pulls together a variety of academic studies and data which show how different types of mental health paraprofessionals can play an important role in relating to mental patients. Their less traditional approach to "mental illness" can become a force for basic changes in the field.

LAMP Information Packet, P.O. Box 822, Berkeley, CA 94701
. . . includes the ROUGH TIMES issue on mental patient rights and organizing, plus articles outlining sterilization and commitment laws which are comprehensively footnoted in order to permit people all over the country to draw up handbooks of the rights and liabilities of mental patients in their jurisdiction. LAMP also offers "YOU AND CALIFORNIA's

MENTAL COMMITMENT LAW," a useful model of an inmate rights handbook; unpublished paper on "SEXISM IN PSYCHOSURGERY," and "WOMEN AND INVOLUNTARY HOSPITALIZATION: AN EQUAL PROTECTION PROBLEM." (*$3*)

PERIODICALS

ROUGH TIMES, P.O. Box 89, W. Somerville, MA 02144. $6/year. Free to GI's and the incarcerated
... an honest, witty, and non-technical monthly magazine emphasizing self-help as an alternative to therapy. It includes position papers, excellent graphics, book reviews, covering such subjects as drugs, rights of children, feminist counseling, and alternative therapies. The listings of groups and general resources aimed at social change in mental health and related areas are invaluable. In 1972 the group changed its name from Radical Therapist because they felt this concept had become co-opted by hip professional middle class therapists. RT is constantly seeking out new directions and undergoing self-evaluation; they are involved in work with mental patients liberation groups, mental hospital workers, and general political and prisoners' groups, to combat psychosurgery and behavior mod. ROUGH TIMES is a prime resource for anyone concerned with mental liberation.

MADNESS NETWORK NEWS, P.O. Box 684, San Francisco, CA 94101, $4/year, monthly.
... monthly journal dedicated to fighting psychiatric abuse and protecting the rights and dignity of people labelled crazy as well as those of workers and others touched by the psychiatric system. MNN draws heavily on literary, historical, and art references to support theories on madness and social-political critique of psychiatry. Poems, arts and essays from mental patients compliment political news. Each edition includes news of psychiatric oppression and control news of those organizing against it, and two special columns, one explaining legal happenings (from LAMP) and the other dealing with medical problems (explaining the effects of drugs, etc.)

ISSUES IN RADICAL THERAPY, The IRT Collective, P.O. Box 23544, Oakland, CA 94623 $4/year
... is a practical political journal serving "as a forum for dialogue and exchange of information among people who are involved in the radical therapy movement. Includes thoughtful articles written by the IRT collective, as well as by therapists and professionals who support the interests of workers and of the incarcerated. They look for materials dealing with political oppression, its relation to psychiatric stress, and people organizing to reclaim power over their own lives. Recent issues have included writings on psychosurgery, sexuality, Wilhelm Reich, men's and women's liberation, bio-energetics and body work (as well as nice photos, poems, and graphics.)

FILMS AND TAPES

The Great Atlantic Radio Conspiracy, 2603 Talbott Rd., Baltimore, MD

Politics of Mental Health I & II, 30 min.
... a clear and powerful presentation, in capsule form, of the consequences of labeling someone as "mentally ill," and how "mental illness" is used as a term of political/personal oppression. Interspersed with relevant songs and statistics, the tapes include brief interviews with Peter Breggin on psychosurgery, with Nancy Henley of ROUGH TIMES, and with members of Baltimore's Mental Patients Liberation Front. A fine public education tool.

Indiana University Audio Visual Center, Bloomington, Indiana 47401
"Fountain House," 29 min. b&w $7.75 (sale: $165)
Fountain House, located in the "Hell's Kitchen" section of New York City, reintegrates patients returning from mental institutions as functioning citizens. It helps people find housing, jobs and provides community services in the House itself.

MENTAL PATIENT SUPPORT GROUPS

MENTAL HEALTH TASK FORCE/MCHR... acts as a national and local clearinghouse, answering general information requests, referring people to groups and activities in their areas of the country, supporting local groups, publicizing atrocities in the field, and acting as consultants to a variety of projects. Organized by a former mental patient, the task force is presently promoting patients' rights and anti/involuntary-commitment legislation in both Missouri and Kansas. Task force members also sponsor a class for mental patients on "Problems in Living." Infused with political overtones, it is intended to urge patients towards action, helping those not used to having a voice figure out how to make the system work for them and how to deal with oppressive situations. Class members often go to legislative groups to give them a consumer voice and "keep them honest." Task Force members also helped teach a seminar on "Mental Health and the Law" for senior medical and law students. They advocate the breakdown of the power structure where the psychiatrist is god; in addition to fighting sexism in the mental health field, it actively supports consumer oriented health services, consumer advisory boards, and (ex-) patient-initiated organizing. Contact MENTAL HEALTH TASK FORCE/MCHR, c/o Sue Budd, 928 N. 62nd 62nd St., Kansas City, KA 66102, (913) 334-3491 or (816) 471-0626.

MENTAL PATIENTS LIBERATION PROJECT/NEW YORK CITY... was formed 2½ years ago by past and present mental patients in opposition to the conditions in mental institutions, and to institutional psychiatry in general. Other chapters exist around the country. They have spoken at colleges, successfully pressured for minimal improvements in area mental institutions, and researched the activities of drug companies. Presently, they operate a switchboard/crisis center, advocate for the incarcerated, work to get them released, find them jobs and housing, and provide them with support. MPLP hopes to become involved in more political confrontations. No psychiatrists are allowed in the group. "We are saying no more shall we pretend that the jailers of the people are the healers of the people." For copies of their fiery consciousness-raising material (including articles on women and psychiatry and a mental patients bill of rights), their newsletter FREE EXPRESSION, or more information on resources they offer, contact MENTAL PATIENTS LIBERATION PROJECT / NEW YORK CITY, 56 E. 4th St., New York, NY 10003, (212) 475-9305.

... We are only interested in being ourselves, being free with our emotions and not conforming to the straightjacket norms that go along with being 'sane'. If all this means we're 'crazy' then we say RIGHT ON! ... We are rising up—no longer will we allow ourselves to be stepped on, to be on the bottom, to be treated as the lowest of the low or to be made to feel that way ourselves. We must take the woro 'crazy' and re-define it as something good and powerful and rise up crazy not afraid of being ourselves—not afraid of feeling our own emotions and not afraid of being different—to be everything that we want 'crazy' to mean.

—RISING UP CRAZY

MENTAL PATIENTS SUPPORT COMMITTEE. . . is a well-established, social justice-oriented group. Composed of students and faculty from Kansas University's School of Social Welfare, as well as professionals, ex-mental patients and other community people, the group originally came together to protest the involuntary incarceration of a student for dating a Black man. They managed to get her released, and then went on to do a 6 month research project on the conditions in Kansas surrounding involuntary commitment; spurred on by the results of another study which disclosed that at that time only 5% of those involuntarily committed appeared at their own commitment hearings. They went on to build a statewide coalition. The group is united in working to end involuntary confinement unless someone is endangering human life, and then she must still receive his/her constitutional rights), and for the treatment of all patients with dignity and respect. Their major activity has been writing up and introducing a progressive mental health bill. Despite an intensive public education campaign, the bill died in committee. Undaunted, they are presently rallying support for new milder legislation to be introduced in the fall of '74. Their efforts have already helped instigate a legislative investigation of all state hospitals, and the overall mental health situation in Kansas, though still atrocious, is much improved over 3 years ago. Members are involved in a variety of activities, from serving as a referral/clearinghouse for the state, to writing articles, speaking to civic and professional groups, teaching consciousness-raising classes in human behavior, and starting a similar group in Missouri. Though desiring to bring class-action suits, they lack the necessary funds and have had difficulty finding lawyers willing to take such cases. Presently they're planning a people-to-people campaign to make the necessary resources available to those going through crises, whether this entails counseling by volunteers or briefly moving into a foster home. The group is also trying to obtain funding for a live-in crisis center, to serve a similar purpose. Soon they hope to do more work in the areas of juvenile rights and rights of the elderly. To receive their information packets, which include copies of their legislation, news clippings, and patients rights materials, contact: MENTAL PATIENTS SUPPORT COMMITTEE, 139 Providence, Laurence, KA 66044, (913) 842-4088.

MENTAL PATIENTS ASSOCIATION. . . is one of the strongest mental patients liberation groups around. Formed in 1971 by patients at a day hospital, they aimed to "alleviate the misery of people incarcerated in hospitals upon their release, and set up a full, human community to prevent further admissions". They operate 5 halfway houses and a drop-in/crisis center, help people with housing and employment, and have moved away from a service orientation into a more political one. This involves consciousness-raising of members and community, and pushing for drastic legislative changes. They also publish a fine monthly paper, IN A NUTSHELL, self-described as "politically dependent. . . standing for the world-wide spread of insanity—namely, peace, love and socialism". Contact MENTAL PATIENTS ASSOCIATION, 1982 W. 6th Ave., Vancouver 9, British Colombia, Canada, (604) 738-5177.

MENTAL PATIENTS LIBERATION FRONT. . . is just completing a patients rights handbook covering legal and civil rights of the mentally incarcerated. MPLF plans to distribute the handbook through sympathetic attendants and has given workshops on the book for legal workers. Recent work has involved working with a group of patients in the state hospital around the issue of patients rights. They were invited to do a workshop there and discussed the complaints of patients, the politics of why they were in the hospital and how they felt about it. They urge patients to focus on changing specific institutional policies that affect them directly—like forced medication, attendants being required to take away their money and private property, or even the poor quality of food—in order to feel that first strengthening of power. Contact MPLF, Box 156, W. Sommerville, MA 02144.

MENTAL PATIENTS RESISTANCE OF WESTCHESTER . . . has brought together people who have suffered at the hands of pychiatrists in institutions. Their goal is to direct their anger and frustration towards eliminating all involuntary hospitalization. People who feel their rights have been abused are offered legal services, alternate housing, and referral service for therapy. A speaker's bureau has been set up with members often guest lecturers in high school, college, and medical school classes. Currently they are negotiating with the NYCLU to file suit against Grosslines Hospital in Westchester because hospital officers refused to permit the distribution of a paper detailing the residents' legal rights. A newsletter is sent to those on their mailing lists. Contact MENTAL PATIENTS RESISTANCE OF WESTCHESTER, PO 185, Croton-on-Hudson, NY 10520, (914) 271-5465.

CLEVELAND PATIENT RIGHTS ORGANIZATION. . . was begun in May, 1972 to promote equal rights for mental patients; they deal with the issues of patients rights (in and out of the hospital), housing and job discrimination against the ex-patient, and community ignorance of what being a mental patient means. Composed mainly of ex-mental patients, membership is open to anyone sincerely interested. Their basic activities have included running a small speakers bureau to publicize their cause to the community, as well as appearing in 20 minute video tape presentation to the Ohio House Judiciary Committee which showed experiences in the state mental hospital. It was used to influence legislators towards voting for Bill No. 984 before the Ohio legislature; the bill, though far from ideal, would drastically alter state mental health law by making it much more difficult to involuntarily commit someone, putting an end to indefinite hospitalization, and generally providing more safeguards in the probate process. CPRO is presently editing a patients rights handbook for the state of Ohio. For their packet of materials or more information, contact LEGAL AID OFFICE, Patients' Rights Organization, 2108 Payne Ave., Rm. 707, Cleveland, OH 44114, (216) 861-6945.

THE COMMITTEE ON HUMAN RIGHTS AND PSYCHIATRIC OPPRESSION. . . came together after a national conference of mental patients, professionals and consumers was held in Detroit in June 1973. They are basically concerned with abolishing involuntary mental hospitalization and counterbalancing "the growing deification of psychiatrists." "We hope to see a future where people are not punished further . . . simply for having suffered." Members of this loosely-knit group have written articles on psychiatric oppression, helped individuals get out of institutions, spoken around the country against human experimentation, inspired newspaper articles on commitment procedures, and written and presented "A Loony-Bird's Eye-View of the State Mental Hospital—a modern comic-tragedy about what life is really like in a state mental hospital paid for by your tax dollars and done in your name." Currently they are setting up a library of resources on psychiatric oppression and are writing a booklet to help people get through and out of mental institutions. To be a member "you need not pretend to be a past or present accredited lunatic or idiot. . . although if you are a genuine holder of such credentials you will be especially welcome." To get on their mailing list, contact THE COMMITTEE ON HUMAN RIGHTS AND PSYCHIATRIC OPPRESSION, P.O. Box 1182, Pontiac, MI 48056 (Anne Mazanka), (313) 366-9456.

HEALTH RIGHTS COMMITTEE . . . of the Suffolk County (NY) Human Rights Commission is trying to pressure the state into providing decent aftercare—particularly in the form of financial assistance and housing—for people released from mental institutions. (Some of whom are often found begging on the streets). This involves trying to get aftercare homes, or halfway houses, licensed by the state to put an end to their financial exploiting of ex-patients. In addition, they're pushing for public transportation facilities (none exist now in this New York City suburb) so that patients can have access to outpatient clinics as well as other community services. They also feel the state criteria for Supplemental Security Income should be changed so that it is based on income needs rather than on disabilities. The committee is composed primarily of people working in the health field who are dissatisfied with the present system. Their efforts, compounded by those of other community groups, helped instigate state investigation of what happens to patients when they leave the hospitals. So far, some aftercare homes have been forced to close as a result. The Committee also serves an ombudsperson function between the county and community groups. They've published and are distributing a Health Bill of Rights which was adopted by the Human Rights Commission as its official statement. It calls for community-worker controlled community health institutions, service-oriented rather than profit-motivated care (a stand which has brought down the wrath of local health institutions), primary health facilities for every community, and more for mental patients. Though they are tied to the county, the committee sees its function as one of constantly prodding the system to change. Contact HEALTH RIGHTS COMMITTEE, Suffolk County Human Rights Commission, Veteran's Highway, Hauptauge, New York 11787, (516) 979-2815.

PEOPLE FOR PATIENTS RIGHTS. . . is a civil libertarian-oriented group of professionals and former mental patients working to produce model mental health legislation that will ensure patients' rights and generally serve to keep people out of mental institutions, yet be moderate enough to get through the state legislature. Working with other interested people in the state to build support for the bill, they are trying to bring Missouri's law into congruence with constitutional decisions and recent regional cases which have set precedents in other parts of the country (for example, Wyatt vs. Stickney which established a patient's right to treatment). A cohesive force for over three years, the group feels strongly that individuals take responsibility for their own actions but that only by having all their rights can they assume such responsibility and maintain the self-determination necessary for mental health. Contact PEOPLE FOR PATIENTS RIGHTS, c/o Dick Jones, 5815 McGee St., Kansas City, MO 64110, (816) 444-6019.

RESOURCES

BOOKS

The Making of a Mental Patient, Richard H. Price, Bruce Denner, eds. Holt, Rinehard & Winston, Inc., 383 Madison Ave., New York, NY 10017, 1973. 378 pp.
. . . a collection of papers that trace the process of becoming a mental patient, with emphasis on social circumstances. this thoroughly documented, fairly technical reader is most valuable as a reference tool.

One Flew Over the Cuckoo's Nest, Ken Kesey, New American Library, P.O. Box 999, Bergenfield, NJ 07621, 1962. 272 pp. $.95
. . . a fictional account of one prisoner-turned-mental patient's attempt to help his fellow patients regain their dignity and self-determination, and of his battle against the entrenched repressive forces of the institution. Earthy, sensitive, uproarious, absorbing—and incredibly powerful. This book says it all.

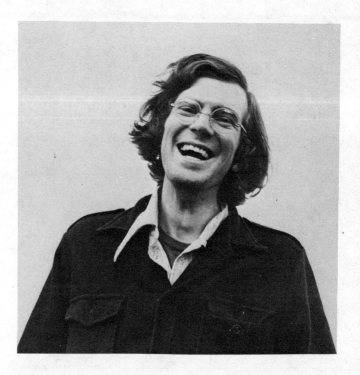

The only freedom which deserves the name, is that of pursuing our own good in our own way, so long as we do not attempt to deprive others of theirs, or impede their efforts to obtain it . . . Mankind are greater gainers by suffering each other to live as seems good themselves, than by compelling each to live as seems good to the rest.

—John Stuart Mill

"The Kansas Experience: An Action Strategy and Its Implementation", order from Mental Patients Support Committee, 139 Providence, Laurence, KA 66044, 1973, 13 pp., send money for xeroxing and postage
. . . an interesting self-analysis of one active group's organizing efforts over a 3-year period. Includes how they worked out strategy decisions, and formulated legislation, as well as major problems and successes. A good resource for groups just getting started.

"REPORT TO THE SENATE HEARINGS ON SENATE BILL 239", Susan Budd, Mental Health Task Force/MCHR, 928 N. 62nd St., Kansas City, KA 66107, 1973. 7 pp. $.80
. . . a justification for the passage of what would have been the most progressive mental health legislation in the country. Though the bill died in committee, this paper can serve as an excellent guide for other groups organizing around similar tactics; it is clearly and calmly written and backs up every plank with sound reasoning. Also helpful for those trying to gain a better understanding of the basic issues of mental patients rights.

"SOME FACTS YOU SHOULD KNOW ABOUT MENTAL PATIENTS RIGHTS IN MASSACHUSETTS," Mental Patients Liberation Front, Box 156, W. Somerville, MA 02114, 1974. 50 pp. Free to mental patients
. . . tells just about every legal aspect of being an institutionalized mental patient. A general political statement is followed by chapters on involuntary admission, rights of minors, civil rights, and treatment. Also includes a valuable explanation on how to file writs. This useful booklet ends with a short peice on what to expect on release and with a mental patients bill of rights. Excellent model.

FILMS AND TAPES

Neal Noelson, c/o Leon Rosenblatt, 333 E. Fifth St., New York, NY 10003

For $50 each (or $25 if tape is supplied) videotapes are available, of and by ex-mental patients who are political activists fighting psychiatric tyranny. Includes tapes on personal experiences of Mental Patients Liberation Project members, an interview with ACLU lawyer, Bruce Ennis, Allen Ginsberg's discussion of his days as a mental patient, and ex-mental patients' poetry, song, and a short drama.

Audio-Visual Center, Indiana University, Bloomington, IN 47401
"To Live and Move According to Your Nature is Called Love," 29 min. b&w $7.75 (sale: $165)
Reverend James Bevel of the Southern Christian Leadership Conference and Almanina Barbour, a Black attorney, are seen in their attempts to organize residents to cope with community mental health problems in Philadelphia. Social problems contribute to mental illness, and it is only when people organize that they can begin finding solutions.

We've been called sick, manic depressive, neurotic. We've never seemed to fit into the roles this society tries to lock everyone in . . . In order to prove we were 'well' we had to conform to the world out there where competition and aggression is what is right for a man—passivity and self-denial right for a woman. And when finally we could fit these roles we were 'cured'. But was it our sickness— our individual inadequacy? Or perhaps it was society. Perhaps our anxieties, frustrations and depressions were the normal reactions to an abornmal society.

—RISING UP CRAZY

TECHNIQUES OF PSYCHIATRIC ABUSE

The advent of new sophisticated forms of psychiatric technology has brought with it a whole new array of psychiatric abuses which are threatening various segments of the population. Psychosurgery, chemotherapy, adverse therapy, sensory deprivation, electrical stimulation, violence screening: these have ceased being codes of a strange, theoretical language to the thousands of mental patients, prisoners, housewives, children, and others who are personally affected by new medical/technological methods of modifying and controlling behavior.

Behaviorist theories have been around for years. Reacting to the psychoanalytical school of psychiatry, the behaviorists basically believe it is not necessary to analyze the past and dig up deep psychological reasons for problem; instead, they concentrate on changing the behavior that is now a problem. This may be a valid approach in some situations, from dealing with autistic children to helping people quit smoking. But it also provides a scientific-sounding rationale for using bizarre and dangerous techniques to produce total conformity, even if those methods severely violate a person's moral, legal, civil, and human rights. Today, the concept and practice of behavior modification has grown to mean living hell for thousands of prisoners, mental patients, and "free" citizens. It is society's newest tool for behavior control, one maintained not only by locks and bars, but by an overwhelming range of pseudo-scientific theories and practices, perpetrated under the guise of humanitarian treatment. As James McConnell, a professor at Michigan State University said in a 1969 speech: "The day has come when we can combine sensory deprivation with the use of drugs, hypnosis, and the astute manipulation of reward and punishment to gain almost complete control over an individual's behavior. We want to reshape our society drastically so that all of us will be trained from birth to do what society wants. I hope the legal profession will help us decide what we should build and show us how to institute the most desirable of building codes." ("A Psychiatrist Looks at Crime and Punishment").

Although many examples of psychiatric abuse can be found in mental hospitals and elsewhere, it is in prisons that the principles of psychiatric control are most blatantly visible. Behavioral scientists have found prisons to be unique and advantageous workshops for testing their behavioral theories: cheap subjects who are already marked as social deviants, controlled conditions, isolated labs. All over the country, special behavior modification centers—euphemistically referred to as "adjustment" units—have sprung up. Some are centralized in one facility and some are decentralized in all the prisons throughout the state. Most are modeled after the sophisticated federal program, START, once a receiving station for all federal prisoners. Though recently abolished as a centralized program, START's hated legacy remains. Behavior modification programs modeled on START act on the principle that to change a person's behavior, it is necessary to take away all support mechanisms that reinforce

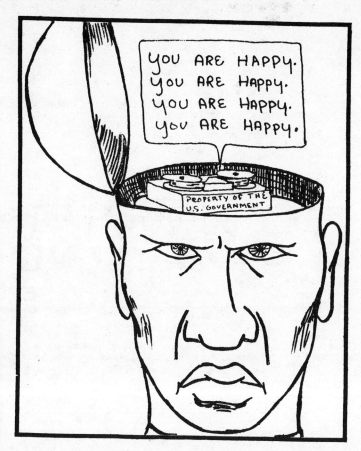

prisoner to be given a quick shot of Thorazine to knock her/him out. And even common psychiatric techniques like **group therapy**, which have use outside of the prison, are destructive in a coercive, total environment. A prisoner forced into such a group, where each participant is encouraged to talk freely, is easily pegged as a "squealer." Often things said in the group can be used against the inmate by guards or fellow cons.

How these practices are perpetuated, who perpetuates them, and who is on the reviewing end is a classic lesson in social control. The START syllabus sums up criteria for choosing participants in behavior mod programs succinctly: "aggressive . . . verbal . . . threatening to the rehabilitation of the less sophisticated offender." This description could actually cover anyone from a prison guard to a politically aware prison organizer. These programs are carried out in the name of therapy, rather than punishment, allowing prison officials to ignore requirements of due process and constitutional guarantees against cruel and unusual punishment. The START syllabus states: "Appropriate behavior can be strengthened by reward and inappropriate behavior can be extinguished by punishment." The task of deciding what is appropriate behavior is left to the wardens and guards, yet neither the prisoners nor the community has elected them to be the safeguards of public morals and social ethics. Furthermore, the scientists in charge of these programs are administratively accountable to no one. Because their practices are classified as being in the field of medicine, they are not directly responsible to the prison system or the courts—a good deal for the accomplice wardens whose similar actions would be dealt with more harshly.

Prisoners and mental patients, along with concerned professionals and public, have successfully brought pressure to stop some of the most sophisticated behavior modification units. Yet the dangers of psychiatric abuse are far from eradicated. They are spreading, from the school room where children are rewarded with M&Ms to conform to certain behavior, to the mental hospital where patients suffer the same indignities as prisoners and must adhere to strict norms if they ever hope to be released. Only continuous monitoring of institutions, and pressuring of legislative and administrative bodies, along with intensive public education and organizing by patient, inmate, and support groups can stop these practices.

Overshadowing even the blatant psychiatric abuse of behavior modification is the upsurge in the irrevocable behavior change known as psychosurgery. **Psychosurgery** is the practice by which sensitive brain tissue is cut away or electrically stimulated to modify behavior (as opposed to neurosurgery, in which tumors are removed or other organic brain damage is repaired.) After the brain mutilation of 50,000 Americans between 1930 and 1950 (most of whom were state mental patients), psychosurgery fell into disrepute as morally, ethically and medically unsound with no lasting positive results. Yet, today psychosurgeons are once again on the prowl. They contend that surgery performance on certain parts of the limbic system which is the seat of higher brain functions and the area believed to control expression of emotion, will "cure aggression and violence", among other things. Yet, a typical reaction to such mutilation is the loss of ability to introspect, to think abstractly, or to express any type of emotion or creativity. Psychosurgeons themselves have described their self-proclaimed successes as becoming ". . . passive and tractable, showing decreased spontaneity. . . patients tend to become more inert. . . less zest and intensity of emotions. . . less capable of creative productivity. . . intellectual capacity deteriorated." (quoted by Peter Breggin in "The Second Wave.") Any scientific base for psychosurgery becomes even more shakey as most psychosurgeons claim that two operations—amygalatotomy and cingulotomy—are the "proper treatment" for everything from schizophrenia to outbursts of hyperactivity in children. It seems simplistically obvious that sufficient cutting away of the brain will block any of these behaviors—at the price of destroying any number of the brain's

previous behavior and then dispense greater and greater token rewards as the subject correctly conforms to the aribitrary norms of the psychiatrist and warden. The more sophisticated behavior mod process consists of a prefunctory "diagnosis"of "agressive"prisoners, who are then integrated into a three part "treatment" procedure. In Stage One, inmates are locked up 24 hours a day in a closet-like cell, sometimes enclosed by chicken wire, and always with minimal communication with the outside world. If the prisoner behaves according to the rules, s/he advances to Stage Two, with a few more privileges, like selected reading material, a little bit of exercise. If s/he does not conform, the inmate remains in Stage One with all privileges revoked. Successful passage through Stage Three entitles the inmate to be released back into the general population of the prison. A special subcategory exists to hold "incorrigibles" indefinitely. Thus whole systems of "Catch 22s" are built into the system of control. The rules invariably reinforce White middle-class values, yet any infraction of them, any protest against what is happening, is thrown back at the prisoner as a sign that more treatment is required. The only way out is complete compliance.

Within the confines of these control units and within the prison as a whole, even more incredible psychiatric abuses to alter behavior are taking place. **Adverse therapy** is a technique that usually involves painful electric stimulation or the use of a drug like Prolixin, or Anectine which produces a feeling similar to drowning. While the drug is taking effect, the authorities describe the behavior the prisoner is supposed to stop. The theory is that the prisoner will cease the forbidden behavior, because it is associated with the death-like sensation in his/her mind. **Sensory Deprivation** means that sense stimuli and support mechanisms are removed, until the subject breaks and conforms to the pattern of behavior the psychiatrist intends. Prisoners going through sensory deprivation are usually placed in solitary confinement, deprived of lights, fresh air, and even the usual noise of other prisoners around them. Over a prolonged period of time, the prisoner becomes a prime target for reprogramming through the gradual increase in supports of a new set of values and behavior. Many prisoners are also drugged into submission.

The use of psychoactive drugs for control, referred to as **Chemotherapy**, is alarming. It is not unusual for a disruptive normal functions. The trouble is that nobody really understands how the brain works or which of its delicate portions controls what reactions. For instance, a woman in Louisville who had recurring violent epileptic seisures was blinded by the severing of her pre-frontal lobes, one of the most sensitive of all brain centers. ("The Second Wave") The psychosurgeon is literally stabbing in the dark when he cuts.

One of the problems the public has had in getting at the truth about psychosurgery is that the surgeons themselves will consistantly proclaim an operation a success within three months of surgery, with no follow-up to see if there is post-surgery deterioration. This presents a grossly distorted picture of the whole issue. The well-known case of Thomas R., whom the notorious Boston surgical team of Sweet, Ervin, and Mark claimed as one of their prime success, is a case in point. Thomas R. was alleged by these leading psychosurgeons to be a violent man; yet, an exhaustive follow-up study investigation of the case by Peter Breggin, a pioneer in the anti-psychosurgery forces, revealed that Thomas R. only became seriously violent after his surgery, and that since his operation this formerly brilliant engineer has become "totally disabled, chronically hospitalized and subject to nightmarish terrors that he will be caught and operated on again. . . ." In another instance, an attending nurse responded to a nationally publicized success story: "I did see pictures of her in LIFE MAGAZINE. . . as an illustration of a person before and after psychosurgery. That article never mentioned her later deterioration, and severe emotional suffering. . . . Her impulsive behavior did not leave her and she began to deteriorate in front of my very eyes. . . She stopped her wonderful guitar playing. She stopped wanting to engage in long, intellectual discussions. She became more and more depressed. Suicidal. . . ."

Selection procedures for subjects is often arbitrary. A mental patient incarcerated for alleged rape-murder in Michigan was chosen to undergo psychosurgery even though he had not shown signs of aggressive behavior for his 18 years in the hospital and furthermore, had undergone no conventional therapy. (Michigan MCHR and DETROIT FREE PRESS). Many of those operated on are people who walk into mental health clinics—rather than long-time inmates of back wards, as might be imagined. Yet, the selection process takes on an ominous political hue when a disproportionate number of women ("a woman's brain is not all that important") and prison activists are chosen to be victims of the knife, and when leading psychosurgeons Sweet, Mark and Ervin state flatly in a letter to the AMA JOURNAL following the Detroit riots in 1967: "It is important to realize that only a small number of the millions of slum dwellers have taken part in the riots. . . . We need intensive research and clinical studies of the individuals committing the violence. The goal of such studies would be to pinpoint, diagnose and treat those people with low violence threshholds." (Sept. 11, 1967, p. 217)

Another trend in psychiatric abuse is to begin modifying the behavior of children who show potential for social deviance. One approach is the proposed mass screening for possible biological and psychological traits which allegedly indicate violent tendencies and possibly using drugs to curb these tendencies. A group of professionals, prisoner groups, and concerned citizens were recently successful in exposing the UCLA proposed Center for the Study and Reduction of Violence, which was to study how to control violence, using methods ranging from mass screening for violence prone traits to psychosurgery. Thousands of school children have been given Ritalin and Dexedrine to thwart hyperactivity. Little is known about the long range effects of these amphetamines on children and there is much to be researched about the nature of hyperactivity (minimal brain dysfunction). But teachers, school psychologists, and others have been stretching this label to include any child who is rebellious or undisciplined. In one midwestern city, 5-10% of the school age children were given their morning pills before heading off to class. (EDCENTRIC) From California comes reports of a doctor who made it his regular practice to expound the glories of chemotherapy at PTA meetings, advocating drugs for everything from a low frustration tolerance level to the inability to postpone gratification. (LNS) A group in Detroit is bringing suit against a state-funded psychiatric clinic for the unauthorized screening of children to see if chemical waste found in the urine could be correlated with aggressive behavior. (MCHR).

None of the above-mentioned examples are isolated incidents or plans of sinister Dr. Frankenstein-like scientists. Rather they are practices and theories developed and perpetrated by government officials and academicians from universities across the country. It was at a three day conference for prison administrators in Washington as early as 1962 that Dr. Edward Stein explained how North Korean brainwashing techniques used American POWs could be applied to convicts in US prisons. The director of the US Bureau of Prisons ended this conference calling on the officials to " . . . undertake a little experimentation with what you can do with some of the sociopathic individuals."

Behavior modification and psychosurgical research and practice have been increasingly funded by federal, state, and local governments over the past decade. Yet, coinciding with this trend has grown a greater prisoner, mental patient, professional, and public awareness and outrage at such practices. Activist individuals and groups have been fighting relentlessly against the new abuses introduced almost daily. They have taken on massive research campaigns, collected mounds of indictive data, embarked on intensive public educational campaigns, testified at legislative and administrative hearings, brought legal suits, and successfully brought pressure to bear in many areas. The Law Enforcement Assistance Agency recently cut off all funds for behavior modification research, while a Michigan court declared psychosurgery unconstitutional and outlawed it in public institutions in the state. Californians were successful in stopping psychosurgery at the Vacaville State Prison and in opposing state funding for the Center for the Study and Reduction of Violence. And three of the most infamous prisoner behavior mod programs have been stopped.

Yet many psychosurgeons and behaviorists are now turning to private funding sources for their projects, while prisons are turning their attention to setting up decentralized "adjustment" centers, ones not so visible as the large ones in the past—and not so easily found and monitored by the community. Yet, indicative of the size of the problem is the scheduled opening in mid-1974 of the $13 million Butner Behavior Modification Research Center. Butner will receive subjects from prisons all over the country and will train technicians in behavior modification. They will then go back to their institutions or communities to "practice".

The real dangers of psychiatric abuse may have only just begun. Only through the continued action and strong organization of those vitally affected and concerned with these issues can the rising tide of psychofacism be stopped in this country.

Psychosurgery was introduced into the United States in 1936 by Walter Freeman, M.D., operating on 4,000 Americans. Freeman describes in his book . . . what he considers to be his best patient. She is 'a negress of gigantic proportions who for years was confined to a strong room at St. Elizabeth's Hospital.' After operating on her the hospital attendants were still afraid of her '300 lbs. of ferocious humanity', so Freeman put on a demonstration of her docility:'Yet from the day after operating (and we demonstrated this repeatedly to the timorous ward personnel) we could playfully grab Oretha by the throat, twist her arm, tickle her in the ribs and slap her behind without eliciting anything more than a wide grin or a hoarse chuckle.'

—"HUMAN EXPERIMENTATION"

DETROIT MCHR/PSYCHOSURGERY PROJECT... has been doing extensive research, speaking, and action around the issue of psychosurgery in mental hospitals and prisons. MCHR, along with the Wayne County Legal Services was the most influential party in a suit to stop psychosurgery experimentation at the state-funded Lafayette Clinic. The court ruled that psychosurgery violates a person's right to privacy and protection under the first amendment and outlawed it in state-funded facilities. The psychosurgery was declared an experiment, not treatment. MCHR has plans to put out a book on the case and expand its action to the issue of control at large. Other important cases involving such control are in the offing. In January MCHR and Legal Aid filed suit related to Lafayette Clinic's use of children in experiments to test if a chemical nutrient supplement can change behavior and if waste material in urine was related to violent tendencies. In both cases, some of the children were not assigned by parents to the experiment; some were sent by the juvenile courts. In neither were provisions made for the child to consent. It is hoped that standards to rule out children for such experiments will be a result of the still-pending case. The project is also giving support to a community group working for a community board to control Lafayette Clinic under state mandate. They put out extensive material on psychological abuse, ethics, and the place of radicals in the psychiatric profession. Contact MCHR c/o Lowinger, 2170 Iroquois, Detroit, MI 48214, (313) 822-4353.

UNITED DEFENSE AGAINST REPRESSION... is "currently involved in a national campaign against programs and projects which relate to the control of human behavior." The Defense educates parents about the use of Ritalin as a control agent on hyperactive, and speaks about the issues of psychiatric abuse. It is beginning to testify about psychiatric repression and along with other such groups is mounting a mass publicity campaign to keep prison officials from sending a noted Chicano jailhouse lawyer, Martin Sostre, to the behavior modification center at Marion, Illinois. United Defense's parent organization, National Alliance Against Racism and Repression, (which grew out of the Angela Davis support committees), sponsored a conference in Michigan covering behavior modification, as well as repressive legislation and prisons in general. United Defense puts out the magazine HUMAN CONTROL AND EXPERIMENTATION REPORT' Contact UNITED DEFENSE AGAINST REPRESSION, 730 S. Wester Ave., Rm. 202, Los Angeles, CA 90005, (213) 388-1288.

NETWORK AGAINST PSYCHIATRIC ASSAULT... grew out of a March, 1974 forum covering the question of forced psychiatric treatment. Composed of present and former psychiatric inmates, mental health workers, concerned citizens and professionals, NAPA is taking a leading role in fighting for legislative and judicial decisions guaranteeing the absolute right to refuse chemotherapy, EST, psychosurgery or any other form of psychiatric treatment. One main focus of the group is education of community and of health workers. NAPA recently gave a workshop on psychiatric abuse to a number of psychiatric technicians. It also does good community education about the issues and steps that can be taken to thwart psychiatric abuse by talking to community groups, making good use of the media and demonstrating at conventions that represent the power of psychiatry. Their pamphlet "FORCED TREATMENT EQUALS TORTURE" provides a good, if frightening, discussion of psychiatric abuse. Contact NAPA, 629 Sutter, San Francisco, CA 94102, (415) 771-3344.

PEOPLE'S LAW OFFICE... does excellent work with political clients in prisons and county jails of Illinois. Focusing on conditions, rights, and atrocities, a prime concern has been behavior modification. A major case has formed around the peaceful work stoppage at the Federal Maximum Security Penitentiary at Marion, Illinois, during which a Latin inmate was brutalized by guards and 150 inmates were locked up, gassed, and put into segregation. The Law Office brought suit against the conditions and unconstitutionality of the lock-up. In the midst of the trial, officials renamed the "hole" as an "adjustment center" and claimed the men were put there for treatment, thus circumventing due process guarantees. Although the Law Office was finally successful in getting most of the inmates out of the center, 50 more have since been shipped there from other prisons in the country. The Law Office has gained access to prison files which reveal that most of those inmates were sent there for political attitudes; it is now filing a second suit to get the rest of the prisoners out. Another suit is the ACLU-initiated case against the Special Programs Unit, Illinois behavior modification plan. Though the suit is still pending, SPU has been officially stopped—for the time being—mostly as a result of pressure from the Black community. Another Law Office suit was brought against the use of Prolixin in the state behavior mod program as a result of an inmate's paralysis and death from the drug. The Law Office's excellent publication on the practice and politics of behavior modification is entitled "CHECK OUT YOUR MIND." Contact PEOPLE'S LAW OFFICE, 2156 N. Halstead, Chicago, IL 60614, (312) 929-1880.

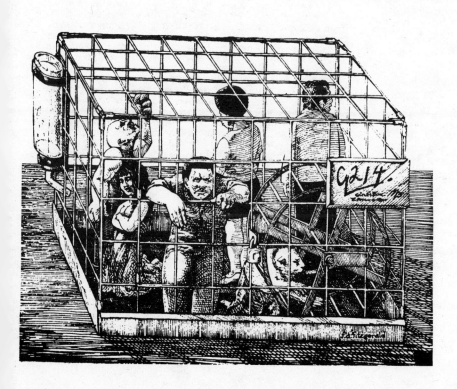

COMMITTEE OPPOSING THE ABUSE OF PSYCHIATRY

... is a group of concerned citizens, mental health and legal workers with the common belief that the tools of psychiatry and biomedical control hold the immediate danger of being used for social control. COAP has taken an active stand against all forms of psychiatric abuse, including behavior modification, and the use of indeterminate sentencing in prisons. It opposes the use of mental patients and prisoners in research because of their economically coercive situations and sees the wide use of drugs in prisons, mental hospitals, and schools as "agents of control." In cooperation with other groups, COAP helped stop project START and the Intensive Programs Unit at the California Institute for Women. One of COAP's most important accomplishments has been stopping the state of California, under the auspices of UCLA's proposed Center for the Study and Reduction of Violence, from using mental patients, children, and other powerless groups for dangerous experimentation. The Committee was concerned that the state ultimately intended to use these techniques for the mass screening of the population. Research, a speakers' bureau, press conferences, lobbying, and public meetings are all part of COAP on-going organizing. Contact COAP, P.O. Box 2278, Station A., Berkeley, CA 94701, (415) 527-7512

NATIONAL PRISON PROJECT

... seeks to broaden prisoners' rights and improve prison conditions through administrative, judicial, and legislative channels and to develop alternatives to incarceration. Besides bringing class-action suits and drafting model legislation and prison regulations, NPP serves as a clearinghouse for information and legal papers on prisoner rights and trains students and legal workers in prison litigation. One of its landmark law suits dealt with the closure of the START behavior modification unit in Missouri. The Project brought suit against the program on grounds of "cruel and unusual" punishment; violation of the first amendment's guarantees of communication, association, and due process; and constitutional guarantees of the right to confront the prosecuter. But before the trial was brought to conclusion, the Federal Bureau of Prisons closed down the unit. Though the project hoped for a court order outlawing such programs, its work will have an effect on deterring future behavior mod programs. NPP lawsuits pending include the right of federal prisoners to correspondence, due process in disciplinary procedures, and the conditions in a local women's detention center. Contact NATIONAL PRISON PROJECT, 1424 16th St., NW, Suite 404, Washington, D.C. 20036. (202) 234-9345.

If the First Amendment protects the freedom to express ideas, it necessarily follows that it must protect the freedom to generate ideas.
—from the 3-judge panel which handed down the decision banning psychosurgery in Michigan, 7/11/73.

THE CENTER FOR THE STUDY OF PSYCHIATRY ... is

an outgrowth of the Project to Examine Psychiatric Technology at the Washington School of Psychiatry. Its founder and director, Peter Breggin, has been one of the pioneering forces in the fight to eradicate psychosurgery; he writes, speaks, and testifies about issues in psychiatric abuse. The Center has taken on research and information-gathering in all areas of behavior modification, large-scale drugging of hyperactive children, massive use of tranquilizers, electro-shock, involuntary mental committment, psychiatric data banks and the use of biological theories to explain political phenomena (such as the alleged inferiority of Blacks due to genetic deficiency.) It distributes its research findings and organizes support to fight against psychiatric abuse through a newsletter, mailings, several books, extensive public speaking across the country, and has helped other groups get started. Largely as a result of the Center's campaign, all identifiable spending on psychosurgery by the federal government has been stopped. Contact CENTER FOR THE STUDY OF PSYCHIATRY, 1827 19th St., NW, Washington, D.C. 20009, (202) 387-6552.

The Truth About Electro-Shock Treatments:
... The attendants come to your cell and tell you you don't get no breakfast that morning. Then they rush you and strap your hands to your sides before you can fight back. Then you're led downstairs to the shock table. A rubber tooth-guard is shoved in your mouth. Two cold steel plates are put to your temples and the doctor ... turns on the juice. A jolt of power jars you into the darkness of temporary death. It's a darkness you can't see or percieve. It's the equivalent of death, except you wake up again. You wake up upstairs in your cell and they feed you breakfast. It destroys some of the cells in your brain and erases your treasured memory ... After my treatment, given to me because I punched an attendant, I couldn't even remember what my mother looked like, and one patient couldn't even remember the names of his kids.
—RISING UP CRAZY

NORTHEAST PRISONERS' ASSOCIATION

... resulted from an April 1973 conference at which 400 ex-cons in the Northeast area shared their experiences and frustrations. The Association's first concerted action was an attempt to end an eight week lock-up in New Hampshire during which all prisoners were prohibited from leaving their cells. NEPA sponsored a court case, organized a six-state demonstration, and spoke on TV and radio; as a result, the lock-up ended. One of NEPA's prime foci has been a campaign against behavior modification in prisons. In 1972 a $188,000 grant was given to leading Boston psychosurgeon to devise a treatment plan for the six northeast states to cover "dangerous special offenders." In 1973-4 the Northeast Correctional Coordinating Council called for the take-over of a New Hampshire naval prison facility and the establishing of a behavior mod and chemotherapy unit. Three hundred and sixty-six convicts, mostly prison organizers and jailhouse lawyers were scheduled to be transferred there. NEPA put together an analysis of the program and organized a demonstration at the Northeast governors' conference in Boston, where recommendations on this program were to be read. The Massachusetts governor was forced to open the hearings and representatives of the 300 ex-cons and supporters spoke about the legal, moral and social points involved; the governors decided not to go along with the proposed behavior mod plan as a unit. However only Massachusetts and Maine pledged not to institute a similar plan in their own states. NEPA helps organize prison and support groups and has produced several films. NEPA NEWS presents accounts of the Northeast and general prison news. The Association is also preparing a resource manual on Northeast prisons and jails, including visiting hours, censorship policy, and details of prison movement groups in the Northeast. Contact NEPA, 116 School St., Waltham, MA 02154, (617) 899-8827.

PRISONER RIGHTS PROJECT/New York Legal Aid...
has been doing legal work around prisons and jails for three years, dealing with inhumane conditions in the institutions throughout the state. The Project was one of the main parties successfully bringing suit against the New York City Men's House of Detention, better known as the Tombs. This monstrous case involved every aspect of the running of the tombs and resulted in a sweeping consent decree covering all jail conditions, including health care. The basic overhaul ordered by the court has not materialized due to administrative delays, in-fighting between the Department of Corrections and the Health Services Administration, so the PRP is seeking to bring a contempt of court citation against offending officials or departments. The group has also been instrumental in stopping the Prescription Program, New York's behavior modification program. Legal workers at the projects visited the program, raised public pressure and threatened a lawsuit so that the state commissioner decided to scrap the program—at least for the time being. The Project also aids prisoners' organizing, provides legal support for prisoner labor unions and argues that prisoners have the legal right to organize under the Public Employees Organizing Act. Contact PRISONER RIGHTS PROJECT' New York Legal Aid, 305 Broadway, New York, NY 10013, (212) 233-2830.

RESOURCES

BOOKS

The Brain Changers, Scientists and the New Mind Control, Maya Pines, Harcourt Brace Jovanovich, Inc., 757 Third Ave., New York, NY 10007, 1973. 248 pp. $7.95
... journalistic report on the relatively new field of brain science. Topics include the effects of mind-changing drugs; the study of memory; and the search for the brain mechanisms that produce violence. The author reports some of the abuses that have come out of research in these areas, such as the idea of "push-button people" (with little black boxes implanted in the brain that respond to computer commands); the Defense Dept.'s development of a different approach to biofeedback, using it as a means to improve combat performance; and the frightening support by a few specialists for direct action on the brain to control fits of violence. Calls for guidelines and for public surveillance.

PAMPHLETS AND ARTICLES

"The Return of Lobotomy," CONGRESSIONAL RECORD, 1735 "K" St., NW, Washington, D.C. 20006, February 24, 1973
... an excellently documented, well-researched case against lobotomy, full of heavily indictive statistics and case-by-case, surgeon-by-surgeon refutation of the whole field. Divided into current psychosurgery around the world, current psychosurgery in the US, and the newest advances in mind control.

It is not, in my opinion, a medical procedure any more than the mutilation of an arm as punishment of a crime is a medical procedure. The mere fact that a physician performs the mutilation does not make it a medical procedure. That was established at Nuremberg. Lobotomy and psychosurgery is an ethical, political and spiritual crime. It should be made illegal.
—Peter Breggin

"The Psychosurgery of Thomas R: A Follow-up Study," Peter Breggin, ISSUES IN RADICAL THERAPY, P.O. Box 23544, Oakland, CA 94623, Autumn, 1973. 3 pp.
... Breggin's classic follow-up study of Thomas R., one of Vernon Mark's "successes" in psychosurgery. Refutes any justification Mark had for operating, including violence or paranoia on the part of the victim. Goes on to tell of Thomas R's post-surgical deterioration and how he is now totally mentally incapacitated.

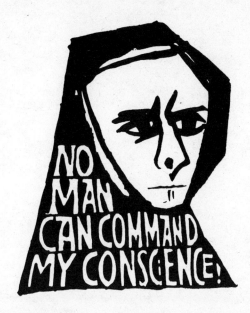

"VIOLENCE ON THE BRAIN," MCHR, 1151 Massachusetts Ave., Cambridge, MA 02138. 24 pp.
... well-done, well-documented paper on all aspects of psychosurgery. The authors draw on various sources to prove that psychosurgery is "scientifically unsound because no one really understands its effects on the brain, medically untenable because there is no accepted criterion for improvement, ethically because it is misrepresented as effective therapy." Warning that we cannot discount these people and their practices as abberations, the book quotes the former head of the President's Task Force on Urban Affairs: "Much of the violence in the ghetto is probably more an expression of mental illness than class culture... the implication... that lower class culture is pathological seems fully warranted."

"CHECK OUT YOUR MIND," People's Law Office, 2156 N. Halstead, Chicago, IL 60614
... really fine overview of the use of behavior mod, psychosurgery, and other forms of psycho-technical control in prisons. Articles by prisoners, legal workers, and others tell about the politics and practice behind these techniques, focusing on their severity, illegality, and double talk. The articles bring together the forms of behavior mod into a system and warn of this threat to the "outside world," as well as its terror for inmates and the need for legal workers and community to provide support. One reason given for the introduction of behavior mod is the growing political awareness and uprisings in prisons, necessitating more sophisticated techniques to maintain the power base. As one behaviorist says about prisoners: "you had no say about what kind of personality you acquired, and there's no reason to believe you should have the right to refuse to acquire a new personality of your own if your old one is anti-social."

"Politics of Psychosurgery," Joe Hunt, REAL PAPER, 10B Mt. Auburn St., Cambridge, MA 12138, May 30, 1973
... a report on the follow-up of the psychosurgery work of three of the most notorious psychosurgeons in the country, Sweet, Ervin, and Mark. Especially significant is discussion of their wheeling-dealing to get funds. They were rejected by NIMH, and then went to Congress where, with support of the head of HEW, they received direct funding through Congress, a very rare occurrence for a research proposal. Because it was not an official grant by NIMH, there were no peer review requirements.

"Shrinks Run Amuck," IRT, P.O. Box 23544, Oakland, CA 94123, Winter 1973-4. 1 p.
. . . thoughtful discussion of the planned UCLA/State of California sponsored Center for the Study and Reduction of Violence, calling it an "unholy alliance in which medical researchers would obtain funding from swollen law-enforcement budgets, while the State gets the promise of sophisticated control techniques. Talks about the Center's plan for chemical castration, long-range surveillance of children said to possess "violence-producing chromosomes," drug experimentation to study female violence associated with menstrual periods, and indiscriminate use of psychoactive drugs for control. The article also reveals how the planners of the Center have changed their proposal to blunt criticism. A few suggestions for practical alternatives to control violence are presented, such as gun control laws and effective drug policy.

. . . Only recently did I come upon one of the best kept secrets of modern times: that German psychiatry began to discuss the extermination of mental patients before Hitler had been heard from, that German psychiatrists were the first to begin exterminating people in Nazi Germany, that they pioneered the gas chamber and crematorium. . . . Wertham, a psychiatrist and the most detailed chronicler of the disaster, observes in A Sign For Cain *that the population of the psychiatric hospitals was between 300,000 and 320,000 in 1939 and 40,000 in 1946. He estimates 270,000 died in the state hospitals. . . The history of the Final Solution confirms what I have more recently found in the campaign against lobotomy and psychosurgery: psychiatry cannot be left alone to police itself. The average psychiatrist has too much personal responsibility for heinous acts of his own: electroshocking people and sending them off to rot in state mental hospitals, to name some of the worst. He cannot afford to point an accusing finger at anyone within his profession, for the finger inevitably points back at himself.*

—Peter Breggin, M.D., "The Killing of Mental Patients"

"FORCED TREATMENT▪TORTURE, NAPA, 629 Sutter, San Francisco, CA 94102, 46 pp.
. . . a diverse, useful introductory packet of political, philosophical, historical, and literary selections covering the principles behind and practice of forced psychiatry and psychiatric abuse. Includes articles by Szasz and Laing elloquently discounting the medical model of "mental illness" and the repression it causes; past and present forms of psychiatric torture-treatment; disconcerting first-hand accounts. Upon discovering electro shock therapy at the time of the Mussulini regime, an Italian scientist stated, "With chronic schizophrenics, as with confirmed criminals, we can't hope for reform. Hence, we must use more drastic measures to silence the dysfunctioning cells and to liberate the healthy cells." Excellent and unusual graphics accentuate the pamphlet.

"The Second Wave," Peter Breggin, MENTAL HYGIENE, National Association for Mental Health, 1800 N. Kent, Rosslyn, VA 22209, March 1973. 4 pp.
. . . a fine introduction covering the scope of psychosurgery and its implications. The title refers to the fact that psychosurgery was discredited in the 50s and has made a recent comeback. Shocking examples of mistakes, procedures ("at the San Francisco Children's Hospital, ultrasonic radiation is sprayed into the frontal lobes of the patient. . . "), and cover-up. One woman who had been operated on several times killed herself; the surgeon claimed her case "gratifying," saying the woman must have been getting over her depression or she wouldn't have had the energy to kill herself. The article discusses the lack of medical base, including the fact that not one controlled study of psychosurgery comparing it to other treatments has been made. Social and ethical questions are also included: "It is one thing for a man to have shallow breathing, another to have a shallow mind. Even if the loss is only partial, we are still dealing with a change in the essence of the person."

"Clock Work Cure in California: Psychosurgery in the Prisons". Venceremos Prison Committee, 1969 University Ave., Palo Alto, CA 94303, 1974. 7 pp. Free
. . . discussion of the proposed use of psychosurgery at the Center for the Study and Reduction of Violence and Vacaville State Prison, what that implies, and a call for action to fight such programs.

"Psychosurgery: The 'Final Solution' to the 'Woman Problem'?", Barbara Roberts, MD, available from Louise Rice, 65 Chestnut St., Cambridge, MA 02139, 4 pp
. . . shows the power of psychosurgery to "silence rebellion while preserving the useful work women do with their hands, their backs and their uteruses." Extreme depression is a major reason for lobotomy, most of which is done in older women; operations are considered successful "if a previously distraught woman is able to return to housekeeping chores." In addition, it's considered more socially acceptable to lobotomize women because the operation destroys their creativity, a trait considered expendable in women. The article also documents psychosurgery on the similarly-oppressed groups of prisoners, the elderly, gay people and children. It concludes with information on the technique of planting electrodes in the brain so people's behavior can be remotely controlled by psychosurgeons. One doctor reports "Some women have shown their feminine adaptability to circumstances by wearing attractive hats or wigs to conceal their electrical headgear."

BIBLIOGRAPHY ON BEHAVIOR MODIFICATION, available from Carleen Arlidge, 505 Alcatraz Ave., No. 15, Oakland, CA 94609, $3.00 for xeroxing, about 40 pp.
. . . put together by a group of radical criminology students, this bibliography includes an overview of the therapeutic state, general behavior therapy, coercive therapy, the adjustment center, psychosurgery (from a legal, ethical, medical and scientific view), important legal decisions, organizations, newsletters, and journals.

BOSTON REAL PAPER, 10B Mt. Auburn, Cambridge, MA 02138, February 6, 27, and April 23, 1974
. . . good three-part investigation of behavior modification, especially in prisons. Includes a brief summary of prison psychiatrists' use of transactional analysis—a technique that is useful in some situations but can be used to divide and manipulate prisoners. According to inmates who submitted a report to the UN Economic and Social Council about behavior mod: "Every effort is made to heighten his suceptibility and weaken his character structure so his emotional response and thought flow will be brought under group and staff control as totally as possible." There is also an excellent characterization of the new Czar of the Butner Research Center, Martin Groder. Groder is a rapidly rising 32 year old psychiatrist who got his start at Marion, Illinois, Federal Penetentiary. There he perfected the use of TA to control prisoner and break the prisoner support system. As Groder says: "It's part of my lengend at the penitentiary what terrible things I did to people."

SCIENCE FOR THE PEOPLE, 9 Walden St., Jamaica Plains, MA 02130, May 1974. 42 pp. $.75
. . . indictive overview of the use of psychotechnology, including how U.S. Marine officers used it in Vietnam, some grueling first-hand accounts by prisoners of their experiences with behavior modification, and a brief history of the development of behavior modification theory in U.S. prisons since the 1700's. Especially appalling is the revelation of plans to implant electrodes into the brain "to maintain a 24 hour a day surveillance over a subject and to intervene electronically or psychically to influence and control selected behavior." Also mentions the use of Ritalin and other psychoactive drugs on school children and the successful efforts of a Boston community to block a $250,000 proposal to examine the effects of psychoactive drugs on children.

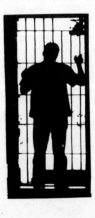

FEMINIST COUNSELING

Feminist counseling grew out of the realization that many women need support in dealing with the contradictions in their changing roles and direction. Often behavior labelled as a woman's personal "neurosis" or "emotional instability" is actually a response to very real oppressive conditions—low paid, dead-end jobs, the pressures of combining a job with childrearing, the constant barriers of situations and attitudes to women's development and use of their abilities. Counseling can help women gain confidence and strength; it can enable them to realize that rejecting traditional feminine behavior is not "sick." When women do have problems in living, they need the support of people—especially other women—who fully respect them, not predominantly male professionals who too often want them to adjust to society's crippling norms.

PHILADELPHIA FEMINIST THERAPY COLLECTIVE...
is a group of professional therapists dedicated to providing non-sexist counseling. The eight women in the collective do not see severely disturbed people on long term medication and prefer to do group counseling. A typical group includes five women and two therapists, meeting one evening per week. Therapy sessions (including one hour individual sessions) cost $10; money is used to cover operating expenses and hopefully will also go towards scholarships and small salaries for the therapists. The collective serves primarily middle class career-oriented women who are trying to assert more control over their lives. Contact PHILADELPHIA FEMINIST THERAPY COLLECTIVE, 2132 Lombard St., Philadelphia, PA 19146, (215) 328-3243.

WOMEN'S COUNSELING SERVICE... began in 1969 when a group of Twin City women formed a feminist collective to work on political/personal goals, discussing topics ranging from a Marxist view of history to their oppression as women. In April 1970, the group split, with one half assuming the Counseling Service as their main focus of attention. The Service offers paraprofessional peer group counseling on birth control, abortion, sex, divorce, feminity, etc. Forty to 70 women, generally between ages 18 and 26, receive counseling each month. Funded by the Freedom from Hunger Foundation, the staff functions as a collective and includes VISTA volunteers, paid counselors, and many volunteers. The overriding goal of the collective is to educate women about their bodies and rights; their literature is very factual and helpful. Contact WOMEN'S COUNSELING SERVICE, 2000 S. Fifth St., Minneapolis, MN 55404, (612) 335-7669.

CLEVELAND WOMEN'S COUNSELING SERVICE...
started as a pregnancy counseling service; it has recently expanded to provide counseling and referral for women seeking psychiatric and legal help. The fourteen collective members view abortion counseling and referral as a function which should be assumed by family planning agencies, freeing the counseling service to offer other programs. They offer workshops, for example, on sexuality and on legal and social/political problems. There is a special interest in reaching middle-aged isolated women. Recognizing that serious depression is common among middle-aged women, the service seeks to help them assert positive control of their lives. The free services are used by Aid-to-Dependent-Children mothers, students and middle class women; funding is from donations. Contact CLEVELAND WOMEN'S COUNSELING SERVICE, P.O. Box 20279, Cleveland, OH 44120, (216) 229-7575.

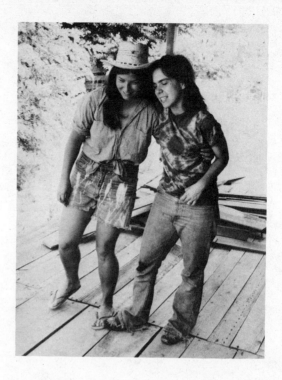

The concept of sickness has all too often made us doubt what we feel— made us hate what is positive in ourselves and made us repress our genuine desires. . . . We need to see ourselves as whole. For too long we've felt our problems were uniquely our own, that no one has felt what we have experienced. . . . Perhaps we can see that it is not us who are at fault but that our feelings are the natural results of living in a society that does everything to thwart our potential. . . .
—RISING UP CRAZY

WOMEN'S COUNSELING AND RESOURCE CENTER...
is a group of 25 women students and workers offering information and non-professional counseling to Boston-area women. The group is divided into 3 teams, each of which has professional supervision and staffs the center for 4 hours a week. While a team is at the Center, it offers individual and group short-term counseling, women's information and referrals. Common problems dealt with in counseling sessions include loneliness, fear of long-term therapy and lack of self-determination. Contact WOMEN'S COUNSELING AND RESOURCE CENTER, 1555 Massachusetts Ave., Cambridge, MA 02138, (617) 492-8568.

WOMEN'S CRISIS CENTER... has a hot line for counselling, rape education, feminist therapy, and problem pregnancy information as well as a speaker's bureau. About 60 volunteers work as counsellors and on the various committees of the center. Policy is decided at bi-weekly meetings headed by 3 rotating general coordinators. Representatives of each committee and each shift attend. New counsellors are constantly being trained to answer the more than ninety calls that come in each week. Some of the workers are women working off court fines, but most of the staff comes from the university. Contact WOMEN'S CRISIS CENTER, c/o St. Andrew's Church, 306 N. Division, Ann Arbor, MI 48104, (313) 761-WISE.

WOMEN'S PSYCHOTHERAPY REFERRAL SERVICE...
originated as a NOW-sponsored monthly discussion group for feminist psychotherapists and has grown into a complete referral service. Each of the thirty-five professional therapists in the group had two years commitment to the women's movement before joining, and currently attends monthly meetings on feminist therapy. Seven to 10 women per week go through the initial interview and are referred to one of the counsellors in the service. Fees are on a sliding scale, starting at $10 per session; the group is unable to accept medicaid until it is successful in its efforts to change its status to that of a clinic. Decisions are made by three coordinators (who started the

group) and approved at the monthly meetings. The Service works largely with women in their 30's who must learn to direct feelings of rage; they also work with a number of older women. No longer affiliated with NOW, the Service is willing to work with feminists in other areas of the country to set up similar programs. Contact WOMEN'S PSYCHO-THERAPY REFERRAL SERVICE, c/o Dr. Susan Schad-Summers, 43 Fifth Ave., New York, NY 10003, (212) 964-0400.

RESOURCES

BOOKS

<u>Women and Madness</u>, Phyllis Chesler, Avon Books, 959 Eighth Avenue, New York, NY 10019, 1972. 340 pp. $1.95
. . . a passionately intense book with a radical feminist per-spective on madness. Phyllis Chesler sees genuine madness as something to be "understood and respected" but never to be romanticized or confused with political or cultural re-volution. Yet the idea of madness in this society has strong political implications for feminists: "What we consider 'mad-ness,' whether it appears in women or in men, is either the acting out of the devalued female role or the total or partial rejection of one's sex-role stereotypes." Women learn to be losers, to be passive, self-effacing martyrs. When they carry this role too far they are sick and when they step too far out-side the role they are sick. Men who are too passive and dependent or who choose other men as lovers are seen as psychotic or neurotic. Those men who carry the male role to its logical extreme end up in prison, not in a mental hos-pital. Thus our society's sex-roles are preserved through its definitions of insanity. Dr. Chesler documents the ef-fects of these definitions in discussions with lesbians, Third World women and feminists. Chesler's style is unique and exciting in that she can write "objectively," but her own emotional involvement in the issues is evident at all times. Indicating directions for the future but reluctant to give pat solutions, she says to the reader: "In bringing you this book, I feel like a time-traveler turned messenger, a bearer of bad news. I wonder how you will receive it, I wonder what will you do?"

<u>Roles Women Play: Readings Toward Women's Liberation</u>, edited by Michele Hoffgung Garskof, Brook/Cole, Belmont, CA 94002, 1971. 210 pp. $3.25
. . . an anthology of feminist readings, dealing with social background and how psychology interacts with that, includ-ing different proposals for change. These twelve articles of-fer a good introductory resource for women in psychology courses.

<u>Getting Clear, Body Work For Women</u>, Anne Kent Rush, Random House/Bookworks, 201 E. 50th St., New York, NY 10022, 1973. 290 pp. $4.95
. . . a feminist book of basic therapy techniques, drawing from Gestalt, Hatha Yoga, Polarity Therapy (based on Chinese acu-puncture). Viewing therapy as a process of "Heightening one's consciousness and mobilizing one's personal powers," the book is filled with ways for women to get in touch with themselves and one another.

<u>The Bell Jar</u>, Sylvia Plath, Bantam Books, 666 Fifth Ave., New York, NY 10019, 1971. 216 pp. $1.50
. . . a gripping portrayal of a successful "bright young coed's" gradual breakdown, suicide attempts and commitment in an asylum. Drawn from the author's personal experiences, the book attempts to "show how isolated a person feels when she is suffering a breakdown. . . to picture her world and the people in it as seen through the distorting lens of a bell jar. . . To the person in the bell jar, blank and stopped as a dead baby, the world itself is the bad dream." Reading Bell Jar helps one understand and feel what it's like to helplessly lose contact with everyday reality.

<u>The Psychology of Women; A Partially Annotated Bibliogra-phy</u>, Joyce Walstedt, KNOW, P.O. Box 86031, Pittsburgh, PA 15221, 1972. 76 pp. $2.25

<u>The Yellow Wallpaper</u>, Charlotte Perkins Gilman, The Fem-inist Press, Box 334, SUNY Old Westbury, Old Westbury, NY 11568, 1973. 64 pp. $1.25
. . . written by the famous turn-of-the-century feminist, is a chillingly precise short story of a woman's journey into mad-ness. Her husband-doctor dismisses entirely her struggles for purpose and self-definition and instead treats the accompany-ing depression as exhaustion. This is the archetypal tale of women attempting to take themselves seriously in a hostile world where men in general and the male-dominated medi-cal profession in particular, treat them as children.

PAMPHLETS AND ARTICLES

"Psychology Constructs the Female or The Fantasy Life of the Male Psychologist," Naomi Weisstein, New England Free Press, 60 Union Sq., Somerville, MA 02143, 1971. 6 pp. $.10
. . . a denunciation of the psychic damage done to women by male psychologists. Weinsstein asserts psychologists have played a major part in preserving the status quo, "describing the true natures of women with a certainty and a sense of their own infallibility rarely found in the secular world." With humor and bitterness, she demonstrates the lack of con-clusive evidence proving any inherent male-female differences beyond the physical.

"THE ANATOMY OF OPPRESSION: A FEMINIST ANALY-SIS OF PSYCHOTHERAPY," by Joyce Jennings Walstedt. KNOW, Inc. P.O. Box 86031, Pittsburgh, PA 15221, 1973. 11 pp. $.60
. . .a feminist view of psychoanalysis. The author points out glaring fallacies and cultural biases in the theories of Freud, Erickson, Theodor Reik and others. She sees the feminist psychotherapist as a kind of midwife, aiding women in their passage from the protected yet confining traditional female role to a life of self-determination. Disjointed in some sec-tions, the concluding section on feminist psychotherapy is of great value to any woman interested in changing the quali-ty of psychoanalysis.

"OPEN LETTER TO PSYCHIATRISTS," Nicole Anthony, KNOW, P.O. Box 86031, Pittsburgh, PA 15221, 1970. 2pp. $.05
. . . an angry account of one woman's experience with a San Francisco psychiatrist. The indictments are common: he destroyed her self-esteem, convinced her that she was sick, and acted in a patronizing and sexual manner. The letter de-mands that psychiatrists listen to women, learn from them, offer reparations for their years of misery and free all prison-ers in mental institutions.

"THE FEMINIST THERAPIST ROSTER OF THE ASSOCIA-TION FOR WOMEN IN PSYCHOTHERAPY," Annette M. Bordsky, 1600 West Freeman, Carbondale, IL 62901, 1973. 14 pp. $.35
. . . an annotated list of feminist therapists in 18 states. Al-though very incomplete, the Roster offers information on training, services offered and position on feminism for each entry. The author hopes to expand, and solicits reader input.

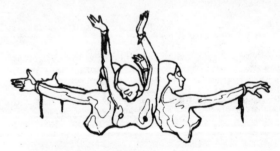

*We are the mad women—
Private property itself rising in rebellion.
The trees and flowers shall join us.
Power is doomed.
—Mary Damon,
Boston Women's Poetry Anthology*

"PSYCHOANALYSIS: A FEMINIST REVISION," Jane W. Torrey, KNOW, P.O. Box 86031, Pittsburgh, PA 15221, 1971. 3 pp. $.15
. . . strives to explain "why it should be that our civilization and most of the others we know about have been so consistently dominated by males." Torrey theorizes that men oppress women to obtain some indirect control over babies. The article ends optimistically, predicting that the decline in birthrates will precede the true emancipation of women.

"Marriage and Psychotherapy," RADICAL THERAPIST, available from KNOW, P.O. Box 86031, Pittsburgh, PA 15221, 1971. 2 pp. $.05
. . .views these two institutions as perpetuating female dependence on men and serving to isolate women. "Each woman as patient, thinks these symptoms are unique and are her own fault. . . . "I wonder what a woman can learn from a male therapist (however well-intentioned) whose own values are sexist, who has been conditioned to view women as inferior, as threatening, as childish, as castrating, as alien to himself?" Good basic analysis.

"DEPRESSION IN MIDDLE AGED WOMEN: PORTNOY'S MOTHER'S COMPLAINT," Pauline Bart, KNOW, P.O. Box 86031, Pittsburgh, PA 15221, 1970. 6 pp. $.30
. . . an academic, yet absorbing study of the causes of depression in middle aged women. "Depression . . . is not due to hormonal changes of the menopause. . .Rather it is due to sociocultural factors that drastically reduce a woman's self-esteem." The article concludes with a strong statement in support of the Women's Liberation Movement.

"WOMEN AND PSYCHOLOGY, ANNOTATED BIBLIO-GRAPHY," 1972 Feminist Studies, Cambridge, MA 02140. $.40

ALTERNATIVES TO INSTITUTIONAL-IZATION

THE TRANSITION COMMUNITY. . . is an outstanding example of a halfway house run by its residents and providing the supportive functions necessary to prepare people to effectively deal "with life and the world." The program aims to counteract the helplessness institutionalized people feel. It helps them to re-learn the skills needed to be on their own, including "social skills and ways of caring for each other"; emphasis is on health, community living and personal interaction rather than on illness. Residents must be adaptable to group living, and show potential for eventually holding down a job. New residents are voted on by present members of the community and all newcomers are given "instant educations" in the women's movement. Everyone takes part equally in household management and in weekly meetings for planning, growup feedback and personal problem-solving purposes. Rent is on a sliding scale, though most people pay about $170/monthly—maximum residency is 6 months. Major policy decisions are made by a board composed of representatives from the house, from the community and from the board of directors (businesspeople who are funding the project). Contact THE TRANSITION COMMUNITY, 3800 Forest St., Kansas City, MO 64109, (816) 931-6977.

HOMECOMING, INC. . . . is a collectively-run community of ex-mental patients who feel they can support each other far better than professionals or social agencies can. They are a recent outgrowth of a 2½ year old group of ex-patients, the Committee of Us, who run a 5-cent-a-cup coffee house and walk-in office for ex-patients in Chicago's uptown community. In this coummunity of street people—mainly poor Whites and Third World—the basic struggle is one of day-to-day survival. The area is referred to as a giant hospital ward, and includes between 8,000-14,000 ex-mental patients who periodically revolve through the doors of the state hospital. As a result, the community is thick with exploitive half-way houses and other social services which reinforce the patients' dependency and in turn feed on them. Homecoming is trying to provide a living alternative to this situation. "What we're really aiming at is control over our own lives, the right to be treated like adults and make our own decisions." One of their first activities was sponsoring a benefit performance of "One Flew Over the Cuckoo's Nest." House residents, of all races, ages, religious, sexes and sexual preferences, and backgrounds see Homecoming as a place to change through living together and through building their own lives. Everyone has a specific function in the house, and emphasis is placed on building self-respect, skills, and not hiding behind job labels. Funded through foundation grants, speaking engagements, welfare/VA checks, and the jobs of residents, Homecoming serves the general mental patient community as well as house residents. They have received a great deal of support from various sections of the Chicago community, yet are essentially making it on their own. Seeing themselves as a social/political prototype, they hope by their existence to encourage others to organize their own communities. Contact HOMECOMING, INC. 1428 W. Jarvis, Chicago, IL 60626, (312) 743-1284.

HUMAN SERVICES. . . is a political commune of former mental patients, social science students and people who've worked in mental institutions who are trying to build a stable, supportive internal community. Generally based on R. D. Laing's Kingsley Hall model, they feel "madness is a sane response to an insane environment." The group initially came together over a year ago at a "Politics of Mental Health" convention at the University of Illinois, at which R. D. Laing spoke. They are currently working on setting up a storefront where people can come and discuss the past openly, as well as teach and learn skills from each other—yoga, psychodrama, etc. Presently, members of the group are doing advocacy for people in institutions, as well as general community education by speaking and writing articles. Contact HUMAN SERVICES, 1238 North Noble, Chicago, IL 60622, (312) 276-4503.

DIABOSIS. . . is a recently opened city-funded residential alternative treatment program for people with "acute psychotic episodes." Formerly a day center, it now houses 6-10 "clients" for up to three months at a time. The staff is largely volunteer and only one has received psychiatric training, though many have undergone psychotic experiences themselves. A major goal of the project is to demonstrate how 'untrained' people can help others. The city pays for those who can't afford the $40/daily fee. No medication is given, and they discourage people coming there who have been mentally incarcerated, however briefly, because they feel the resulting internalized labeling is too damaging for them to work on eradicating at this time. Emphasis is placed on helping people better understand themselves and fully "express their psychosis." Contact DIABOSIS, 1128 Pine, San Francisco, CA 94109, (415) 928-1078.

RESOURCES

PACIFIC INSTITUTE FOR RESEARCH AND EVALUATION... is a recently initiated project presently trying to identify effective primary prevention programs all over the country, from those working on alternatives to drug abuse to prevention of mental problems. Funded by the state of Pennsylvania, and representing a network of 20 professionals and paraprofessionals in psychology, they plan to visit, videotape and package the best programs they uncover, and distribute these materials to communities. Contact PACIFIC INSTITUTE FOR RESEARCH AND EVALUATION, 2229 Lombard St., San Francisco, CA 94123, (415) 931-0176.

CENTER FOR THE STUDY OF PRIMARY PREVENTION ... has been successful in obtaining $¼ million from the State of Oregon to use in instituting experimental primary prevention programs in Eugene. Presently this involves hiring child development specialists to work in the public schools and "teach young people how to respond to stress, and to generally make more informed choices. Community taskforces have also been set up to identify those things in the community that cause unnecessary stress and to determine ways to get rid of them. This involves focusing on the areas of home, school, social services, church, recreation, justice, media, health care and government which are seen as major leverage points in the community that effect people's lives. The center itself is currently writing "a catalog of simple things to improve the quality of life for people". It hopes to soon bring together a national conference of people and groups developing primary prevention projects in their communities, from designing school curriculums to improving the health care delivery system. The Center also acts as a clearinghouse for primary prevention ideas, resources and programs, and does community education and organizing. Contact CENTER FOR THE STUDY OF PRIMARY PREVENTION, c/o Richard Ingraham, Box 451, Star Route 1, Kingston, WA 98346.

OPERATION FRIENDSHIP... is a social agency "offering services directed toward resocialization, rehabilitation and problem-solving for adults with emotional, mental deficiency, psychological and/or social disturbances or problems." This community based mental health program is primarily intended to provide support in an informal, personal setting, to help people readjust to the community after being institutionalized, and helps others avoid hospitalization. People pay $5/year to become members and participate in the daily activities all over the city which range from recreational projects to discussion groups, skills development, and counseling. Presently, most funding comes from the state mental health department. Most of the staff are social workers and a strict policy is maintained on confidentiality. The concept of membership is an important one, whereby those seeking service are seen as active participants in the problem-solving process. Contact OPERATION FRIENDSHIP, Detroit and Wayne County, 8530 W. McNichols, Detroit, MI (313) 864-5550.

"CRISIS HOSTEL: AN ALTERNATIVE TO PSYCHIATRIC HOSPITALIZATION FOR EMERGENCY PATIENTS," Bryan D. Brook, Southwest Denver Community Mental Health Services, 3052 W. Mississippi, Denver, CO 80219, 1973. 4 pp. ... describes a five-month experiment to place clients in a crisis hostel for emergency intervention instead of putting them in inpatient facilities. During the five month period, 49 people (half diagnosed as schizophrenic; ¼ as having depressive reactions; alcohol and drug abusers, and those with miscellaneous problems) went through the hostel. Stays were limited to seven days and there were no regular full-time staff people assigned to the hostel. The outcome of the experiment was compared to an in-patient control group of 49 people. Results were impressive: six of the control group were re-admitted, while only one hostel person was. Hostel residents were able to leave the hostel for work, none made attempts at suicide, and no attempts were made to go AWOL. Nice support for a non-medical model above a medical model of care.

Currents, Horizon House Institute, 1019 Stafford House, 5555 Wissahickon Ave., Philadelphia, PA 19144, Free ... reviews strengths and weaknesses of innovative mental retardation programs, as well as current federal legislation affecting the mental disabilities spectrum. The Winter /73 issue includes information on self-governing communes of "chronic mental patients", model day care programs for the aged, and geriatric crisis teams (which find old people community alternatives to hospitalization). The Spring /74 issue mentions advocacy programs for mental patients, an NIMH-funded training program for medicine men, and programs in which carefully-screened landlords/ladies provide housing and support for groups of ex-mental patients.

FILMS

Vision Quest, Inc., 325 W. 86th St., New York, NY 10024

"**Asylum**" feature length cl.
This is filmed in a non-exploitive way by a crew who lived for six weeks with the residents and therapists of Kingsley Hall. This therapeutic community was formed by R. D. Laing and a few colleagues who believe schizophrenia to be a strategy for survival in a "soffocating and anti-human society." Kingsley Hall aims to provide a place where people can live with "equality and respect and help each other explore their 'schizophrenia.'" Laing claims this is "the only thing we have in film that shows what we think works for people who feel society is destroying them.

Indiana University Audio Visual Center, Bloomington, Indiana 47401

"**They're Your People,**" 29 min. b&w $7.75 (sale: $165)
The Singer Zone Center in Rockford, Illinois, is seen aiding short-term patients and helping local communities develop their own mental health facilities. The objective is to keep people out of hospitals, since this often hinders rather than aids, the progress of the patient.

"**Horizon House,**" 29 min. b&w $7.75 (sale: $165)
Horizon House helps patients stay out of hospitals. Because a patient's rehabilitation cannot be separated from where and how s/he lives, the community must be part of the reintegration process. Scenes show community teams making visits and acting as ombudspeople.

CRISIS CENTERS

The wide-spread use of drugs in the 1960s resulted in the founding of many "hotlines" to keep information and communication flowing between adults and youth. To the surprise of many hotline staff, most of their calls were not bad trips or drug-related, but were youth and other people in need of open and honest dialogue with non-judging, caring peers and adults.

Each year, close to one million young people between the ages of 12 and 18 run away from home. They run away for a variety of reasons, but their actions usually represent a call for help. A few find their way and achieve a state of independence; others find help in a runaway house or crisis center. But a large proportion remain on the streets, directionless and afraid, until the police force them to return home. More and more runaway houses and crisis centers are coming into existence but they are too small and few to meet the needs of great numbers of runaways and troubled young people.

Confidential health and mental health facilities for minors in this country are limited. For all practical purposes, a minor is the private property of her/his parents and treated as such: property must be immediately returned to its owner, with limited legal rights. Over the last 10 years concerned adults and young people have developed a number of ways to deal with the low status and special problems of youth.

The hotlines, crisis centers, and runaway houses listed here are oriented toward serving youth, their physical and mental needs. They act as advocates by helping point out all the possible solutions to a problem, allowing the person to make a choice, and then providing support while the youth moves in her/his chosen direction.

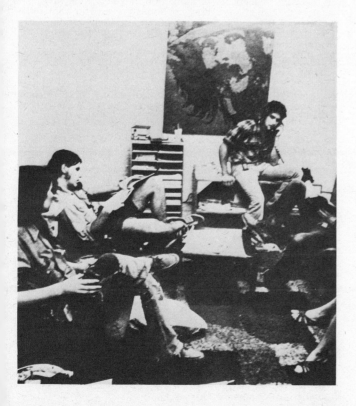

COMMUNITY CRISIS CENTER. . .provides all types of counseling, medical, drug, and referral services to the Atlanta area. The Center began as a "youth-oriented, drug-centered, hip organization in the heart of the counter-cultural street scene" four years ago and has moved "towards becoming a true community center for the whole city." They have developed a Crisis Center Collective to run the facilities and specialize in crisis intervention counseling. There are now four major areas: a hotline, a free medical clinic, a psychological clinic, and a walk-in outreach service. The Center also has two projects in development: a drug analysis program and a 24-hour mobile-crisis unit. Contact COMMUNITY CRISIS CENTER, 40 Peachtree Pl., NW, Atlanta, GA 30309, (404) 892-2492.

SUICIDE PREVENTION CRISIS CENTER. . . provides emergency services for people with problems they cannot cope with. All of the work is done over the phone by a staff of paid and volunteer workers. The Center has its own training program for staff and an experienced counselor is on duty 24 hours a day. Since the Center is a telephone service only, much of the work is making referrals to a walk-in counseling service located in the same building. Contact SPCC, 801 Prudence Rd., San Francisco, CA 85710, (602) 296-5411.

YOUTH EMERGENCY SERVICE, INC. . . is a volunteer organization that has been helping young people in crises since 1969. A small paid staff and volunteers maintain a 24-hour, seven days a week telephone answering service. The service provides crisis counselling, information, and referral to other community services for over 190 callers a day. Volunteers receive 24 hours of intensive training in interpersonal communications and referral skills. Y.E.S. also maintains an educational program and a consultation service for professionals and community groups in the areas of alienation, youth values, drugs, and sexuality. For more information on one of the oldest and most successful community counseling services, contact Y.E.S., Inc., 1429 Washington Ave. South, Minneapolis MN 55404, (612) 339-0895.

LOWER KENSINGTON ENVIRONMENTAL CENTER. . . is putting together a "multiple service center which is effective for the community." It grew out of an alternative high school as a response to the needs of the surrounding working community, especially the young. The Center now involves a drug abuse program, an alcohol abuse program, and a 24 hour crisis intervention center. It handles housing, employment, and family problems as well as medical counseling. Current projects include eye exams to spot problems caused by a particular drug, and a health survey program to screen for lead paint poisoning and other common health problems. When a problem requires medical treatment, the person is sent to a local hospital or clinic. Contact LKEC, Fourth and Somerset, Philadelphia, PA, (215) 426-0900.

PROJECT PLACE. . . in Boston, began as a runaway house in 1967. Since then Place has developed a runaway house, a 24-hour switchboard and drop-in counseling center, a 24-hour emergency counseling van, and a farm. It also has a group locating alternative living situations, and a drug education program with in-staff training and a parent counseling group. Although runaways must secure parental permission to stay over 24 hours, they can remain for almost an indefinite period of time. Staff, which operates on a collective basis, provides individual, group, family, employment, and educational counseling. The Place Legal Aid Cooperative provides legal services. Contact PROJECT PLACE, 32 Rutland, Boston, MA, 02118, (617) 267-9150.

YOUTH EMERGENCY SERVICE... was begun in 1968 by high school students who felt the need to aid community youth in the drug, health, and family problems they encountered. They set up a hotline and runaway center where the emphasis is on youth helping youth. The Service has four paid administrative staff, but most of the volunteers are youth under 20 who do one-to-one counseling. Anyone under 17 (the age of majority in Missouri) can come to the service for confidential counseling but they must contact their parents within three days. Ideally the person returns home within four days to two weeks; when this is not possible the Service can arrange for foster care on a work exchange basis. Contact Y.E.S., 9307 Olive St., Olivette, MO, 63136, (314) 993-2292.

HUCKLEBERRY HOUSE... is an old and experienced runaway house open 24 hours a day, seven days a week. Huckleberry can provide both short and long-term housing arrangements in their "licensed facility" or in foster homes, live-in jobs, or group situations. Counseling services include family therapy, psychiatric help, group meetings, and individual assistance. Informational and educational services are also available on medical, drug, birth control and pregnancy, job and other topics. Legal services are provided by two lawyers on the staff of Huckleberry's sponsoring agency, Youth Advocates Incorporated. Contact HUCKLEBERRY HOUSE/YOUTH ADVOCATES, 3830 Judah St., San Francisco, CA 94122, (415) 731-3921.

OZONE HOUSE... provides housing, counseling, and referrals for transient youth and runaways from the local area and institutions. The House is staffed by a collective of four who do one-to-one, family, and sometimes group counseling. Staff boasts about its alternative foster care arrangements: homes include gay and unwed couples and single individuals. The House is working with Detroit Transit Alternative and other Michigan youth services to establish new legislation that gives minors more rights and is developing its own residential care center. Other interests include improving the quality of care the House staff delivers and providing more personal training. Contact OZONE HOUSE, INC., 719 Arbor St., Ann Arbor, MI, 48104, (313) 769-6540.

RUNAWAY HOUSE... provides short term crisis intervention housing and counseling for runaways. Viable working relationships have been established with the police. Since most of the young people coming to the house are from the area, counselors try to arrange meetings with families as soon as possible. Working with various social service agencies, counselors and back-up professionals try to do whatever is necessary to deal with the problems which caused people to run away in the first place. SAJA, Inc. (Special Approaches in Juvenile Assistance) sponsors the house and has its own recruitment and placement service for foster homes, under the approval of the Jewish Social Services. Contact RUNAWAY HOUSE, 1743 18th St., NW, Washington, D.C. 20009, (202) 462-1515 or SAJA, 1830 Connecticut Ave., NW, Washington, D.C. 20009, (202) 234-6664.

VOYAGE HOUSE... serving mainly low-income inner city families, provides a wide range of shelter and counseling services for young people under 18. Voyage runs its own group homes for long term placements, along with an alternative school. In the future it also hopes to acquire another house for interval stays and half-way housing. When necessary, staff is willing to help those over 16 fight for status as emancipated minors. Legal, employment and medical services are also available and counseling is on an individual or family level. Two staff members act as outreach workers, making contacts on the street. Contact VOYAGE HOUSE, 2041 Walnut St., Philadelphia, PA, 19146, (215) 567-0990.

NATIONAL HOTLINE AND SWITCHBOARD EXCHANGE
... is the central clearinghouse for information on hotlines, switchboards, and other youth-oriented and alternative crisis centers. Various materials on setting up and maintaining programs are available. Of particular interest and value are:

National Directory of Hotlines and Youth Related Services.

Published twice a year in January and July, this useful booklet lists over 1,200 hotlines, switchboards, free clinics, information and referral centers, runaway houses.

The National Exchange. A monthly newsletter for hotlines and youth services, the Exchange includes announcements of conferences and legislation, jobs, and articles and reviews on relevant topics.

Crises Information Centers: A Resource Guide. This annotated bibliography has 300 listings with a brief description of the item, where to obtain a copy, and cost, if any. A few of the topics covered are: drugs, free clinics, radical therapy, sexuality, suicide, telephone techniques, volunteers, many more.

For more information on these and other services, Contact THE EXCHANGE, 311 Cedar Avenue South, Minneapolis, MN 55404, (612) 341-2793.

> *it's very hard to adolesce*
> *one is given a number of years*
> *and told that within this time*
> *he must pubert all the way to maturity*
> *this enormous charge*
> *would not seem so unbearable*
> *utterly impossible*
> *were it not given*
> *when one has not yet learned*
> *how to child ...*
> —Jayne West, NO MORE FUN AND GAMES

RESOURCES

National Directory of Runaway Centers, National Youth Alternatives Project, 1830 Connecticut Ave., NW, Washington, DC 20009, 1974. 60 pp. $1.00
... provides information on centers all over the country, and includes an overview of all the different categories of centers, their programs, funding, etc.

Toward A Radical Therapy, Alternate Services for Personal and Social Change, Ted Clark and Dennis Jaffe, Gordon and Breach, One Park Ave., New York, NY 10016, 1973. 187 pp. $12.50 (cheap paperback version available soon)
... was written by two community organizers/radical therapists who helped start Number Nine—a crisis telephone line which expanded into various other services—in an attempt to discover the needs of young people and develop programs to meet those needs. This collection of essays were written to facilitate social change; they are about "crises and transitions in personal life and society and about building communities and alternate services to help people live through these crises." (Note: Dennis Jaffe is a good resource person in this area, and can now be reached at the University of Pennsylvania's Dept. of Psychiatry, Philadelphia).

Nothing Left to Lose Jeffrey Blum and Judith Smith, Beacon Press, 25 Beacon Ave., Boston, MA 02108, 1972. 142 pp. $2.95
... account of two workers at the Sanctuary, "a storefront counseling center, a hotline, and a hostel" for streetpeople and youth in the Boston area. In an effort to "develop an overall view of the problems and questions which Sanctuary's kids had to face," the authors explain, in depth, many of the cases Sanctuary's counselors have dealt with. "The Sanctuary staff views psychiatric problems not as symptoms of mental illness but as the signs of what might be called "difficulties in living." An important resource for hotlines, crisis centers, and all counseling programs.

CRISIS INTERVENTION RESOURCE MANUAL, Patrick Mills, Coordinator, The Vermillion Hot Line Program Office, University of South Dakota, Vermillion, SD 57069, May, 1973. 170 pp. $4.00
...a model manual compiled from 86 crisis intervention manuals from various parts of the country. Generally well-done, the book covers drugs, suicide, sexuality counsellor training programs, and screening of applicants. The drug section is pretty comprehensive, although the glossary of slang terms is quickly out-dated. The sexuality is a bit questionable in its treatment of homosexuality and its virtual lack of any treatment of rape, but the book as a whole demonstrates an orientation towards noncondescending, nonjudgmental supportive counseling.

LEGAL ADVOCACY

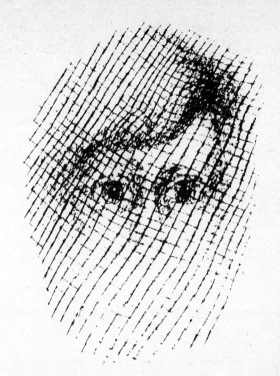

THE CENTER FOR THE STUDY OF LEGAL AUTHORITY AND MENTAL PATIENT STATUS (LAMP)... has been doing research and education in the field of psychiatry and law since 1971. The Center was formed in response to the following problems: 1) lack of accurate information about the question of "mental illness" 2) irrational public fear and distrust of alleged mental patients 3) absence of legal defense tor those accused of mental illness; 4) unsupervised and inhumane use of psychiatric technologies (such as psychosurgery). Acting as a national/local clearinghouse, the Center is working on collecting, organizing, writing and disseminating information concerning various aspects of legal control of psychiatric technology, to students, lawyers, organizers, and the general public. LAMP wants to arouse legal interest in the procedures and practices involved in involuntary mental institutionalization and generally introduce people to the issues. The Mental Patient Law Project, recently formed in the Bay Area, has grown in large part out of LAMP's educational efforts. Through an international correspondence and largely Western Regional telephone work, the Center puts people in touch with information on legal developments in the area of psychotechnology and law, and is developing a bibliography on specific issues. Development of a community switchboard to inform people of alternatives to institutionalization is a priority for future work. Operating with a small core staff of mostly volunteers, LAMP welcomes people coming to work with them for school credit. They request that a self-addressed stamped envelope be enclosed with all inquiries "and include a donation if possible." Contact LAMP, P.O. Box 822, Berkeley, CA 94701, (415) 526-5415.

MENTAL HEALTH LAW PROJECT... does test case litigation on behalf of mental patients. It has been successful in precedent-setting cases covering the right to education, treatment, right to compensation and minimum wage. The last was a nationwide class-action suit against the Department of Labor. MHLP holds training sessions and conferences for bar groups, helping them gain access to wards. Two publications cover the basic rights of the mentally handicapped (written for consumers), and the legal rights of the mentally handicapped (primarily for legal workers.) Contact MENTAL HEALTH LAW PROJECT, 1751 "N" St., NW, Washington, D.C. 20036, (202) 872-0670.

MENTAL PATIENTS CIVIL LIBERTIES PROJECT... is a legal services center organized to protect the legal rights of those incarcerated in mental hospitals. Suits include one against forced labor on constitutional grounds, and a consent decree is expected from the Department of Public Welfare, which means the Department agrees to stop the offending behavior but does not admit guilt. The plaintiff is sueing for 35,000 hours in uncompensated labor. Another deals with the rights of juveniles (including the right to a hearing and representation by attorney). MPCLP brought a $1 million lawsuit in behalf of a man wrongfully committed for 30 years and whose only treatment was unauthorized shock and drug treatment. After doing an exhaustive and indictive study of Haverford State Hospital, MPCLP signed a contract with the institution to serve as advocate for its inmates. An in-house organizer co-ordinated the project work with a patients rights organization and a newsletter had been started when the hospital threw the organizer out in fall, 1973. A suit to regain access to the hospital was then filed and moving slowly. MPCLP is now doing preliminary work in organizing Philadelphia State Hospital, talking to patients, finding out what their needs are, and trying to establish trust with the patients,

who are inherently distrustful of those connected with the court system. The project offers consultation and referral service, including requests for interpretations of the Pennsylvania Mental Health and Retardation Act of 1966, a speaker's bureau, and a research service for agencies in the mental health law field. Publications include a report of the Haverford struggle and a patients' rights leaflet. A more extensive patients' rights book is in the offing. Contact MPCLP, 1315 Walnut St., Suite 1407, Philadelphia, PA' 19107, (215) 735-8409.

ST. LOUIS UNIVERSITY LAW SCHOOL... currently offers a pilot program in mental health law, a new trend in all too few schools. Included is a seminar on Law and Psychiatry, which requires of each student a major piece of litigation on mental patients' rights, as well as a clinical course called "The Lawyering Process." To give them greater familiarity with the issues, students work at the Malcolm Bliss Mental Health Center in St. Louis, devoting at least one-third of their energies to patients rights. For more information on this program, as well as on similar programs thoughout the country, contact Jesse Goldne, ST. LOUIS UNIVERSITY LAW SCHOOL, St. Louis, MO 63103, (315) 535-3300.

PUBLIC DEFENDER SERVICE FOR THE DISTRICT OF COLUMBIA... represents free of charge approximately 2,200 District residents a year who are incarcerated for mental reasons and unable to hire an attorney. The service has operated full-time out of St. Elizabeth's Hospital since early 1972, but it also serves those confined in the D.C. hospital system. Although funded out of the federal budget, they function independently of government restraints; for example, they have sued hospital staff and even judges. Once people are involuntarily hospitalized, the Public Defender Service is appointed to them automatically and is often able to get people out almost immediately. Consequently the number of patients involuntarily committed at St. Elizabeth's has significantly dropped. In addition to a small core staff of lawyers and a social worker, the service is revitalized by an influx of 25 area law students each semester. They make it a point to float around the wards constantly, where they are accessible to all patients with problems or complaints. Every 90 days patients are counseled briefly about their rights. Contact PUBLIC DEFENDER SERVICE, Mental Health Division, St. Elizabeth's Hospital, Washington, D.C. 20032, (202) 562-2200.

MENTAL HEALTH LEGAL SERVICES PROJECT... provides free day-to-day civil legal services to people in the Chicago area, particularly to the 240 patients a month at Reed Mental Health Center. They concentrate on patients rights work and on releasing those held at Reed on an emergency basis before they can be committed. Most people stay at Reed only three weeks, and the project does follow-up legal services for those needing continued assistance when they've left the hospital, as well as dealing with job discrimination and landlord/tenant disputes. The project receives 85% of its funding from the city Mental Health Department, since it is the only area group providing these services, but is a private organization and has even sued the state on occasion. The staff consists of two full-time lawyers as well as area law students and paralegal advocates. They occupy an office at Reed daily, and spend much time on the wards with patients. Contact MENTAL HEALTH LEGAL SERVICE PROJECT, 73 W. Monroe, Chicago, IL 60603, (312) 641-0767.

MENTAL PATIENT LAW PROJECT... is a newly-formed group of attorneys, legal workers, psychiatrists and students involved with cases to secure the release of persons from psychiatric facilities and to resolve problems resulting from mental hospitalization—child custody questions, confidentiality of records, employment discrimination, etc. MPLP is also involved with protecting the rights of mental patients through test cases and legislation. Recently a bill drafted by the MPLP was introduced into the California State Senate and Assembly, establishing a right to refuse treatment (specifically, psychosurgery, shock, and chemotherapy) for inmates in California's psychiatric facilities. Other MPLP projects include investigating sex and racial discrimination in commitment, researching "mental illness" and "dangerousness"—which are the criteria for commitment, and investigating other psychiatric abuses in prisons, hospitals for the criminally insane, and mental hospitals. Contact MENTAL PATIENT LAW PROJECT, 2637 Fulton Street, Suite B, Berkeley, CA 94704, (415) 849-1483.

MENTAL HEALTH INFORMATION SERVICE/1st DEPARTMENT... is one of the few state-funded legal services for the mentally incarcerated (including the mentally retarded and alcoholics). Authorized in 1965, the service spans the entire state and is divided into 4 departments which inform patients of their rights and advise the court. The First Department serving Manhattan and the Bronx, is the only one that actually represents patients in court. Patients are seen automatically upon their admission to an institution (both state and private, as well as psychiatric wards of hospitals). Twenty lawyers and 4 social workers spend the bulk of their time trying to get people out of the hospitals, and devising alternatives for them. State laws are also challenged and recently a right-to-treatment case was won in the New York Court of Appeals which will set a precedent for the state. Contact MENTAL HEALTH INFORMATION SERVICE, Appellate Division, 1st Department, 27 Madison Ave., New York, NY 10010, (212) 876-3522.

RESOURCES

The Rights of Mental Patients: An American Civil Liberties Union Handbook, Bruce Ennis and Loren Siegel, Avon Books, 959 Eighth Ave., New York, NY 10019, 1973. 336 pp. $1.25
... this clearly-written, useful resource describes the laws and court decisions that affect mental patients and includes a state-by-state outline of statutes covering voluntary and involuntary admissions, counsel, release procedures, rights in the hospital, financial and property problems, rights upon discharge, and penalties. Appendices cover information on trial techniques, which give lawyers some general tips on how to successfully interrogate psychiatrists on the witness stand; an extensive bibliography of cases; and a list of minimum constitutional standards for adequate treatment of mental patients.

Prisoners of Psychiatry, Mental Patients, Psychiatrists and the Law, Bruce Ennis, Harcourt, Brace Jovanovich, Inc., 757 Third Ave., New York, NY 10017, 1972. 232 pp. $6.95
... hard-hitting book about Ennis' experience defending men and women whose lives were changed and often destroyed by the label "mental illness," and the fight to change the laws that stripped them of their liberty and dignity. For example, one man 88 years old has been in a hospital for the criminally insane for 20 years, long after someone else confessed to and was electrocuted for the crime. The stories are shocking because they are not unusual examples; he chose them because they are typical. Calling for the abolition of involuntary commitment, Ennis concludes: "Even if all the abuses of the mental hospital system could be eliminated, the system would still remain, and it is the system that must be changed."

Santa Clara Lawyer, School of Law, University of Santa Clara, Santa Clara, CA 95053, Spring, 1973. 623 pp. $3.50
... is a special symposium on "mental illness, the law, and civil liberties." The fine collection of articles includes "Into the Abyss: Psychiatric Reliability and Emergency Commitment Statutes" (a thorough critique of mental illness theory), "Loosing the Chains: In-Hospital Civil Liberties of Mental Patients," and a discussion of the Rosenhans study.

CLEARINGHOUSE REVIEW, National Clearinghouse for Legal Services, Northwestern University School of Law, 710 North Lake Shore Drive, Mezzanine Floor, Chicago, IL 60611. $2 each or $10/year
... a monthly newsletter which covers current cases in outline form; includes a constantly expanding section on mental health law, as well as occasional articles.

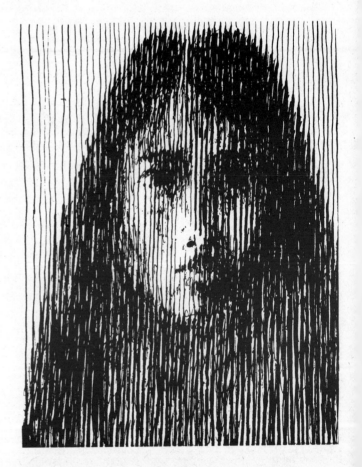

Every human person is a mystery that must be learned slowly, reverently, with care, tenderness, and pain . . . never learned completely.

—OFF OUR BACKS

COMMUNITY MENTAL HEALTH

THE WASHINGTON HEIGHTS-WEST HARLEM-INWOOD MENTAL HEALTH COUNCIL, INC. . . . is a grass-roots group of residents of northwest Manhattan who organized to challenge the traditional research and training oriented approach to community mental health services. The Council runs a Mental Health Center which is directly answerable to the community through the Council and a community elected board of directors. Membership in the council is open and free to all community residents. Basically the Center provides treatment, crisis intervention, preventive programs, consultation and educational services to the community through clinic-based and outreach programs. It actively promotes collaboration between receivers and providers of these services, emphasizing extending service "to those whose mental health needs are traditionally unmet" and to catalyze improvements in the community." The Council deals with business of the Center as well as with mental health related community issues—this has included a police-community dialogues working with a cable tv project on marital relationships and compiling an inventory of recreational summer programs for community youth. The Mental Health Center itself is staffed mainly by mental health workers and social workers, as well as by some psychologists and psychiatrists. Their work includes advocacy with other agencies from daycare to union compensation review boards, and general follow-up; giving individual/family/group therapy to both outpatients and those few receiving short-term hospitalization within the community (as well as setting people up in group homes in the community); providing supportive, socializing general skills-improving and prevocational training activities for those recently released from state institutions; and putting energy into combating community problems which promote stress. Staff of the latter team have fought to save an area hospital, helped improve the conditions of a single room occupancy hotel which had become a focal point of crime and human misery, and worked with public housing programs for the elderly as well as day care centers. Their "Operation Doorbell" is especially significant, consisting of canvassing areas about their concerns and helping bring residents together to organize around a common issue and work for dramatic improvements. They also work closely with schools, health service agencies, churches to develop community-related network of mental health services and have given workshops between community and area lawyers about how to make the law work for them. This is a fine model of what community mental health services can and should be. Contact COUNCIL'S MENTAL HEALTH CENTER, 558 West 158th St., New York, NY 10032, (212) 781-5000.

SOUTHWEST DENVER COMMUNITY MENTAL HEALTH SERVICES, INC. . . . is staffed by about 50 volunteers together with paid professionals. With state revenue-sharing funds they have initiated an Alternative Community Settings Program. This involves placing people undergoing acute crises in area family homes for about 10 days in order to avoid hospitalization. Disruption in the clients' lives is minimized, and they can stay in touch with everyday activities and participate in family life while working with SW Services staff to resolve the cause of the problem. Families in the 30% Chicano and Anglo community are carefully selected and prepared for their role, and are paid for their services. These "sympathetic people with a spare bedroom and time to listen to human problems" often continue social contact with the clients long after the crisis has subsided. Clients pay for room and board on a sliding scale, ranging from 50 cents to $16 daily. The program, which is unusual in that it aims to provide institutional alternatives before incarceration rather than afterwards, has been effective for about 85% of clients in "acute psychiatric emergencies" (though they always have hospital back-up). Also part of the Mental Health Services is a center which offers 24-hour service and is developing similar alternatives for drug addicts, alcoholics and

youth. Workers at the center also do on site consultation at areas around the country which want to implement similar programs. Contact: ALTERNATIVE COMMUNITY SETTINGS PROGRAM, Southwest Denver Mental Health Services, Inc., 3052 W. Mississippi, Denver, CO 80219, (303) 922-3673.

RESOURCES

The Madness Establishment, Ralph Nader's Study Group Report on the National Institute of Mental Health, Franklin D. Chu and Sharland Trotter, Grossman Publishers, 625 Madison Ave., New York, NY 10022, 1974. 232 pp. $7.95. All Royalties to the Center for Study of Responsive Law
. . . shows how the "bold new approach" intended by the 1963 Community Mental Health Centers Act never fulfilled its expectations, because the centers have remained tied to the self-interest of the psychiatric profession, perpetuate different standards for rich and poor, and lack consumer input at all levels of decision-making as well as any built-in means of evaluation. The report analyzes the structure of the federal program and includes descriptions of five centers around the country (including the Lincoln Hospital Revolt) which highlight critical but common problems. Interestingly, the authors found that the most innovative and responsive centers avoid federal money, and the best of the federally-funded ones tend to ignore some federal guidelines. Calling for humane care given by sympathetic people (and placing mental health problems outside the realm of medical responsibility), they conclude: "In retrospect, the community mental health centers program was vastly oversold, the original goals quickly perverted—possibly because of the contradictory assumption that revolutionary change could be successfully wrought by those professionals and politicians with a vested interest in maintaining the status quo." A thoughtful, informative analysis.

Evaluation of Community Involvement in Community Mental Health Centers, Health/PAC study available from U.S. Dept. of Commerce, National Technical Information Service, 5825 Port Royal Rd., Springfield, VA 22151, 1971. 360 pp. $6.00
. . . case-study of six community mental health centers focusing on degree of community participation. The sites were chosen for racial, economic and regional variety. Each study analyzes population served, services, outreach, treatment, effectiveness of community involvement, and more. Concludes that community involvement was mostly token and ineffective, that the outreach was poor (most was to other social service agencies), and access often was bad. A useful study for understanding the concepts and practice of community mental health centers.

"The Aged and Community Mental Health: A Guide to Program Development," Committee on Aging, Group for the Advancement of Psychiatry, 419 Park Ave., South, New York, NY 10016, 1971. 96 pp. $2.00
. . . sets guidelines for establishing services for old people in community mental health centers, including giving them opportunities to participate in groups with patients of all ages, and providing counseling to deal with their special needs such as retirement and bereavement. They should be encouraged to become part of social action groups, to combat feelings of helplessness and low esteem.

HEALTH/PAC BULLETIN, Barbara Ehrenreich and Maxine Kenny, 17 Murray St., New York, NY 10007, May, 1969, and December, 1969. $.60 each
. . . two-part expose of the whole community mental health field, drawing on the experiences of New York City, particularly Columbia University.

SPECIAL HEALTH NEEDS

This section covers the health needs of the elderly, blind, deaf, handicapped, retarded and prisoners. This diverse group of people are all, to some degree, dependent on society to meet their special needs. Yet society's response has been consistently inadequate, and often inhumane. Our present system has, at best, only a wavering commitment to the health and human needs of the economically unproductive—and the blind, deaf, handicapped, retarded and elderly are all classified as unproductive; even prisoners, who work long hours for negligible wages, are put into this category.

Ironically, the non-productivity of which they are accused is reinforced and perpetuated by the ways they are treated. Societal stereotypes of helplessness and lack of adequate training programs deny access to many jobs the elderly, blind, deaf and handicapped could easily handle. Few training programs exist and those that do are sorely underfunded and more geared toward making small crafts than learning economically valued skills. Prisons may offer token vocational training, but the skills taught are rarely useful in the outside world. The fact is that our economy does not provide enough jobs for those who are seeking them, and those people seen as marginal are often shunted aside.

This often means being warehoused—crowded into institutions isolated from the normal life of the community. The elderly end up in nursing homes, prisoners in vast "pens", the retarded in huge institutions giving only minimal custodial care. Such institutionalization is actually necessary in only a small percentage of cases; yet families trying to deal with a handicapped child or elderly relative may find that they have no other financially feasible alternative. Most public money goes to support warehouses rather than programs that allow people to stay in the community—day programs for the elderly, community centers for prisoners, group living situations, half-way houses, etc. Such programs allow the participants to continue to relate to their family and community, in many cases to hold down jobs, and generally to lead much less restricted lives. In the long run, community-based programs may often be cheaper and more efficient than warehousing; but setting up such programs requires initial expenditures and commitment that public office-holders have rarely tried to muster.

Those services which are offered are often limited in their usefulness by the fact that they are defined and controlled by professionals rather than the people supposedly being served. Deaf people know their own problems best, and what approaches are most helpful. Elderly people, clearly, are most in touch with their own needs. Yet one repeatedly finds such contradictions as organizations "for" the blind, with boards made up entirely of sighted people. There is a widespread assumption that certified professionals can speak and decide for deaf people, handicapped people, etc. This assumption implies that those society preceives as handicapped or past their stage of economic usefulness, or prisoners who have in some way violated social norms, are judged to be totally incapable of significantly thinking, speaking, and acting on their own behalf. They are to be the wards of society rather than continuing participants in it.

Such attitudes--patronizing at best, scornful at worst--underlie the neglect and inadequate care described in the following pages. This section should not exist as a seperate unit; groups such as the old, prisoners, and the handicapped should all be included under community health--their needs should be integrated into the normal life of the community. The present conditions of isolation and neglect will change only as we build toward a society which values human life first and economic productivity second, and which has a greatly increased respect for the worth and self-direction of all people.

PRISONERS

Prisoners in this country have long been among the most ignored and abused segment of the population, routinely denied human, economic and civil rights and dignities. Prisons have been used to intimidate, isolate, and punish social and political outcasts. Eighty years ago poor European immigrants comprised the main population of prisons; often their only crime was to steal enough to stay alive. Today, the prisons are full of poor Whites, Blacks, Chicanos and other Third World people. While suburban youth are given suspended sentences and probation for minor crimes, poor and Third World youth are sent to prison.

Inmates live in the roughest, filthiest, most frightening conditions immaginable with every aspect of prison life mitigating against a sound body and mind. Most prisons house at least twice as many prisoners as originally intended; rodents run rampant through the tiers; insects infest bland, non-nutritious food (some states spend as little as 11¢/day per inmate for food); sanitation is minimal, often consisting of an open drain in the middle of the cell; and fresh air is a rarity. Prisoners are told when to eat, sleep, talk, walk, exercise and use the toilet. Work is slave labor, with wages averaging less than $1 for 8 hours of work. Gang rape is a grim reality. Lock-up (prisoners are not allowed to leave their cells, even for meals), the hole (solitary confinement) and beatings are commonly used by authoritarian guards to keep prisoners "in line".

Under such conditions, health care is almost impossible to deliver; and when provided, it is grossly inadequate. Initial screening (intake) consists of a few general questions and a cursory VD exam. Blood tests, urinalysis and X-rays are rarely give, and sick call is limited to a few patients each day. With medicine distributed haphazardly and the threat of withholding sick call used to keep prisoners in line, power plays are rampant. Since prisons are built far from population centers, hospitals are also usually miles away. Medical records are seldom well-kept and rarely transferred from one facility to another; follow-up care is disastrously poor.

Most prison health care is delivered by incompetent doctors who aren't successful on the outside ("I just had too many (malpractice) suits before I came here") or by foreign doctors who often do not speak English. Many prison doctors are in it for the money. For instance, one doctor in Oklahoma makes $30,000/year for part-time prison work; many such docs have a thriving private practice besides their token prison one. With most prison doctors hired by and answerable to the Department of Corrections, it is no surprise that many are more obsessed with the need for security than the need for good health care.

The special needs of women prisoners are commonly ignored. Pregnant women seldom receive adequate nutrition or prenatal care and are often not allowed to see their babies, once born. (Programs are being instituted to allow mothers to keep their children.) Women are also subjected to incredible indignities, such as undergoing vaginal exams for contraband every time they leave the tiers. Women in prison quickly learn that the fastest way out is to become a "lady", with all the oppressive sex-role stereotyping it implies.

All in all, the prison system virtually guarantees ill-health. Every year scores of prisoners die from serious or chronic illness not properly diagnosed or treated. Overcrowding, unsanitary conditions, and deficient diets make prisons a prime

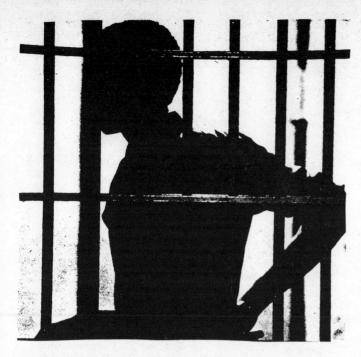

target for communicable disease and poor mental health.

Lack of decent care and indifference by the medical profession are themselves bad enough. But the use of prisoners' minds and bodies for human experimentation is deplorable. The American medical profession has thwarted every effort of international medical societies to end experimentation on prisoners. After all, prisoners are the cheapest, most efficient subjects for testing new drugs and medical procedures; the drug companies can buy these human subjects for a fraction of the free world price; and results are easier to tabulate because all the subjects are in one place.

Many drug tests done on prisoners would never be sanctioned for student subjects at any price because of the risk and pain involved. Prisoners have very little recourse when things do go wrong. Few records are kept and most prisoners are forced to sign papers releasing virtually everyone connected with the test from responsibility. Because of recent outcries, an abundance of guidelines for human experimentation have come about in the past few years; but when asked if any action to enforce the new regulations had been taken, and HEW official responded, "None, to date." Nowhere is there a comprehensive list of which prisons are allowing human experimentation, what the experiments are, and what drug companies and physicians are involved. One HEW official explains, "We do give some research grants that involve prisoners. But there is no convenient way of recovering the information as to whether our guidelines are being followed. That responsibility lies with the principle investigator." Leaving the responsibility to the companies whose profit depends on ignoring those guidelines is insufferable.

Inmates are very vulnerable to the wooing of the drug companies. To a person denied all dignity, material possessions, and most things that the "free world" considers necessities, the few dollars a week the drug corporations dole out in return for use of a prisoner's body and mind, seem like a goldmine. Free choice and informed consent cannot exist under such economically and psychologically coercive conditions. Furthermore these drug company experiment wages—inflated by prison standards—feed into the destructive aspects of the prison sub-economy. A prisoner making five or six times as much as fellow-inmates can use her/his advantage to bribe, control, or extort other inmates.

Society has done its best to ignore prisons. Yet the recent wave of prison riots has forcibly brought public attention to prison conditions and demands. Attica, San Quentin and McAlister are prime examples. A resurgence of prison unity has resulted, with inmates forming unions, striking for recognition and negotiating for their rights. Prisoner newspapers keep cons aware of the action and outside support groups offer essential legal, community education and publicity assistance.

Because bad health care cannot be separated from the other oppressive conditions in prisons, we are presenting both those working for health care and general prisoner organizing and support groups. Almost all of the groups listed are drawn together by the belief that the prison system as we know it must be abolished, for the only real way to 'deter crime' is to change political and economic conditions. As Jessica Mitford points out in Kind and Usual Punishment, the overwhelming majority of experienced corrections officials consider only 10-15% of the inmate population dangerous to the public. Some of the groups listed are working to develop alternatives to incarceration; others are taking measures to increase inmate power to end such repressive practices as the indeterminate sentence (a convict is incarcerated for an indefinite period of time), the discretionary power of the parole board, the discriminatory bail system, human experimentation, forced "rehabilitation" through behavior modification, and the general denial of inmates' rights.

(For more information on prisons, see subsection on Techniques of Psychiatric Abuse in Mental Health.)

PRISON HEALTH GROUPS

The following groups are working for improved health conditions. They call for systematized intake and sick-call procedures; the hiring of competent doctors and outside paraprofessionals (using inmates feeds into the internal power plays of prisons); transfer of responsibility for prison health from the Department of Corrections to the Department of Health or other non-security-oriented branches of government; and the creation of prison wards in "free-world," general hospitals. Some are also pushing for prison health courses to be taught by medical schools.

BAY AREA MCHR PRISON TASK FORCE...does exemplary prison health work on a local, state, and national level, as well as serving as a national coordinator for MCHR prison projects. Their successful entry in the prisons and investigation of health care at California's Soledad, San Quentin and Folsom prisons resulted in access to the prisons by medical teams; legal suits and a legislative investigation followed, although no direct action has been taken. MCHR work in the San Francisco area includes a 1968 city and county jail investigation, culminating in a court decision that prison health

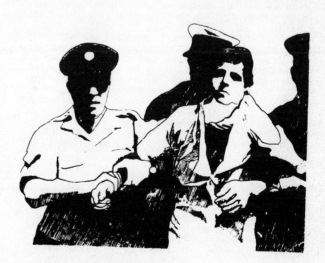

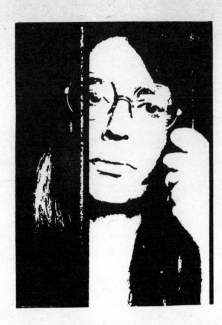

care is "cruel and unusual punishment." Along with hospital workers, cons and the local sheriff, MCHR successfully pressured San Francisco General Hospital into using a 20 bed ward for prisoners; this is particularly important since prisoners are not segregated from the general hospital population. Plans are to have medical and nursing students rotate through the jail as part of their training. In non-health related work, the Task Force monitors the Bureau of Prisons; travels nationally, collecting information on policy and conditions; and has, with other prison support groups, successfully stopped the construction of a new California penitentiary, part of a proposed $700 million expansion of the federal prison system. A member of the Task Force was appointed to the Mayor's Commission to study the expansion. Contact BAY AREA MCHR PRISON TASK FORCE, 588 Capp St., San Francisco, CA 94110 (415) 824-5888.

PRISON HEALTH TASK FORCE/NEW YORK URBAN CO-ALITION...works to improve health care for prisoners in New York City. A 1971 court case to which they were party, resulted in an order to clean up New York's Mens House of Detention (the Tombs); subsequently, responsibility for prison health was transferred from the Department of Corrections to the Health Services Administration (HSA). After visiting local prisons and jails, the Urban Coalition Task Force met with HSA to negotiate the use of Bellevue Hospital's 18th floor for inmate care. The Task Force hopes to improve treatment by placing inmates in general medical facilities rather than inadequate prison and jail infirmaries. Working with prison support and legal groups, the Task Force has been striving to get health workers for all city institutions and to organize an inmate health council on a state level. It sees itself as a liason and arbitrator between inmates and provideers and has taken a very active role testifying at hearings, publicizing conditions and organizing support. Committees of the Task Force investigate and review behavior modification, mental health, women's health, and contracts between hospitals and prisons (to protect inmates from experimentation, research and general abuse). Comprised of professionals and ex-cons, they visit prisons; check the implementation of changes in detention homes; and keep tabs on HSA. Contact PRISON HEALTH TASK FORCE/NEW YORK URBAN COALITION, 55 5th Ave., New York, NY 10003, (212)

If the researchers really believe these experiments are safe for humans, why don't they try them out in their labs on students? Because they know the University would never permit this—and furthermore it would never occur to them to do these things to people they regard as colleagues and social equals. They look on men behind bars as something less than human.
— Dr. Sheldon Margen, Chairperson of Nutritional Sciences Dept., Univ. of California

COOK COUNTY PRISON TASK FORCE...was formed to assist the 55,000 people passing through the infamous Cook County Jail each year. (Only 7% are found guilty of the alleged crime). With the back-up of Cook County Hospital and employing military-trained medical corpsmen, the Task Force is slowly developing programs to improve prison health care. The corpsmen work closely with prisoners, bringing services to the tiers; meanwhile the hospital provides specialist services. Attempts are being made to have highly qualified doctors rotate through the prison health system and to create a structure to insure continuity of care for those released (i.e. passing prison health records on to neighborhood clinics). Of particular significance is the fact that Cook County Hospital is quasi-independent and not under the direct control of the Chicago political machine. Contact COOK COUNTY HOSPITAL, Department of Medicine, 720 Wilcott, Chicago, IL 60612, (312) 633-6702.

PRISON LEGAL SERVICES PROJECT...provides civil, legal services to the Illinois prison population. With a strong interest in prison health care delivery, the Project has recently filed 5 federal suits in this area. One such suit grew out of the death of a diabetic inmate and challenges the prison's inadequate attention to diabetics, poor food and hygiene, sick call procedure and distribution of insulin treatment. Other legal work includes a class action suit on behalf of epileptics and defense of a prisoner suing the prison doc, wardens and officers for withholding medication. In the latter case, the officials were found liable and the con awarded $500. The Project would like to act as a clearinghouse on the barbaric conditions in Illinois prisons and feels that the judgements won, although presently applying only to Illinois prisoners, will provide useful precedents for other court cases. Although funded by the Law Enforcement Assistance Administration, they are doing constructive and important prison legal work. Contact PRISON LEGAL SERVICES PROJECT, 73 W. Monroe, Chicago, IL 60603, (312) 641-0767.

MASSACHUSETTS PRISON HEALTH PROJECT... began in 1972 as an OEO-funded demonstration project to fell in the gaps existing in state prison health services and to design a model program to be duplicated in other prison systems. It has been successful in building up a core staff of medics—mostly ex-military corpsmen—and doctors at most of the state's prisons and in developing inmate medical committees at three. Project funds helped renovate Norfolk Prison Hospital and a training program for inmate lab technicians was prepared. The project got surplus equipment from the Civil Defense Agency and outdated supplies from civilian hospitals. Regulation forms for incoming patients have been developed. A project staff person regularly goes out to monitor prison health conditions and monthly review meetings are held for prison health staff. Recently, the project has had internal problems and has shifted to a more traditional corrections top-down philosophy. It has quit speaking out on such issues as drug experimentation, "special offenders" units, and other prison abuses. Implementation of some of its original, innovative plans has either slowed down of ceased altogether. Half of the project staff has resigned in response to this change of orientation. Contact PRISON HEALTH PROJECT, 80 Boylson St., Rm. 1201, Boston, MA 02116, (617) 423-1548.

DADE COUNTY MEDICAL SERVICES...began in 1967, using doctors from Jackson Memorial Hospital to provide inmate medical care. One of the most significant features of the program has been the training and upgrading of nurses to become nurse practitioners for three Dade County jails and prison facilities. They have been found to be just as-if not more-effective than fellows from the hospital. Each of the dispensaries is accessible 16-24 hours/day; the prison has a 12 bed infirmary and 11 disease isolation cells, as well as a suite of rooms at Jackson Memorial for emergency and specialty cases. A new experimental system will be instituted using a closed-circuit video camera at the dispensaries, hooking them up with the hospital for consultation with doctors there. When a prisoner enters the jail, s/he is given a brief screening; women also get pap smears, and if they want, VD tests. If an inmate is sent to the blockade, a more extensive physical and history is taken. PMS feels its main achievement has been to set up a system of training, monetary, and organizing health care to insure good delivery. Contact PMS, c/o Dept. of Medicine, Jackson Memorial Hospital, Miami, FL 33136, (305) 325-6338.

GENERAL PRISON GROUPS

Listed below are a few of the many prisoner organizing and support groups. Inside organizing can only thrive with strong outside support.

THE PRISONERS UNION. . .grew out of state-wide meetings of cons, ex-cons and community people following a series of prison strikes and riots in 1971. Viewing unionization as a vital first step toward convicts obtaining civil rights, minimum wages and benefits, abolition of indeterminate sentences, etc. this excellent group will help inmates anywhere to unionize. Much the same as a labor union, a prisoner's union can confront the economic power structure within the institution through refusal to work in prison industries; thus the administration (management) is forced to negotiate with the prisoners (labor). Only when inmates receive just compensation for their labor will they be economically free to refuse to sell their bodies for drug company experimentation, etc. Tactics used by Prisoners Union include: educating community groups, churches, and schools through speaking tours; publication of a newspaper, "The Outlaw"; challenging the lack of due process (right to a trial or hearing) through administrative and court proceedings; and creation of grievance procedures. The union files 3-4 lawsuits each year on behalf of inmates. One such suit involves $22,000,000 in the Inmates Welfare Fund (profits from prison labor) which authorities refuse to release for recreational supplies. Prisoners Union has been successful in forcing prisons to allow distribution of "The Outlaw" and is now collecting data on how the federal system arbitrarily denies inmates access to information and support people. Contact PRISONER'S UNION, 1315 18th St., San Francisco, CA 94107, (415) 648-2880.

Shortly after I arrived at Raiford, a supervisor told me, 'Mr. Roberts, before you are here one year you'll hate a convict worse than anything on earth.' An officer at Raiford is expected to feel that a convict is the lowest thing on earth.
—a guard's testimony before the Select Committee on Crime

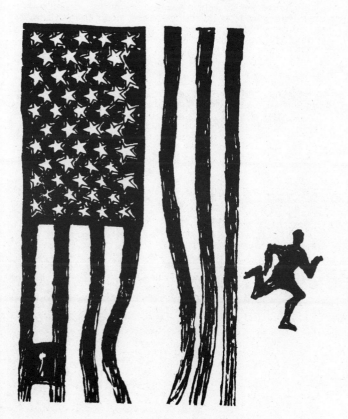

CHICAGO CONNECTIONS. . .has a staff of cons, ex-cons, and community people doing service and activist-oriented work in support of Illinois prisoners. Volunteers answer inmate requests for administrative and legal help, such as assistance in obtaining credit for time served; access to law libraries and drug programs; legal referrals; and housing and job referrals. As one member put it " . . .take a big rock and start chipping 'til nothing is left but a pebble." Connections monitors and pressures court-appointed attorneys and agencies, forcing them to live up to their duties and to protect the rights of inmates. It has done some legislative work and testifying on prison conditions. Connections is now putting together an information packet in preparation for any possible future rioting at Illinois prisons, including legal rights, arrangements for the press, and transportation. They want to avoid reprisals and promises of amnesty which are later retracted. Contact CONNECTIONS, 21 E. Van Buren, Room 605, Chicago, IL 60605, (312) 939-4227.

UNITED PRISONERS UNION. . .aims to unionize all California prisoners and then use the power of a state-wide strike to achieve basic civil rights (including health care) and fair wages for inmates. Their bill of rights calls for: an investigation into the role of guards in racial conflicts; end to indeterminate sentencing and slave labor; cessation of censorship; and exposure of prison industries. UPU has participated in class-action suits over prison officials refusal to allow copies of the "Anvil" (UPU newspaper) and ex-cons into the prison. A Women's Committee exists within UPU to deal with the special needs of women prisoners. The Union supports prisoners strikes; holds rallies in behalf of prisoners; embarks on letter-writing and petitioning campaigns; testifies at hearings of the legislature; educates about prison conditions; and organizes the outside community to sponsor and pass on communications to prisoners. In addition, UPU provides survival services such as counseling on employment and housing and transportation to nearby prisons for the families of cons. A multi-national organization, UPU sees prisoners as the most oppressed sector of the working class and prisons as a microcosm of the classism and economic contradictions of the society as a whole. UPU does considerable work in defense of political prisoners. Contact UPU, 3077 24th St., San Francisco, CA 94110 (415) 285-3100.

MINNESOTA PRISONERS UNION. . .began in 1971 in an effort to unionize Stillwater State Prison. A non-inmate organizer is elected by the cons and supported by the Union to do work within the prison. The Union is committed to economic change with the prison structure and is working to gain control over all profits from inmate's labor. Currently 10% of the profits go into an institutionally administered fund for inmate's recreational supplies and 90% goes to guard benefits. The Union takes advantage of their relatively good access to legislators and state officials as well as the "progressive" reputation of Minnesota's corrections officials to pressure the Department of Corrections into change. Minnesota Prisoner Union believes that the unionization of prisoners provides a new institutional power base from which to challenge Department of Corrections programs in the community. They are currently trying to limit Corrections control of non-prison institutions, such as therapeutic communities, which are less physically brutal, but can still be very manipulative. Contact MINNESOTA PRISONERS UNION, 1427 Washington Ave. S., Minneapolis, MN 55404 (612) 339-8511.

THE PRISON LAW COLLECTIVE. . .has been doing fine prison work since 1971, focusing on legal action against brutality and arbitrary confinement in solitary as well as bringing class action suits to secure prisoners rights. In the field of health, the collective is using legal tactics and working with medical people to end barbaric treatment (i.e. operations without anesthesia). One of the few legal groups concerned exclusively with prison work, the Collective receives an overwhelming volume of requests; they would like to find groups to whom they can do referrals. The Collective played a strong role in supporting the 1973 strikes at California prisons, getting information to and from inmates and coordinating outside support. They have written and distribute "The Jailhouse Lawyer." Contact PRISON LAW COLLECTIVE, 558 Capp St., San Francisco, CA 94110 (415) 282-3983.

AMERICAN FRIENDS SERVICE COMMITTEE... has been working in support of prisoners and ex-cons since 1971. The major activity of AFSC has been to assist in the organization and development of Prisoners and Community Together (PACT), a prisoners' resource center. PACT provides employment and housing assistance; counseling; emergency services for people recently released, such as clothing, medical care and transportation; and temporary housing. In addition, PACT has initiated emergency first aid training in prisons and community-prisoner dialogue groups. AFSC provides legal services to directly support such prisoner organizing efforts as work stoppages and rebellions. A major prisons rights case, to which AFSC was party, resulted from the publication (by AFSC) of a booklet of prison letters from a Black prisoner who spent 3½ years in the hole. The Court found the seclusion unit to be cruel and unusual punishment and ordered it closed. AFSC directly assisted in the formation of "Indiana Prisoners for Progressive Action", which represents over 60% of the inmates at two maximum security prisons; currently, the Committee is working to rejuvinate a state-wide citizens hearing committee on criminal justice. Community education centers around such issues as behavior modification, the dangerous discretionary control implicit in indeterminate sentences, and the god-like power of the parole board. Contact AFSC, 8 North Washington St., Valparaiso, IN 46383, (219) 872-9139.

CHICAGO WOMEN'S PRISON PROJECT... started in 1972 to educate around and act on the problems of women prisoners, particularly those at Dwight prison, a women's penitentiary in the Chicago area. After much letter writing, press conferences, and general public presure, the ex-cons and professionals in the project were finally able to gain access to Dwight. Joining forces with everyone from the ACLU to the Black Panthers and a wide range of the women's movement, the Project worked through a Task Force to present 4 pages of demands to the Department of Corrections. In fall 1973, a decision was arbitrarily made by the Department to convert Dwight into an all-male prison and move the women into the more deteriorated county jail. The Task Force is now seeking to guarantee that conditions will be improved before the move. Two of the group's main successes have been to establish a "Women and Their Bodies" course, and along with the Chicago Lawyers Guild, a legal course for women at Dwight. Contact CHICAGO WOMEN'S PRISON PROJECT, c/o Chicago Women's Liberation Union, 852 W. Belmont, Chicago IL 60657, (312) 929-5004 or 348-43004.

LEAVENWORTH BROTHERS OFFENSE/DEFENSE COMMITTEE... formed after a January, 1974 uprising at Leavenworth Prison. Twenty-six inmates were segregated (after amnesty had been promised) and indicted on charges ranging from assault to murder; most were leaders of the rebellion and political activists, including members of VVAW. The Committee, which is organizing a legal defense, includes the Leavenworth Brothers, ex-cons, lawyers, and community people. Repression has been heavy with prison officials banning correspondence with the accused, the denial of due process, the selection of an all-White jury to hear the cases of Black defendants, etc. Offensively the Committee is educating community groups around the conditions in Leavenworth and prisons in general, puts out a newsletter and actively supports local struggles such as a city-wide teachers' strike and United Farm Workers organizing efforts. Contact LBO/DC, PO Box 5818, Kansas City, MO 64111, (816) 753-1619.

ATTICA BROTHERS DEFENSE COMMITTEE... is composed of the inmates indicted for the 1971 Attica uprising plus legal and community support people. The Committee's actions center around preparing a legal defense for the Attica Brothers and public education around the issues of Attica and prisons in general. Repression has been rampant with a biased jury, infiltration, and denial of information to inmate defendants; a recent proposal to drop charges because of the impossibility of a fair trial has been filed. The Committee supports other liberation struggles and puts out a newsletter. They are in dire need of financial and personnel help. Contact ATTICA BROTHERS DEFENSE COMMITTEE, 1370 Main St., Buffalo, NY 14209, (716) 884-4423.

NATIONAL PRISON CENTER... has been researching prisons, supplying legal help for prisoners, doing referrals on jobs and housing, and sponsoring workshops and community services for 3 years. Their main activity is publishing PRISONERS' DIGEST INTERNATIONAL. Recently, NPC has put together a proposal for a new community, run by and for prisoners. In 1974, the NPC-PDI collective split up. Some members, disillusioned with their limits as a medium, joined with the Church of the New Song, begun by inmates at an Alabama penitentiary. The Church believes in dealing with the whole person—personal, political, spiritual—and that brutality in prisons can only end when the cycle of violence is stopped. Members see the Church as a way to enter the prisons from the outside and to build solidarity and effect change from the inside. Although a recent court case ruled that a chapter could be set up in Iowa State Penitentiary, repression has

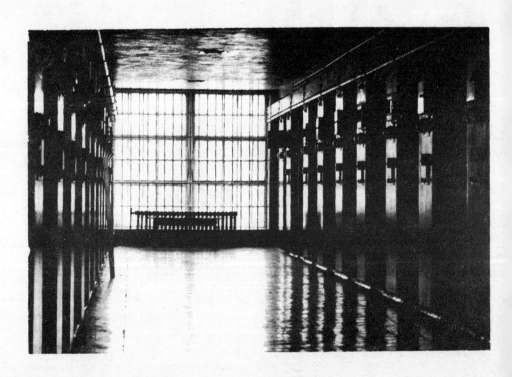

been great. Other members of NPC have formed a prison law collective and PDI has been taken over by a group in Eastern Iowa. For more information on NPC and the law collective, contact LAW COLLECTIVE, Dey Building, Iowa St., Iowa City, Iowa 52240, (319)337-3702; for information on THE CHURCH OF THE NEW SONG, contact c/o Copeland, 835 Ave. F, Ft. Madison, Iowa 52627.

HELP OUR PRISONERS EXIST... does needed support work at McAlister state prison and other Oklahoma institutions. All money and authority for the Oklahoma prison system are centered in McAlister, an illegal condition which HOPE is working to change. It is also pressuring for a full-time, elected parole board free from the political influence of the government and lower-level functionaries. HOPE has instituted a grievance form and mechanism and will keep track of the success of this procedure. Community education around the repressiveness of prison conditions and a transportation system to assist inmates and their families maintain contact are also HOPE projects. In addition, they are studying the public defender and parole system and trying to get a full-time prison doctor. Contact HOPE, 431 SW 11th St., Oklahoma City, OK 73103, (405) 236-0521.

COMMITTEE FOR PRISONER HUMANITY AND JUSTICE ...has a small paid staff and large volunteer contingent, who divide their energies between helping individual prisoners with conviction, confinement, and due process problems and researching and exposing prison conditions and parole alternatives. They are currently gathering information on prison adjustment centers (a fancy new name for barbaric maximum security units). The group works to get inmates paroled and has joined with other prisoner professional and community groups to stop psychosurgery in California prisons. The Committee contends that prisoners have a contractual relationship with the state, with certain rights inherent in that arrangement. CPHJ opposes the warehouse institutionalization of prisoners and believes that the criminal justice system does not have the right to forcefully 'rehabilitate' inmates. Rather, it believes, social, educational and community services should be available to cons and ex-cons if they want them, but should not be a "requirement". Viewing parole as just an extension of prison, with the convict responsible to the government, CPHJ would like to see a system of community half-way houses set up where prisoners are directly responsible for their own lives and to the community in which they live. Contact CPHJ, 1029 4th St., Rm 37, San Rafael, CA 94901 (415) 454-5700.

RESOURCES
BOOKS

Health Care in Pennsylvania Prisons, Health Law Project, University of Pennsylvania Law School, 133 S. 36th St., Rm. 310, Philadelphia, PA 19104, 279 pp.
... perhaps the most comprehensive study of prison health delivery to date. The report begins with a general description of Pennsylvania prisons and then covers environmental health conditions, including physical conditions, food, recreation, industrial safety and health. The meat of the report deals with the health care delivery process, presenting what the system is supposed to be and what, in fact, it is. Catagories deal with every aspect of prison health and prison conditions. The report concludes that the system needs an independent office of medical care in the DOC or better yet, in another agency; that external review bodies be set up to oversee prison practices; and that prison grievance procedures be set up. The methodology model of this report is invaluable for community groups studying their state or municipal corrections system.

It's just that the walls are not there to keep us from getting out. They're there to keep people from coming in. As long as they can keep us isolated from the community, nobody knows what's happening.
Richard X. Clark, Attica

Soledad Brother: The Prison Letters of George Jackson, Bantam Books, Inc., 666 Fifth Ave., New York, NY, 1970. 250 pp. $1.50
...is a plunge into the pain, fear, hatred and courage of a man who spent his entire adult life in solitary confinement. Incredibly, he was still capable of intense hope, love and trust, as evidenced in some of these letters to his parents, his brother Jonathan, Angela Davis, and others.

Kind and Usual Punishment: The Prison Business, Jessica Mitford, Alfred A. Knopf, New York, 1973. 340 pp. $7.95
...an outstanding expose of the penal system. Jessica Mitford cuts through hypocrisies and doubletalk to reveal the total failure of prisons to deal humanly with prisoners, or even to protect society from crime. In her controlled yet intense writing style, she attacks the farce of prison reform and therapeutic communities which couple professional psychological abuse with the usual physical punishment. A chapter called "Cheaper than Chimpanzees" documents dangerous drug experiments that are being performed on prisoners with increasing frequency. A strong sense of righteous anger pervades the book from beginning to end, where Mitford calls for the abolition of the penal system as part of the radical restructuring of social and economic institutions. She demands this not simply from a humanitarian viewpoint, but out of her awareness that the prison is an integral part of our society. "Those of us on the outside do not like to think of wardens and guards as our surrogates. Yet they are, and they are intimately locked in a deadly embrace with their human captives behind prison walls. By extension so are we."

Jessica Mitford on behavior predictors:
Their recurring refrain: "If only the clearly discernible defects in Oswald's psychological make-up had been detected in his childhood — had he been turned over to us, who have the resources to diagnose such deviant personalities — we would have tried to help him. If we decided he was beyond help, we would have locked him up forever and a major tragedy of this generation could have been averted." They refer, of course, to Lee Harvey Oswald, who allegedly gunned down President Kennedy — not to Russell G. Oswald, the New York Commissioner of Corrections who ordered the troops into Attica, as a result of which 43 perished by gunfire."

Struggle For Justice: A Report on Crime and Punishment in America, prepared for the American Friends' Service Committee. Hill and Wang, 72 Fifth Ave., New York, NY 10011, 1971. 179 pp. $1.95
... a compelling, action-oriented book which dissects the practice and theories behind prison reform to show the fallacies of most proposals for change. "After more than a century of persistent failure, the reformist prescription is bankrupt." Decrying the whole idea of "rehabilitation, the authors (several of whom are ex-cons) call for an end to indeterminate sentencing, implementation of a Prisoners' Bill of Rights, a reduction in the number of acts considered crimes, and uniform application of criminal laws. A book of unusual strength and worth.

Transitions to Freedom, Transitions to Freedom, Inc. 1251 Second Ave., San Francisco, CA, 1973. 130 pp.
. . . presents "a model for an urban program designed to improve the employment situation for men and women returning to metropolitan areas from prisons and jails." The book describes the work of Transitions to Freedom, an organization that concentrates on opening the job market for ex-prisoners, and helping them learn the skills they need. A detailed and pragmatic guide, the book covers job counselling, training, public relations, and more.

PAMPHLETS AND ARTICLES

"Prison Doctors," Tommas Murton, THE HUMANIST, available from Louise Rice, 65 Chestnut St., Cambridge, MA 02139, 1971. 6 pp., $.27
. . ."documents complicity by prison doctors in prison brutality." It is absolutely devastating to read of case after case where doctors either ignored or actively participated in the atrocities. The author was Commissioner of the Arkansas Department of Correction in 1968 and discovered three human skeletons buried on a state prison farm. After charging that these were the remains of inmates murdered by prison officials, he was quickly fired. The state pathologist reported that he found no evidence of violent death although two of the bodies were decapitated and "the skull of the third has been crushed to the size of a grapefruit." Filled with horror and a growing rage, Murton raises an important question: what meaning has the Hippocratic Oath when physicians tolerate and participate in medieval torture and murder?

"PRISON HEALTH," HEALTH/PAC BULLETIN, 17 Murray St., New York, NY 10007, September, 1973. $.60
. . . a necessary resource for anyone trying to understand the facts and politics behind prison health—or, more accurately, the lack of it. This bulletin provides an excellent overview and indictment of "medicine behind bars"; what constitutes a good prison health program; and an indepth case study of the struggles for decent prison health in New York and San Francisco. The last two pages discuss the chain of events and political intrigues leading to a cut-off of state funds for the UCLA-sponsored Center for the Study and Reduction of Violence research project which would have used prisoners in behavior modification and screening experiments without prior legislative approval. The need for a strong community organization to keep such centers from receiving future funding is discussed. The bulletin concludes that ". . . living conditions in prison, as well as the oppressiveness and meaninglessness of prison life mitigate with extraordinary force against good health care. Those who would improve health care cannot avoid these larger issues."

The Jailhouse Lawyer's Manual: How To Bring a Federal Suit Against Abuses in Prison, Prison Law Collective, 558 Capp St., San Francisco, CA 94110, revised 1973. 48 pp.
. . . well-written, packed with information, this book tells how "how a person in a state prison in California can start a lawsuit in a federal court, without the help of a lawyer, to fight against mistreatment and bad conditions." Based on Section 1983 of the US Code, it explains who can use Section 1983, basic procedures and information about the US legal system. The graphics are excellent; so are the appendices, which are filled with useful information, such as which law libraries will lend books to prisoners.

"The Captive Patient: The Treatment of Health Problems in American Prison," Susan Alexander, CLEARINGHOUSE REVIEW, National Clearinghouse for Legal Services, Northwestern University School of Law, 710 North Lake Shore Dr., Chicago, IL 60611, May 72, pp. 16-27
. . . a comprehensive survey of court cases dealing with prison health.

"Women Locked Up," WOMEN: A JOURNAL OF LIBERATION, 3028 Greenmount Ave., Baltimore, MD 21218, Vol. 3, no. 3, 1972
. . . fine collection of articles on women in mental institutions and prisons, dealing as well with other ways that women are phychologically imprisoned—through oppressive schools and psychologists. Reading this issue, one is brought face to face with the author's conviction that mental and penal institutions are integral parts of this society; any major movement for change must challenge the economic basis for this society: capitalism.

"ATTICA: MURDER BY OMISSION," Marcia Sollek, Health-PAC Bulletin, November, 1971, pp. 7-10. $5/year for students, $7 for others
. . . explores the roles of the University of Buffalo Medical School in the September 1971 Attica rebellion. During the uprising doctors and nurses were denied entry on several occasions. Although the dean of medical school and the director of surgery both took a very passive stance when faced with evidence of medical negligence and cruelty inside the prison, the eye-witness accounts of medical students who were allowed inside brought important facts out to the public. Thus "the medical school and its affiliates can and should play a prominent role in opening the prisons to public view and accountability."

"PRISONER YELLOW PAGES," Outmates, P.O. Box 174, Storrs, CT 06268 . . . national listing of prisoner organizing and support groups; legal, employment and educational resources; prisoner unions; and prison literature and periodicals.

The following are examples of prison newspapers written by and for prisoners and devoted to building a strong movement. The conditions and torture in prisons and the anger, sensitivity, and strength of the inmates is portrayed in terms not easily forgotten. Free to prisoners.

PRISONERS' DIGEST INTERNATIONAL, Box 390, Bettendorf, Iowa 52722 . . .

The Midnight Special, c/o National Lawyers' Guild, 23 Cornelia St., New York, NY 10014.

The Outlaw, Prisoners' Union, 1315 18th St., San Francisco, CA 94107.

NEPA News, New England Prisoners' Association, Franconia College, Franconia, New Hampshire 03580.

Chicago Connections Newsletter, 21 E. Van Buren, Chicago, IL 60605.

FILMS

North East Prisoners' Association, 116 School St., Waltham, MA, 02154

> **"3000 Years and Life"** 16mm, 50 min. color
> Captures series of events that took place when inmates at Warpole State Prison set up a self-governing structure during a strike by prison guards.

Third World Newsreel, 26 W. 20th St., New York, NY 10011
"The Attica Film," 80 min. cl.
Powerful, deeply disturbing study of the American character as revealed by those officials who participated in the Attica massacre of 1971.

> **"Teach Our Children,"** 35 min. b&w $50
> Interviews with brothers inside Attica during the rebellion, and Carlos Feliciano and his family. A film about Third World struggle in this country.

> **"We Demand Freedom,"** 55 min. b&w $75
> Prisoners describe their growing awareness of themselves as a potentially powerful political force. Contains footage from prisons, labor struggles, Japanese Detention Camps of WW II, Birmingham, Alabama, Vietnam, and other historical events.

THE ELDERLY

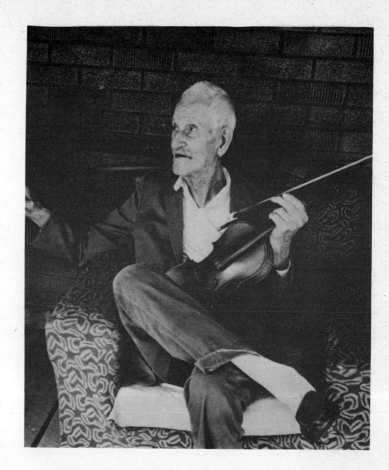

"In 1969, the American people spent five billion dollars on preparations to keep them looking young; in 1970, the Federal government spent one and a third billion dollars on Old Age Assistance." (Old Age: The Last Segregation). These statistics accurately describe the priorities of your youth-oriented culture where the elderly are cast aside, ignored and abused. Industry has little use for older workers (especially in time of high unemployment) and most people are forced to retire at 65. Many are capable of working much longer but will jeopardize their meager social security benefits (averaging $161/month) if they earn more than $1,680/year. So the elderly are forced to depend on Social Security benefits, pension plans, and an array of confusing and shockingly inadequate social services provided by state and local governments.

The principal government health program for the elderly is Medicare. Two plans exist under this program: hospital insurance, which is available to anyone over 65 who is covered by Social Security; and medical insurance, which costs $6.30 per month. Both have considerable deductables (on plan A, the consumer must pay the first $84 of yearly expenses and on plan B, $60) and neither one covers check-ups, hearing aids, eyeglasses, dental care and many home care services. Out-of-pocket expenses (costs not covered by Medicare) have doubled since 1966, when Medicare was started. Those Seniors with low incomes are also eligible for the Medicaid program, although it too ignores out-of-hospital foot, eye, ear and dental care. In a country where three fourths of older people suffer from at least one chronic illness (Gray Panther statistic), this lack of preventive care is an extremely serious omission. Long waits, confusing forms and intimidating bureaucracy further limit the usefulness of Medicare and Medicaid. (See Health Plans)

One out of every five US citizens below the poverty line is 65 or over with the percentage higher for Third World people and women. Old people in rural areas are also particularly hard hit since they often work in agriculture and have no pension plans. The indignities of welfare are increased in less populated areas, where anonymity is impossible and self-sufficiency a strong value. Inaccessibility of doctors, clinics, and social services increase the hardship.

Poverty is the source of other major problems of the elderly. Medical expenses shoot up as income drops, and a balanced diet becomes a mere fantasy on a subsistence income. Many old people cannot see well enough to drive, cannot afford the bus and are asking to get mugged if they go out alone. This powerlessness combined with poverty inevitably results in feelings of loneliness, alienation and dangerous physical isolation. For many the most terrifying question is: What happens when you can no longer care for yourself? Too often the the answer is frighteningly simply—you go into a nursing home and wait for death.

While nursing homes are often a destructive experience for older people, businesspeople recognize them as a very profitable investment. The helplessness of nursing home patients and the anxieties of relatives make them easy marks for nursing home owners. Sometimes patients are required to sign irrevocable entrance contracts which entitle the owner to all their funds, even if the patient later decides to leave. After signing their lives away, too many Seniors find themselves living in a dirty firetrap or a sterile, antiseptic environment.

Even the "best" nursing homes do little more than keep the patients clean, fed, dry and quiet. In an effort to increase Medicare payments and keep patients drugged into acquiescence, such powerful sedatives as Mellaril and Thorazine are often prescribed. The over-use of addicting drugs, coupled with the total lack of rehabilitation programs and facilities are all secondary to the overwhelming mental and sometimes physical degradation suffered by nursing home residents. At best they are treated as children in need of advice and guidance; at worst, as mindless animals. In the nursing home it becomes more evident than ever to the elderly that they are useless, unwanted, even actively resented by overworked aides and guilt-ridden relatives.

Older people are getting angry. In the words of Maggie Kuhn, convener of the Grey Panthers, "Our oppressive, paternalistic society wants to keep the elderly out of the way, playing bingo and shuffleboard. But we're challenging it. We're putting our bodies on the line." As the elderly begin exercising "Senior Power", solutions to current problems emerge. One of the most crucial areas is alternatives to institutional care. Adult day care facilities, "Meals on Wheels", foster home programs, homemaker services, programs to check on shut-ins and neighborhood groups to run errands all help the aged to stay in their own homes as long as possible. Nursing home ombudsperson programs protect the rights and human dignity of nursing home residents while other groups pressure for changes in nursing home regulations. Meanwhile groups like the Grey Panthers push for long term legislative changes regarding national health care plans, and adequate income for all. Perhaps most important is the fact that older people are realizing that they have a right to self-determination and a decent life. "Once we have understood what the state of the aged really is, we cannot satisfy ourselves with calling for a more generous 'old-age policy', higher pensions, decent housing and organized leisure. It is the whole system that is at issue and our claims cannot be otherwise than radical—change life itself." (The Coming of Age, Simone de Beauvoir).

GREY PANTHERS... is a group of old and young people struggling "to build a new power base in our society, uniting the people presently disenfranchised and oppressed." Recently merged with Ralph Nader's Retired Professional Action Group, their priorities include health issues, housing, ending the war in Indochina, mass transportation, social security reform, and court reform. With the support of organized workers, ethnic minorities and religious groups, the Panthers fight the system through demonstrations, lobbying and testimony at public hearings. They encourage elderly citizens to write their congresspeople concerning various health care bills, and stand ready to go en masse to Washington when an important bill comes up for a vote. The health issues they work with include upgrading of nursing homes, protection of patients' rights, preventive medicine, alternatives to institutional care, and accountability of doctors. Viewing medicare and medicaid as woefully inadequate, the Panthers have written their own proposal for a comprehensive National Health Care plan. They also distribute a model nursing home contract, a nursing home action proposal and a study on the hearing aid industry. Contact GREY PANTHERS, 3700 Chestnut St., Philadelphia, PA 19104, (215) EV2-6644.

NATIONAL URBAN LEAGUE ADVOCACY PROJECT... works to educate and assist aged members of minority groups fight for their rights under the law. Senior paraprofessional advocates and professional intermediaries pressure social, health and welfare agencies for more and better services. Operating in San Diego, Chicago, and Columbia, South Carolina, the project helps Black, Brown and White elderly citizens get the most out of present programs while developing more comprehensive plans for the future. In two cities, monies were generated on a local level for a multi-service senior center as a result of the project. HEW funds the project and has the right to approve the staff director. Contact NULAP, 55 East 52nd St., New York, NY 10022, (212) 826-6340, San Diego (714) 263-1423, Chicago (312) 666-7351, Columbia (803) 779-8010.

CITIZENS FOR BETTER CARE... focuses on all problems of the elderly with special emphasis on improvement of nursing homes and related facilities. Since its formation in 1969, the CBC has dealt in publicity, litigation and legislation to force state officials into action. "In one instance CBC sued the (Michigan) State Health Department and successfully forced action on a Detroit nursing home with a long history of poor care." Other actions center around the misuse of patients' funds in nursing homes and the tendency of HEW to retroactively deny benefits to Medicare nursing home patients. CBC also operates the HEW-funded Nursing Home Ombudsman Program through a contract with the National Council of Senior Citizens. Membership meetings are held monthly and the Board is dominated by senior citizens. Contact CBC, 960 East Jefferson Ave., Detroit, MI 48207, (313) 963-0513 or 963-8563.

SENIOR CITIZENS COALITION OF THE CITIZENS ACTION PROGRAM (CAP)... represents over 350,000 senior citizens in the Chicago area. An anti-corporate, anti-corruption group, the senior members of CAP work for self-determination in their neighborhoods. Recently they got a bill introduced into the Illinois legislature enabling pharmacists to sell drugs by the generic name rather than by expensive brand names. Over 200 seniors then forced the president of Abbot Laboratories to see them, demanding that he withdraw his lobbyists against the bill; he refused to comply. Undaunted, the group went to the Board of Directors of Abbott to repeat their demand. Although no definite commitment to withdraw the lobbyists has been made yet, the pressure is on: there's been a great deal of publicity and the coalition plans to attend the next Abbott stockholders' meeting. In the past the group was instrumental in the passage of a bill that allows property tax and rent rebates for the elderly and disabled and successfully opposed the building of the Crosstown Expressway, which would have destroyed the homes of many old people. A steering committee makes policy decisions with the advice of the research staff and leadership committee of CAP; seniors support the group through raffles, bingo games and crafts. Contact SENIOR CITIZENS COALITION OF CAP, 2200 N. Lincoln, Chicago, IL 60614, (312) 929-2922.

GERIATRIC EVALUATION SERVICE... is a state and federally funded pilot program to prevent unnecessary commitments to mental institutions through preadmissions screening of older people. When people call the Service, a doctor and social worker are sent to try to find an alternative solution: counseling, boarding homes, nursing homes, etc. In a typical month of 32 calls, only 3 people are actually admitted to mental hospitals. Contact GERIATRIC EVALUATION SERVICE, Baltimore Health Department, Montebello Hospital, Argone Dr., Baltimore, MD 21239, (301) 396-6006.

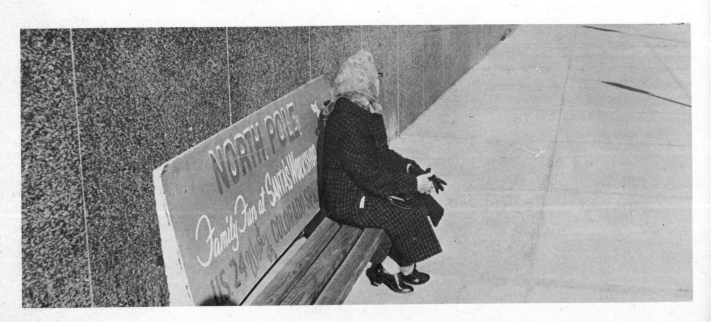

NATIONAL CENTER FOR THE BLACK AGED...collects, evaluates, and disseminates information on the elderly Black community. The Center works with the problems of income, health, housing, retirement and employment. Because the situation of the Black elderly is systematically ignored, the Center is working for change by developing technical, consultative, and training services to increase the awareness and effectiveness of public and private agencies dealing with the Black elderly. It is a national clearinghouse, funded by a government grant and staffed by people experienced in research and social services. Contact: National Center for the Black Aged, 1725 DeSalle St., Suite 402, Washington, DC 20009 (202) 785-8766.

SELF HELP FOR THE ELDERLY...offers a wide range of services to the Asian community: translation at social service agencies and on the telephone; portable meals, meeting dietary restrictions; Home Health Aids to care for home-bound people; visits to Asians in convalescent homes; and recreational outings. Weekly meetings are held at three locations for information about social security, public health and discussions about socialism and community. SHE is also developing a Mental Health Day Center for elderly and a Senior Consumer Discount (5-20%) with local merchants. Building low income housing above a library and church are further priorities. No one needing help is turned away. Contact SHE, 3 Old Chinatown Lane, San Francisco, CA 94108, (415) 982-9171.

COUNCIL OF ELDERS...concentrates on returning the elderly to useful positions in the community and improving the care of those who are no longer able to work. Part of Boston's Model Cities Program, the Council has over 500 senior members. The Council's legal services department has contested the licensing of nursing homes charged with inadequate patient care. The elderly who wish to remain in their homes are encouraged and assisted by home aides who do light housekeeping and errand-running. For the nursing home patient, there is opportunity to attend lectures, concerts and other outside activities through the Nursing Home Program. Other projects of the Council of Elders are a nutrition program and supportive services which center around medical assistance, social security, income maintenance and job referral services. Cooperation with the Roxbury Comprehensive Health Center has resulted in bringing a doctor, nurse and physical therapist to the Center, offering free services. Contact COUNCIL OF ELDERS, 1990 Columbus, Boston, MA 02119, (617) 442-1091.

Because the attendants had to physically care for, handle the aging bodies of these old people, they began to treat them as if they were infants, unhearing, uncaring, unable to speak or communicate in any way. The patients were uniformly called honey or dearie or sweetie—or sometimes naughty girl if they soiled their beds—just as one tends to call children pet names... The bodies were kept clean, fed, powdered, combed and clothed. They awere as infants, without modesty or sex or privacy.
—Nobody Ever Died of Old Age

OVER 60 COUNSELING AND EMPLOYMENT SERVICE...finds jobs for the elderly in the Washington-Maryland area. A free service administered and financed by the Montgomery County Federation of Women's Clubs, the program offers job training as well as placement. "Over 60" also develops specific programs to create jobs such as the "Good Neighbor" Family Aid Program which trains older people to care for shut-ins and small children. Other programs employ pruners, woodcrafters and seamstresses. Serving between 50 and 75 people each month, they offer group and individual pre-retirement counseling. Contact OVER 60 COUNSELING AND EMPLOYMENT SERVICE, 4700 Norwood Drive, Chevy Chase, MD 20015, (301) 652-8073.

COORDINATING COUNCIL FOR SENIOR CITIZENS...organizes government and independent organizations to better serve older citizens of Durham. One project, Attendant Corps for the Elderly, trains "the energetic elderly in care of the frail elderly." Other services in this comprehensive program are: job placement, counseling and discussions for residents of nursing homes; education on health, nutrition, income tax preparation, safe driving, wills and legacies; SenCit Mediport, which provides transportation to medical appointments; and SenCit Check, which coordinates neighbors to look in on shut-ins or others who live alone. A United Fund Agency, the CCSC publishes the SENIOR CITIZENS POST ($1.50/year for non-members), which covers national and local legislation and has articles on retirement. Contact CCSC, c/o Senior Citizen's Memorial Center, 519 E. Main St., Durham, NC 27701, (919) 682-8104.

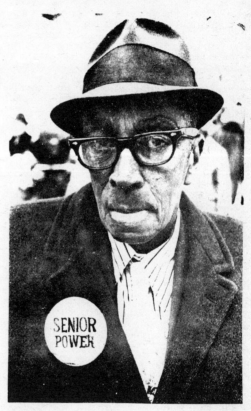

The aged are of low priority in the culture as a whole. Besides, they are not very interesting medically. When you are 65 or so, you find your complaints are no longer listened to; you meet the impenetrable barrier of glazed eyes and careless hands, anxious to take care of someone younger, someone who seems to have a higher potential for complete recovery... So at precisely that time of life when adequate medical care means the difference between being independent and gradual physical debilitation, many old people cannot get the help they need.
—testimony of Sharon Curtin, R.N., before the Subcommittee on Health of the Elderly

NATIONAL COUNCIL FOR SENIOR CITIZENS...led the fight for Medicare and stronger Social Security and now seeks a guaranteed annual income, comprehensive health coverage, property tax relief, satisfactory housing and improved low-cost transportation. Through the political power of its 3 million members, the NCSC works at federal, state and local levels of government to "restore the dignity and independence of older Americans." NCSC sponsored projects include a Nursing Home Ombudsman Program and the Senior AIDES Program which provides part-time community service jobs for poor older Americans. NCSC Goldcard membership is $3/year and entitles seniors to SENIOR CITIZEN NEWS, a monthly publication on legislative information; discount mail-order drug service; and low-cost health insurance. Contact NCSC, 1511 "K" St. NW, Washington DC 20006, (202) 783-6850.

ON LOK DAY HEALTH CENTER... aims to provide comprehensive health care to the elderly, primarily those who do not speak English well and are of Chinese, Filipino or Italian background. Offering day-time care to the isolated, confused and physically handicapped, the Center provides medical services; counseling; physical and occupational therapy; speech and hearing therapy; one balanced meal each day; recreation; foot care; laundry and grooming services; and dental referral. The Center also helps old people in hospitals prepare for their return home. This is an exceptionally fine example of an alternative to institutional care. Funded by HEW, it is part of the Chinatown-North Beach Health Care Planning and Development Corporation's plan to offer comprehensive health care for the aged. Future plans include a geriatric clinic, adequate housing and other supportive services. Contact ON LOK DAY HEALTH CENTER, 140 Mason St., San Francisco, CA 94133, (415) 989-2578.

ACTION ALLIANCE... is an umbrella organization with representatives from 200 groups working to improve conditions for the elderly in the Philadelphia area. By pressuring public officials and institutions, they have successfully reduced bus fare for the aged to 10¢, lowered gas and water rates by 20%, and persuaded banks to offer the elderly free checking accounts. Present concerns are nursing home and boarding home conditions. Using extensive education and research as aids to political action, the group meets regularly with local political leaders and public officials to push for legislative changes as well as better enforcement of present regulations affecting the aged. A Board elected at an annual convention makes the policy decisions of the Action Alliance. Determined to stay independent of the government, the Alliance gets all funding from small grants and donations. Some labor organizations give them financial help. Contact ACTION ALLIANCE, 1213 Race Street, Philadelphia, PA, (215) 568-3897.

NURSE OMBUDSMAN PROGRAM... "exists to provide a platform for consumer advocacy on behalf of the nursing home patient." Two local units in Detroit and Menominee, Michigan, work through individual nursing homes and if necessary, through local government agencies. Volunteer ombudspeople visit nursing homes once or twice a week, talking with both patients and staff, as well as organizing community interest groups to work with nursing home patients. The state and national offices of the program deal mainly with government agencies on long term care issues such as changes in state nursing home regulations. Contact NURSING HOME OMBUDSMAN PROGRAM, National Council of Senior Citizens, 1511 "K" St. NW, Washington DC 20006, (202) 783-6850 or the state unit in Lansing, MI (517) 482-7048.

GERIATRIC SERVICES OF DELAWARE... uses private and foundation funds to keep the elderly in their own homes as long as possible. Trained aids help the handicapped and old with light housework, give limited bedside care and offer companionship, counseling and referrals. Five days a week Meals on Wheels brings a full course meal and a bed supper to convalescents and older people. For those who can't live alone but do not need special medical attention, the program has asked local citizens to open their homes, placing between one and three elderly people in each home; the cost is $188/month, with a sliding scale for those of low income. Contact GERIATRIC SERVICES OF DELAWARE, 1300 N. Broom St., Wilmington, DE 19806, (302) 658-6731

RESOURCES

BOOKS

<u>Old Age: The Last Segregation</u>, Claire Townsend, Project Director, Bantam Books, Inc., 666 5th Ave., New York, NY 10019, 1971. 229 pp. $1.95...this Ralph Nader Study Group report describes in graphic detail the treatment of the aged in nursing homes. The extent of the abuse is overwhelming. Clearly one of the best books in the field, the book documents government dealings with the elderly, the reasons behind substandard nursing homes, general problems of old people in the US as well as programs in other countries. It ends with an urgent call for the "emergence of a retired people's liberation movement" to fight against the economic, governmental and social injustices suffered by the elderly each day.

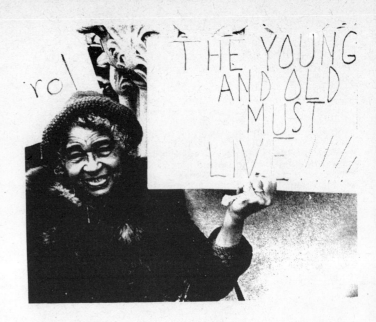

<u>The Coming of Age</u>, Simone De Beauvoir, Warner Paperback Library, 315 Park Ave., South, New York, NY 10010, 1973. 864 pp. $2.25...breaks the "conspiracy of silence" surrounding the plight of the aged. Simone De Beauvoir paints a depressing and hopeless picture of the lives of old people and demands nothing less than a total change in a society that "cares about the individual only in so far as he is profitable." Her book states the case with eloquence and desperation as she speaks of old age historically, biologically and sociologically. This is a work of conviction and committment to radical social change.

<u>Nobody Ever Died Of Old Age</u>, Sharon R. Curtin, G. K. Hall & Co., Boston, MA, 1973. 270 pp. $7.95...is a beautiful book written in anger and love. Sharon Curtin is a nurse who has spent a lot of time talking and living with old people. Full of disgust for our youth-worshipping culture, she describes the elderly she met with great compassion and respect for their adaptability and will to survive. Yet most of them are stripped of any dignity or self-determination by their forced dependence on social welfare services. Ms. Curtin tells of a social worker who brought some older people together to live communally. Everything was going well until one of them was discovered to have terminal cancer. Although the other people in the house wished to care for the dying woman, the social worker decided it was too depressing and sent the woman to a nursing home where she died alone. This is typical of the attitudes Sharon Curtin is fighting. Her book in its eloquence and urgency will hopefully be a tool in bringing about the change she sees as so essential.

<u>Tender Loving Greed: How the Incredibly Lucrative Nursing Home Industry is Exploiting Old People and Defrauding Us All</u>, Mary Adelaide Mendelson. Knopf, Inc., Random House Building, 201 E. 50th St., New York, NY 10022, 1974. 245 pp. $6.95
...important coverage of the business aspects of nursing homes. Controversial and enlightening, it will force people to deal with the painful realities of aging and of the poor care available to older people.

<u>A Practical Guide to Long Term Care and Health Services Administration</u>, ed. Monroe Mitchel. Panel Publishers, Greenvale, NY, 11548, 1973. 400 pp. $24.50
...contains a wide range of thoughtful essays on long term care facilities, particularly nursing homes. With a deep respect for older patients and their unique needs, the authors discuss medical problems, administrative approaches, the role of nurses and other personnel and more. Useful resource for administrators and those trying to humanize long term care facilities.

Older Americans: Special Handling Required, Marjorie Bloomberg Tiven. National Council on the Aging, 1828 "L" St., NW, Washington, DC 20036, 1971. 118 pp. Free
. . .describes the conditions of the aged in the US: poverty, inadequate health care, malnutrition, impersonal institutional care, and more. Government programs (Social Security, Old Age Assistance, and Medicare) are overly bureaucratic, confusing and limited. Often times, older people must sell their homes and give up all their savings before qualifying for state or federal assistance. Those with mental disorders or no close relatives are shuttled between state institutions, mental hospitals, and nursing homes, left to die in isolation and despair. The indictments are well-documented and clear. The book also includes suggestions on how to improve care but lacks a strategy for organizers.

PAMPHLETS AND ARTICLES

"LEGAL PROBLEMS INHERENT IN ORGANIZING NURSING HOME OCCUPANTS," Health Law Project, 133 S 36th St., 6th Floor, Philadelphia, PA 19174, August-September 1972. 9 pp. Free
. . . tells the possible legal problems in organizing toward a patient's rights group in a nursing home. The article discusses, in practical, technical terms, what to do if the home tries to force patients to leave for siding with the organizer.

Access to Nursing Home Services of Spanish Speaking Aged in the Southwest, National Council of La Raza, 1025 15th St. NW, Washington, D.C. 20005, 1973. 30 pp. Free
. . .presents the results of a study focusing on nursing home services for the Spanish speaking elderly. The underlying concern is the total disregard by the majority society for the cultural tradition and distinct lifestyle of the elderly Spanish speaking in federal nursing homes. The proposed model is a board-and-care home, consisting of 2-5 beds, located in el barrio; in this way the elderly may remain in a familiar, supportive environment. The study is quite comprehensive, listing the numerous problems the board-and-care homes face and suggestions for improving relationships between home operators and the government. Presents the need for clear, concise information for nursing home operators, taking into consideration linguistic and cultural differences. An excellent introduction to some of the problems faced in setting up programs for the Spanish speaking elderly.

THE CRUSADER: MORE THAN TEA AND TOAST, Sallie Ruhnka and Vicky Spiegal, Food Research and Action Center, 25 West 43rd St., New York 10036, Winter/Spring 1973. 12 pp. Free. . ."a guide for community groups organizing nutrition programs for the elderly." Tells how to get government funding, plus examples of current nutrition programs. Detailed descriptions of government regulations, where to apply for money, general resources and necessary equipment make this newspaper a must for health organizers.

FILMS AND TAPES

Center for Mass Communication of Columbia University Press, 1365 S. Broadway, Irvington, NY 10533

"The Old Ones," 29 min. b&w (sale: $174)
Since 1891 when the first old-age assistance act was passed, Denmark has tried many different approaches from free medical care to rent subsidies and old people's "estates." In this film, the older Danes discuss the successes and failures of the welfare measures.

If you are over sixty-five, you are forced to retire. If your hair grays, you must dye it. If your physical condition deteriorates— as it must—you will enter an institution. If you look for an apartment, people may refuse to rent to you; old people smell and can't take care of themselves. If you stop to watch children playing, you're suspected of being a dirty old pervert. . . If someone wishes to pay you tribute, they say you're so young—considering your age. That is as grievous an insult as telling a woman she 'thinks like a man'.

Nobody Ever Died of Old Age

THE DEAF AND HEARING IMPAIRED

Hearing loss is presently the most prevalent health handicap in the US, affecting approximately 15,000,000 people, over one million of whom are totally deaf. These people are routinely denied adequate education tailored to their needs, sufficient job training and placement, reasonable insurance rates, easy access to services and, most of all, the right to self-determination. The general public simply refuses to accept the deaf as people worthy of dignity and respect, avoiding them in embarrassment, or blatantly ignoring them.

The deaf child's—and ultimately the deaf adult's—greatest handicap is the educational system into which s/he is forced. This system is geared toward hearing people and reinforces oral communication. Deaf children are pressed into this mold, whether or not they are able to communicate by reading lips or using hearing aids. As a result, children grow up totally void of basic information about the world around them. Professionals encourage parents to develop the child's residual hearing (which often doesn't even exist), and rarely level with them about the extent of the child's deafness, or counsel them to deal with it as a handicap in communication, not in intelligence or in ability to learn and grow.

However, many parents are beginning to insist that a concept of Total Communication be taught to their children and themselves. This involves using every means available to communicate—auditory aids, lipreading and speech, as well as manual communication or "signing" and fingerspelling. One tremendous advantage to this system, is that signing is usually picked up easily by children, often as early as 8 months of age.

In the past "oralists" who disdain manual communication, perpetrated the myth that once children learn sign language they would never try to speak vocally. But parents, deaf people, and educators attest to the fact that the more tools a child is taught, the greater the desire to communicate and the more spontaneous and total the communication. Once a child realizes s/he is understood, the gates are down, self-confidence is gained and progress and adjustment of children

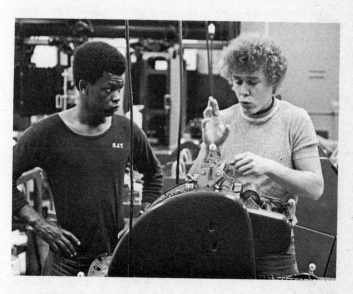

exposed to Total Communication as compared to those using only "oral" methods.

Higher education and job training are limited for the deaf; there are only 30 community colleges and vocational schools nationally. Funds for vocational rehabilitation are very limited and 80% of deaf clients see vocational counselors who cannot communicate with them. Yet Nixon twice vetoed a new Vocational Rehabilitation Bill, and only allowed a greatly watered down version to pass which cuts out most funding for education and training for the handicapped, including wiping out several successful government programs.

Widescale discrimination against deaf people is hardly subtle. Despite studies to the contrary, the deaf are marked as "accident prone" and are consequently charged higher than average insurance rates. Housing complexes for the aged have been known to bar the deaf from living there on the premise that they can't hear a fire alarm. Employment is another prime example of anti-deaf discrimination, with private industry the greatest offender, often falsely claiming that hiring the deaf increases insurance rates. Although the government employs more handicapped people than private companies do, many of its job descriptions include a hearing requirement that is actually unnecessary for effective job performance.

For the elderly, gradual hearing loss is a natural by-product of age, yet such loss creates major changes in people's lives, causing them to withdraw from former activities and hampering their interchange with others. Through highly questionable sales practices, unqualified hearing aid hawkers convince the old that hearing aids will solve all their problems. Unfortunately, many who buy such aids have either permanent nerve damage, or medical problems indicative of disease, which can sometimes be successfully treated. Several states are presently working on legislation that will require a health exam before hearing aid purchase. In addition, new federal regulations require that intermediary care facilities which provide rehabilitative services also provide speech and hearing services to qualify for matching funds. Disturbingly, Public Health Service Studies show that 4/5 of those able to effectively use aids don't wear them because of high prices, lack of public education about hearing loss, the shortage of qualified physicians and the stigma our society associates with hearing loss.

Recently there have been token gains for some of the deaf. The government has financed an experiment in 10 East Coast cities where captioned (subtitled) daily news is broadcast through the public television system. Teletypewriters (TTY), although expensive are becoming more widespread, enabling the deaf to use telephones and related services.

Increasingly the deaf are becoming more assertive, demanding the right to set up group living situations, to communicate freely anywhere and to institute deaf studies programs in schools. Teletypewriters must be made more accessible and more research must be devoted to serving the needs of all all the deaf. Forceful, autonomous community action campaigns, deaf groups and parents groups must form coalitions, holding professionals accountable and demand that the institutions provide support services responsive to individual deaf needs. Anti-discrimination suits must be brought against local industries and signing classes must be accessible to all. Comprehensive testing of the newborn for hearing disabilities must become routine, and doctors must deal realistically with parents and counsel them about all available options. Most significantly, the deaf must gain control of their own services and lives.

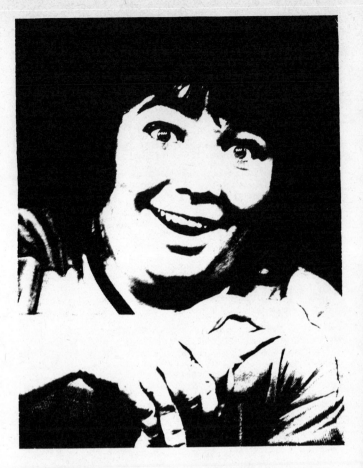

NATIONAL ASSOCIATION OF THE DEAF... is a leader in the struggle for first class citizenship for deaf people in this country. Run by and for deaf people, the Association acts as a clearing-house for services to the deaf, works closely with deaf interest groups and has member organizations in every state which act as advocates for the deaf. Through letter writing, speaking tours, personal contacts and the publication and dissemination of a wealth of materials, they pressure for Total Communication, special communications devices, and education geared specifically for the deaf, claiming that present "education for the deaf is education for the hearing with patches in it." For more information and a list of their excellent publications, contact NAD, c/o Fred Schreiber, 814 Thayer Ave., Silver Spring, MD 20910, (301) 587-1788.

DEAFPRIDE, INC.... "aims to promote the development of leadership capability in the deaf community and in parents of deaf persons so that they can work for change in the institutions that serve deaf persons." An action-oriented, non-profit umbrella group working actively with Parents for Deaf Pride, the Capitol City Association of the Deaf, and the Concerned Parents Task Force, Deafpride is "dedicated to working for the human rights of deaf persons.", particularly equal educational opportunity. Past projects have included holding a series of communications workshops for the deaf and their community, the development of a basic course in American Sign language (AMESLAN), and the formation of a revolving loan fund enabling the deaf to obtain TTY machines. This program provided the first TTYs to black deaf residents of D.C. Contact Deafpride, Inc., 2010 Rhode Island Ave., NE, Washington, D.C. 20018, (202) 635-2050. (Voice and TTY).

THE DEAFNESS RESEARCH AND TRAINING CENTER OF NEW YORK UNIVERSITY... is currently doing research on education, psychology, sociology, rehabilitation and communication, to assist the deaf community in becoming a stronger source of its own advocacy. They took the first national census of the deaf in this country since the 1930's, and have researched improving visual acuity (the heightening of vision in compensation for hearing loss) and deafness and the mentally retarded. In an effort to train people in deaf education and rehabilitation, the program accepts anyone already study-ing at NYU who can justify applying their own specialty to deafness. Presently program participants (deaf and hearing) represent 16 different fields and conduct workshops on com-munications and on orienting people to deafness. The Cen-ter provides free, temporary referral and counseling service to deaf people in New York. Contact DEAFNESS RESEARCH AND TRAINING CENTER OF NEW YORK UNIVERSITY, 80 Washington Sq. East, New York, NY 10003, (212) 598-2308.

PARENTS FOR DEAF PRIDE. . . was begun in 1972 to edu-cate parents about deafness and encourage communication between parents and deaf children. They fought to get more deaf teachers at Kendall School for the Deaf and volunteers are presently teaching signing to anyone who wants to learn it. An advocacy program is being developed so that deaf people going to the store, hospital or lawyer can call them for an interpretor. The group feels strongly about educating everyone to sign, particularly those who serve the public, in order to facilitate more total communication between the deaf and hearing—above all they strive to develop in their children a sense of pride and confidence rather than paranoia and shame. Contact: Parents for Deaf Pride, 2010 Rhode Island Ave., NE, Washington, D.C. 20018, (202) 889-7771.

INTERNATIONAL ASSOCIATION OF PARENTS OF THE DEAF . . . is a national catalyst for change, demanding that professionals, legislators and educators work with them to provide the best available opportunities for their deaf children. Backed up by statistics indicating that pre-sent educational methods are miserably inadequate (30% of deaf children leave school at 16 or older still function-ally illiterate) these active parents are fighting for the use of Total Communication techniques. The group present-ly numbers over 6,000 and includes 35 affiliates. Working closely with the National Association of the Deaf, IAPD is struggling to develop political clout, primarily by re-cruiting key people to set up intensive letter-writing and phone-calling campaigns in their area so that parents can speak out as a unified voice over issues affecting their children. This non-profit group acts as a personal re-source center, request-answerer, advice-giver, and advo-cate for deaf people and parents, letting them know that they are not alone. They are involved in everything from helping with the adoption of deaf children to setting up a variety of community education programs, working with a local library to set up a story-telling hour for deaf children to developing special kits to "generate parent/ child communication". They are committed to exposing incompetency, inefficiency and dishonesty, to demand-ing change from the bureaucrats, the media, educators and legislators. For more information, including a pub-lications list of books, films, and toys, contact IAPD, 814 Thayer Ave., Silver Spring, MD 20910, (301) 589-7928.

NATIONAL TECHNICAL INSTITUTE FOR THE DEAF/ ROCHESTER INSTITUTE OF TECHNOLOGY. . . is the nation's first post-secondary technical program for the deaf, serving 450 deaf students, with a soon-to-be filled capacity of 750. Though government funded, NTID is situated on a private institution's campus, giving students the option of cross-registering into RIT and working toward a BS degree. Admissions are very individualized and the college offers interpretors, tutoring, notetaking, personal and social coun-seling, vocational placement (96% are successfully placed), manual communication training and supervised housing. All students are required to take several courses from the communication center to strengthen skills necessary for job placement and community involvement. Summer programs include preparatory courses for in-coming students and an interpretor training program for hearing students and com-munity people who want to provide services in hospitals and courts. They recently sponsored a highly successful "Listen to the Deaf" week, including films, mini-sign lan-guage classes and the fitting of certain school officials with binaural ear molds so that they could have a taste of the deaf experience. Contact NTID, Public Information Office, RIT, One Lomb Memorial Drive, Rochester, NY 14623, (716) 464-2038.

CONCERNED PARENTS TASK FORCE. . . grew out of dis-satisfaction with the hiring of teachers at Kendall School for the deaf. Organized in early 1973, the parents have worked with professional organizers to protest the hiring of teachers who can not even communicate with the children. The en-suing struggle uncovered mass misappropriation of funds by administrators and general underhandedness and lack of ac-countability. The parents aroused the indignation of the campus community and teachers at the school, and four administrators resigned. A year after the formation of the Task Force and after much compromise, a parent&teacher advisory board has been established on a one-year trial basis. The Task Force has become a powerful recognized force at the school, which is under the supervision of Galludet Col-lege, and present administrators are held publicly account-able for every action. Parents participate on a screening com-mittee which interviews and hires new teaching staff as well as pushing for raising the reading level and getting more de-tailed report cards which tell parents just what to work on with their children at home. Contact CONCERNED PAR-ENTS TASK FORCE, c/o Elethea Heddin, 1330 Hemlock St., NW, Washington, D.C. 20012, (202) 726-2977.

MENTAL HEALTH PROGRAM FOR THE DEAF. . .pro-vides comprehensive mental health services to the deaf through programs in dance, education, psychodrama, speech and recreational therapy, family group and individual counseling, vocational rehabilitation and industrial training. In three years this federally funded program has developed from a group psychotherapy experiment to a comprehensive mental health program based in a 30-bed facility. Over half the participants are outpatients, some holding down jobs and remaining active in the community. Contact MENTAL HEALTH PROGRAM FOR THE DEAF, Saint Elizabeth's Hospital, Washington, D.C. 20032, (202) 574-7215.

THE COMMUNITY SERVICE CENTER FOR THE HEARING DISABLED...is run by deaf Black people and serves hearing impaired residents of the District of Columbia. Services in-clude individual, group and family counseling, social work, advocacy for the deaf when misunderstandings occur as a re-sult of the communication barrier, education of various agen-cies on how they can more effectively serve deaf people, in-terpreting service for encounters with courts, doctors, and po-lice, referral to other agencies, limited job placement and the dispensing of public health information on drugs, sex, hygiene, and public housing. The center is sponsored by Galludet Col-lege with funds from the DC Title I Higher Education Act of 1965. Contact THE COMMUNITY SERVICE CENTER FOR THE HEARING IMPAIRED, 2010 Rhode Island Ave., NE, Washington, DC 20018, 202-635-2139, TTY 635-2131.

PROJECT ACCOUNTABILITY. . . is an alternative media group putting together a production focusing on a day in the life of (a) deaf Black, in Washington, D.C., "Brother Can You Hear Me". The captioned show deals with specific problems such as employment, education, discrimination and general services for the deaf, as well as with creativity in the deaf com-munity, including a deaf poet and dancers. For more informa-tion on how to order the film or put together your own, con-tact PROJECT ACCOUNTABILITY, 3109 Martin Luther King Ave., Washington, D.C. 20032, (202) 727-2540.

PRINCE GEORGES COUNTY HOTLINE...has a TTY mach-ine so that deaf people with TTY's can call them in a crisis situation. This is a vital service, both in cases of "normal" emergencies and in situations particular to the deaf—for in-stance, if someone can't make it to work and has no way of informing people that s/he won't be there. In operation since 1972, the hotline for the deaf receives over seven calls daily. Deaf people are being trained to staff the deaf section of the hotline four nights a week; further services will be expanded depending on response. Meanwhile, all hotline workers are learning signing to enhance communication among them-selves. Call 301-864-7271, TTY 301-864-4488.

THE NATIONAL THEATER OF THE DEAF...rollics across the professional stage, ablaze with talent and vitality, to provide entertainment and to display to the world the beauty, grace and skill of deaf people. Formed in 1965, the NTD presently exists through federal funding, outside grants and touring income. Most of the company comes from Galludet College. One of two such professional acting groups in the world, the 14-member troupe has given over 1,000 performances (including two Broadway runs) in 38 states and around the world. Two Little Theaters of the Deaf have formed from their ranks, which perform for children with reading/learning problems as well as in ghetto schools and job camps. The company communicates in sign language, while three hearing members speak the lines, creating the magical effect of hearing the signed language. "You've got to remember," their producer adds, "that deaf people are born actors. Their lives are a constant struggle to communicate." Contact NATIONAL THEATER OF THE DEAF, The O'Neill Center, 1860 Broadway, New York, NY 10023, 212-246-2277.

NATIONAL FRATERNAL SOCIETY OF THE DEAF...provides an alternative to established insurance companies who generally charge deaf people higher rates, claiming their life expectancy is shorter and that they're more accident-proned. Run by and for deaf people, the Society has over 100 divisions in principal cities and supplies equitable rates to approximately 12,000 people in the U.S. and Canada. Contact NFSD, c/o Frank Sullivan, 6701 W. North Ave., Oak Park, IL 60302, (312) 383-4626.

THE AMERICAN SPEECH AND HEARING ASSOCIATION ... is a professional organization lobbying for federal licensure statutes which would only permit trained people to provide audiological services (thus cutting down on the hearing aid racket). They are also working to get hearing aids and other related services covered by medicare/Caid, larger federal budget allotments for hearing and speech services, adequate care for the prisoners' hearing and speech needs, and more effective noise pollution controls. Contact ASHA, 9030 Old Georgetown Rd., Washington, D.C. 20014, (301) 530-3400.

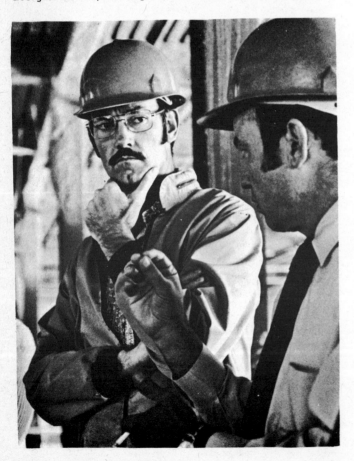

NATIONAL ASSOCIATION FOR HEARING AND SPEECH AGENCIES...is a professional organization providing communities with consultants to help set up programs (particularly infant screening) and upgrade existing facilities for the deaf. The Association certifies administrators of hearing, speech and language centers, sponsors education and training workshops (such as on the effect of industrial noise on hearing loss), acts as a clearinghouse, assists professionals with job placement, carries out an active public awareness campaign and tries to influence legislation. NAHSA distributes various films as well as "Hearing and Speech News", a bi-monthly covering news on developments in hearing, speech and language, and "Washington Sounds", an excellent newsletter giving up-to-date accounts of action in Congress and other government agencies. Contact NAHSA, 814 Thayer Ave., Silver Spring, MD 20910, (301) 588-5242.

RESOURCES

BOOKS

Paying Through the Ear: A Report on Hearing Health Care Problems, Public Citizen's Retired Professional Action Group, Public Citizen Inc., P.O. Box 19404, Washington, D.C. 20036. ...records the results of an extensive sixteen month study of the hearing aid industry. The Retired Professional Action Group (RPAG) talked with over 1000 individuals and 200 state, local and federal offices finding an appalling lack of quality services, products and information on hearing problems. Government agencies, with the exception of the Veteran's Administration, seem to have little interest in regulating the hearing aid industry. Universities promote speech therapy to the neglect of hearing therapy and medical schools graduate students with minimal training and little knowledge in the field. All these factors tend to leave the hard-of-hearing at the mercy of the hearing aid industry, an incredibly high profit competitive business. Salespeople have a monthly quota to meet and have few qualms about making extravagant claims the hearing aids never fulfill, or selling people two or three hearing aids when they may need none at all. RPAG suggests several alternatives to the present fiasco including a non-profit corporation in each community with a board of directors made up of hard-of-hearing consumers and representatives of various social service agencies. This corporation would purchase hearing aids from manufacturers and make them available to hearing specialists, clinics, etc.

They Grow in Silence: The Deaf Child and His Family, Eugene D. Mindel and McCay Vernon, National Association of the Deaf, Silver Spring, MD, 1971. 118 pp. ... an outstanding book designed to sensitize the hearing person to deaf people's problems. The authors talk honestly about the plight of deaf children's parents who are often torn by the conflicting advice of professionals concerning their child's needs. The emphasis is on total communication but also covers causes of deafness, and vocational and educational problems. Excellent introductory material.

Answers, ed. James A. Little. New Mexico School for the Deaf, Santa Fe, New Mexico. 87501, 1970. 183 pp. Free ... a diverse collection of writings on deafness, some intensely personal and some academic. For the most part, the articles emphasize the inadequacies and prejudices inherent in traditional approaches, although two are exceptionally effective in conveying the frustration and alienation of the deaf and their parents in a society geared for the hearing.

Services for Elderly Deaf Persons: Recommended Policies and Programs, Report of the Conference in Columbus, Ohio June 15-17, 1971. National Association of the Deaf, 814 Thayer Ave., Silver Springs, MD 20910, 1971. 86 pp. $3.00 ... a good listing of major problems of the elderly deaf, although the programs are mostly small scale and do not deal with the economic roots of the problems of people who are no longer productive members of our capitalist society. The report is somewhat useful in pointing directions for change.

American Annals of the Deaf: Directory of Programs and Services, Ed. by William N. Graig and Helen B. Craig. 5034 Wisconsin Ave., NW, Washington, D.C. 20016, 1973. 407 pp. $5.00
. . .lists education, community, rehabilitation, research and information services, and more. An excellent resource, including such useful information as where to find housing for deaf senior citizens, lists of periodicals relating to deafness and where to find summer camps for deaf children. Published yearly by the Conference of Executives of American Schools for the Deaf and the Convention of American Instructors of the Deaf.

A Guide to Clinical Services in Speech Pathology and Audiology 1973, American Speech and Hearing Association, 9030 Old Georgetown Rd., Bethesda, MD 20014. 158 pp. $3.00
. . . lists "all known facilities which provide services to the general public throughout the United States." Includes both clinics and general practitioners.

Operation Tripod: Toward Rehabilitation Involvement by Parents of the Deaf, sponsored by the Department of Special and Rehabilitative Education, San Fernando Valley State College. Available from HEW, Social and Rehabilitation Service, Rehabilitation Services Administration, Washington, D.C. 20201, 1971. 100 pp.
. . . proceedings of a workshop that brought together vocational rehabilitation workers, deaf adults and parents of the deaf. Some of the topics discussed were problems of setting up a parents' organization, how parents can best help their children to grow strong and independent, and how to improve education for the deaf. A must for parents of the deaf and highly recommended for anyone concerned with the issues.

PAMPHLETS AND ARTICLES

"What You Should Know About Hearing Aids," Linwood Mark Rhodes, National Association of Hearing and Speech Agencies, 814 Thayer Ave., Silver Spring, MD 20910, August, 1969. 6 pp. Free
. . . a summary of essential information for the prospective hearing aid consumer.

A Guide to College/Career Programs for Deaf Students: Post Secondary Programs, 1973, E. Ross Stuckless and Gilbert L. Delgado. International Association of Parents of the Deaf, 814 Thayer Ave., Silver Springs, MD 20910. 73 pp. $.75
. . . lists liberal arts, technical, and vocational schools, with information on possible majors, preparatory activities, and services offered, such as tutoring and interpreting.

"WHAT'S AVAILABLE FOR DEAF PEOPLE IN REHABILITATION?" McCay Vernon and Judith Ann Snyder. National Association of the Deaf, 814 Thayer Ave., Silver Springs, MD 20910, 1972. Available as part of Rehabilitation Literature Packet, $1.00
. . . lists colleges, rehabilitation facilities, vocational and technical schools and mental health services for the deaf.

FILMS AND TAPES

Total Communications Laboratory of Western Maryland College, Westminister, MD 21157.

"We Tiptoed Around Whispering," 30 min. cl. $15, 1973
A powerful dramatization of what a family goes through from the birth of their child until deafness is diagnosed. Especially good for families with deaf children and for professionals needing to better understand the parents' experience. Available with captions.

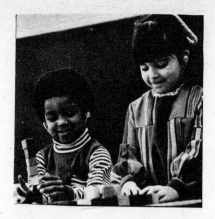

"Listen," 30 min. cl. $15, 1973
a documentary providing "an exciting orientation to the problem of hearing loss in today's society." Includes approximations of what hearing loss is like for the profoundly deaf as well as those exposed to hard rock music. Available with captions.

"Total Communication," 15 min. cl. $8.00, 1973
Explains and demonstrates Total Communication for parents and professionals. Available with captions.

"Swan Lake: Conversations with Deaf Teenagers," 15 min. cl. $6.00, 1973
"A unique look at life from the viewpoint of deaf youth" including their attitudes about racism, family relationships, education and the future. In sign language with a spoken narrative interpretation.

"Intolerable," 10 min. b/w $4.00, 1973
an experimental education entertainment film performed by two National Theater of the Deaf actors. Using classic silent movie techniques and slapstick comedy, it is "intended to teach basic vocabulary to deaf children and be entertaining to deaf and hearing persons of all ages."

The Maryland Center for Public Broadcasting, Bonita Ave., Owings Mill, MD 21117

"They Grow in Silence: An Evening of Deafness," 3 hrs. cl. 1973 (sale: $480.) (½ inch video tape or video cassett) A Special television program including the first four films listed above as well as a nationally prominent panel answering the deluge of phoned questions and response to the films. The program, which received the Community Service Award of 1972 is available as a set of 16 mm prints which local commercial TV stations can use to transfer the program to tape in their studios.

THE BLIND

Pity and condescension form the basis of public attitudes toward the blind. Such attitudes are manifest in assumptions that the blind are not only visually disabled, but totally incapacitated and abnormal, capable of only such monotonous tasks as mop making, chair caning, and piano tuning.

One would expect the institutions and agencies concerned with educating and rehabilitating the blind and disseminating facts about blindness to be unyielding in their opposition to such stereotypes of incapacity and degradation. Yet, ironically enough, the public and private agencies claiming to serve the blind are most responsible for perpetuating this oppressive view of blindness.

The population of the visually disabled in the U.S. is predominantly made up of the aged blind, the multiply-handicapped, the poor and low skilled, and persons with some residual vision. Yet agencies for the blind are disproportionately geared toward children with single handicaps and adults of working age. The gap between services and needs is so great that only 20% of those eligible receive any benefits—the others are ignored, deceived, pushed into other agencies, or given minimal income maintenance and custodial care. Even agencies which appear most enlightened are seldom effective because their programs reach only a small portion of the blind.

Agencies dominated by professionals (seldom blind themselves) seem to believe that they understand the problems of the blind and how to deal with them. In truth many of these professionals are more interested in making their jobs secure than in actually helping the blind. Like many other oppressed people, the blind are now struggling against those who make decisions which affect their lives. An example of this quest for self-determination is displayed in the controversy over the National Accrediting Council (NAC).

The NAC was established to accredit, index, and publicize agencies and workshops employing the blind. The people chosen to establish these standards are an "impressive" array of public officials, business executives, and officials of the American Foundation for (not of) the Blind—all of whom are also high ranking officials of agencies serving the blind, with their own vested interests to guard.

Opposition to NAC has principally come from the National Federation of the Blind (NFB), an organization of the blind, active in such areas as anti-discrimination cases, public education, etc. Their list of grievances is long: closed meetings with only token representation of the blind; accreditation of sheltered workshops which ignore the workers' rights to collective bargaining, grievance committees, minimum wage (some are paid less than $.50/hour), and participation in policy making; certification of schools which maintain academic standards lower than public schools; exclusion of qualified blind people from the staff of accredited agencies; and lack of community input into decision making.

To act on these grievances the blind have organized themselves against NAC. Spirited campaigns in several states have discouraged agencies from seeking accreditation and in getting accredited agencies to drop their association with NAC. Hundreds of blind people mobilize themselves annually to appear at the NAC convention to demonstrate against its repressive attitudes and call for open meetings and a minimum of one-third of the governing body from organizations of the blind.

In addition to confronting the NAC, the blind are also challenging public attitudes toward them. In some states the blind are not considered competent enough witnesses to bring charges into court. To be blind can also mean that only a ground floor hotel room or apartment can be rented; that as an education student, one cannot student teach; that both civil service and private employment can be refused; that train and airplane transportation can be denied; that higher insurance premiums must be paid (even though there is no evidence that the blind are more prone to accidents); that compensation cannot be sought for an injury while working in a state-sheltered workshop; and that as a prisoner parole

can be denied. Nevertheless, in recent years there have appeared some discernable cracks in the stereotypes and restrictions. Today there are blind lawyers, judges, doctors, school teachers, professors, and chemists—the number of jobs that a blind person can fill are limitless. The blind have found some success in filing complaints with the Interstate Commerce Commission and with individual travel companies to combat discrimination in travel. Insurance premiums have been reduced by appeals to the state insurance commission and to the insurance agencies themselves. And, "White Cane Laws" which extend basic civil rights to the blind have been enacted in some states.

A new pride of the blind is awakening. Historians have uncovered a rich "blind history" which was altered or conveniently forgotten. Napoleon once said that history is a legend agreed upon; if this is true, then the blind are organizing to negotiate a new agreement, one which is more nearly true.

The integration of blind people into society hangs largely upon their assimilation as equals, deserving of dignity and respect. Kenneth Jernigan, President of the NFB has said, "We will never go back to the ward status of second class citizenship. There is simply no way. There are blind people aplenty—and sighted allies too—who will take to the streets and fight with their bare hands if they must before they will let it happen."

NATIONAL FEDERATION OF THE BLIND...is the largest organization of blind people in the US. This dynamic and progressive group holds that the real problem of blindness is not the loss of sight but misunderstanding on the part of the public and the media. The Federation does not ask permission for the blind to work along with the sighted in all occupations and activities. Instead it demands this as a right and is prepared to take whatever action may be necessary to secure it. Established in 1940, the federation has affiliate chapters in almost every state; state and national conventions provide blind citizens with an opportunity for collective self-expression. NFB assists any blind person who has experienced discrimination through demonstrations, court action, negotiations, and publicity. New state and federal laws and regulations concerning the blind are researched, and the blind are informed of services available to them and of their rights under the law. NFB consults with Congressional committees, state legislatures, federal and state administrators. Their major fight is against governmental agencies, private charitable organizations and foundations providing services to the blind who falsely claim to speak for the blind. The Federation's stand is that only the blind (acting through their own organizations) are able to speak for the blind. The Braille Monitor, NFB's communications organ, is published monthly. Contact NATIONAL FEDERATION OF THE BLIND, 218 Randolph Hotel, Des Moines, Iowa 50309, 515-243-3169.

BLIND OR DEAF GAY INDIVIDUALS...started in 1973 out of a gay men's peer group to conquer the social isolation of blind and deaf gay people. Created as an alternative to the frustration of meeting in bars, this discussion group is now a place where blind and deaf gay people can feel comfortable and meet other gays. A core group of 10 meets regularly to explore their special needs and discuss how to deal with them. Contact BLIND OR DEAF GAY INDIVIDUALS, 1907 3rd St., N.W., Apt. 302, Washington, DC 20001, 202-332-6952.

INDEPENDENT 920 INDUSTRIES OF THE BLIND...is one of two unions in the United States that represents workers in "sheltered workshops." Theoretically sheltered workshops are necessary to provide work opportunities to people with disabilities such as blindness, who will be ignored by the profit-oriented businesses in this country who are not even concerned with employing non-disabled workers. In truth, sheltered workshops like Industries of the Blind generate large profits due to fat defense contracts—a Congressional act channels a percentage of defense money to industries for the blind. Instead of returning this money to the workers or using it to develop more jobs and better work conditions, sheltered workshops use it to pay administrators and agency heads inflated salaries. These businesses are exempted from allowing their employees even basic labor rights such as minimum wages and recognition of workers' organizations. Independent 920 grew out of the struggle against such inequities at the Greensboro Industries of the Blind, which employs over 100 people. In 1970, workers there struck to increase wages from $1.22 to $1.60 an hour. In late 1973, the workers organized again to act on several other problems at Industries of the Blind, including management's refusal to give raises to workers who qualified under the company's merit system, the powerlessness of the worker-elected Employee Advisory Committee and the Grievance Committee (which represents workers in disputes with management), fire hazards within the factory, and the refusal of the General Manager to meet with the workers. Ninety five workers signed union authorization cards (indicating they wanted the union to represent them): a press conference was called to publicize the grievances and several local newspapers covered the events at the workshop. Workers began a work stoppage to express the strength of their feelings on the necessity of a general meeting between the employees and the management. The General Manager refused to call such a meeting until they went back to work. Work was resumed, but the General Manager still refused to meet; his only action was to initiate monthly fire drills. But the biggest defeat for the workers came when the National Labor Relations Board denied their petition to unionize even though they had more than enough employee signatures to qualify. Independent 920 was formed anyway to provide what workers hope will become an organization through which workers at the Greensboro Industries of the Blind can negotiate for their rights. Contact INDEPENDENT 920, Industries of the Blind, 211 North Cedar St., Apt. 35, Greensboro, NC 27401, 919-275-3159.

SCIENCE FOR THE BLIND...is the only organization offering technological services to the blind community that is geared to work on an individual project basis. Science for the Blind started in 1955 with a $2000 grant to make taped scientific data available to blind scientists and students. The tape service now reaches 1000 listeners in the United States and Canada, and the project has expanded to the point where it is capable of communicating general or specific technical data on virtually every scientific level. A whole line of standard electrical instruments for the blind have been devised and stocked, such as multimeters, thermometers and continuity checkers. Science for the Blind claims that the chances are they can develop and provide any special instrumentation requests for the blind. They offer consultation on any problems relating to work by blind people in science or technology. Contact SCIENCE FOR THE BLIND, 221 Rock Hill Rd., Bala-Cynwyd, PA 19004, 215-664-9429.

BLINDED VETERANS ASSOCIATION...was organized by the war-blinded of World War II so that "the blinded veteran may take his (sic) rightful place in the community of his fellows and work with them toward the creation of a peaceful world." Since no other agency, public or private, seeks out the blinded ex-service person and makes him or her aware of the benefits and services available, the Blinded Veterans Association has undertaken this responsibility through its field service program. The Association aids veterans in getting jobs by contacting employers and analyzing the various positions to determine suitability of the jobs for the blind. Work demonstrations are set up to expose employers to the possibilities of hiring the blind. Field representatives and service officers of the Association visit blinded veterans to provide motivation for rehabilitation; help with adjustment to blindness; encourage attendance at the Veterans Administration's blind rehabilitation program for prevocational adjustment training, including foot travel; assist in securing vocational training; assist in obtaining veterans' benefits; and encourage participation in community activities. The services are not limited to members; they are available to all blinded veterans. The Association can truthfully say it is an organization of the blind, not for the blind. Contact BLINDED VETERANS ASSOCIATION, 1735 De Sales., N.W., Washington, DC 20036, 202-347-4010.

RESOURCES

"The Right to Live in the World: The Disabled in the Law of Torts," Jacobus TenBroek, Chandler Publishing Co., San Francisco, 1966. 79 pp.
...a detailed review of the Law of Torts with regard to the 1965 Rehabilitation Acts. The author, a blind lawyer, explores important laws affecting the handicapped, concluding that the courts do not actively support the national policy of integrating the handicapped into the community socially, economically, and physically.

<u>Blindness and Services to the Blind in the United States,</u> Organization for Social and Technical Innovation, Inc., 83 Rogers St., Cambridge, MA 02142, 1971. 212 pp.
...the best part of this study is the summary of findings and proposed directions of change. It outlines the failings of present services to the blind in their inefficiency and misplaced priorities. Most services are directed towards blind children and blind adults with potential for employment, whereas the majority of blind citizens are aged or multiple handicapped with less potential for vocational opportunities. The summary also recommends areas for research, experimentation, and program development. The material that follows is factual and well-documented, but tedious.

Aids and Appliances, American Foundation for the Blind, Inc., 15 West 16th St., New York, NY 10011, 1973-4. 72 pp. Free
. . . a catalogue of products made especially for the blind, such as writing equipment, tools, clocks and mathematical aids. Most of the prices are fairly reasonable although some items seem over-priced.

The following pamphlets are available from the **National Federation of the Blind,** 218 Randolph Hotel, Des Moines, Iowa 50309, 515-243-3169.

"Blindness—Handicap or Characteristic," Kenneth Jernigan, free
...a refutation of the belief that blindness is a handicap that sets a person apart from the society of the sighted. The article points out that normality is determined by the majority in a given society. For example, in our country, Black skin is a definite handicap. Jernigan asserts that blindness itself is not psychologically crippling, but attitudes toward blindness are.

"Jargon and Research—Twin Idols in Work with the Blind," Kenneth Jernigan, 1971. 11 pp. Free
...a humorous, yet urgent treatise on the effects of meaningless jargon and trivial research on the problems of the blind. These two often become barriers between blind people and the rehabilitation they want and need. Jernigan concludes "Let the high flown jargon and pseudo-research go the way of the dinosaur, and let us as blind people move forward with determination and vigor to our rightful place in the mainstream of social and vocational achievement."

"Blindness—Discrimination, Hostility, and Progress," Kenneth Jernigan, 9 pp. Free
...documents the types of discrimination suffered by the blind in public transportation, insurance programs, and employment.

"Beginning a Transcribing Group," by Florence Grannis, 19 pp. Free
...tips on organizing and sustaining a group of volunteers to transcribe material for the blind in any of 3 ways; taping, large typing, and Brailling.

"Model White Cane Law," Russell Kletzing and Jacobus tenBroek, 1966, 3 pp. Free
...a draft proposal written by two blind lawyers concerned with eliminating discrimination against the blind in transportation, employment and housing.

"Handbook for Blind College Students," June, 1970, 25 pp. Free
...some questions for blind students to consider when entering college, such as how tests will be taken, how material will be obtained from the blackboard and how state and federal rehabilitation services can best be used.

"A Left-Handed Dissertation: Open Letter to a Federationist," Kenneth Jernigan, 6 pp. Free
...compares being blind to being left-handed; i.e., the handicap stems mainly from being different in a society based on normality.

"Blindness: The Triple Revolution," Kenneth Jernigan, 9 pp. Free
...a call for the blind to join together in attacking "three great bastions of our society: public opinion, official ideology, and the minds of the blind themselves." Jernigan describes the oppression of the blind: "We are the hapless subjects of a benevolent dictatorship of public opinion, which holds us in a kind of colonial status of halfway membership and second-class citizenship."

THE RETARDED

It was over 100 years ago that Dorthea Dix observed New England institutions where the retarded were placed "in cages, closets, cellars, stalls and pens! Chained, beaten with rods and lashed into obedience." In 1972 a television documentary awakened the public to the fact that conditions have not changed all that much. The cameras at Willowbrook State Hospital (Staten Island, New York) recorded "naked, neglected humans lying in their own excrement in huge unfurnished rooms" (HEALTH RIGHTS NEWS). Investigations into other institutions revealed the widespread existence of parasitic diseases, epidemics of hepatitis, serious nutritional deficiency and over-use of tranquilizers.

But the issues around retardation are broader than institutionalization. The first questions must be: who is considered mentally retarded? and on what basis is that decision made? Generally the retarded are first classified as a result of intelligence tests. Hypothetically these tests measure IQ, but because of their social and economic bias they only measure performance and past exposure to learning experiences. Guidelines for classification are overly broad and all too often insufficient evidence permanently categorizes people as retarded with no means of appeal or retesting. Indeed, some people have mental impairments, but the built-in prejudice of IQ tests guarantees that the classification of retardation will be inequitably placed on the poor and racial minorities.

For those whose low IQ test scores aren't a one-way ticket to a state school for the retarded, the scores are often the key that locks the door to public school facilities. Some states flatly specify that education is for the "socially adjusted and the economically useful"; the result is that, on a national level, 1.5 to 2 million children classified as retarded are denied access to public education. For the 95% of those classified as retarded who are capable of entering the job market, the denial of education often ends any hope of self-sufficiency and results in life long dependence on others for support. Ironically, the government (and ultimately the public) ends up paying far more in long term support and institutionalization than it would in special education programs for the retarded.

Only a small minority of institutional residents require the constant supervision and care that is, in theory, provided. For example, 68% of the residents in a Washington, D.C. hospital are confined for no reason other than the lack of less restrictive and more appropriate community facilities such as adult/child day care, personal care homes, foster homes and half-way homes. Yet virtually all of government funds for the retarded go to warehousing institutions—perpetuating a system of dependence and supporting a network of administrators, psychiatrists, etc. The non-policy making workers in these institutions also suffer by being placed in a villian-victim role—villian in that they knowingly administer the archaic policies and are immediately responsible for the resident's care, but also victim, powerless to affect policy and working in overcrowded, understaffed warehouses.

Currently, the principle alternative to institutions is state-funded local agencies. Generally they are poorly administered, under-financed (in comparison to institutions) and reach only a fraction of those needing assistance (e.g. only 10% in New York state). Local agencies have been characterized as "bureaucracies run for the benefit of the administrators; using largely public funds to operate what amounts to private businesses and taking care of only the easier people.

against the state which resulted in the hiring of more MD's, nurses and custodial care. Training and development programs as well as recreation programs and staff remain insufficient and result in cruelty through neglect. Currently the Benevolent is fighting to keep open Willowbrook's best building which has been condemned due to administrative neglect. In the future the Benevolent plans to organize for laundry improvement, hiring of mroe supervisors, and ultimately de-isolation and the end of ware-housing of the mentally disabled. Contact BSRCWC, 39 W. 32nd St., New York, NY 10001, (212) 244-6837.

CHILDREN'S DEFENSE FUND (CDF)... is a national advocacy group for children that "seeks reform in the education, classification, treatment, and care of children who are served by a variety of public and private institutions." CDF strives to reach children from racial and ethnic minorities, poor children, children whose first language is other than English, children without parents, and migrant, handicapped and institutionalized children. Initial areas of focus are: the right to education for those excluded from school; classification, labeling and placement in special education classes and specialized institutions; the right to treatment and education for institutionalized children; care and treatment of children by juvenile justice systems and other agencies affecting children; the right to adequate medical care; the use of children as subjects for medical and drug research. CDF also does work against the use of drugs to "treat" hyperactive children. Contact CHILDREN DEFENSE FUND, Washington Research Project, 1763 R St., NW, Washington, D.C. 20009, (202) 483-1470.

CENTER ON HUMAN POLICY... is an outstanding group striving to raise general consciousness about the potential for dehumanization in closed, isolated institutions, and to promote alternatives to such segregation. The Center is interested in developing normal and non-stigmatizing services and life patterns for all people, but especially those with unusual needs (i.e., the mentally retarded and handicapped). As one alternative, the Center, which operates out of Syracuse University, has worked to set up model group homes for people who have been institutionalized. An advocacy and information service is available for parents of children with special needs and anyone who has been or is now in an institution. They train teachers, community people, physicians, institution staff and social workers to better understand the full implications of such disabilities as mental retardation. The Center publishes a variety of pamphlets including "CHILDREN WITH SPECIAL NEEDS AND THE NEW YORK STATE EDUCATION LAW" and "THE FUTURE OF SOCIAL POLICY FOR CHILDREN"; they have also published several books. Recently the Center developed a system for evaluating social service programs, which is explained in pamphlet form. A slide and tape show has been produced which explores some of the disastrous conditions in institutional care. Contact CHP, 216 Ostrum Ave., Syracuse, NY 13210, (315) 476-5541.

Communities are striving to improve services and the delivery system. Across the country, consumer groups consisting of the retarded, their parents and friends have organized. Some groups formed out of the frustrations encountered in trying to obtain services in their community; others organized after institutional atrocities were exposed. Often groups develop their own public education, referral and therapy services and most are involved in lobbying on the local, state and, in some cases, the federal level. One of the consumer groups most important functions is to force public and private agencies to fulfill their obligations. To do this, the groups use the courts as a tool with the aid and advice of the several law projects established for the retarded and handicapped. This is how such basic rights as education (Mills vs. Board of Education) and adequate treatment (Wyatt vs. Stickney) were affirmed. Advocacy work is important for the many issues which can be solved out of court.

Not all consumer groups are content to reform the present services for the retarded. Rather, they seek to create new attitudes and systems within the community. Many take ideas from the progressive Scandinavian countries where comprehensive health, housing, recreation and education services, integrating the retarded into the society, are provided from birth. Some people in the U.S. prefer to create new alternative communities, structured to integrate and utilize the abilities of all members.

BENEVOLENT SOCIETY FOR RETARDED CHILDREN, WILLOWBROOK CHAPTER... has taken a militant stand against the administration of Willowbrook State School. Originally a traditional, charity-oriented organization, in recent years its conciliatory position has been reversed by young, angry parents concerned with the human rights of Willowbrook's residents. In a class action suit on behalf of the residents, the Benevolent gained an injunction in federal court

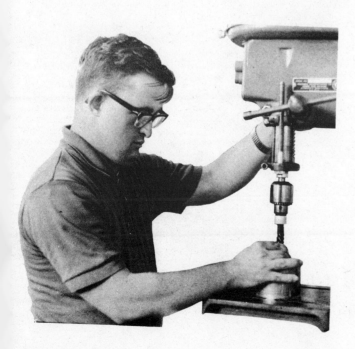

LEGAL ADVOCACY FOR THE DEVELOPMENTALLY DISABLED OF MINNESOTA... operates and advocacy program for mentally retarded, epileptic, and cerebral palsied citizens in the State of Minnesota. The project advises and represents individuals on legal matters, distributes materials on the legal rights of the disabled and writes model legislation. A reference collection of law-related materials is now available, although the group's future is somewhat tenuous due to funding. Workshops are conducted on the fundamentals and enforcement of legal rights and on advocacy training. Contact LADDM, 501 Park Ave., Minneapolis, MN 55415, (612) 338-0968.

CAMPHILL VILLAGE... is a community of over 200 people, slightly less than half of whom are retarded. Based on the model of Rudolf Steiner, (an Austrian philosopher and social theorist), Camphill Village provides a creative and positive alternative to institutionalization for mentally retarded adults. Retarded people who are accepted into the community—called villagers—must be at least 18 years old, physically healthy, and able to adopt to the community's work schedule. Each member of the community belongs to a "family" which consists of a married couple, their children and several villagers and community workers. The Village is supported through donation, villager fees, and the community industries of farming, wood-working, ceramics, doll-making and baking. Each member of the community participates in this work which is structured to allow sufficient diversification to avoid monotony or over-specialization. No guidelines are set as to how much work a member of the community does: each person, staff and retarded alike, works according to his/her ability and receives according to her/his needs. A negative aspect is that traditional male-female roles are upheld both in the workplaces and in the individual families. Contact CAMPHILL VILLAGE, Copake, N.Y. 12516, (518) 329-4851.

INNISFREE VILLAGE. . . is a non-profit, non-sectarian community established in 1971 to serve as a dynamic alternative to dehumanizing institutionalization. Innisfree, modeled after an English community called Camphill Village, serves as an innovative example of non-institutionalized care by absorbing mentally retarded people over the age of 17 into a community of non-handicapped children, women and men. Occupying four hundred acres of farmland, this refreshing community will ultimately reach a population of 150. Houses are shared by house-parents, their own children, co-workers, and retarded citizens; there is no division between patients and staff. All members of Innisfree Village live at a subsistance level and work daily in the farm and garden doing woodworking, weaving, and baking bread. Contact INNISFREE VILLAGE, Route 2, Box 506, Crozet, VA 22932, (703) 823-5088;

NATIONAL ASSOCIATION FOR RETARDED CITIZENS . . . is a well-known group working with retarded people. NARC coordinates state Associations for Retarded Citizens to combat the humiliating paternalism found in programs for the retarded. Specific programs include research into the treatment and prevention of retardation (i.e. improved nutrition and pre-natal care) and advocacy for improvement of existing facilities. NARC is consciously striving to reach Third World and poor people with their programs. In accordance with a national trend away from institutionalization, NARC is developing plans and lobbying for community-based care for the retarded. NARC helps parents find local services and works with ARCs to improve their programs. The administrative office is in Texas, with a Washington, D.C. office doing lobbying and legislative work. Contact NARC, 2709 Ave. E., East, Arlington, TX 76011.

FAMILY CARE PARENTS ASSOCIATION. . . was formed in 1971 to upgrade New York State's Family Care Program. Through the Family Care Program people with mental handicaps are taken from public institutions and placed with families in an effort to offer more personalized care. The FCPA formed to protest the low daily allotment paid by the state, to force formal certification of homes and generally improve the quality of the program. Instances of abuse of the handicapped boarders equal to the mistreatment found in large institutions have been reported. The greatest success of the Association is in the attention focused on the Family Care Program and the services it delivers. Contact FCPA, P.O. 445, Unionville, NY 10988, (914) 246-6394.

75% of the total (of retarded Americans), an incredible three out of four, were not born handicapped; they were born with healthy minds. They were made irreversibly retarded by the failure of society to provide what they needed to survive.
—Milton Brutton, <u>Something's Wrong With My Child</u>

CENTER FOR LAW AND EDUCATION. . . is an OEO-funded group providing legal services to community organizations and low-income people. Work centers almost exclusively around the public school system: exclusion of the mentally and physically handicapped and misclassification of students. The Center objects to the cultural bias of IQ tests and classification of students with learning disabilities as retarded. Their periodical, "INEQUALITY IN EDUCATION" discusses current legislation and litigation concerning education inequities. Contact CLE, 14 Appian Way, Cambridge, MA 02138, (617) 495-1000.

WASHINGTON STATE MENTAL HEALTH LAW PROJECT . . . is an OEO-sponsored project which provides legal services to the mentally ill and handicapped who often have criminal problems, guardian difficulties, or feel that they have been discriminated against by employers. In a fashion similar to groups in other states, the Project has developed a right to education suit. Future plans include challenging the right of state institutions to bill residents for all their savings in excess of $200, a common practice in some areas. Contact WSMHLP, 110 Cherry St., Seattle, WA 98104, (206) 622-8125.

HAVERN CENTER. . . teaches children between the ages of 5-10 years "who have definite learning disabilities due to a psycho-neurological dysfunction"—a comprehensive term covering perception and coordination difficulties. Their goal is to eventually place the child back in a regular classroom. This is a difficult task since the children have very low self-esteem, are easily distracted, have cognitive and perceptual problems, and in some cases suffer from almost total lack of muscle co-ordination. A specially trained faculty works in programs aimed at academic and social development of motor skills and sensory perception to help each student attain full self-realization. Contact HAVERN CENTER, 4000 South Wadsworth Blvd., Littleton, CO 80120, (303) 986-1541.

CALIFORNIA ASSOCIATION FOR THE RETARDED. . . is an umbrella organization for California's 78 community-based Associations for Retarded Citizens (ARC). Because the staff is small, CAR works through the local ARCs and other volunteer groups. They follow legislation which effects the retarded, educate parents and other concerned people about rights and services for the retarded, and provide administrative assistance and supervision to legislators and government officials. Watchdog and advocacy services such as aiding the retarded in disputes with state agencies are offered, and litigation is sometimes used. Contact CAR, 1225 Eighth St., Suite 312, Sacramento, CA 95814, (916) 441-3322.

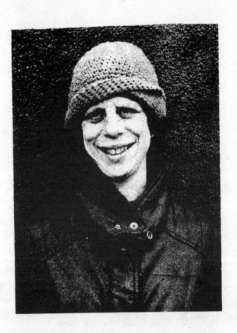

WASHINGTON STATE ASSOCIATION FOR RETARDED CITIZENS. . . uses lobbying to better conditions for the mentally retarded. Their specific goals include: improvement of housing; guarantee of legal rights, especially regarding involuntary confinement and criminal cases; increased job training, placement and educational opportunities; and expanded research into prevention of mental retardation. Successes have come in lobbying, and their efforts were the main impetus behind a referendum for construction of a $25 million primary health facility for the developmentally disabled. They are also creating a booklet to be used by the retarded which explains their legal rights. The other responsibilities of the Association include the monitering of state agencies and the coordination of efforts of the local chapters of the Association for Retarded Citizens. Contact WSARC, 213½ East 4th Ave., Suite 10, Olympia, WA 98501, (206) 357-5596.

"If we are unable to form a coalescence between our bricks and money, on one hand, and our philosophies and practices on the other, I know that the community centers planned for our future will differ from current 'human warehouses' only in size and, for awhile, in smell—but not on the per capita harm they will promote unwillingly and the wasted lives they will not be able to salvage."
—Exodus from Pandemonium,
Burton Blatt

RESOURCES

The Way We Go To School: The Exclusion of Children in Boston, Task Force on Children Out of School, Beacon Press, 25 Beacon St., Boston, MA 02108, 1971. 85 pp. $2.95
. . . a dramatic indictment of the Boston school system's failure to provide an education for a growing number of children. Among the excluded are the retarded, Spanish-speaking, pregnant girls, the crippled, and children with "behavior problems". As a result of this report, Spanish-speaking people now have the right to bilingual classes and pregnant girls can attend classes as long as they choose. This is a good model for other communities to work with: it's concise, yet angry, with excellent examples to illustrate points and an extensive list of demands.

HEALTH/PAC BULLETIN, 17 Murray St., New York, NY 10001, January, 1973. 18 pp. $5/year for students, $7/others. . .
. . . includes "The Politics of Mental Retardation," by A. Sandra Abramson and Constance Bloomfield, and "Willowbrook: From Agony to Action," by Ronda Kotelchuck. The first documents the lack of "Federal commitment to provide any form of program to the retarded." The states provide only dehumanizing institutions and community services are private and middle-class-oriented, tending towards segregation of the retarded from society. The second article discusses the struggles around Willowbrook State Hospital for the mentally retarded on Staten Island. Recently parents have begun organizing to change these conditions with some success and many problems. The workers at Willowbrook feel threatened by parents' demands, because they fear this will mean more work or loss of their jobs; the administration has used these fears to good advantage. But communication is improving somewhat and parents are hopeful about a class action suit on its way to the Supreme Court. Both articles are highly recommended.

"LEGAL RIGHTS OF THE RETARDED CITIZEN OF WASHINGTON," prepared by George A. Brock, Catherine Morrow, James Causey, 712 Carlyn Ave., Olympia, WA 1973. 17 pp. Free
. . . a report on a retarded citizen's legal rights in the state of Washington, covering property holding, education, institutionalization, rights to marry and bear children, and social security benefits. Complete and clearly written, the report is a good model for people in other states to follow, as well as providing necessary information for friends and family of the retarded.

SCIENCE FOR THE PEOPLE, Scientists and Engineers for Social and Political Action, 9 Walden St., Jamaica Plain, MA 02130, March, 1974
. . .the March issue covers the concept of IQ and how it has been used to keep poor and oppressed people "in their place". Reputes the theories of such people as Jensen and Hernstein, who imply that Black and poor people are genetically inferior. The various articles offer convincing proof that social class and economic status, not IQ, determine success in this society.

Basic Rights of the Mentally Handicapped, Mental Health Law Project. Available from National Association for Mental Health, 1800 N. Kent St., Roslyn, Arlington, VA 22209, 1973. 123 pp. $1.25
. . . focuses on the rights of the mentally retarded and ill to treatment, education, and compensation for work done in institutions. The report cites specific court cases that have clarified these rights and is a good general introduction although it's view of mental health is weak.

THE HANDICAPPED

OFFICE TO COORDINATE SERVICES TO THE HANDICAPPED...is unique in that it is part of the executive branch of the county government and thus has total freedom to use all other pertinent county agencies. The result of over two years of community complaints about the difficulty in locating available programs for the handicapped, this recently formed interagency program aims to better utilize existing resources in the county by compiling and publicizing a comprehensive list of available services; it also has hopes of developing plans for group living situations for every major disability area. The office uses public hearings to inform people of its existence and raise people's consciousness about the handicapped. Community committees determine priorities of the program and problems are worked out with an advisory committee of consumers, parents and private agencies. In addition, the office works closely with the Prince Georges County Coalition, a group of 16 voluntary organizations for handicapped children. Eventually the office hopes to organize a similarly administered program on the state level. Contact OFFICE TO COORDINATE SERVICES TO THE HANDICAPPED, Courthouse, Upper Marlboro, MD 20870, 301-627-3000, Ext. 216 or 217.

COORDINATING COUNCIL FOR HANDICAPPED CHILDREN. . .is a Chicago-based coalition of 55 parent and professional organizations concerned with the special needs of all handicapped children. In 1973, the Council was able to win over $24 million in city and state funds for programs for the handicapped. The Council works to implement special education laws, thus providing a "direct means through which parents can obtain services for their children from public and private agencies." Other activities include the facilitation of communication between parents of the handicapped, a telephone assistance service which handles over 2,000 calls a year, and distribution of fact sheets. "Parent Helper Workshops" instruct parents on what services are available for their handicapped child, and how to get them. Contact CCHC, 407 S. Dearborn, Chicago, IL 60605, (312) 684-5983.

NATIONAL CENTER FOR LAW AND THE HANDICAPPED
. . . strives to guarantee all handicapped people their full rights. This HEW-funded Center is staffed by four attorneys who work with other organizations on litigation, negotiating with the local bureaucracies, and performing speaking engagements. In some states welfare is unjustly denied to handicapped people whose condition, according to the government, is expected to get worse. The Center has gone to court to win welfare benefits in such cases; they are also working to eliminate architectural barriers in public institutions and to affirm the states' obligation to provide education to all, including the handicapped. Contact NCLH, 1235 Eddy St., South Bend, IN 46617, (219) 288-4751.

United Cerebral Palsy, 910 17th St., NW, Washington, D.C. 20006, (202) 785-1066

Muscular Dystrophy Association, 810 Seventh Ave., New York, NY 10019, (212) 586-0803

Disabled American Vets, 1221 Massachusetts Ave., NW, Washington, D.C. 20005, (202) 737-2434

National Multiple Sclerosis Society, 257 Park Ave. South, New York, NY 10010, (212) 671-4100

RESOURCES

Help For the Handicapped Child, Florence Weiner, McGraw-Hill Book Co., 1221 Ave. of the Americas, New York, NY 10020, 1973. 221 pp.
. . . an extremely worthwhile and comprehensive guide for parents with a handicapped child. Part one gives a brief description of the nature, treatment and availability of services for all common handicaps. In Part Two, valuable state, community and government services are listed as well as insurance information.

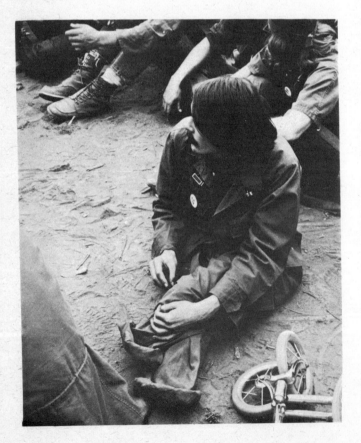

How to Organize An Effective Parent Group and Move Bureaucracies, Charlotte Des Jardins, Co-ordinating Council for Handicapped Children, 407 South Dearborn, Chicago, Illinois 60605, 1971. 112 pp. $1.50
. . . "this booklet is written specifically for parents of handicapped children and their helpers to show them how to move bureaucracies and get services for their children." Unfortunately, the focus is exclusively on middle class families and the approach is somewhat traditional. Nevertheless, it offers some good ideas and models.

"Right to Education: Handicapped Children," Harriet Katz Berman, CIVIL LIBERTIES, 22 E. 40th St., New York, NY 10016, January, 1974. pp. 2-3. $1/year
. . . reviews the "class action suit being brought in federal court on behalf of all children in Colorado who are not receiving an education at public expense." This includes at least 20,000 children in Colorado who are retarded, perceptually or physically handicapped, autistic and emotionally disturbed. Often these children are misdiagnosed and put in inappropriate public special education programs or excluded from school altogether because no program exists or their IQs are too low.

Federal Programs for the Handicapped, Edward R. Klebe, Education and Public Welfare Division, Congressional Research Service, Library of Congress, April 16, 1971. 108 pp. Free
. . . lists all federal programs designed specifically for the handicapped as of 1971, with a brief description of each program, type of grant available, authorizing legislation, fiscal data, and the federal agency administering the program.

"YOUR RIGHTS AS PARENTS OF A HANDICAPPED CHILD," James O. Crary, Charlotte Des Jardins, Catherine Condon, Co-ordinating Council for Handicapped Children, 407 South Dearborn, Chicago, IL 60605, 1969. 37 pp. $.50
. . . informs parents of their legal rights both nationally and in the state of Illinois. The booklet tells what provisions the schools are required to make for the handicapped, as well as the basis on which they can exclude a child. Information on rights, social security benefits, and tax exemptions make this a useful tool for parents of the handicapped in all states where bureaucracy and buck-passing run rampant.

Therapy in Music for Handicapped Children, Paul Nordoft and Clive Robbins, St. Martin's Press, Inc., 175 Fifth Ave., New York, NY 10010, 1971. 176 pp. $6.50
. . . explores the possibilities of group and individual music therapy for children with physical and emotional handicaps. Various types of programs are explained in considerable detail. This is a refreshing account filled with hope, excitement, and a great respect for the children with whom the authors worked.

FILMS AND TAPES

Audio-Visual Center, Indiana University, Bloomington, IN 47401
"Everybody's Handicapped," 17 min. b&w $5.25
Presents the case for wider employment of the physically handicapped in jobs for which they are qualified. Uses graphs to show the lower accident rates and absenteeism of handicapped workers.

Perennial Education, Inc., 1825 Willow Rd., Northfield IL 60093.
"Like Other People," 37 min. cl. $37.50, 1973. (sale: $375)
. . . powerful statement on societal attitudes toward the handicapped, particularly in the area of sexuality. This documentary filmed in an English residential treatment center focuses on the relationship of two cerebral palsy victims, with cameras following the couple through a typical day. A good consciousness-raising film.

DRUGS

PROBLEM

We live in a culture permeated by drug use. Increasing numbers of people look to chemicals to relax and enjoy themselves, to wake up, to go to sleep, to lose weight, to calm a fidgety child, soothe the strains of alienation, find God, or escape. Our medical system is highly drug-oriented; there is presumed to be a drug to help almost every ill. . . and increasingly, almost every personal and social need.

ILLEGAL DRUGS AND DRUG ABUSE

To be sure, drug use is not unquestioningly accepted in all its forms. For example, people can be given 10 or 15 year sentences, or more, for selling a weed much less toxic and incapacitating than alcohol—a barbarism that confounds all reason. New York recently took a giant step backwards by passing a law that is almost surreal: possession of one fourth to one ounce of marijuana for first time offenders is a felony with a maximum prison sentence of seven years. Second-time offenders face a maximum 15-year sentence.

Drugs are a complex reality: potent for healing, pleasure and insight, with equal potential for control and destruction. To an extent, it is not surprising that our culture's reaction to drugs is confused and contradictory. Few people are seriously interested in giving up the solid benefits of modern medical drugs, and most US citizens will continue to turn for social enjoyment to such drugs as alcohol, tobacco, and marijuana. Yet anyone who has seen the havoc heroin works in a community, or watched a growing political awareness dissipated by speed and strychnine-laced trips is likely to have anti-drug feelings as bitter, if not as hysterical, as any judge throwing people in jail to stop killer marijuana. Illegal drugs have come out of the inner city to cut across all class lines, from the Vietnnam vet to the high school-aged daughter of a wealth suburbanite. Feminists are keenly aware of the role alcohol, tranquilizers, and other drugs play in pacifying women and reinforcing acceptance of repressive roles. The increasing use of drugs (under the guise of rehabilitation) to coerce, manipulate, and punish prisoners and people defined as mentally ill is a horror story arousing growing protest.

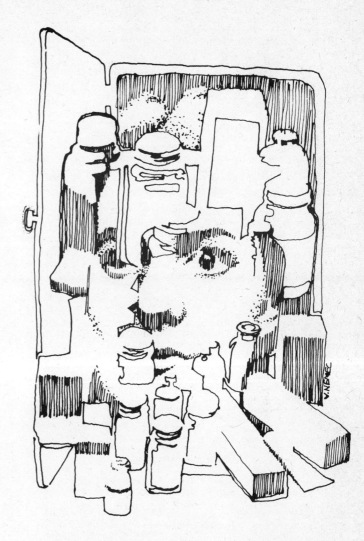

Drugs open up grey areas of ambiguity, where decisions are hard to make, and even the principles on which decisions should be based are sometimes difficult to define. Does the positive potential of hallucinogens—increased perception of self and the world, exploration of altered states of consciousness—outweigh the risks of bad trips, the apathy of an ingrown drug culture? How much rights does a society have to decide that certain drugs are too dangerous for individuals to consume? Obviously the illegality of marijuana makes no more sense than the prohibition of alcohol. But it is equally clear that legalizing heroin while perpetuating social conditions that create joblessness, poverty, and despair would be simply legitimizing the mass destruction of lives, primarily in poor White and Third World communities. Where then can the lines be drawn, and on what basis?

But if judgments about drugs and their role in society are inherently complex, they are further complicated and distorted by several aspects of our society and its reactions to drugs.

Most basic, of course, is the overall failure to deal with economic injustices, racism, alienation, and other conditions that foster the misuses of drugs, from tranquilizers to alcohol, speed, or heroin. The US has relied on criminal, psychiatric, and medical models to deal with a social problem. This is not to say no one involved in drug traffic should go to jail, or that drug dependence does not, often, go along with serious personal problems in living. But to deal with drug use by tossing users in jail, or by trying to change individuals' personalities through such programs as therapeutic communities, is by itself futile. To deal with it through programs of methadone maintenance—legalized addiction—without any attempt at opening up jobs, education, etc.—as in in the methadone maintenance programs now gaining in popularity—is a confession of failure and a sell-out of these peoples' lives.

An important factor in this country's drug problem is the official toleration of organized crime—a booming business which finds one of its highest-profit items in drugs, and which has intimate connections with government and legal business at many levels. Nixon's administration announces with great fanfare "Project Intercept," a shiny new strategy to keep marijuana from crossing the Mexican border while heroin continues to pour into the cities. . . after all, who wants to take on the mafia? And the drug companies continue to produce many times the amount of barbituates needed for legitimate medical purposes, while the government coyly pretends not to notice where those pills end up.

There there is the pervasive commercialism that promotes drug use with complete disregard for the social and human costs. Alcohol, which vies with heroin as the nation's most serious drug abuse problem, is promoted endlessly, along with a chemical cure for every bad mood. Drug abuse is not just a matter of illegal drugs; it also includes the whole society's overreliance on legal drugs, and the drug industry's misuse of drugs as a means to profit and control rather than health.

THE DRUG INDUSTRY

The drug industry has been characterized as "one of the most powerful, influential, and richest segments of the American economy" (Retail Drug Price Competition). In the last decade, the drug industry has held either first or second place among all US firms in terms of profitability. In 1971, drug manufacturers had a profit of 19.3%, double the average for all manufacturing corporations; at the same time, taxes on these earnings dropped 9.5% (Retail Drug Price Competition). Some 2000 companies in the US deal in some way with pharmaceuticals; 115 of these (comprising the Pharmaceutical Manufacturers Association) account for 95% of prescription sales, and nine of these alone control 50% of the total. The markets into which the drug industry has been broken down are separate and generally non-competing.

Well over half of the chemical entities produced have only one manufacturer, forming a virtual monopoly. These monopolies are created by the 17 year patents granted by the government to the drug's discoverer which prohibits the unlicensed production by other companies and leaves the holder of the patent "free to charge what the traffic will bear" (Kefauver Report). A monopoly can be extended past 17 years by patenting the same drug in new dosage forms (chewable rather than liquid), by making minor modifications in the chemical structure of the old drug, or combining it with another old drug. Seven per cent of the drug industry's sales is invested in research; up to 90% of the drug products introduced each year are in the form of these essentially meaningless elaborations.

The major component of drug profits results from extensive promotion and advertising aimed at institutions, health providers, and students. Medical students receive black bags, teaching aids, and other odds and ends as "gifts" from drug companies. Near the end of medical students' training, "detail men" begin bombarding them with free drugs, journal advertisements and even color TVs, and Caribbean tours. The industry's yearly promotion budget of about a billion and a half dollars comes to over $5000 spent on each physician (including psychiatrists) in the country.

These exorbitant promotion practices cause major problems for the patient-consumer. The costs of promotion (nearly three times the amount spent on research) is inevitably passed on to the consumer to the tune of 25 cents out of each prescription sales dollar. There is no uniform arrangement for the distribution of objective drug information in the US. Medical education only touches on pharmacology, and over 65% of physicians admit that salespeople are their "most effective" source of information on new drugs. Yet, over 70% of the drugs now marketed are not effective for all the ailments advertised; 15% are ineffective for all ailments advertised; and in case after case, harmful side-effects are underplayed and contraindications neglected by promotion campaigns. As a result, an estimated 76% of all doctors prescribe drugs for unsound reasons. The results of this unwarranted prescribing are shocking: 1.5 million are hospitalized and 30,000 die annually from adverse drug reactions; "an additional 50,000 to 100,000 Americans will die from resistant forms of killer bacteria whose emergence has been contributed to by misuses of antibiotics." (Kennedy Subcommittee Hearings).

Drug advertising and promotion is also aimed at getting the patient to buy the drugs on which the highest profits can be made. A common approach is to get the physician in the habit of brand name prescribing. Each company's version of a drug (assuming no monopoly exists) will usually have a different brand name, and each name carries a different price. More often than not, drugs sold under their generic name are the same price or cheaper than their brand name counterparts Yet nine out of ten doctors prescribe brand name drugs, resulting in high profits for the manufacturers of the drugs and an avoidable expense for the consumer. Because of industry pressure, most states have passed "anti-substitution" laws requiring the pharmacist to fill the prescription with the brand of drug indicated, even if the same drug exists under a cheaper name. Even without these laws, there is still no guarantee that the pharmacist will fill the prescription with the least expensive drug.

To circumvent the anti-substitution laws, many people have begun to ask their doctors to write their prescriptions using the generic name. A word of caution is in order here, for generic prescribing is not the panacea consumers seek. Studies have shown that 50% of time, the pharmacist does not fill a generic prescription with a generically labelled product. Also, the drug under its generic name is not always the cheapest. This is because approximately 60% of each type of drug

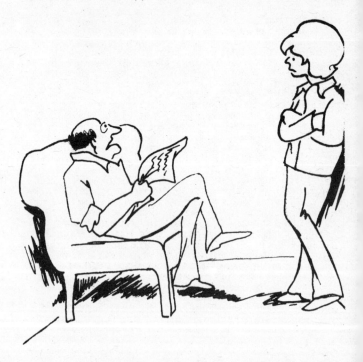

Crime, inflation, corruption. . . if it weren't for tranquilizers I think I'd be on drugs by now.

has only one manufacturer, so the cost is the same for both the brand name and the generic name; in several cases, the generically labelled drug is more expensive than an available brand name labelled one.

Another serious problem is the drug companies' role in pushing the use of psychotropic drugs (drugs that alter moods). Women disproportionately bear the brunt of this. Advertisements picturing them as demanding, crabby, and depressed conclude that the best solution is some drug rather than a changed life-style. Or drugs are used to prevent people from confronting and perhaps coming to terms with situations which are genuinely fearful or sad: one ad, for example, promotes the use of mood elevators to eradicate the depression of people threatened with invalidism. This wholesale application of drugs to any troubling situation is even more pronounced, of course, in ads discussing the elderly, or people in counselling or in mental hospitals. In the last ten years, the use of psycho-active drugs has more than doubled.

Doctors, and the medical professions in general, are well aware of how lucrative the drug business is, and a mutual back-scratching alliance has been forged between the two. The present yearly amount paid to the AMA by drug companies for advertisements is nearly $9 million or over one quarter of the Association's total budget. Much of this money is returned to the drug companies: in September 1972, the AMA announced it had invested $10 million from its retirement fund in pharmaceutical stocks. Physicians' investments in drug stocks are also reportedly widespread.

The drug industry has been busy forming alliances with medical teaching centers. Departments of pharmacology, schools of pharmacy and individual scientists at these centers have come to rely on the industry's support through grants, contracts, and so on. The drug industry-medical center alliance is further deepened by the fact that they have interlocking directorships. Each of the largest drug companies has at least one director at a medical center, or at a university with a medical school, who is in a position to make major policy decisions.

The Food and Drug Administration is the federal government agency responsible for regulating the drug industry. But the large number of former drug industry employees in high FDA administrative positions makes it unlikely that the consumer will be adequately represented or protected. FDA officials often return to industry with an intimate understanding of FDA's inner workings and a knowledge of FDA's future plans.

The contradictions between good health and the demands of drug industry for maximum profit are clear. It is in the drug companies' interests to keep prices high even though that denies medication to people who need it. It is in the drug companies' interests to tenderly nurture our culture's excessive dependence on drugs, using every possible tool of persuasion to discourage us from honestly confronting the problems of our lives which may demand painful growth—and political action.

In one case, a firm manufacturing a well-known mouthwash was accused of using a cheap form of alcohol possible deleterious to health. The company's chief executive, after testifying in Washington, made this comment privately: 'We broke no law. We're in a highly competitive industry. If we're going to stay in business, we have to look for profit wherever the law permits. We're not in business to promote ethics. Look at the cigarette companies, for God's sake! If the ethics aren't embodied in the laws by the men who made them, you can't expect businessmen to fill the lack. Why, a sudden submission to Christian ethics by businessmen would bring about the greatest economic upheaval in history!'
—Albert Z. Carr in HARVARD BUSINESS
REVIEW

PLATFORM

1. Rational and realistic drug education should be taught in all schools.

2. Growth, sale and use of marijuana should be legalized.

3. All drug and alcohol advertising should be abolished, including over-the-counter psychotropic drugs.

4. Penalties for possession of hallucinogens such as LSD and mescaline should be greatly reduced and unbiased research on the physical and psychological effects of hallucinogens should be publicly funded to examine the pros and cons of legalization. This would assume controlled distribution and no advertising.

5. A tax on alcoholic products should be established and used to fund rehabilitation programs for alcoholics and research on the effects of alcohol.

6. Public funding should be withdrawn from methadone maintenance programs and made available to decentralized, community controlled detoxification units, therapeutic communities, and social change-oriented rehabilitation programs. Such programs must include educational and job training programs, and be related to on-going efforts to win adequate housing, health care, jobs, schools, and self-determination in the communities affected.

7. Funding must be made available to study the arguments for and effects of programs to supply free heroin to addicts, on the model used in Great Britain. Such research programs must be directed by representatives of the whole of spectrum of communities affected by heroin addiction—that is, primarily Third World and poor White.

8. The Justice Department and local police departments must be pressured to crack down on organized crime and the heroin traffic in particular—focusing on entry of heroin into the country and its large-scale distributors. But because the government's and police systems' response will be partial and sporadic at best, the major anti-heroin thrust must come through community-based education and rehabilitation, and through battling to change the conditions on which heroin use thrives.

9. Quotas for production of barbituates, amphetamines, and other dangerous drugs must be set and strictly enforced. Illegal channeling of such drugs by the companies should be investigated immediately and those responsible should be indicted.

10. Physicians should keep informed of all aspects of the drugs they prescribe; they must prescribe the least expensive drug that is safe and effective.

11. Medical school curriculums should include courses in clinical pharmacology as well as the economics of prescribing and comparative prices of drugs with similar efficacy; drug company promotional activities should be kept off school property. HEW and NIH should halt the dependence of health science schools' departments of pharmacology on drug company grants and "gifts" through major funding for research and training.

12. Drug testing should be contracted by the government to non-profit, independent institutions or to an industry-financed, publically operated, quasi-governmental organization whose researchers should not know who manufactured the drugs being tested, nor would the manufacturers know who was testing their drugs. The FDA should forbid manufacturers to patent a new drug unless the drug is significantly more effective or safer than those already on the market; Congress should amend patent laws to greatly reduce the period during which a manufacturer enjoys a monopoly on a new drug, either through mandatory licensing after a set time or by shortening the patent life.

13. FDA officials must be required to wait five years before working for a company which that official had dealings with on behalf of the FDA.

14. All unsolicited descriptive advertisements for prescription drugs should be banned; the FDA should periodically distribute a compendium listing prices and providing objective guidelines for use of drugs.

15. Pharmacists should charge a fixed fee rather than a proportional mark-up; state laws should be amended to require the posting of the prices for the 100 most frequently prescribed scribed drug entities; state anti-substitution laws should be repealed or amended to permit the pharmacist to only substitute, with the consumer's consent, a lower priced, but equally effective and safe drug.

16. Health professionals, medical educators, and lay people should get in the "one-name, one-drug" mindset; all medications must be labelled with the generic name of the active drug within.

17. Drug costs should be included under medical insurance; reimbursements under Medicare and Medicaid must be limited to the lowest costs at which a drug is available; pharmacists must be required to charge no more than the lowest price so that there are no out-of-pocket expenses.

18. Doctors, pharmacists, medical educators, health institution administrators, and their professional organizations should not hold stock in any pharmaceutical companies or in ancillary companies, nor should they serve as consultants or policy-setting board members of these same firms. Likewise, these people and their associations, except for pharmacists, should not hold stock or own any part of pharmacies.

19. None of the above demands necessarily insure that drugs will be available on an equal basis. In the long run, drug production should be controlled by the government, either through nationalization or as a public utility; drugs should be free or extremely low in price.

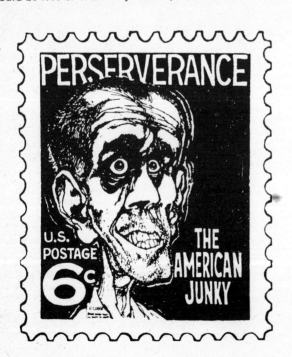

PROGRAM

1. Formulate a drug education curriculum, covering everything from alcohol and marijuana to addicting drugs, psychoactive drugs, and the role of the drug industry. Organize for its acceptance by schools in your community. Use other institutions—community organizations, churches, etc.—to carry drug education into the community

2. Where there is need, set up a drug crisis line and analysis center. Ideally, such a center should not only handle bad drug experiences and cut down on deaths and injury by analyzing the contents of street drugs; it should also make referrals to addiction treatment programs and should educate people about general drug use.

3. Organize local referendums to greatly reduce or abolish the penalty for possession or use of marijuana. Use these campaigns as a basis for community education, building toward state-wide legalization drives.

4. If there are therapeutic communities in your area, research their programs (are they sexist, do they use methadone maintenance, who controls their board). Push for community representation on their governing boards, for job training programs, and for awareness of the social context of drug use.

5. Educate community people to demand the elimination of methadone maintenance programs, and the funding of community-controlled, social change-oriented drug treatment centers—including centers for alcoholics.

6. Research drug companies: their advertising practices, profit levels, overproduction of drugs for illegal distribution, domination of such supposedly regulatory groups as the Food and Drug Administration, and general promotion of a drug-dependent culture. Don't stop with research! See that your information and conclusions are distributed as widely as possible. Use your research as a basis to lobby for stricter regulation, and eventually public ownership of drug companies. Use information on drug companies to promote a better understanding of the role of big industry in general.

7. Research the alcohol and tobacco industries—their economic power, the government agricultural subsidies they receive, and the massive advertising campaigns they carry on. Research hospital and AMA collusion with these and other drug industries. Use all this information to build demand for the abolition of advertising and an end to subsidies.

8. Health science students: start with drug industry abuses as organizing issues. Refuse to accept drug company "gifts", gather and publicize indictive material on the drug industry, and time its release to coincide with the appearance of drug company representatives; organize a boycott of your school

DRUG
EDUCATION
AND
INFORMATION

"drug days"; expose your school and faculty's dependence on the drug industry for funds, e.g., look for investments, conflicts of interest among trustees and administrators, faculty on retainers from the industry, research grants; organize alternative classes and seminars on pharmacology, the economics of drug prescribing, and the use of nonstandard medicines such as herbal remedies and homeopathic preparations.

9. Doctors: survey pharmacies in your area for prices of drugs you commonly prescribe, and ask drug company representatives for precise information on wholesale prices and pass this information on to patients; prescribe generically, but include the name of the least expensive generically labeled product; join with other doctors in refusing all drug company "gifts"; use your position to investigate and expose any vested interest between the drug companies and institutions or professionals with whom you are in contact.

10. Pharmacists: post the prices of the 100 drugs you sell the most frequently and quote prices over the phone or in person; charge a fixed fee for your services rather than a proportional mark-up; when a customer brings in a prescription for a high priced drug, suggest a cheaper substitute and call the physician for permission; fill all generic prescriptions with the lowest priced product available and pass the savings along to the customer; organize support in your profession to voluntarily remove barriers to consumer information; use your place of business to educate people about how they can save money on their prescriptions, the drug industry, and alternatives to drugs.

11. Conduct a prescription drug survey to document and publicize pharmaceutical abuse. Typically such a survey begins by filling prescriptions for the same drug at different pharmacies or by filling both a brand name prescription and a generic one at several pharmacies. A survey can examine only price variance in brand name and generic drugs at the various pharmacies, or may look for misbranding, substandard packaging, and unethical (often illegal) substitutions. The survey approach does have its limitations, since it leaves the drug problem untouched at the manufacturers' level.

12. Organize a community owned, community/worker directed, anti-profit pharmacy, This will serve to provide low cost, high quality prescription and non-prescription drugs, provide educational information for physicians and the community, coordinate actions against the drug industry, as well as irresponsible doctors and pharmacists, and to act as an alternative to capitalist businesses. The most effective of these pharmacies will be those that allign themselves with other health struggles.

Drug education and information programs are tailored to a wide variety of audiences. Some are directed toward the general public; they provide realistic information and encourage open, non-hysterical discussions of drug use. Others are directed toward street people and the (primarily young White) drug culture. These often include programs to analyze samples of street drugs and identify mislabeled, possibly dangerous drugs. Such analysis programs can cut down on unnecessary deaths and bad trips, and provide a focus for educating those who use illegal drugs about some of the risks they face (arsenic-laced acid, for example). Many drug programs also offer crisis counselling for people experiencing bad trips, advice in dealing with overdoses, etc. Crisis centers and hotlines often offer similar services.

Most drug-culture oriented information programs are strongly-opposed to such destrictive drugs as heroin, speed, and barbituates, while maintaining a positive or non-judging attitude toward such substances as marijuana and hallucinogens. With some exceptions, they do not analyze the social and political implications of drugs. But they provide important immediate services and a grassroots force opposing addictive, physically damaging drugs.

DO IT NOW FOUNDATION. . . is an energetic and prolific organization for "realistic street drug education." DIN has produced dozens of informative and pointed brochures on barbituates, heroin, street psychedelics, sniffing, quaaludes, etc. Lots of facts, humorous and hard-hitting graphics, and straightforward language make their publications highly useful. DIN offers how-to material on setting up crisis and referral centers, training medical technicians, and more, with some material available in Spanish. Entirely funded by the sale of their publications, DIN runs a large-scale analysis program in Hollywood/Los Angeles, and a rehabilitation center for drug users in Santa Cruz, CA. For a complete price list, contact DO IT NOW, National Media Center, P.O. Box 5115, Phoenix, AR 85010, (602) 957-9617.

NATIONAL COORDINATING COUNCIL ON DRUG EDUCATION. . . is America's largest private non-profit drug education network. The 100 national organizations in the Council are making a coordinated effort to find rational approaches to drug abuse prevention through organizing community action programs, evaluating drug education materials, and disseminating factual drug information. They offer a variety of good resources, including THE NATIONAL DRUG REPORTER newsletter. This is the most comprehensive resource for realistic drug education. Contact NCCDE, Suite 212, 1211 Connecticut Ave., NW, Washington, D.C. 20036, (202) 466-8150.

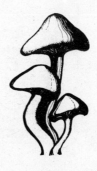

STUDENT ASSOCIATION FOR THE STUDY OF HALLU-CINOGENS. . . disseminates unbiased information about psychoactive drugs and their use. The STASH Library is the most complete collection of the published literature on hallucinogens in the country, with the possible exception of the National Library of Medicine. Bibliographic searches and selected loans are available to members. Publications include: SPEED: The Current Index to Drug Abuse Literature, Directory of Drug Information and Treatment Organizations, occasional pamphlets, and bibliographies and (in cooperation with the Haight-Ashbury Clinic), the Journal of Psychedelic Drugs. Over 80 professional consultants are available to advise on research and education. Contact STASH, 638 Pleasant Street, Beloit, WI 53511, (608) 362-8848.

DRUG INFORMATION CENTER. . . was initiated in the Spring of 1972 at the University of Oregon to provide factual answers on the physiological, psychological, and sociological aspects of drug usage, whether they be prescription, over-the-counter, or illegal street drugs. Since its inception this agency has completed over 250 major research projects and answered over 4000 telephone calls requesting information about drugs and related topics. The DIC also sponsors accredited under-graduate and graduate courses on psychoactive drugs, open to the community as well as to students and faculty. The DIC contains one of the most comprehensive drug libraries on the west coast. Drug Analysis Project is a free, anonymous service providing factual information on the street and exploding common drug myths. Contact DIC, 1 EMU, University of Oregon, Eugene, OR 97403. (503) 686-5411.

DRUG EDUCATION CENTER. . . started as a volunteer detoxification and counselling service for the local community and Michigan State University; it is now supported by municipal health funds and controlled by a community mental health board. Street drug analysis is provided through the State Department of Public Health. They have offered East Lansing's fire department training in handling overdoses and relating to the drug subculture. DEC, along with a free clinic that grew out of the Center, has worked with students, teachers, and local residents in drug education, and they are constantly involved in trying to improve emergency room procedures in local hospitals. Contact DRUG EDUCATION CENTER, 405 Grove St., East Lansing, MI 48823, (517) 351-4002.

STRAIGHT DOPE ANALYSES CENTER. . . is a clearinghouse for street drug analyses programs. They have 14 centers around the country, and have compiled information on 200 analysis centers. Their resources consist of a newsletter, an essay on starting a street drug analysis program, a list of high quality, inexpensive labs, and information on analytical standards. In exchange for expenses, Straight Dope will provide on-the-site assistance to groups trying to set up a drug analysis program. Contact STRAIGHT DOPE, 612 Clayton, No. 1, San Francisco, CA 94117, (415) 864-1179.

BOARD OF CHRISTIAN SOCIAL CONCERN OF THE UNITED METHODIST CHURCH. . . has produced a series of drug education material excellent for use with parents, educators, church people, and others unfamiliar with drug culture. The material's tone is concerned and credible, outlining the types of drugs from alcohol and tobacco through marijuana, uppers, downers, psychedelics and narcotics. The Board recognizes drug use as a human problem related to poverty, poor health care, alienation, and other social problems, and recommends non-punitive treatment of addicts and abusers. While not recommending legalization of marijuana, their publications undercut most of the myths of its harmfulness; they also show a surprising openness to the positive potential of psychedelics. In keeping with Methodist traditions, they recommend abstenance from alcohol and tobacco; they emphasize, however, that these should be personal decisions, made without selfrighteousness and accompanied by compassionate concern for alcoholics. A list of their drug-related publications is available. Contact BCSC/UMC, Service Department, 100 Maryland Ave., NE, Washington, DC 20002.

RESOURCES

Common Sense Lives Here, A Community Guide to Drug Abuse Action, A Project of the National Coordinating Council on Drug Abuse, Suite 212, 1211 Connecticut Ave., NW Washington, D.C. 20036, 1970. 104 pp
. . . a useful guide for beginners to community organizing. Tells how to look at a town (power structure, resources, goals, etc.) and determine the drug abuse program(s) best suited to the town's specific conditions. Other guidelines explain how to get information, how to coordinate on-going programs, and how to ready and organize the community for action. Its weaker aspects include a fairly simplistic, inconclusive analysis of the drug scene itself and an over-emphasis on the various drug-related government agencies. Includes a glossary of slang drug expressions.

Understanding Drug Abuse, An Adult's Guide to Drugs and the Young, Peter Marin and Allan Y. Cohen. Harper and Row. 49 E. 33rd St., New York, 10006, 1971. 157 pp.
. . . depicts the problem of drug abuse as one "deeply rooted in our abuse of one another and ourselves"—a problem which can be alleviated only by a feeling of community, a radical transformation of our cities and society. This gives a sympathetic, understanding view of what it is like to be young in America.

In January 1968 . . . nationwide front-page stories appeared stating that LSD had blinded six college students. This was supposed to have occurred when the six young men stared fixedly at the sun under the influence of LSD and was presented as established fact . . . by the State Commissioner for the Blind. . . . It was some days later, after the story had been accepted as "fact" by millions of people, that the Governor of Pennsylvania, under pressure from the federal Food and Drug Administration and others . . . publicly announced that the charge had been a deliberate lie ("fabrication") . . . . No instances of blindness have been shown to result from LSD use. . . . The propensity of the mass media uncritically to accept lurid and sensationalistic stories emanating from generally untrustworthy and uninformed government sources is probably far more dangerous to our social fabric than LSD

—*The Pleasure Seekers*
Joel Fort, MD p. 139-40

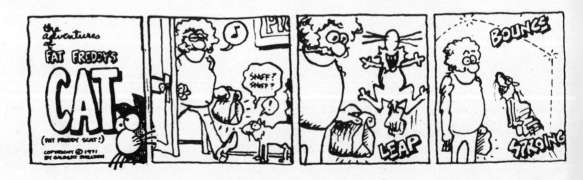

Drug Abuse Films, National Coordinating Council on Drug Abuse, Suite 212, 1211 Connecticut Ave., NW, Washington, D.C. 20036, June 1973. 117 pp. $5.00
... an invaluable, honest report on over 220 drug abuse education audio-visuals and films, evaluated for their "scientific accuracy and conceptual integrity" by panels of students, experts, ex-drug addicts, professionals, drug counselors, people with a political orientation (RAP), and workers from a wide range of fields and experiences. The explanation of reviewal criteria is an education in itself, and the entire report exhibits a high political consciousness of what our 'drug problem' is indeed about. Included is a synopsis of each film, its rental and purchase price, and the panel's evaluation of its strong and weak points. In addition, the procedure of determining the value of a film for a specific group is discussed. "Unfortunately the quality of drug information in this report reflects the confusion, hysteria and misconceptions that characterize the majority of existing drug abuse education programs."

The Pleasure Seekers: The Drug Crisis, Youth and Society,
Joel Fort, MD. Bobbs-Merrill Cl., 4300 W. 62nd St., Indianapolis IN 46268, 1969. 255 pp.
... a good primer on drug abuse, one of the earliest to view the problem in a holistic light. Fort even dares to proclaim that drugs do not necessarily cause any significant changes in the lives or personalities of their users. His chapter on "Better Living Through Chemistry?" explains in detail exactly how an extensive list of mind-altering drugs affects body systems, as well as other related factual information. The traditional scare myths about marijuana and LSD—instant insanity, brain damage, chromosome damage, etc.—are smashed. Fort perceives drug abuse as a socio-cultural rather than legal problem. Comes down hard on public officials, police, educators, advertisers, etc., for their power-hungry, profit-making, punitive approaches, and stresses the necessity for a variety of different treatment methods, as well as the importance of moving society beyond all drugs altogether.

PAMPHLETS AND ARTICLES

"Education and Drugs," EDCENTRIC, P.O. 10085, Eugene OR 97401, March 1972, $60
... double-issue of generally outstanding articles on drugs. Includes information on the widespread and condoned use of drugs in organized athletics; a biting analysis of conventional 'drug education programs' as well as suggestions for making such programs more viable; a hard-hitting slam at use of Ritalin on "hyperactive" children,' a sketch of one free clinic's primary prevention approach; an excellent directory of drug education resources, and more. Indispensable.

Facts About Commonly Used Drugs, A Non-Abuser's Guide to Pharmacological And Non-Medical Use of Drugs, by David P. Jenkins and Robert Brody, DO IT NOW, P.O. Box 5155, Phoenix, AZ 85010, June 1973. 67 pp. $1.25
... "if you are an initiate into the world of illicit drugs, this is a book which won't boggle your mind." This pamphlet tries to reduce the hysteria often surrounding the subject of drugs without "polemical arguments about the merits or hazards of the drug experience." Non-condescending.

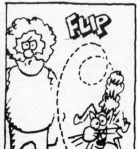
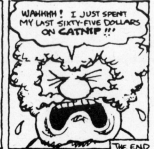

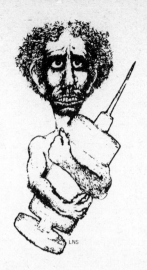

Drug Abuse: Summons to Community Action Eunice Jones Matthews, by North Conway Institute, 8 Newbury Street, Boston, MA 02166, 1970. 56 pp. $.50
... honestly analyzes why white middle class youth seek drugs and what communities can do to effectively and comprehensively deal with this.

"DOING IT: COMMUNITY ACTION ON DRUG CONCERNS," Thomas E. Price and Lawrence Wayman, Service Dept., Board of Christian Social Concerns, 100 Maryland Ave., NE, Washington, D.C. 20002, 1971. 59 pp. $.60
... short guide for churches organizing their communities to set up effective drug abuse programs. "Jesus is not the only answer for a person who takes 8 reds a day." Calls on churches to deal with the drug problem from a Human Problems approach and advocates radical revision of drug laws. Emphasizes the necessity of community coalitions to tackle the drug situation, as well as specific suggestions regarding the churches' role in such coalitions. Also included are brief funding tips.

"CONSCIENTIOUS GUIDE TO DRUG ABUSE" Vic Pawlak, Do It Now, P.O. Box 5115, Phoenix, AZ 85010, 1973. 48 pp. $1.00
... this "crash program in drug survival" is one of the very best of its type around. Written expressly for 'drug users and abusers', it covers everything from marijuana and glue-sniffing to opium and barbituates. Old drug myths are exposed as well as the very real and dangerous physical effects of certain drugs (mixing barbituates and alcohol for example). Practical information is offered on what to do in case of overdoses, what your rights are if busted, etc., and great emphasis is placed on the importance of having pills analyzed before taking them.

DRUG ABUSE: A REALISTIC PRIMER FOR PARENTS," Vic Pawlak and Do It Now staff, P.O. Box 5115, Pheonix, AZ 85010. 1973. 14 pp. $.35
... briefly covers speed to downers to acid to grass, etc., including each drug's overdose potential and possibility of physical addiction. Also listed are steps parents should keep in mind when communicating with their children on drug issues ("Arguing that marijuana causes harmful psychological reactions has proven itself fruitless, and if anything shows your kids how little you know.") Non-alarmist, common-sense approach.

Educating and enlightening young people and adults to the part they play in the total scheme of things politically, socially and economically is drug prevention. Relating to the basic needs of the people in terms of food, shelter, and clothing is drug prevention. Medical assistance, legal aid (welfare rights, tenants rights), day care, job opportunities and relevant and adequate education for young people in our community is drug prevention."
                              —United Front for a Drug Free Community.

"THE SNIFFING SPECTRUM," Do It Now, P.O. Box 5115, Phoenix AZ 85010. 10 cents
. . . a biting brochure on the effects of sniffing aerosol sprays, paint-thinner, glue, etc.—the most notable effect being the destruction of brain cells.

"WOMEN AND SMOKING," Jane E. Brody and Richard Engquist, Public Affairs Pamphlet No. 475, 381 Park Ave., South, New York, NY 10016, 1972. 24 pp. $.35
. . . provocative, well-documented discussion of why more and more women are smoking (and at an earlier age), health risks involved, effects during pregnancy, and quitting the habit.

"What Educators Can Do About Cigarette Smoking", Physical Education and Recreation Guide for Leaders in Smoking and Health Education, 201 16th Street, NW, Washington, D.C. 20036, 1971, 24 pp.
. . . urges educators to actively participate in smoking education programs in the schools and community, and to get faculty, parents, and youth involved as well. Lists a wide variety of possible projects and ideas along this line, and recommends helpful resource groups.

"DRUG EDUCATION BIBLIOGRAPHY," National Coordination Council on Drug Education, Suite 212, 1211 Connecticut Ave., NW, Washington, D.C. 20036, 1971. 45 pp.
. . . offers a fine comprehensive selection of materials on drugs (including alcohol, glue sniffing, etc.) representing a wide spectrum of opinions. For specialists as well as for those just desiring a basic orientation. It is presently being updated.

"HARD DRUGS AND THE MOVEMENT," Joe Axton, Do It Now, P.O. Box 5115, Phoenix, AZ 85010
. . . bitter denunciation of the cop-out hard drugs represent for radicals.

More than 80 percent of existing drug abuse education films contain scientific or medical misstatements about drugs and drug effects. . . one-third of them contain so many errors that NCCDE has classified them as scientifically unacceptable.
—quote by Peter Hammond, exec. dir. of National Coordinating Council on Drug Education

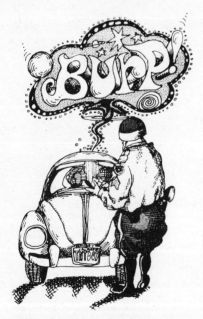

Never carry more than you can eat.

LEGISLATIVE GROUPS

NATIONAL ORGANIZATION FOR THE REFORM OF MARIJUANA LAWS (NORML)... works for state and federal legislative reform, focusing on education and lobbying for the decriminalization of marijuana. Well-funded by private foundations, NORML is also supported by sale of buttons, posters, and bumper stickers, and by the distribution of the 1936 propaganda film "Reefer Madness". Current legal efforts are reported in their newsletters, THE LEAFLET. Contact NORML, 1237 22nd St., NW, Washington, D.C. 20037, (202) 223-3170.

COMMITTEE FOR A SANE DRUG POLICY... was formed in December 1970 by a group of citizens who believe that criminal punishment for the non-medical use of drugs is inappropriate. Through public speaking, lobbying, and affiliation with other groups, the Committee works for the reform of laws on marijuana and other drugs. They advocate treating heroin addiction as a medical condition requiring professional supervision. Contact CSDP, 302 Berkeley St., Boston, MA 02116, (617) 267-3526.

AMORPHIA, THE CANNABIS COOPERATIVE... is a national organization for psycho-active drug research, education, and public policy reform. Funded entirely through the sale of ACAPULCO GOLD rolling papers, AMORPHIA was the largest single contributor to marijuana legalization campaigns in California, Michigan, Oregon, and Washington in 1972. Other reform projects include the publication of the Marijuana Review, contributions to a legal aid group for marijuana prisoners, as well as presentations to and research for influential groups like the National Commission on Marijuana and Drug Abuse. AMORPHIA is one of the best sources of information and action on the elusive cannabis plant. Contact AMORPHIA, 2073 Greenwich St., San Francisco, CA 94123, (415) 563-5858.

ACTION ON SMOKING AND HEALTH... takes legal action against smoking and tobacco companies. In the past they have worked on banning cigarette commercials and in establishing separate sections for smokers and non-smokers on airlines. They are now working on legal actions to force tobacco companies to pay for the death and disability they cause and on increasing protection for non-smokers on all means of transportation. They produce a bi-monthly newsletter on their programs. Contact ASH, 2000 H. St., NW, Washington, D.C. 20006, (202) 659-4310.

I guess I just don't think it's right to make a profit out of killing people
—Fairfax Cone, on leaving advertising agency with cigarette accounts

RESOURCES

<u>Marijuana: A Signal of Misunderstanding, First Report of the National Commission on Marijuana and Drug Abuse,</u> Superintendent of Documents, US Government Printing Office, Washington, D.C. 20402, March, 1972. 184 pp. $1.00
. . . this is the study that Nixon authorized and then ignored when the results were not to his liking. A readable, rational (but hardly radical) examination of known facts resulting in, among other things, the recommendation that possession of marijuana for personal use no longer be an offense.

"COUNCIL ON HEALTH ORGANIZATIONS STATEMENT ON DRUG USE AND ABUSE," Paul Lowinger, Council on Health Organizations, c/o Physician's Forum, 510 Madison Ave., New York, NY 10022, April 1971. 2 pp.
. . . radical perspective on drug laws, proposing that the US "Deal with the social pathology of poverty, racism, war, repression and deteriorating quality of American life for everyone. Attacking drugs alone is of limited value. We should be making necessary changes in the values and conditions of family and community life in America, especially for the young, the black, brown, and poor who are the most alienated groups." Appropriately reminds the reader that "the largest drug abuse problems in the United States are with alcohol and tobacco."

ALCOHOL

Alcohol is the nation's most widespread drug abuse problem. It kills thousands yearly through damage to the liver or other organs, and through driving accidents. Over 50% of all car accidents are caused by drunk drivers. Alcoholism affects all segments of the population somewhat, but thrives especially on conditions of deprivation and alienation. Liquor stores concentrate in poor urban areas. Native Americans, often impoverished, faced with racism and the erosion of traditional lifestyles, find alcoholism is a problem of major dimensions. Women caught in the housewife role make up a large—and largely ignored—alcoholic population.

In spite of the magnitude of the problem, there are not many programs to deal with alcoholism. Usually family, friends, and possibly a counsellor or clergyperson consulted individually must help the alcoholic as best they can. Many areas do have an Alcoholics Anonymous chapter, which offers a supportive group of other alcoholics. Some live-in therapeutic communities, similar to those set up for heroin addicts, have been created for alcoholics, as well as other types of group living situations and detox units. Occasionally, heroin-oriented programs will take alcoholics as well (see Addiction Treatment subsection and drug education).

NATIONAL COUNCIL ON ALCOHOLISM. . . was founded to "combat the disease of alcoholism." They are active in providing community education and referral services, stimulating labor-management alcoholism programs, and pushing for inclusion of alcoholism training in med schools and in physicians' post-graduate training. They also have a large library and resource center of alcoholism materials, including a number of their own books and pamphlets. Contact NATIONAL COUNCIL ON ALCOHOLISM, 2 Park Ave., New York, NY 10016, (212) 765-0990.

ALCOHOLICS ANONYMOUS. . . is one of the oldest and most widespread organizations for alcoholics. "The only requirement for membership is a desire to stop drinking." Funded solely through donations, AA's "primary purpose is to stay sober and help other alcoholics achieve sobriety." Contact ALCOHOLICS ANONYMOUS, 2660 Woodley Rd., NW, Washington, D.C. 20008, (202) 332-1933.

CASA ADELANTE. . . opened in February 1974 to serve the particular needs of the male Chicano alcoholic. The staff of 7 is bilingual, with a hiring preference for ex-alcoholics. Although Adelante views alcoholism as a sickness and not a crime, they are selective in whom they accept as residents in the 29 bed house; participants in the program must how a desire to help themselves. The daily schedule includes group and vocational counseling, recreation, and responsibility for house maintenance; residents are permitted to hold outside jobs after a three week probation period, although Adelante has a difficult time finding employment in non-agricultural seasons. A strong feature of the program is the resident's council which can, among other things, expel program participants for returning to Casa Adelante drunk. Casa Adelante strives to provide a more constructive, concerned environment than the abundant profit-making programs for alcoholics in the area; meals are high protein (to meet the special dietary needs of the alcoholic) and often include Chicano dishes. Initial funding is from the local Model Cities program, with Aid to the Disabled providing continuing source of revenue. Contact CASA ADELANTE, 2212 Quimby Rd., San Jose, CA 95122, (408) 274-6210.

UNITED INDIAN COALITION ON ALCOHOL AND DRUG ABUSE. . . includes representatives from 32 Native American alcohol and drug related programs in 9 upper mid-west states. The paid and volunteer staff assist the coalition members with proposal writing, managerial assistance and announcements of available grants, as well as initiating some programs. UICADA recognizes alcoholism as the number one drug problem, and believes that any realistic solution must deal with the root causes: unemployment, poor education, inadequate housing, etc. The whole membership meets annually, with interim decisions made by a Board of Directors representing each of the states. Contact UICADA, c/o American Indian Services, 800 W. Baltimore St., Detroit, MI 48202, (313) 871-5330.

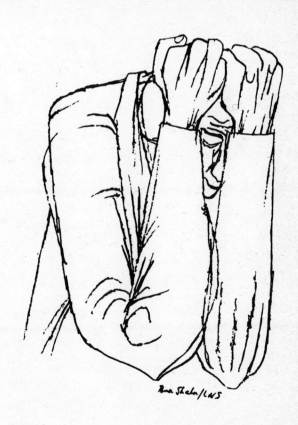

WESTERN REGIONAL INDIAN ALCOHOLISM TRAINING CENTER... has a one year program for people actively involved in alcohol projects. Participants spend a total of two months at the University of Utah campus and the remaining 10 months working with on-going projects. Tuition is free and credit is transferable. The Center is funded by NIAAA and approximately 85% of the students are Native American. Contact WRIATC, University of Utah, 1400 E. 2nd St., Salt Lake City, UT 84112, (801) 581-6244.

ANISHINABE WAKI-IGAN... is a half-way house for Native Americans released from prison. The house serves 16 men, many of whom have drinking problems. Average stay is 48 days and a full-time employment counselor assists residents to find work; those employed are encouraged to save ¾ of their income. The all Native American staff of 7 provides individual and group counseling in an effort to strengthen cultural and Indian pride. Funding has been from the Governors Crime Commission, although the over-bureaucracy and demand for statistics and data have presented problems. Contact ANISHINABE WAKI-IGAN, 3033 Portland Ave. South, Minneapolis, MN 55407, (612) 823-6236.

NATIVE AMERICAN REHABILITATION ASSOCIATION ... is an outreach program and half-way house for Native American women and men with drinking problems. The average age of house residents is 42 and stays range from one day to one year. The function of the home is to: reduce alcoholism, improve nutrition and general health, and strengthen personal, family and community relationships. Individual, group and family counseling, education on alcoholism, food and lodging are all provided, although vocational training is done by the Urban Indian Program for Employment. The outreach program works with Native Americans in hospitals and prisons to educate, counsel, and assist in finding employment upon release. Contact NATIVE AMERICAN REHABILITATION ASSOCIATION, 3303 SE Division St., Portland, OR 97202, (503) 233-7643.

Other native American alcoholism programs and half-way houses:

INDIAN GUEST HOUSE
3020 Clinton Ave. S.
Minneapolis, MN 55407
(612) 824-5501

JULES FAIRBANKS AFTERCARE RESIDENCE
806 N. Albert St.
St. Paul, MN 55104
(612) 646-2749

INDIAN NEIGHBORHOOD CLUB
1401 E. 24th St.
Minneapolis, MN 55404
(612) 721-5329

1971: Experts figure that alcohol-related traffic deaths amounted to over 27,000. If in comparison if ocean-going vessels were sinking with a loss of approximately 538 lives per week, or airliners were crashing with a loss of 538 lives per week, or if this tragedy were occuring in any form of public transportation, this country would be up in arms.

AMERICAN INDIAN COMMISSION ON ALCOHOL AND DRUG ABUSE
5775 Everett St.,
Arvada, CO
(303) 423-7800

NATIONAL INDIAN BOARD ON ALCOHOL
c/o United Southeastern Tribes
1970 Main St., Sarasota, FL 33577
(813) 955-0281

RESOURCES

"ALCOHOL," Department of Health, Education and Welfare. US Government Printing Office, Washington, D.C. 20402, 1971. 14 pp. $.15
... brief introduction to alcohol: how it effects the body, degree of danger, causes of alcoholism and dealing with it. The concluding section on "How Can We Prevent Alcoholic Problems" strongly urges preventive education, although it does not discuss the social and political conditions which cause people to seek escapes.

ENGAGE, Board of Christian Social Concerns of The United Methodist Church, 100 Maryland Ave. NE, Washington, D.C. 20002, August 1972
... collection of articles on alcohol and alcoholism. Written as part of an effort to redefine the position of the Church on drinking (which is total abstinence), the magazine includes two interviews as well as pieces on the prevention of alcoholism, the role of the federal government and more. Of particular interest is "The Alcohol Industry," which points out: "The industry's contribution to research into alcohol problems amounts to a mere $100,000 annually. By contrast, it spends 9000 times that much to advertise its wares. That $100,000 spent must be termed a public relations 'rip off'."

ADDICTION TREATMENT

This section deals mostly with heroin addiction, though programs may also include heavy users of amphetamines, cocaine, barbituates, or hallucinogens. No type of program has a clear record of success. Few even attempt follow-up studies, and they're difficult to do. So "Success" is hard to estimate. Attempts to "treat" drug use rather than punish it, on any significant scale, have not been going on for many years, and continue to be minimally funded.

Addicts, the people who care about them, and courts that are not satisfied to simply throw addicts in jail face the harrowing decision of what to try that might work. At this time there are no really satisfactory answers—no way in sight to deal with addicts as fast as new ones are being created.

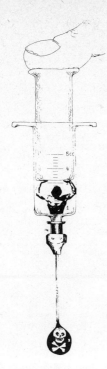

METHADONE

Methadone Maintenance, the fastest-growing form of addiction treatment, views heroin addiction as primarily a physical problem, to be treated medically. Proponents of this plan claim that heroin usage causes changes in the addict's body, creating a permanent physiological need that must be satisfied by heroin or a substitute drug. Methadone allegedly fills this need without producing euphoria or "nodding," so the addict can function normally. Supporters also claim that methadone prevents the addict from getting a heroin high and so removes the motivation to use illegal drugs. The addict is expected to get a daily dose of methadone for the rest of his/her life. There are now approximately 60,000 people in methadone maintenance. Most government funding is going to these programs, leaving little money for alternative approaches.

Methadone maintenance may be briefly described as a farce. Methadone is a synthetic, drug, four times as addictive as heroin, and causing more severe withdrawal symptoms. Many studies, including those done in the federal drug facility in Lexington, KY as far back as 1948, show methadone produces the same euphoria and nodding as heroin. When either is taken orally (as in the maintenance programs) the effect is milder, but it does not generally leave the addict functioning "normally". Other studies show that methadone does not block a heroin high, and that many addicts on maintenance us use other drugs. Side effects of methadone may include constipation, constant sweating, sexual impotence, sleepiness, nightmares and insomnia, pre-natal addiction, and brain damage. Widespread distribution of methadone has—naturally—led to its entering the illegal market; in Washington, D.C., by 1971, more people were dying of methadone overdose than of heroin overdose.

One scientist doing research on methadone recalls that heroin was first introduced as a cure for morphine addiction, before doctors realized how dangerous the new drug was. The way methadone is being used today, he said, is "so similar it sends shivers up my back."

—Southeast Asia: The Opium Trail

Sometimes, it is true, the availability of a free, reliable fix allows addicts to maintain a more stable life, including jobs and family relationships. For some long-time addicts, a maintenance program (preferably using heroin as a less harmful drug) may be necessary. But the present eagerness to substitute one addiction for another, and create a whole new illegal drug market, without ever dealing with the causes of addiction or making any attempt to create meaningful alternatives for addicts indicates an intolerable disregard for people's lives.

RESOURCES

Methadone Maintenace: A Technological Fix, Dorothy Nelkin. George Braziller, Inc., 1 Park Ave., New York, NY 10016, 1973. 164 pp. $1.95
... shows that the growing sense of urgency concerning drug addiction (increasing crime) results in an increasing tendency to use an efficient technological solution, such as methadone maintenance, which overlooks the implications of such social control.

"METHADONE MAINTENANCE—PART OF THE SOLUTION OR PART OF THE PROBLEM?" United Front for a Drug-free Community, South End Drug Council, 674 Tremont St., Boston, MA 14 pp.
... part of a "massive grass-roots education campaign" by the United Front, written by and for the people, particularly urban blacks. The pamphlet thoroughly attacks the heroin/methadone drug scene: how pushers are busted but importers go free; how methadone clinics rarely provide help in re-integrating ex-users into society (and have even been known to bar addicts with black liberation insignia); how methadone producers successfully lobby in Washington. Methadone maintenance as such is soundly condemned for all but 'last resort' cases. Demands are made to stop economic aid to opiate-producing countries, to eliminate legal addictive drugs for maintenance purposes, and to build programs which bring people together to create the kind of communities where drugs (heroin) aren't needed. Strong and convincing.

"METHADONE, THE FACTS," Barry Festoff, MD, available from RAP, Inc., 1904 "T" St., NW, Washington, D.C. 20009, 1972. 4 pp.
... dramatic indictment of the use of methadone maintenance with strong emphasis on clear (but usually ignored) facts of the effects of methadone. An example is the fact that the dosages received in maintenance clinics can cause electrical seisures of the brain. Higher dosages can stop brain waves.

"METHADONE: FEDERAL DRUG ADDICTION," Available from Louise Rice, 65 Chestnut St., Cambridge, MA 02139. 8 pp. $.30
... scathing attack on government-sponsored methadone maintenance programs, pointing out that methadone "accumulates, primarily in the brain, whereas no such cumulative effect is seen with the natural opiates, heroin or morphine." The people who gain from methadone maintenance programs are not the addicts—but the drug manufacturers (particularly Eli Lilly and Mallinckrodt Chemicals), the laboratories who process the mandatory urinalysis tests, the professional administrators who operate the programs and individuals involved in black market sales of methadone.

Federally-funded methadone clinics are already using this power to impose restrictions on the activities of the patients. Some forbid patients to enter particular parts of their communities or to associate with particular individuals. In New York, clinics have barred addicts who wear black liberation buttons. The usual penalty for violating these regulations—methadone being withheld for 3 days—just long enough for the agony of withdrawal to begin to peak.

—United Front for a Drug Free Community.

THERAPEUTIC COMMUNITIES

These live-in communities, focused around group therapy sessions and highly structured lifestyles, regard addiction as the result of a sick lifestyle. Therefore, they focus on long-term individual rehabilitation. Programs usually follow the same general pattern. Treatment begins when a prospective member enters the house and goes into a period of containment, during which s/he has little or no contact with the outside world (mail, visitors,—etc.). During this period—which may last as long as six months—the addict must usually demonstrate to the staff enough motivation to be accepted as a full program member, at which point s/he enters the lowest level of a strictly hierarchical society. S/he has few privileges, usually does menial work, and will participate, from one to several times weekly, in a group session composed of other program members and led by ex-addicts or psychologists. These sessions are designed to break through the defenses and rationalizations of addicts, and build self-awareness, self-confidence, and the strength of personality to maintain a drug-free lifestyle. The person will presumably advance thru various levels of the program, each entailing more privileges and a more responsible position within the community. Later stages involve increased contact with the outside world, culminating when the ex-addict leave the community. Many programs last up to two years.

Serious questions have been raised about therapeutic communities. Their effectiveness has been challenged by claims that many "graduates" who do not remain in the program as staff people return to drugs. Other critics attack the values inherent in the therapy. Advancement within the program is linked to conformity to the given standards of behavior, and that in turn is equated with "health" or "character development." Such "health" may include unquestioning obedience, stifling of any criticism of the program leadership, and unswerving conformity to traditional sex roles. Women are routinely expected to do all housekeeping chores, while men are only required to do them as punishment. The group sessions can be experienced as exercises in oppression, in which a group uses ridicule, humiliation, and social pressure to shatter an individual's personality, and then attempts to re-assemble it according to specifications.

Therapeutic communities, it seems, may be helpful or worse than useless. The strict structure of such a community can help addicts recover some order and stability in their lives. Good therapy groups can lead to an understanding of drug-use as an escape, and to the renewed self-confidence necessary for a changed life-style. But therapeutic communities can be a totalitarian environment, all the more questionable because many perhaps most—participants are not volunteers, but have entered the program to avoid being jailed. Even the best therapeutic communities send people back to unchanged social conditions which makes return to drugs likely. Yet, for many people, therapeutic communities remain the best available option. . . better than jail, better than being out on the street waiting to OD.

The programs below are listed because of particular strengths—such as job training, programs for Spanish-speaking addicts, or some commitment to involvement in the larger community —or because they have houses in regions where addiction programs are rare or non-existent. None use methadone maintenance. All are free or charge on a sliding scale. Programs which openly express condescension towards addicts or attribute addiction solely to individual immaturity or "illness" have been excluded; but others have been excluded simply for lack of space. Since courts often refer addicts to therapeutic communities, houses in a given city can usually be located through the city government.

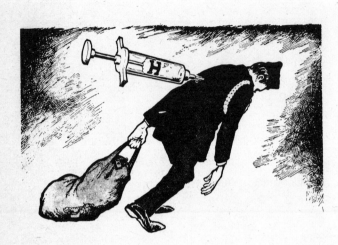

Sam Stone came home
to his wife and family
after serving in the conflict
overseas;
and the time that he served
had shattered all his nerves
and left a little shrapnel
in his knee.
But the morphine eased the pain,
and the grass grew round his brain,
and gave him all the confidence he lacked
with a purple heart
and a monkey on his back;
there's a hole in daddy's arm
where all the money goes . . . .
                    —John Prine

SERA... is a well-respected, comprehensive program for Spanish speaking addicts and youth. Although Puerto Ricans have the highest addiction rate in New York City (30% of all addicts are Puertoriqueños), Sera is the only drug program for and by Spanish-speaking people, housing 700 residents. This multifaceted project has 6 facilities in the South Bronx. At the Induction Center, staffed by ex-addicts, drug-users are oriented to the concept of a therapeutic community and encouraged to detox; this process takes about one month, with actual detoxification done through Lincoln Hospital or Morris Bernstein Institute. Stage two is a 3-6 month involvement in Sera's 24 hour therapeutic community. Group therapy, encounter sessions and role-playing are mandatory as well as informal classes in English. A gynecologist, 2 general practitioners and several nurses provide medical care. At the day care center (stage 3), the participants devote their time to academic activities, vocational training and job placement, culminating in employment and gradually decreasing involvement in Sera. This facility is equipped with a carpentry shop, garage, huge appliance repair shop and secretarial school. Two other Sera projects are: a youth treatment center, which is a therapeutic community, a day care center and preventive education program for youth who might be tempted to experi-... nt ment with drugs; and a community development component. The latter is comprised of bilingual ex-addicts working in an outreach capacity to organize the community around drug use and community problems. Sera accepts women and men and has a daycare center for the children of the members of the therapeutic community. People come to Sera from the streets court referrals, prison and other city programs. Eighty % of the 185 staff members are ex-addicts. Sera's million dollar plus budget is paid by city, state and federal funds. Sera is a fine example of a therapeutic community aimed at the Spanish-speaking people. Contact SERA, 1771 Andrews Ave., Bronx, NY 10453, (212) 583-9813.

TODAY, INC.... is a therapeutic community based on feminist principles. The 70 full-time residents participate in all-female or all-male therapy groups in an effort to come to grips with the depth of their sex-role stereotyping. Only at the end of the program are groups coed. Women are encouraged to express their anger (also to control it when necessary), and men to express vulnerability and emotions. Residents are given considerable responsibility for program upkeep and it is not uncommon for a woman to head the maintenance and repair team while a man leads the kitchen crew. Since most participants are 19-21 years old, work toward a high school degree and resolving family conflicts are stressed. The therapeutic community was started in 1971 by three professionals who were concerned at the growing incidence of heroin use. Local advisory boards have input into policy decisions. Contact TODAY, INC., P.O. Box 317, Newtown, PA 18940, (215) 968-4713.

PROJECT RETURN... is a multi-dimensional therapeutic community directly serving approximately 230 women and men. With five drug-free homes, a community orientation center and a youth coliseum, the program offers many services: a full-fledged therapeutic community, with stays averaging 8-16 months; ambulatory program for people kicking addiction; community education around the dangers of drug use; sponsorship of health fairs and community gatherings; and a home for delinquent youth. Participants in the therapeutic community go through a six point program, including encounter group sessions, education toward a High School Equivalancy Diploma, and vocational training. All graduates of Project Return must have a job or be in school. The strongest feature of the Project is its community involvement, which includes a prison outreach program, speakers bureau, choral group, block parties, etc. Funding is from city, state and federal agencies and all staff members at the therapeutic community are ex-addicts. Contact PROJECT RETURN, 141 East 34th St., New York, NY 10016, (212) 725-2656.

EXODUS HOUSE... started doing drug work in 1948 and became a full-fledged drug free residential community in 1968. Unlike most therapeutic communities, therapy sessions are non-attack oriented and vocational training is heavily stressed. The residence houses 24 men for 3-5 month periods, with another 66 women and men participating on an ambulatory basis. Following the therapy and counseling period, participants enter an extensive vocational training program. Stage one is an evaluation workshop during which time people can dabble in areas such as ceramics, carpentry, and printing in an effort to define skills and interests. Personal Adjustment training follows, with participants assigned to one of three shops: printing, ceramics, and carpentry. The final and most thorough stage of training requires specialization in one area: house management and therapeutic community type counseling; return to prior vocation; academic education; or practical skill studied through the State Office for Vocational Rehabilitation. English is taught and tutoring for the General Equivalency Diploma is available. The program is intentionally small, and will help other groups with technical assistance. Decisions are made by the Board of Trustees (1/3 of whom are from the community) and staff of 22, seven of whom are trained ex-addicts. Contact EXODUS HOUSE, E. 134th St., New York, NY 10037, (212) 876-8775.

ODYSSEY HOUSE... has a residence program supervised by psychiatric professionals and ex-addicts, followed by gradual re-entry into society, and after-care group therapy sessions. Addiction is considered "sociopathic"—the lifestyle, rather than the person, is sick—and is challenged through intensive group therapy. Odyssey welcomes court referrals, believing that, though addicts often do not have the motivation to change, motivation can usually be built once they enter the program. Odyssey has special programs in NY for pregnant women, adolescents, addicted parents, Spanish-speaking addicts, and those with unusually high IQ's. Contact Odyssey House, 207 E. 52 St., New York, NY 10022, (212) 371-9470; 61 Lincoln Park, Newark, NJ 07102, (201) 642-6550; 30 Winnacunnet Rd., Rte. 1, Hampton, NH 03801, (603) 926-5200; 68 South Sixth East, Salt Lake City, UT 84102, (801) 322-1001; 1225 Detroit St., Flint, MI 48503, (313) 238-0483; 1125 North Tonti St., New Orleans, LA 70119, (504) 821-9211.

SYNANON FOUNDATION... is one of the oldest, largest, and best known therapeutic communities, with a wide influence on other groups. Its program for addicts—and every other facet of the organization—is built around the Synanon Game, a verbal free-for-all designed to facilitate honesty, confront each person with how others see him/her, and thus provoke personal re-evaluation and growth. Most addicts come to the program as parolees. Synanon people see themselves creating not just a drug treatment program but a model community—racially integrated, ecologically sound, and based on a strong ethic of honesty discipline, constant learning, and achievement. Those addicts considered successfully treated usually stay on in the Synanon community; a high percentage of the people who leave return to drug use. Increasing numbers of non-addict "lifestylers" are joining Synanon as an alternative way of life. Contact Synanon Foundation, 1910 Ocean Front Walk, Santa Monica, CA 90401, (213) 399-9241; Detroit Intake Facility, 18940 Sheaffer Rd., Detroit, MI 48235, (313) 341-2944; New York Intake Facility, 338 W. 84th St., New York, NY 10024, (212) 877-2912.

RESOURCES

"FEMALE PATIENT AS BOOTY", Jeanie L. Peak, Peter Glankoff, available from Jeanie Peak, P.O. Box 1000, Escondido, CA 92025, 1974. 6 pp. Free
... insightful article on the unique position of the female addict. The author contends that in our sexist society, "when a woman openly begins using drugs for pleasure she becomes considerably more of a deviant from social norms than her male counterpart." The female addict is made to feel more guilty for deviating from her role as daughter, wife or mother than for using a destructive and dangerous drug. The article also centers on the way female addicts are exploited in therapeutic communities. Therapeutic communities are extremely hierarchical. The counselor, who is often an ex-addict, is at the bottom in both salary and status. Because the counselor has few privileges or powers, "sexual exploitation becomes one of his/her spoils of War;" the female addict is his booty or price. Calls for the elimination of sexist behavior in drug treatment programs, and a genuine commitment to training and advancement for ex-addict counselors.

"Radical Feminist: A Treatment Modality for Addicted Women," Ardelle M. Schultz, P.O. Box 317, Newtown, PA 18940, 1974. 30 pp. $1.50 to cover xeroxing
. . . story of one woman's growth from a fashion model to an alcoholic to a commited feminist. In this honest and insightful article, Schultz draws on her own experiences to develop a feminist model for treating addicts, in particular women. Therapeutic communities in general use women addicts to fill male addicts'need for a mother, wife or daughter image upon whom to vent frustrations and anger. Because there are relatively few women in therapeutic communities, they are divided among the therapy groups, leaving women unsupported, without positive role models and unable to confront their own anxieties about sex-role stereotyping. Schultz proposes all-women's groups with a strong feminist bias, as well as breakdown of sex-roles in therapeutic community job distribution. Conveys the anger, love, courage and sensitivity of one woman struggling to develop non-sexist structures to deal with addiction.

We Mainline Dreams, Judianne Densen-Gerber. Penguin Books, 7110 Ambassador Rd., Baltimore, MD 21207, 1974. 421 pp. $2.95
. . . tells the story of one therapeutic community that had some degree of success and the people who have passed through it.

FILMS AND TAPES

University of California Extension Media Center, Berkeley, CA 94720

"Or Die," 18 min. b&w 1966 $10
Brief look at some of the activities of Synanon—a unique social movement run by former drug addicts—made over a period of six months by a filmmaker participating in the daily life of Synanon.

The mission in Laos was to make friends with the Meo people and organize and train them to fight the Pathet Lao. One of the main tasks was to buy up the entire local crop of opium. About twice a week an Air America plane would arrive with supplies and kilo bags of gold dust. Paul gave the gold to the Meo in return for their bags of opium which were loaded on the plane. Each bag was marked with the symbol of the tribe. There was no mistaking the bags since the symbols were quite complicated.

—Southeast Asia: The Opium Trail summation of testimony of former Green Beret, Sgt. Paul Withers at Winter Soldier Hearings in Boston October 9, 1971

POLITICAL PROGRAMS

In the past few years, a number of groups have emerged which recognize drug addiction as a political problem rather than simply a matter of individual weakness or maladjustment. Some of these groups have adapted the techniques of therapeutic communities. Politically-oriented programs "don't deny that the individual junkie needs to change. But they understand that the best hope for a long-range solution to the whole problem is a mass movement fighting against racism and poverty" (Opium Train). They offer addicts a broader view of their position in society and the forces that fostered their addiction. Rather than simply returning ex-addicts to an alienating and oppressive social situation, they offer a program of ongoing involvement in the struggle for political change—a lifestyle with a sense of pride, direction, and meaning.

Like most anti-drug groups, these are experimental, and their long-term effectiveness in keeping ex-addicts off drugs has yet to be measured. Often, they are so severely restricted by lack of funds that they must give up the effort to deal with addicts directly, and move into programs of education and community organizing. Yet they are the most hopeful signs in the grim picture of drug addiction and dependence.

REGIONAL ADDICTION PROGRAM (RAP). . . is "a completely drug-free counter-culture concerned with revolutionary concepts in education, community activity and political commitment." RAP's 15 month to 2 year residential program draws on the techniques of therapeutic communities, but does not aim to "cure" individual hang-ups. Rather, they want people to understand the social conditions that encourage them to turn to drugs, and to find new pride and sense of direction in working to change those conditions. Around 70 people in their residential program learn skills for survival and social change (mechanics, public relations, construction, drama, etc.) and participate in community service programs such as legal aid referral and community

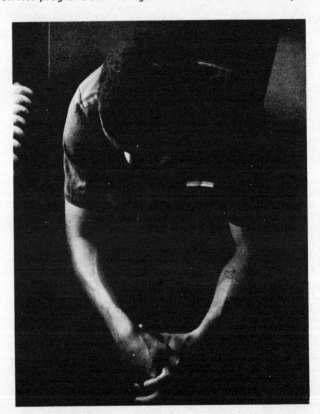

education around drugs as a method of social control. Their graphics shop provides leaflets and brochures on RAP programs, methadone, drug, education, etc. Accepting no government funding, RAP manages to stay a few months ahead of the bills through community contributions and a sophisticated program to get church and foundation grants, contributions and gifts in kind from businesspeople. Currently about 70% Black and drawn mostly from DC's inner city, RAP will soon be opening a second facility in suburban Maryland. Contact RAP, 1904 "T" St., NW, Washington, D.C. 20009, (202) 462-7500.

LINCOLN DETOX UNIT. . . is a very unique program in the drug field. The unit operates from a political base: teaching classes in the politics of heroin, operating collectively and insisting on local community control. They oppose methadone maintenance and therapeutic communities, believing that neither confronts the economic and societal causes of addiction, but only perpetuates a new form of dependence. Detoxification is done through twice daily administration of gradually decreasing dosages of the drug; for heroin users the process takes 10-15 days, while methadone addicts spend 3-4 months detoxing. The Unit is currently experimenting with the use of acupuncture for detoxification, since it has been found helpful in combating sleeplessness and depression. During the detoxification period, individuals are exposed to political education around the economics of heroin, assisted in getting on welfare and Medicaid and provided money for transportation. Yet, for the 61% who successfully complete the detox program (6 times the city's rate) the real problem is in finding a job. The predominantly Third World, ex-addict staff of Lincoln Detox operate through five collectives such as legal, medical and clerical; each collective chooses a representative to sit on the governing council. Working out of a large auditorium and 2 offices, it is amazing that Lincoln Detox can treat 250 people/month. However, since the New York Health and Hospital Corporation has reneged on a promise to fund complete in-and-out-patient care, the Unit has been forced to do its best in extremely inadequate facilities. Funding is from the state and city government. For information on this prototype project, contact LINCOLN DETOXIFICATION UNIT, Lincoln Hospital, 333 Southern Blvd., New York, NY (212) 960-5151.

BLACK FEMINIST ADDICTION COMMITTEE/NATIONAL BLACK FEMINIST ORGANIZATION. . . challenges the sexist orientation of therapeutic communities and drug programs. Most of the eight women on the Committee are actively involved in New York drug programs, working from within to affect change. In addition, the Committee is establishing a network of Black feminists involved in drug treatment; doing consulting and staff training for on-going projects; and advocating for change. Virtually all therapeutic communities treat women as second class participants who are responsible for house cleaning, are objects for male hostility; and are qualified to learn only secretarial and other traditionally women's jobs. Gynecologists are not available at therapeutic community clinics nor is there day care for children of addicts. And, if straight women are treated poorly, lesbians are far worse off. In 1973 Committee members visited 30 New York therapeutic communities finding all but two unresponsive to the particular needs of women addicts. A proposal is being written to fund a Black feminist treatment collective and center, and the Committee is putting out a newsletter. It is a real inspiration to talk with these women. Contact BFAC, c/o Ashaki Taha, 40 Stone Gate Rd., Ossining, NY 10562, (914) 762-4291.

WHITE LIGHTENING. . . was founded by residents of a standard therapeutic community called Logos, who began to develop a radical political consciousness linking drug use with oppressive social conditions. Directors of the house objected to this trend and tried to keep political literature and radical speakers from the house. Eventually, 70 of the 150 residents left. Some of them eventually formed the White Lightening collective and began putting out a paper by that name, a lively radical periodical with news on economics, ecology, sexism, Third World struggles, as well as anti-drug education. They hope to build a broad community organization that can move back into direct work with drugs. All White and working in a basically White working class neighborhood, WL considers anti-racism work one of its focuses. They see the courts as the most obvious way people in their community encounter injustice, so they run a legal aid program concentrating

on criminal and housing law. WL does all investigation and preparation of the cases; lawyers do only the court presentation. WL also works to expose the inadequacy of therapeutic communities which treat addiction as an individual psychological abberation for which the addict must beg forgiveness. WL believes that therapeutic communities should be run on a basis of community action, by residents, staff and community representatives, not by directors or for profit. Contact WHITE LIGHTENING, 109 E. 184th St., NY, NY 10468, (212) 584-5984.

WOMAN'S ORGANIZATION TO MOVE AGAINST ALCOHOL AND NARCOTICS (WOMAN). . . is a collective of 15 working class and professional women who believe that drug use is not the result of individual psychopathology but a response to oppressive conditions. They work in Cass Corridor, a racially mixed, skid-row area marked by low income, high drug use, and many transients. They are currently involved in drug education, stressing that drugs are one small part of the problem of community   . WOMAN also pushed for the formation of a woman's caucus in Detroit's drug abuse co-ordinating council and is lobbying for the hiring of more women to work in the drug programs. They are considering bringing a class action suit against the city's therapeutic communities because only one of them will accept women. Future plans, dependent on funding, include detoxification and out-patient treatment for drug users, day care, and further community organizing around drugs. Contact WOMAN, 145 W. Alexandrine Drive, Detroit, MI 48201.

In many cities, police may arrest addicts for stealing or other crimes, but show no interest in challenging the open sale of heroin, so long as it is confined to poor White and Third World areas. In growing frustration and anger, community people have at times begun to take over police functions themselves. In one New York neighborhood, women tired of having their children exposed to street-corner heroin peddlers got together and began chasing the pushers out of the neighborhood every day when they showed up. Some Black and Puerto Rican communities have established "Drug-free zones"; pushers entering such areas are likely to be beaten and thrown out. In Baltimore, several killings have been carried out by the Black October Organization. Statements released by the group explained that notorious pushers had been given several warnings, and were shot upon their refusal to quit pushing.

RESOURCES

BOOKS

The American Heroin Empire: Power, Profits and Politics, Richard Kunnes, MD, Dodd, Mead & Co., 79 Madison Ave., New York, NY 10016, 1972
. . . exposes the large number of government, military and industrial officials who covertly participate for power and profit in the production, transportation and sale of illegal heroin.

National Directory of Drug Abuse Treatment Programs, Deena D. Watson, National Clearinghouse for Drug Abuse Information, Suite 212, 1211 Connecticut Ave., NW, Washington, D.C. 20036, 1972. 381 pp.
. . . an incredible inclusive inventory, by state, of all types of drug abuse and addiction treatment and rehabilitation facilities (approximately 1300 in all). Each listing includes the name and address of the center, the contact person, the type of program involved, services offered, who is (and isn't) served and staff composition.

Strong at the Broken Places: Women Who Have Survived Drugs, Barbara Kerr. Follett Publishing Co., 201 N. Wells, Chicago, IL 60606, 1974. $8.95
. . . story of six middle class women who turn to drugs to escape the emptiness of their lives. The Villain of the piece is a society whose sexism and narrow range of roles for women too often cripples both those who remain confined and those who have 'escaped'.

"THE SMACK BRIGADE," Available from National Clearinghouse on Post Vietnam Syndrome, 439 N. Fratney, Milwaukee, WI 53212, December 1972. 9 pp.
. . . deeply provocative article on heroin use by Vietnam Veterans and the involvement of the US government. In 1969 military officials began to crack down on marijuana use, while ignoring the influx of heroin on US bases. Because the ruling elite of South Vietnam, Laos, Cambodia and Thailand benefited from increased sales, the US government did nothing. "Thus in the last months of 1970, more American soldiers were evacuated from Vietnam because of drug addiction than because of combat wounds." Compelled to do something, the government set up ineffective detoxification and counseling centers. "At the end of the 'program' the addict was then simply returned to duty, in the same working conditions, the same combat environment, the same proximity to drugs that had led to his addiction in the first place." Back in the States, the government continues its policy of neglect and false promises. VA treatment has been minimal and geared toward methadone maintenance. Thoroughly condemning the Nixon administration and the VA, this is a most important resource.

"THE OPIUM TRAIL: HEROIN AND IMPERIALISM," written for the Committee of Concerned Asian Scholars, New England Free Press, 60 Union Square, Somerville, MA 02143, 1972. 84 pp. $.25
. . . an excellent overview of opium use, which includes heroin and morphine—who and how it profits and oppresses. Tracing the origins of heroin and morphine addiction, it blames capitalists here and elsewhere for the massive international narcotics network. ". . . the US government firmly supports the same people who bring heroin to the GI's in Vietnam. By turning their eyes away from the obvious official corruption, American authorities have effectively used opium profits to reward Asian elites for their support of US goals in Southeast Asia." Particularly notable is the realistic evaluation of therapeutic communities—how they usually view the addicts' problem as individual rather than social, and how their long, expensive, strictly-disciplined programs often do not prepare ex-addicts to re-enter their native environment. Though not totally discounting therapeutic communities, the authors stress political activism as the most successful therapy.

"The Political Economy of Junk," Sol Yurick, MONTHLY REVIEW, available from Louise Rice, 65 Chestnut St., Cambridge, MA 02139, Dec., 1970. 15 pp. $50
. . . "The addict is a social type generated in response to changes in the social economy in a time of world crisis. A mistake frequently made is to view drug consumption merely as an indulgence, a gratification, an escape rather than a market response to economic and social dislocation." The author holds that "the junk industry serves three useful functions for the capitalist economy: it employs an otherwise unemployable sector of the labor force, it creates spin-off industries and it suppresses the righteous anger of oppressed and alienated people. The junk industry directly employs people as pushers and creates a wealth of jobs in the areas of prostitution, fencing, law enforcement, drug rehabilitation, etc." A complex, angry article.

"Heroin in the Suburbs," Robert Levengood, Paul Lowinger, Kenneth Schooff, AMERICAN JOURNAL OF PUBLIC HEALTH, 1015 18th St., NW, Washington, D.C. March, 1973 pp. 209-213
. . . dispels the myth that addiction is only a problem of the inner city by reporting on a study in Grosse Point, Michigan. The rate of heroin used in one public high school reached 4.1% in 1970. The article is statistical, drawing exclusively on a study conducted through a local clinic. Although somewhat outdated, the conclusions are grim.

"THE BRITISH NARCOTICS SYSTEM," Report Series 13, National Clearinghouse for Drug Abuse, Suite 212-1211, Connecticut Ave., NW, Washington, D.C. 20036, April, 1973. 12 pp.
. . . one of a series of fact sheets written by STASH, this surveys the workings of the British Narcotics System from 1924 to the present. The British system assumes that narcotics dependence is a medical problem for medical professionals rather than a criminal problem. Cites some problems, such as non-addicts becoming addicted through free doses at the clinics, and users selling their excess on the black market, because doctors are unable to determine necessary dosage, or even if someone is really addicted. However, statistics suggest that the system has cut down on the extent of the British black market involvement with narcotics.

"NEONATAL NARCOTIC ADDICTION," Jane S. Lin-Fu, Children's Bureau, Welfare Administration, HEW, Government Printing Office, Washington, D.C. 1967. 9 pp.
. . . summarizes the problems of pregnant women who are addicted to narcotics.

FILMS AND TAPES

Radio Free People, 133 Mercer Street, New York, NY 10002

"Capitalism Plus Heroin Equals Genocide," 28 min. cassette or reel to reel, $6, $10 for institutions
This tape is a vivid analysis of who's reponsible for "the plague" in the ghetto and why, by Michael Cetewayo Tabor, a former addict and Panther 21 defendant. In 1969 at least 25,000 youths in New York City, mostly Black or Puerto Rican, were addicted to heroin—210 of those died that year. Government concern was only expressed when the epidemic significantly invaded the "inner sanctums" of the middle class. Seeing heroin as "a form of genocide in which the victim pays to be killed," Tabor points out the complex interconnections between "legitimate" and "illegitimate" (such as the mafia) capitalism citing two different dope deals in particular, "sponsored" by reputable business-people. In powerfully-flowing oratory, he describes the cycle of despair of the heroin addict, including the dope pusher who issues "death on the installment plan" and police who take payoffs from drug peddlers. Since drug abuse is a "social phenomena that grows organically from the social system," Tabor calls for nothing short of revolution to eradicate it. This is also available in article form from Louise Rice, 65 Chestnut St., Cambridge MA 02139, 11 pp. $.38

Newsreel, 26 W. 20th St., New York, NY 10011.

"Smack the Enemy—Get High Off the People," still in production but available soon. A film about hard drugs and how they are used to repress the Third World communities in New York City.

LEGAL DRUGS

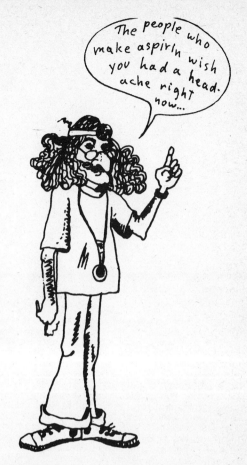

The people who make aspirin wish you had a headache right now...

COUNCIL ON ECONOMIC PRIORITIES. . . disseminates unbiased and detailed information on the practices of US corporation in such vital areas as equal employment, environmental quality, military production, consumer practices, and foreign affairs. CEP is conducting an in-depth study of the pharmaceutical industry, examining the safety and effectiveness of prescription drugs and the effects of advertising on drug prices. Special focus is on the price structure of the antibiotic market. Contact CEP, 35 Fifth Ave., New York, NY 10011, (212) 691-8550.

DRUG ADVERTISING PROJECT. . . has recently been funded by the Drug Abuse Council for indepth research into drug advertising. The study proposes to explore the economics of drug promotion, media impact on drug taking patterns, the problems of self-regulation within the industry, advertising codes and other relevant areas of concern. So far, the Project has produced a "Selected Bibliography on Drug Promotion" and an excellent slideshow which points out various controversial medical journal advertising practices and illustrates the emotional appeal to physicians and advertising's influence upon prescription patterns. Contact DRUG ADVERTISING PROJECT, National Council of Churches, 100 Maryland Ave., NE, Washington, D.C. 20002, (202) 546-1401.

In a speech entitled 'They're Shooting at Us,' Jonah Gitlitz, executive vice president of the American Advertising Federation said . . . that the issue of greatest concern to his group is the current trend to question the social and economic values of advertising. . . . Among the consumer protection proposals opposed by the AAF, warning in advertising is the most significant, according to Gitlitz. Poison warning on household products and pollution warnings on detergents containing phosphates are 'opposed to the whole concept of advertising,' he said. 'We are opposed to the whole concept of warnings in advertising because our primary purpose is to sell. If we do inform, it is only in order to sell,' Gitlitz said.

—THE NEW ORLEANS TIMES-PICAYUNE

PUBLIC COMMUNICATIONS, INC. . . . "is the country's first joint public interest law firm and advertising agency. Public Communications was founded to attack the problems of public interest groups in disseminating important information and the media's self-censorship which often blocks attempts to discuss controversial material. While none of their litigation pertains to drugs or the drug industry, they have developed several public service messages which deal with pharmaceutical problems. These include a 30-second TV spot on aspirin, an ad for print media urging generic prescribing, and a 30-second radio spot on prescription drug pricing. The firm also distributes research papers on prescription durg prices, the FDA and hazardous drugs, aspirin and combination analgesics, and cold remedies. Copies of these research papers and the media spots can be obtained by writing PUBLIC COMMUNICATIONS, INC., 10203 Santa Monica Blvd., Los Angeles, CA 90067, (213) 553-0648.

SAN FRANCISCO CONSUMER'S ACTION. . . has surveyed 178 pharmacies in the Bay Area examine whether or not the pharmacies complied with the California mandatory drug price posting laws, the price of their prescription drugs, and their services (such as whether they deliver prescriptions.) The results were compiled into the "SHOPPERS GUIDE TO PHARMACIES" which has been used by San Francisco residents to find the best pharmacy. Contact SAN FRANCISCO CONSUMER'S ACTION, 312 Sutter, San Francisco, CA 94108, (415) 982-4660.

COMMUNITY PHARMACY. . . combines low-cost, high quality prescription drugs and "health and beauty aids" with community education projects. The pharmacy was started in 1972 with the aid of the Wisconsin Student Association who placed it on the campus of the University of Wisconsin and staffed it with volunteers. Much of the money required to open the store was obtained by borrowing from other campus organizations and by selling non-redeemable bonds to students and community people. The pharmacy is open every day, and currently employs three part-time pharmacists and nine other paid workers. The Community Pharmacy staff members also are involved with VD and drug education projects, and hope to expand this dimension of the store. Seeking to make the pharmacy independent of the Student Association, the staff plans to ultimately place it under worker control. Organizers of the pharmacy warn that it is very important for groups planning to set up alternative pharmacies to work with someone that is experienced in small businesses and to enlist the aid of a lawyer. Contact COMMUNITY PHARMACY, Wisconsin Student Association, 511 N. Lake St., Madison' WI 53703, (608) 251-3242.

PEOPLE'S PHARMACY COOPERATIVE. . . was created by a group of Milwaukee community people who believed that quality medication could be obtained at a low cost. The goals of this community-owned-and-operated pharmacy are, selling prescription and non-prescription drugs on a non-profit basis; giving community education programs about drugs, the drug industry and health, legislative analysis; and most importantly, establishing the power of people to control their own lives. The pharmacy staff includes three pharmacists who volunteer time and a paid VISTA worker. To fulfill their community education goals, the cooperative has taken over responsibility for a drug abuse education program in Milwaukee public schools, is sponsoring a class in the local Free University on mystification and drug misuse, and publishes a monthly newsletter. Contact PEOPLE'S PHARMACY COOPERATIVE, c/o David Laluzerne, 820 E. Locust St., Milwaukee, WI 53212, (414) 962-2459 or 562-3300.

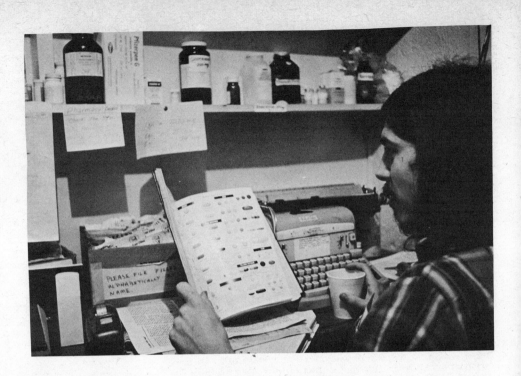

ADAMS-MORGAN COMMUNITY PHARMACY... is currently planning and constructing a pharmacy in one section of a community, anti-profit food store. The collectively-run pharmacy now only sells over-the-counter items and educational material while they are searching for a pharmacist to work with them. Money to open the pharmacy has been raised through loans from community people and by selling redeemable bonds. All decisions are made by concensus and the pharmacist will have no more policy-making power than other collective members. The pharmacy has literature available on the side effects of drugs, the economics of generic-prescribing, educational materials from FDA, and general health resources. After the pharmacy is operating it will enter into a delivery service with the food store for old people and others who cannot easily get to the store. Contact ADAMS-MORGAN COMMUNITY PHARMACY, 2447 18th St., NW, Washington, D.C. 20009, (202) 483-3884.

RESOURCES

BOOKS

The American Connection: Politicking and Profiteering in the 'Ethical' Drug Industry, John Pekkanen. Follet Publishing Co., 201 N. Wells St., Chicago IL 60606, 1973. 348 pp. $7.95
. . . vivid account of the corporate drug concerns' opposition to legislation to control dangerous drugs in order to gouge the public for some of the highest profits in the US economy. The books tells how the Nixon Administration pushed tough Omnibus Drug Abuse Prevention and Control Act (the no-knock provision) while lobbying against stricter controls of amphetamine production records. John Dean was a representative of the Justice Department at the time, lobbying for loose controls on the industry. In the wake of the Watergate scandal, it has been disclosed that Nixon accepted a trust fund for his daughter from Elmer Bobst, a drug industry big-wig. Industry and politicians, the prestigious Washington law firms and their well-connected super-attorneys, and federal administrators come across as an intermeshed system working to the disadvantage of the uninformed consumer. This is a primer of American capitalism in its most pernicious form. Although the author consistently understates the case, the mentality of drug-advertising leaves little doubt as to who the 'pusher' has been all along.

The Great Drug Deception, Ralph Adam Fine, Stein and Day, 7 East 48th St., New York, NY 10017, 1972
. . . examines the blatant manner in which a pharmaceutical company disregarded negative test findings on one of its drugs; misrepresented the product to the medical profession and public; submitted falsified information to the FDA. It thus increased its profits at the expense of patients' well-being. The book underscores the need for an independent group with no financial stake in the results to do all testing and for the totality of a company's experience with a drug to be disclosed to the public.

The New Handbook of Prescription Drugs, Richard Barack, MD. Ballantine Books, Inc., 101 Fifth Ave., New York, NY 10003, 1970. 362 pp. $1.25
. . . an excellent reference for both doctor and patient. It offers some sound proposals for separation of the medical profession from the pharmaceutical industry—such as a mandatory labeling law and a national drug-testing center. The book contains a Prescription Drug List (PDL), listed by brand-name and cross-listed by generic name; a list of the 60 basic drugs used in treatment of at least 90% of adult patients, divided into 21 therapeutic categories; comparative price lists of drugs; several informative appendices on prescribing for children; and a list of some distributors of generic drugs with addresses and phone numbers. The drug lists are highly informative, with annotations on history, effectiveness and safety for most of the drugs listed. The PDL includes certain non-prescription drugs; notes on which ones qualify for Medicare; and notes on how much senior citizens use.

MYSTIFICATION AND DRUG MISUSE, Hazards in Using Psychoactive Drugs, Henry L. Lennard and Associates. Jossey-Bass, Inc., 615 Montgomery St., San Francisco 94111, 1971. 133 pp.
. . . an extremely well-written, perceptive analysis of the general mystique surrounding drug-taking in our culture. . . how we are manipulated and misled into taking drugs by the pharmaceutical industry and the medical profession (as well as by educators who encourage the use of drugs to control unmanageable children). They urge us to depend on drugs to mask our anxieties rather than to deal with them. Gives solid recommendations to doctors, drug companies, educators, community organizers, and the like.

PAMPHLETS AND ARTICLES

"PUT HER DOWN ON DRUGS: PRESCRIBED DRUG USAGE IN WOMEN," Linda S. Fidell, Dept. of Psychology, UCLA, 405 Hilgard, West Los Angeles CA 90024, 1973
. . . a highly documented study of why women take 60% of nonpsychoactive and 68% on psychoactive drugs in the US. Fidell contends that doctors view women as "neurotic hypercondriacs," thus not taking their illnesses seriously; doctors respond by prescribing long lists of tranquilizers, stimulants, depressants, etc.

"THE DRUG INDUSTRY" and **"THE MEDICAL PROFESSION-DRUG INDUSTRY ALLIANCE,"** Rick Barnhart, available from Louise Rice, 65 Chestnut St., Cambridge, MA 02139, February 1970. 20 pp. $.68
. . . factual articles revealing the extent of profiteering and drug company-doctor collusion. Dispels drug industry myths that prices are kept high due to research and development, strong competition, superiority of name brands and the cost of quality control. The information on drug industry advertising is appalling: The primary purpose of the detail man is to make a sale even if it involves irrational prescribing and irrational combinations. "During my time in the drug industry I had a close ongoing relationship with detail men. It was from them that I learned the simple maxim: If you can't convince them, confuse them."

"DRUG COMPANY GIFTS," available from Louise Rice, 65 Chestnut St., Cambridge MA 02139. 7 pp. $.27
. . . informal notes by medical students on the implications of receiving drug company gifts. They see the gifts as bribes that ultimately cost the consumer; receiving gifts promotes a lack of price consciousness on the part of doctors. Also, doctors are among the financial elite in the US and least need free goods. Excellent organizing literature.

·PEDDLING DANGEROUS DRUGS ABROAD: SPECIAL DISPENSATION," Stanford Sesser, available from Louise Rice, 65 Chestnut St., Cambridge MA 02139, March 6, 1971. 2 pp. $.10
. . . infuriating account of the overseas sales of US manufactured drugs found to be dangerous by the FDA. The most cogent example is Chloromycetin, which can result in aplastic anemia ("Aplastic anemia means that the bone marrow stops manufacturing blood cells; if treatment fails, as it often does, the patient dies.") After the FDA forced Parke, Davis and Co., producers of Chloromycetin, to warn doctors and consumers of the side effects, the Defense Department "purchased 10,642,300 capsules of Chloromycetin from Parke, Davis last year. Almost ten million capsules were given to South Vietnam for use on South Vietnamese."

"VPIRG REPORT," Vermont Public Interest Group, 26 State St., Montepelier, VT, July 1973. 6 pp.
. . . valuable guide to Vermont's pharmacies. The report lists, in chart form, 96 of the state's 99 pharmacies and price each charges for 50 drugs. The drug stores are divided into geographic regions and the highest and lowest price per drug per region is indicated. A must for Vermont residents and an excellent model for other states.

"In Whose Hands," ECONOMIC PRIORITIES REPORT, Council on Economic Priorities, 84 Fifth Ave., New York, NE 10011, August/November 1973. pp. 2-52
. . . explores the irresponsibility of the drug industry: profits, effectiveness of products, safety of drugs and more. It includes a thorough profile of the top 16 drug manufacturers (accounting for 68% of all sales) as well as a useful glossary of drug-related terms.

"DRUG ADVERTISING AND PERCEPTION OF MENTAL ILLNESS," KNOW, P.O. Box 86031, January 1971. 10 pp.
. . . highly documented account of the role of the drug industry in defining mental "illness," particularly in women. "600-800 million dollars is spent yearly for the advertisements and promotion of all drugs. This is a little less than the total spent on all medical schools in the United States in

1956. We might estimate that 200 million dollars is spent in promotion of psychotropic (mood-altering) drugs." The article identifies seven areas where the drug industry is trying to convince doctors that medication will "cure" the individuals, such as women, distressed by tedious housework, or an older person bothersome to his/her family. Includes many glaring examples of sexism in drug industry advertising.

"Company Town at FDA," Michael Jacobson and Robert White, THE PROGRESSIVE, 408 W. Gorham St., Madison WI 53703, April 1973, pp. 48-53
. . . exposes the extent of collusion between the food and drug industries and the Food and Drug Administration. The authors report case after case of former industry employees making high level decisions within FDA on products of their prior employer. Equally common are FDA officials moving on to lucrative food and drug industry jobs, well educated in the decision making process of FDA and the trade secrets of their competitors, not to mention well known to influential government officials and policy makers.

"Health Information During a Week of Television," Frank A. Smith, et al, NEW ENGLAND JOURNAL OF MEDICINE, 10 Shattuck, Boston, MA 02115, March 9, 1972, pp. 516-520
. . . reports the results of an experiment whereby "a commercial network television channel in Detroit was monitored during a typical 130 hour broadcast week." Three medical students evaluated health-related content as to its usefulness and accuracy; they found "10 times as many. . .messages urging the use of pills or other remedies as there were against drug use or abuse."

"How to Lower the Price of Prescription Drugs," in A Public Citizen's Action Manual, Donald K. Ross. Citizen Action Group, 2000 P Street, NW, Washington, D.C. 20036, 1973 238 pp. $1.95
. . . good, brief examination of why "Americans spend over five billion annually on prescription drugs alone. Also included is a brief, step-by-step process for concerned people to eliminate this sophisticated form of thievery.

"THE CASE OF RITALIN," Alan F. Charles, available from Louise Rice, 65 Chestnut St., Cambridge MA 02139, October 31, 1971. 3 pp. $.14
. . . more accurately titled the case against ritalin, this article explains how the drug is commonly used and the inherent dangers. In essence, Ritalin is given to children who do not conform to the norm, although "parents and teachers may want to consider the proposition that it is the schoolroom atmosphere and not the child's behavior which is pathological." Often there is no medical basis for prescribing the drug and little energy is invested in discovering the real causes of the child's behavior: hunger, emotional stress, poor teaching and overcrowded classrooms to name a few. The drug's "manufacturer admitted that Ritalin accounts for 15% of his gross profits, or about $13 million a year."

Children have a great deal of energy; they live and learn with their muscles and bodies, not just their eyes and ears. When adults try to compel them to remain still and silent for long periods of time they resent and resist it. Most of them can be cowed and silenced by various bribes and threats, 5 to 15% cannot. These we diagnose as suffering from a learning malady called "hyperkenesis" and so they are drugged into submissiveness.
—John Holt

WOMENS' HEALTH

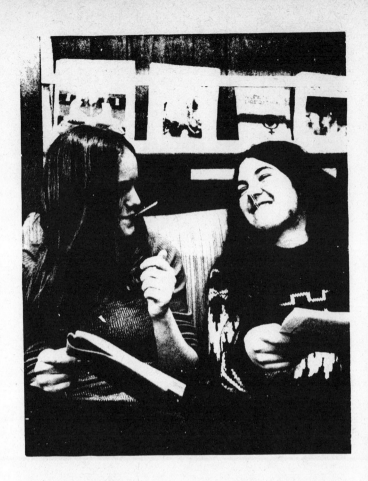

The emerging women's movement has found one of its major focuses in the field of health. Many of women's health needs are unique to them as women: menstrual problems, choices in forms of birth control, vaginitis, abortion, care during pregnancy, childbirth, menopause. Such specifically female concerns inevitably become focal points revealing society's (and doctors') sexist attitudes towards women. The combination of women's special health concerns and dominance by men makes health care a logical area for women to organize and assert their new demands for self-determination.

Medicine, like US society in general, is male-controlled; 92% of all doctors and 97% of the gynecologists are men. Medical schools are reluctant to accept women, claiming that they will marry and give up their careers. Women who convince admissions committees they are serious and committed find their problems are not over. One cardiologist reports: "If you complain, you're a bitch; if you don't, you're too passive. If a woman has some idiosyncrasy, like brashness or aggressiveness, she has a personality problem; if a man has the same trait—he's probably a surgeon."

The health industry routinely treats women in patronizing and demeaning ways. Women find doctors have no time to answer questions or explain what's being done to them. Third World and poor women, especially, receive inadequate and impersonal care—including such obvious violations of their rights as sterilization without their consent. Women have been used as guinea pigs to test birth control and morning-after pills, often without their knowledge, or without warning of the dangers involved. For example, in one birth-control pill study done on poor Chicano women, some of the women were given placebos (pills which actually contain no active ingredient). The purpose was to find out if the side effects women complain of are psychosomatic. Of course, a number of the Chicano women who thought they were on birth control became pregnant—a "side effect" that apparently did not concern the researchers.

In many ways our culture leads women to live unhealthy lives. The myth of femininity discourages the building of physical strength, and demands that women use "sex appeal" tooth pastes that corrode enamel from teeth, starve themselves into shapes they were never meant to be, and use cosmetics that are bad for skin, hair and general health. The National Commission of Product Safety reported in 1970 that cosmetics "injured 60,000 persons, mostly women, annually, so seriously as to restrict activities for one day or require medical attention." Feminine deodorant sprays, for example, can cause irritation, infection, swelling and other adverse reactions. A classic case of manufacturers creating demand for a useless product (soap and water is as effective and safer), feminine deodorant sprays were first introduced in the US in 1966. By 1969, sales exceeded $19 million, and by 1974 were nearly three times that. (FDA Consumer, Oct. 1973)

In opposition to such degrading commercialization, the women's movement is creating new, healthy and self-affirming life-styles. And women have begun the long process of eliminating sexism in health care, particularly in those areas of concern unique to women. They are creating their own services to provide direct medical care through women's clinics, self-help training, contraceptive services, etc. Other programs serve women through referrals, education, advocacy, lobbying, litigation and doctor-clinic monitoring (evaluating area health services). The first groups listed below are general resource groups or projects that cover a variety of areas. (See also Feminist Counseling in section on Mental Health.)

CHICAGO WOMEN'S LIBERATION UNION (CWLU)...includes about 20 work-groups throughout the city, involved in programs ranging from rap groups to study and service projects. The Health Evaluation and Referral Service of the CWLU provides referral, information and counseling on health care. Other health-oriented projects include an Abortion Task Force, Southside Women's Health Collective, and the Rape Crisis Line. CWLU publishes an internal newsletter for member groups and a feminist newspaper, Womankind, which includes extensive coverage of feminist health issues. Cost is 25 cents/monthly issue. Contact CWLU, 852 W. Belmont, Chicago, IL 60657, 312-348-0430 or 312-528-2736 for the Health Evaluation and Referral Service.

FEMINIST WOMEN'S HEALTH CENTER...has projects in Los Angeles, Oakland, and Santa Ana, California, with two new offices in formation. The centers exist to help women take decisive control of their bodies through self-help clinics, paramedic training, free well-women clinic services including pregnancy screening, birth control information, counseling and referral, abortion counseling and advocacy services, a speakers' bureau, and advanced self-help research. The centers offer summer school programs in medicine, feminism, social politics and business skills. In the future they hope that women will be able to get college credit for the courses. Women needing abortions can simply call the Center; all appointments and arrangements are made for them, and a patient's advocate accompanies the woman through the entire procedure. Using their influence as a referral agency, the Center is able to make effective demands on doctors and hospitals. The Oakland Center hopes to open an abortion clinic staffed by a feminist doctor and paramedics. Literature on feminist health and self-help are distributed by the Centers as part of a strong emphasis on sisterhood and demystifying medicine. Contact FEMINIST WOMEN'S HEALTH CENTER, 746 S. Crenshaw, Los Angeles, CA 90005, 213-936-7219; 429 S. Sycamore, Santa Ana, CA 92701, 714-547-0327; 444 48th St., Oakland, CA 94706, 415-653-2130.

YALE UNIVERSITY HEALTH PLAN...is a prototype campus group offering extensive gynecological services for women students, employees and families. A gynecologist and psychiatric social worker are available for counseling on birth control, abortion and human sexuality. OB/GYN services are free, including abortions and surgical expenses. Maternity costs are covered if the baby is delivered at Yale-New Haven hospital; if not, the Health Plan pays all doctor bills and $350 towards hospital costs. Contact YALE HEALTH PLAN, 17 Hillhouse Ave., New Haven, CT 06520, 203-436-2203.

BERKELEY WOMEN'S HEALTH COLLECTIVE...has about 75 members, all of whom are involved in smaller function groups, centered around a specific interest. Some women paramedics offer a weekly women's clinic and baby's day at the Berkeley Free Clinic. Other collective members maintain a storefront office, providing birth control and abortion counseling, information on nutrition, and monitoring of doctors. A third group within the collective has written a book on nutrition, Feeding Ourselves. Funding from the Berkeley City Council and donations pays a small group of women to do administrative work. The collective strives to demystify medicine and help women control their own bodies. Contact BERKELEY WOMEN'S HEALTH COLLECTIVE, 2214 Grove ST., Berkeley, CA 94704, 415-843-6194.

PHILADELPHIA WOMEN'S HEALTH COLLECTIVE ... began in 1970 and currently has 12 members. The major thrust of their energy recently has been toward the creation of a 45-minute slide show, focusing on women as health workers. It covers a brief history of women and the health care system, and evidence of sexism, racism and classism directed at women health workers. Past projects of the collective are the compilation of experimentation and abortion guidelines and involvement in the Harvey Karman case. The latter involved medically unsafe abortions performed on 20 Chicago women (brought to Philadelphia before abortion was legalized), resulting in a high incidence of complications. The collective has done some writing around the incident as well as considerable analysis of the politics of butcher abortion and subsequent trials. Meetings are held weekly at collective members homes. Contact PHILADELPHIA WOMEN'S HEALTH COLLECTIVE, c/o Amy Brodkey, 5427 Wayne Ave., Philadelphia, PA 19144, (215) 844-5122.

SAN FRANCISCO WOMEN'S HEALTH CENTER . . . offers a wide range of services including self-help demonstrations and classes, a menopause rap group, the beginnings of a medical referral system, a birth center (working toward good hospital and home pre-natal, labor and post-natal care), and excellent literature and information on other health projects. In addition, women are doing research into herbal medicine, premenstrual tension and making a self-help film. Acting out of a strong feminist consciousness, the group is concerned with challenging the health delivery system as it presently exists. Contact SAN FRANCISCO WOMEN'S HEALTH CENTER, 3789 24th St., San Francisco, CA 94114, (415) 282-6999.

WOMEN'S HEALTH FORUM...promotes and implements programs to "educate and support women in their struggle for quality health care." They offer courses on such subjects as menopause and teen-age sex education, while maintaining a literature center and speakers bureau. The literature center has been particularly successful as a consciousness-raising tool. WHF staff includes three full-time and two part-time women plus fifteen volunteers, many of whom are involved in teaching WHF courses. Contact WOMEN'S HEALTH FORUM, 156 Fifth Ave., Suite 1228, New York, NY 10010, 212-691-1140.

ASIAN WOMEN'S CENTER...grew out of a student group, Asian Sisters, which worked with young Asian women hooked on drugs. With HEW funding, the Center provides full-time counseling on drug abuse and prevention, family conflicts and pregnancy. The staff consists of paid and volunteer women, many of whom are ex-addicts. The Center exists to help Asian women fight the double oppression of racism and sexism and be more forceful in demanding their rights. Contact ASIAN WOMAN'S CENTER, 722 South Oxford, Los Angeles, CA 90005, (213) 387-1347.

RALEIGH CITY WOMEN'S HEALTH COMMITTEE...developed when a group of 30 West Virginia women decided to organize for better health care in their area. Dissatisfied with the local doctors, they helped bring in a new doctor so that people would have more of a choice. They have distributed pamphlets on "What is a Good Gynecological Exam" and give support to local people working on health issues. Some women in the group have organized a self-help class, and 3 people teach prepared childbirth classes in a local church. Pregnant women and their partners travel from surrounding counties to learn about their bodies and share experiences. Contact RCWHC, c/o Ruth Yarrow, Cool Ridge, WV, 304-787-5872.

NATIONAL BLACK FEMINIST ORGANIZATION...confronts the dual racist and sexist oppression of Black women. Members participate on committees directed at addiction, Black lesbianism, creative writing, rape, media image of Black women, and more. In addition, general monthly meetings focus on sex role stereotyping and the Black child, female sexuality, and Black women as consumers. The First Eastern Regional Conference on Black Feminism was sponsored by NBFO and attracted over 500 participants. NBFO is setting up a mechanism for affiliation of local chapters and will help Black feminists establish contact with sisters in their area. Contact NBFO, 370 Lexington Ave., NY, NY 10017, (212) 685-2344.

KNOW, INC...began as a group of women "who believed you can't have a revolution without a press — and bought one." KNOW functions as a collective and carries a large variety of articles and books, covering all aspects of the women's movement. Their health literature topics range from vaginal infections and abortions to feminist psychotherapy. Other projects are KNOW NEWS, an irregular bulletin, and periodically up-dated lists of feminist periodicals and "Reporters You Can Trust." Contact KNOW, INC., PO Box 86031, Pittsburgh, PA 15221, 412-241-4844.

RESOURCES

BOOKS

Our Bodies Ourselves, Boston Women's Health Book Collective. Simon Schuster, 630 Fifth Ave., New York, NY 10020, 1973. 275 pp. $2.95.
...a lot of love went into this book. It's full of hope, courage, and a strong sense of struggle—besides being packed with much needed information. It's a great relief to read a health book by women who assume some intelligence on the part of the reader, and who are not afraid to let their feelings show in their writing. There is much in this book that all women need to know: information on reproduction, childbirth, exercise, menopause, lesbianism, contraception, venereal disease, abortion, nutrition and self-defense. Discussions of more general topics, such as sexuality, personal relationships and the US health care system make this book the most comprehensive health resource to date. Our Bodies Ourselves combines personal experience with practical information, the realities of the US health empire with programs for change. With ample graphics and charts, it is a sensible, passionate work for women of all ages striving to understand and control their own bodies.

New Women's Survival Catalog, Kirsten Grimstad and Susan Rennie .Coward, McCann & Geoghegan, 200 Madison Ave., New York, NY 10016, 1973. 224 pp. $5.00
... top-notch national directory of feminist groups, services and resources. The excellent use of graphics and design give one a real sense of the strength and energy of the women's movement, although the lack of an index makes the book somewhat difficult to use. Includes information on lesbians, communications, art, health, children, learning, self-defense, work and justice.

The Rights of Women: The Basic ACLU Guide to a Woman's Rights, Susan R. Cross. Discus Books/Avon Books, 250 West 55th St., NY, NY 10019, 1973. 384 pp. $1.25
...strongly recommended guide to women's rights under the law and suggestions on how to change them. Written in question and answer form, the book covers: Constitutional rights, employment discrimination, education, mass media, crimes and juvenile delinquency, health care, divorce, names and name changes, and more. The section on health focuses on abortion, birth control and sterilization.

Women's Medical Directory, Feminist Mental Health Project, AFSC, 2160 Lake St., San Francisco, CA 94121. 68 pp. $ .25.
...prototype guide to medical facilities for women in one area (San Francisco, Berkeley, Oakland). Each entry includes name, address, phone, who the program serves, hours, fees, and services offered. The directory covers a wide range of straight and alternative facilities. Occasionally it includes subjective descriptions, although more would be valuable, particularly when covering straight institutions. Strong feminist consciousness, good graphics and quotes.

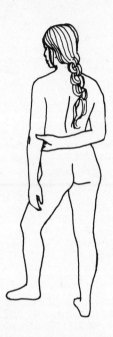

I want a women's revolution like a lover.
I lust for it, I want so much this freedom,
this end to struggle and fear and lies
we all exhale, that I could die just
with the passionate uttering of that desire.
Just once in this my only lifetime to dance
all alone and bare on a high cliff under cypress trees
with no fear of where I place my feet.

--Robin Morgan

What Women Should Know About the Breast Cancer Controversy, George Crile, Jr., MD. Macmillan Publishing Co., Inc., 866 Third Ave., New York, NY 10022, 1973. 179 pp. $4.95
...asserts that radical mastectomy as a treatment for breast cancer is no longer necessary. The author feels strongly that women must be informed of all possible treatments and the risks that accompany each one. He describes the range of possibilities, from a simple mastectomy to radiation, and points out the fact that doctors may be tempted to do unnecessary radical mastectomies because they make the most money that way. This book will help women make informed decisions about their bodies.

Women's Organizations and Leaders, Myra E. Barrer, ed., Today Publications, National Press Building, Washington, DC 20004, 1973. $25
. . . national listing of more than 8000 women and women's organizations. Each entry gives an address, phone number, and very sketchy description. Not limited to feminists, the book's major value is as a library reference since the cost makes it prohibitive for individuals.

PAMPHLETS AND ARTICLES

"COMPLAINTS AND DISORDERS: THE SEXUAL POLITICS OF SICKNESS," Barbara Ehrenreich and Deirdre English, Glass Mountain Pamphlet No. 2, The Feminist Press, Box 334, Old Westbury, NY 11568, 1973. 96 pp. $1.50.
. . .a revealing study of the relationship of medical practice and beliefs to women's oppression. The authors stress the power of doctors to keep women down with the rationale that it's all "for their own good." Tracing medical history from the nineteenth century to the present, the authors point out that because of their fragility, upper class women were prevented from any kind of meaningful work while working class women could do nothing but work under conditions hazardous to both physical and mental health. The history in this pamphlet is fascinating—its main point extremely well presented: women's oppression does not stem from biology, but from a "social system based on sex and class domination." Women must seize control of the technology that defines their biology if they hope to change that social system.

"HEALTH RESEARCH GROUP REPORT ON THE MORNING AFTER PILL," DC PIRG, 2000 P SL., NW, Suite 708, Washington, DC 20036, 1972, 8 pp. Free
. . .documents the dangers involved in Morning After Pill (MAP) usage, the lack of adequate research, its rate of effectiveness, the irresponsible manner in which it is prescribed and recommendations for action. This article is enough to convince anyone not to use it!

"Afterthoughts On The Morning-After Pill," Kay Weiss, MS, Nov., 1973. pp. 22-26
...angry, frightening article on DES (diethylstibestrol), chief component of the morning-after pill. Traces the history of DES usage as an anti-miscarriage drug between 1945 and 1965, resulting in about 200 cases of a rare type of vaginal or cervical cancer in the daughters of the women. "When Charles Edwards, Commissioner of the Food and Drug Administration was asked in November, 1971, why he did not alert those young women whose mothers had taken DES during pregnancy to have immediate medical examinations, he responded that the FDA had to be 'careful not to create an emotional crisis on the part of American women.' " In a powerful indictment of the morning-after pill, the author explains "any woman who takes the 50-milligram dose daily for five days, which constitutes the morning-after pill, is ingesting 835,000 times the amount of DES that the FDA has declared 'unfit for human consumption' in beef." Analyzes why DES (which resulted in sales of nearly $2 million for the Lilly Co. alone in 1972) is still on the market: "If the FDA were less protective of the profits of large drug companies, and the medical profession were less eager to do competitive research, we might assume that neither would want to repeat the mistakes of the 1940s and 1950s with a new DES drug."

"Those Vaginal Deodorants," Judith Ramsey, MS, November, 1972, pp. 28-33.
...expose of the vaginal deodorant industry: how advertisers set out to convince women to be ashamed of their bodies, side effects and dangers, lack of adequate testing and more. "Last year some 24 million women spent a cool $50 million on these products...Since deodorants are considered cosmetics, neither the manufacturers nor the government is legally obliged to conduct the kind of intensive studies mandatory for new drugs. Furthermore, the manufacturers don't even have to list the ingredients." Ramsey cites articles written by several gynecologists warning of the effects of vaginal deodorants, such as bad cases of vulvitis (infection of the vulva). Good factual coverage, although lacking in righteous anger.

"THE GYNECOLOGICAL CHECK-UP," Health Organizing Collective of NY Women's Health and Abortion Project, 36 W. 22nd St., New York, NY 10010, 1971, 8 pp.
...perfect for women who have never had an internal exam (or for those of us who were never too sure what was happening). Diagrams name the organs and demonstrate how the examination is done. Besides explaining what will happen, the pamphlet lists what should be covered in a thorough examination (weight and blood pressure, general medical herstory, gynecological herstory, external and internal exam, pap test, test for infections and VD, bimanual exam).

"YOUR BREASTS: INFORMATION AND SELF-EXAMINATION," San Francisco Women's Health Center, 3789 24th St., San Francisco, CA 94114. 12 pp. $.25
. . . written with a pervasive feminist bias, this pamphlet covers the anatomy of the breast, how-to-do self-examination, types of breast lumps, patients' rights, and treatment for malignant tumors. Since 6% of US women get breast cancer, this pamphlet is well worth reading and sharing.

"Menopause: A Rite of Passage," Joan Solomon, MS, Dec., 1972, pp. 16-18
...brief introduction to menopause: biological changes, medical response, and psychological implications. Views estrogen pills with due suspicion, quoting a woman who worked with one of the biggest producers: "The drug companies are tremendously excited by the notion of 'estrogens forever.' Permanent medication means permanent money in their pockets. So they urge physicians to give estrogen to their patients for the rest of their lives." The article also notes that in societies where the status of women rises in middle age, menopausal depression has not been reported, according to Dr. Pauline Barl, a sociologist at the University of Illinois."

PERIODICALS

OFF OUR BACKS, 1724 20th St., NW, Washington, DC 20009. $5/year individual, $15/institutions

WOMANKIND, Chicago Women's Liberation Union, 852 W. Belmont Ave., Chicago, IL 60657. $4/year, individual; $12/year, institutions

THE SECOND WAVE, Vol. 2, No. 3, Box 344, Cambridge, A, Cambridge, MA 021391. $3/year

HERSELF, 225 E. Liberty, Suite 200, Ann Arbor, MI 48108. $4/year, $10/institutions

SISTER, The Women's Center, 218 South Venice Blvd., Venice, CA 90291. $3/year. $.25/copy

THE WORKING MOTHER, Maternal Services, Inc., Suite 1E, 46 W. 96th St., New York, NY 10025. $3/year (individuals) $10/year (organizations)

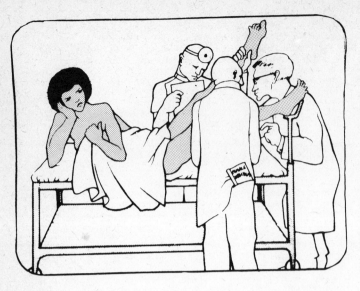

WOMEN'S CLINICS

Clinics run by and for women provide an immediate alternative to a sexist medical system. Generally, such clinics are not large enough to directly challenge the medical establishment. But they offer immediate assistance to some women and serve as a valuable educational tool by demystifying medicine and demonstrating that medical care need not be hierarchical or sexist. Women's clinics are a concrete way for women to assume power over their lives. Learning about their own bodies, and turning for help to other women rather than to a condescending and alienating male system, can be a powerful builder of pride and self-confidence. Many women first entered the women's movement through women's clinics, which often act as centers of information on a whole spectrum of women's issues.

To increase women's understanding of their own bodies, many clinics are initiating self-help groups where women perform their own pelvic exams. Through self-help exams women can catch early symptoms of vaginal infections and often successfully treat them, and detect signs of pregnancy. Through self-help and self-education women gain the understanding and confidence to challenge the patronizing and closed-mouthed attitudes of most doctors. Women learn to question doctors directly about examinations and diagnosis, insisting on understanding what is happening to them and what the doctor proposes to do.

At the same time, women's clinics provide support and encouragement for those clinic workers who decide to become full time health workers. As doctors and other workers, these women will challenge the sexist and profiteering aspects of the whole health system. So women's clinics act as a nucleus of change, building forces both inside and outside the medical system.

The following clinics are only examples. No comprehensive listings of women's clinics exist, but local women's centers can usually provide contacts.

FILMS AND TAPES

Newsreel, 26 W. 20th St., New York, NY 10011
  "The Women's Film," 45 min. b&w $60
  One of the first films to come out of the Women's Movement, it is still distinguished by its documenting of Third World women who unite to change their oppressed condition. Reveals the relationship among sexism, racism, and class structure.

Impact, 144 Bleecker St., New York, NY 10012
  "Growing Up Female," 60 min. b&w $70 1971 (sale: $375)
  An honest and persuasive film about the socialization and sex role of the American woman, realized through a personal look into the lives of sex females of varying ages, background, and race.

Feminist Woman's Health Centers, 746 Crenshaw Blvd., Los Angeles, CA 90005
  "Radical Mastectomy," 30 min. b&w $30 (sale: $50)
  Every year, 50,000 women in the US undergo radical mastectomies, many of them unnecessary. In this tape older women share their knowledge and feelings as well as their astute political analysis of this situation.

Video Women c/o Minda Bikman, 535 Hudson St., New York, NY 10014
  "Women Talk About Sex," 30 min. b&w
  Women speak about heterosexuality, bisexuality, lesbianism, older women's sexuality, and the relationship between economics and sexuality.

Great Atlantic Radio Conspiracy, 2743 Maryland Ave., Baltimore, MD 21218
  "Women and Health Care," 30 min. cassette tape No. 06-1173-70 (sale: $5). An informative, entertaining tape covering such subjects as feminist therapy, nursing, self-help, women hospital workers and a brief history of women in medicine. Interspersed with bits of song, the tape is an excellent introduction to women's health issues. The self-help discussion is particularly engaging.

(See also Health Education in section on Community Health.)

WELL WOMAN CENTER...serves Chicano, White, and some Black women, mostly between 25 and 35. The collective of eight women works with two doctors, offering self-help classes, birth control, menopause counseling, pap smears and pregnancy tests. One of the doctors delivers in his office, and the Center itself hopes to be licensed for child delivery soon. The Center offers educational programs on preventive medicine in local schools, factories and homes, as well as in the Center. Funding comes from a bank loan and patients' fees. The minimum request for a service is $5; beyond that, patients are asked to pay the cost of services provided if possible or make a donation. Contact WELL WOMAN CENTER, 1050 Garnet Ave., San Diego, CA 92109, 714-488-7591.

SOMERVILLE WOMEN'S HEALTH PROJECT...is a collective of 40 women serving a predominately White working-class community. The project sponsors medical nights for women and children twice a week, classes in "Women and Our Bodies" and first aid, and counseling on drugs, birth control and abortion. Affiliated with the Project is a mental health collective, dealing with short-term counseling. The project has received some foundation funding for the drug counseling center and hopes to get enough support in the future to expand to a full-time women's clinic and counseling service. The Project, in an attempt to effectively serve the local community, will only accept Somerville residents. Contact SOMERVILLE WOMEN'S HEALTH PROJECT, 326 Somerville Ave., Somerville, MA 02143, 617-666-5290.

ARADIA CLINIC...exists to offer women free, quality medical care and to challenge established medical practices. It began in 1971 when the women of the University of Washington YWCA decided to act on the lack of responsive medical care for women. Using a loan from the YWCA, and led by a woman architect, 60 women learned the necessary skills to transform a warehouse into a clinic. The Clinic is completely staffed by women; patients are encouraged to ask questions and to understand the treatment and the expected results. Services offered include: information on menstruation, conception, menopause and sexuality; detection and treatment of vaginitis, urinary infections and VD; pregnancy detection and counseling; routine pelvic exams including pap smears; and breast exams. Women seeking non-gynecological services are referred to an area clinic and accompanied by a patient's advocate from Aradia. Aradia is run collectively, with six paid staff and many volunteers. Training for paramedics and lab workers is offered jointly by Aradia and three other Seattle women's clinics. Women from many other states have visited Aradia, to get ideas on training and other programs. Contact ARADIA CLINIC, 4224 University Way NE, Seattle, WA 98105, 206-634-2090.

THE WOMEN'S HEALTH CLINIC...is a free health care clinic run collectively by and for women. The 40 volunteers (including several RN's) serve about 150 lower-income women from Southeast Portland each month. Emphasizing preventive medicine and education, the clinic offers blood pressure checks, pregnancy tests and counseling, pap smears, and gynecological referrals. Patients are taught basic anatomy and are given explanations of their examinations as they happen. Training of the volunteers is being expanded to include complete pelvic exams and first aid. In the future they hope to bring preventive health care programs, including preventive dental care, directly into the community. Contact the WOMEN'S HEALTH CLINIC, 4160 SE Division St., Portland, OR 97202, 503-234-9774.

WOUNDED KNEE WOMEN'S HEALTH COLLECTIVE...consists of 18 Native American women in the Porcupine Ridge district of the Pine Ridge reservation who came together to learn and share knowledge of their bodies. Currently, their energies are devoted to study and community education around birth control VD, vaginitis, prenatal care, self-help and pap smears. In addition, the Collective is surveying the health needs of local women and attitudes toward birth control. For women unable to travel or reach a central location, the Collective arranges "home clinics," although they hope to use the proposed Wounded Knee Free Clinic as a base of operations. The work of the Collective is important not only as an expression of women understanding and controlling their own bodies, but also as a direct medical service in an area incredibly short of doctors and health personnel (4 doctors serve the entire Pine Ridge reservation of 13,000). Contact WOUNDED KNEE WOMEN'S HEALTH COLLECTIVE, c/o Larelei Means, 807 Fariview St., Rapid City, SD 57701, (605) 348-5629.

VERMONT WOMEN'S HEALTH CENTER...resulted from a 1972 Vermont Supreme Court ruling which liberalized state abortion laws. A group of women came together—including committed feminists, two physicians, single and married women, and women with children—to develop a clinic. The staff currently includes two female OB/GYNs, four full-time and eight part-time paramedics, and volunteers from the community. The Center does vacuum aspiration abortions and early uterine evacuation (an early abortion that can be used 35-65 days after the last menstrual period). They also provide gynecological check-ups and treatment, counseling and health education. Open every weekday, the clinic serves about 100 patients per week. Fees are set on a sliding scale. The Center is a fine example of a feminist owned and run clinic offering a wide range of services in a positive atmosphere. Contact VERMONT WOMEN'S HEALTH CENTER, Box 29, Burlington, VT 05401, 802-655-1600.

We are rising, powerful in our unclean bodies; bright glowing mad in our inferior brains; wild hair flying, wild eyes staring, wild voices keening; undaunted by blood we who hemorrhage every twenty-eight days; laughing at our own beauty we who have lost our sense of humor; mourning for all each precious one of us might have been in this one living time-place had she not been born a woman.... We are rising with a fury older and potentially greater than any force in history, and this time we will be free or no one will survive.
POWER TO ALL THE PEOPLE OR TO NONE.

--Robin Morgan

RESOURCES

PAMPHLETS AND ARTICLES

CIRCLE ONE SELF-HELP HANDBOOK," Vicki Ziegler and Elizabeth Campbell, 409 E. Fontanero, Colorado Springs, CO 80907, 1973. 34 pp. $.75
... a warm and beautiful book on women reclaiming their bodies. With a sprinkling of poetry and personal testimony, it covers pelvic exams, bi-manual exams, breast exams, vaginal infections and their treatment, the physiology of sex, masturbation, childbirth and more. The intent is to provide a broad base of information for women entering (or involved in) the self-help movement. Excellent how-to guide with lots of graphics; a real high to read.

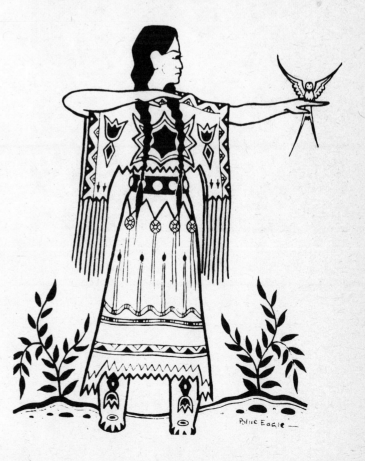

"INFECTIONS OF THE VAGINA," Health Organizing Collective of NY Women's Health and Abortion Project, 36 W. 22nd St., New York, NY 10010, or KNOW, PO Box 86031, Pittsburgh, PA 15221. 11 pp. 10 cents.
...explains the symptoms and causes of common vaginal and urinary infections as well as effective treatment. Offers suggestions on where to get help and a brief discussion of problems women face in the health delivery system. Short and clear.

FILMS

Feminist Women's Health Centers, 746 Crenshaw Blvd., Los Angeles, CA 90005

"Self-Help Clinic," 30 min. b&w $30 (sale: $50)
The innovation which inspired a worldwide women's health movement was the concept and practice of self-help. This tape is a documentation of a Self-Help Clinic including discussion and self-examination.

Herstory Films, 17 E. 97th St. (3D), New York, NY 10029
"Know Your Body,"
Slide series designed to be used in a self-help group.

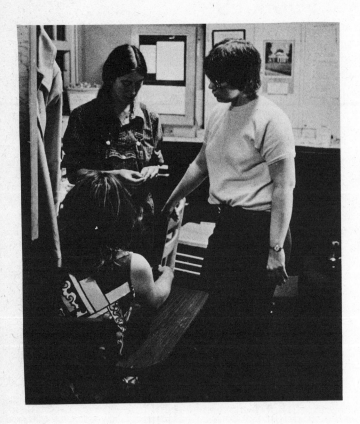

BIRTH CONTROL AND ABORTION

Women's control of their own bodies is the basic issue in both birth control and abortion. Traditionally women have been considered incapable of making responsible decisions in these areas, and so have been regulated by laws and (male) doctors.

Birth control should be the responsibility of both partners, yet the brunt of it falls on the woman, who will suffer the side-effects of dangerous birth control methods and the consequences of an unwanted pregnancy. We are including birth control in the section of women's health because virtually all birth control projects are closely related to women's health groups and because most forms effect women's bodies, not men's.

Women's health groups devote considerable energy to education and counseling on birth control, largely because there is no form of contraceptive which is completely acceptable. The pill and IUD, the most effective methods, can produce uncomfortable or dangerous side effects. Other forms of birth control produce fewer negative side effects, but with the exception of sterilization they are less effective.

Contraceptive drugs have repeatedly been distributed to women after inadequate and careless testing. Enovid, the first oral contraceptive marketed in the US, was given a trial run in Puerto Rico in 1956...Five women in this group died from 'heart attacks;' no autopsies were done. The handling of such experiments could help explain why British studies linked the pill to blood clotting risk two years before US studies. Similar irresponsible drug distribution is currently being carried on in the case of the Morning After Pill (MAP). College health clinics freely dispense the MAP containing Diethylstilbestrol (DES), although daughters of women who have taken the drug run a high risk of developing vaginal cancer. The pills are, in at least some instances, distributed without warning women of the dangers involved, without testing to see if the women are already pregnant from earlier intercourse (in which case the fetus may be affected), and without follow up to see if pregnancy continues in spite of the pill and whether the child is adversely affected. Incidents like this will continue as long as drug production and research continue to be dominated by corporations whose interest is in profits, and who have an obvious investment in finding their own products "safe."

The January 23, 1973 ruling of the Supreme Court on abortion, seen as a victory by the women's movement, abolished all restrictions on abortion during the first trimester, except the requirement that a licensed physician perform the abortion; during the second trimester the state can limit abortions to protect the woman's health and during the third trimester to protect the fetus.

The Supreme Court ruling is certainly a gain, and yet it is far from enough. Restrictions that exclude paraprofessionals from performing abortions are likely to limit their availability, keep the price artificially high and discourage the development of simpler procedures. Some hospitals still refuse to perform abortions, and Right-to-Lifers are fighting to pass highly restrictive legislation on state and federal levels. Foremost is the drive to outlaw abortion through a Constitutional Amendment. Well-financed lobbying groups and massive campaigns to gain public support (often paid for by tax-exempt Catholic Church money) make the anti-abortion movement a continuing threat.

Commercial abortion referral agencies are legal in almost all states. It is not uncommon for them to charge a substantial referral fee and then receive a kick-back from the doctor, thus doubling the cost of an abortion. One thrust of the women's movement is to provide an alternative to these commercial set-ups.

As with most health services, poor and Third World women face special problems. The cost of an abortion (minimum of $100-$125) may be prohibitive, and too many women wait until the second trimester, when the abortion is more expensive. Third World women often do not feel comfortable approaching White-dominated feminist groups for referrals, but it is difficult for women to investigate abortion services on their own.

Fewer women today request abortion counseling; as abortion becomes more accepted it carries less emotional stress. It is still important that counseling be available for women who are unsure of their own feelings about abortion, or who want to explore other options. But abortions should be viewed as a medical procedure which does not ordinarily require special counseling or legislation.

NATIONAL ABORTION RIGHTS ACTION LEAGUE (NA RAL)...has long been a leader in the struggle to guarantee safe and accessible abortions. The Association, formed in 1969, has used a variety of tactics, including education, litigation, lobbying, and direct confrontation; nevertheless, membership is broad based, encompassing a loose coalition of over 90 state and national groups involved in women's liberation, civil rights, professional and religious areas. Currently energy is focused against a proposed constitutional amendment to outlaw abortion and legislation to prohibit the use of Medicaid funds for abortions. Two members are working as lobbyists in a newly opened Washington office. NARAL is also legally challenging public hospitals which do not provide abortions and encouraging private hospitals to expand thier facilities. The Association, nationally recognized and respected, serves as a clearinghouse for ideas and literature on abortion and publishes a regular newsletter. NARAL staff includes two full-time and four part-time employees; funding is from donations. Contact NARAL, 250 W. 57th St., New York, NY 10019, 212-265-5125.

WOMEN'S HEALTH ADVOCACY GROUP...offers early, accurate pregnancy testing and pregnancy counseling, including a 24-hour phone line. Abortion and all other alternatives are thoroughly discussed once pregnancy is confirmed. The group will provide adoption agency referrals for women who wish to continue the pregnancy, or financial and housing assistance if the woman decides to keep her baby. Unmarried mothers are informed of their legal and welfare rights. Both Black and White women use these services. The only charge is $4 for pregnancy tests. The all-volunteer staff, made up of RN's and other concerned women, will train new volunteers for any of three different jobs: receptionist, pregnancy tester, and counsellor. Contact WOMEN'S HEALTH ADVOCACY, 5323 Oxford Ave., Philadelphia, PA 19124, 215-824-0161 or 331-7260.

CHOICE...is a multi-service project, committed to making safe and comfortable abortions available to all women. Choice programs include an Abortion Counseling Service, research and writing a manual on Abortion Counseling Services, development of a resource center on abortion and women's health, and a consultation service. The women at Choice realize that one abortion counseling service cannot serve their area, so through the consultation service, Choice plans to train other groups in providing abortion counseling and setting up health care facilities. Training or consultation does not necessarily lead to Choice endorsement. Their resource center will include a notebook and bulletin (available by subscription) on abortion facilities in the Philadelphia area as well as a hotline offering immediate information and referrals and eliciting feedback on area clinics and doctors. Choice, funded by foundation grants and donations, is staffed by a small group of paid coordinators and patients' advocates, and over 80 volunteer counselors. Most women served are single, under 30, and pregnant for the first time. Choice is aware of legislation to limit abortion in Pennsylvania and works to educate and unify people against such bills. Contact CHOICE, 2027 Chestnut St., Philadelphia, PA 19102, 215-567-2904.

Going one step further than the old Marxist dictum that workers must seize the means of production, we say women must seize the means of reproduction.

--Robin Morgan

POPULATION CONTROL FUND...of the University of Maine loans money to any student seeking an abortion. The project, started in the spring of 1971 with $5000 from the student senate, requires that a student sign the promissary note, although it can be used for a non-student. Written confirmation of pregnancy is requested when the students administering the loan feel doubt. Strict confidentiality is maintained, with a maximum of two people knowing the identity of the woman seeking a loan. In two years of operation, 85 loans have been given, 75% of which have been paid back. Contact Karen Edgecomb, POPULATION CONTROL FUND, 12 Lord Hall, Student Senate Office, University of Maine, Orono, ME 04473, 207-581-7801.

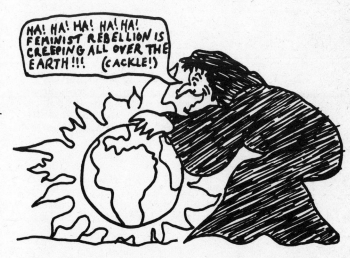

CLERGY CONSULTATION SERVICE ON ABORTION...is a loose national federation of clergy and lay counselling services to help women deal with problem pregnancies. The service was started in New York City by 20 ministers and rabbis, back in 1967 when such activities were still illegal; it has since spread to every state. A service affiliated with the national office cannot charge for counselling and must make referrals to responsible agencies. The Clergy Consultation Service hopes to increase its advocacy role and spend more energy making poor and Third World women aware of abortion possibilities. Though sometimes criticized as male-dominated, and certainly not strongly feminist in its orientation, the Service often offers counselling where other projects are not available. Contact CLERGY CONSULTATION SERVICE ON ABORTION, 55 Washington Square, S., New York, NY 10012, 212-477-0034.

PLANNED PARENTHOOD FEDERATION OF AMERICA
...has been instrumental in shaping birth control services in the US. PP also spent $25 million in 1972 on controlling the population in Latin America, Asia, and Africa. In many Third World countries, PP has been accused of pushing permanent or unsafe, experimental forms of birth control on unsuspecting women. PP is associated with the often-unpopular Agency for International Development, so some overseas towns are refusing their services. (AID is the US agency responsible for channeling most civilian foreign aid.) In the US, PP has been accused of genocide by Third World people who feel PP concentrates on controlling non-White birth rates, and pushes the pill above other, safer means of contraception. Some PP affiliate clinics have a reputation for prescribing birth control pills without adequately explaining the hazards, checking medical history, explaining preventive precautions, or treating the gynecological problems (such as vaginitis) that result. Nevertheless, PP is the largest US family planning organization, with 695 affiliate clinics. When used by women who already know the form of birth control best for them, PP clinics are an inexpensive or free source for birth control, pregnancy and VD testing and pap smears. Most of these clinics will serve women under 18 and give abortion referrals. Recently PP has sponsored several experimental programs: a vasectomy clinic in New York City, programs to train paraprofessionals and nurses in tasks traditionally reserved for doctors, and an experimental program for migrant workers. For a list of publications, films, and posters, contact PLANNED PARENTHOOD FEDERATION OF AMERICA, 810 Seventh Ave., NY, NY 10019, (212) 541-7800.

Abortion II: Making the Revolution, Lawrence Lader. Beacon Press, 25 Beacon St., Boston, MA 02167, 1973. 225 pp. $7.95
...relates the drama of courageous women and men fighting for the right to control conception. The list of heroines and heroes is long: Margaret Sanger, crusader for contraceptives in the early 20th century; Dr. W.J. Bryan Henrie of Grove, Oklahoma, who performed 5,000 abortions before 1962 for a maximum fee of $100 (despite an otherwise unblemished reputation and great support from the community, he was eventually arrested and jailed for two years); Patricia Maginnis, founder of the Society for Humane Abortion, and many more. Exciting and inspiring.

The Pill, Morton Mintz, Beacon Press, 25 Beacon St., Boston, MA 02167, 1970. 132 pp. $3.95
...sharply questions the safety of the birth control pill, while indicting the drug industry, medical establishment, and US government for withholding information on dangerous side effects. Mintz writes of the correlation between the pill and incidents of blood clotting, cancer, depression, nausea, loss of sexual interest and other adverse effects. Birth control pills are a big money maker for the drug companies, who invest heavily in promoting them to doctors. "In 1968, for example, net earnings after taxes (for G.D. Searle & Co., chief producer of the pill) were...more than 18%." Somewhat technical in its language at times, this book offers valuable information for questioning your doctor and making a personal decision on birth control.

PAMPHLETS AND ARTICLES

"IT'S ALL RIGHT DOC, I'M ONLY DYING," Susan Bondurant, available from KNOW, PO Box 86031, Pittsburgh, PA 15221. 3 pp. $ .10
...a brief, powerful statement by a Seattle woman who nearly died after being sterilized. The doctors involved refused to acknowledge the physical basis of her pain (blaming it on "guilt feelings") until women friends had repeatedly demanded X-rays, medication for pain, and a complete exam. After 18 hours, the doctors discovered that her large intestine had been perforated during the sterilization, a condition that would have been fatal if left untreated.

RESOURCES

BOOKS

Abortion Rap, Diane Schulder and Florynce Kennedy, 1971, McGraw-Hill, 239 pp. $3.95
...examines the abortion fight's relevance to the fight for women's freedom. It follows the case of Abronowicz vs. Lefkowitz, a challenge of abortion laws in New York State, 1969. Personal testimonies set forth the courage and suffering of women who endured the consequences of "compulsory pregnancy" laws—back-alley abortions, shot-gun marriages, being forced to "slink away." Experts examine the privileged access of the wealthy to safe abortions, the different emotional reactions to wanted and unwanted pregnancies, population control, and a theological position on abortion. Later chapters also direct attention to the Black genocide charge, the population explosion claim, the Friends of the Fetus, the hospital scene, and the church-state conflict. A strongly political perspective on abortion.

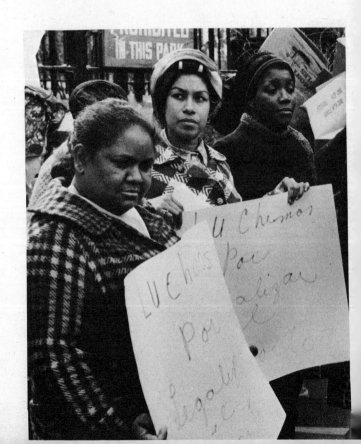

"BIRTH CONTROL HANDBOOK," Donna Cherniak and Allan Feingold, McGill University, 1970, $ .25, 47 pp.
...is an excellent presentation on the effects of different birth control methods. Included is a full bibliography (up to 1971) on Population and Birth Control, IUD's, and Hormonal Contraception. In a highly political introduction Zero Population Growth and Paul Ehrlich's THE POPULATION BOMB are sharply condemned for their support of forced sterilization. "I am sometimes astonished at the attitudes of Americans who are horrified at the prospect of our government insisting on population control as the price for food aid (to India)." (Ehrlich) This guide is the forerunner of the many birth-control handbooks distributed at US colleges; it is still the most complete and accurate birth control handbook in its price range.

"THE ABORTION GAME," Women's Health and Abortion Project, PO Box 136, Times Plaza Station, Brooklyn, NY 11217, 1972. 77 pp. $ .75
...excellent guide for women seeking abortions in New York City. Explains what happens during an abortion, gives information on all the city abortion clinics (address, type of abortion, cost, hours, Spanish-speaking staff, airport pick-up and fee, payment system, and much more). They also include subjective descriptions of the facilities and staff attitudes, a few brief essays on women's right to control their bodies; and a section on the abortion industry: "Abortion Bonanza—for Doctors," "Reform and Repeal," Abortion Counseling (and how the male capitalists use it for their benefit), and a limited bibliography. Practical and useful—a good model for other cities.

"Abortion and the Catholic Church; Two Feminists Defend Women's Rights," Evelyn Reed and Claire Moriarty. Pathfinder Press, 410 West St., New York, NY 10014, 1973. 14 pp. $ .35
...informative essays tracing the Catholic Church's stance against abortion, birth control and the liberation of women. Has continuing significance in light of the Church's massive contributions to continuing anti-abortion campaigns—such as the campaign to outlaw abortion by a constitutional amendment.

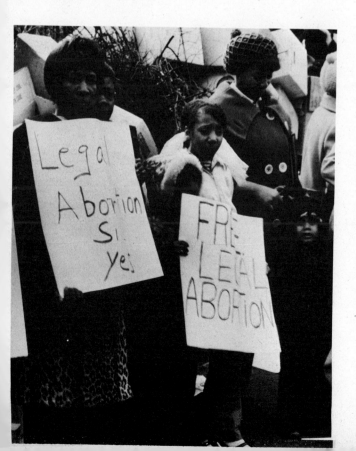

"HERNIA," Sarah Wernick Lockeretz, KNOW, PO Box 86031, Pittsburgh, PA 15221, 1972. 2 pp. $ .05
...amusing satire on abortion, with female legislators, doctors, and experts confronting male militants who demand legalization of hernia operations. "The strident males—mostly jacketless and tie-less, many not wearing athletic supports—puzzled and alarmed the legislators, medical experts, and others present." Cleverly and effectively reveals the absurdity of males controlling women's right to abortion.

"VACUUM ASPIRATION ABORTION," Health Organizing Collective of NY Women's Health and Abortion Project, 36 W. 22nd St., New York, NY 10010, 1971. 7 pp. $ .10
...clear, sensitive explanation of vacuum aspiration abortion, including step-by-step procedure and pictures of instruments used. Describes possible complications (hemorrhage, infection, perforation and incomplete abortion) and aftercare.

"SALINE ABORTION," Health Organizing Collective of the NY Women's Health and Abortion Project, 36 W. 22nd St., New York, NY 10010, 1971. 8 pp. $ .10
...diagrams and explains in detail how a saline abortion is performed, side effects and complications, who should have a saline abortion and how the woman should expect to feel. Prepares women for the abortion in a sympathetic and articulate manner.

"Study Packet on Abortion," United Methodist Church, 100 Maryland Ave., NE, Washington, DC 20002, 1972. $1.00
...complete, useful resource for study groups on abortion, particularly those religiously oriented. Packet includes: "Letters from Three Women," "Responsible Parenthood," locations of Clergy Consultation Service on Abortion, magazine articles, information on counseling, statements of churches concerning abortion, and much more. In a non-moralistic way, it poses questions for discussion, offers further resources and a plan of action (research, education, lobbying, coalition building, counseling). Although written before the Supreme Court ruling, most of the information is still relevant.

"The Philadelphia Story: Another Experiment on Women," Philadelphia Women's Health Collective. 5030 Newhall St., Philadelphia, PA 19144, 1972.
...describes illegal abortions performed on 20 Chicago women bussed to Philadelphia. Although asked to help with the weekend plans, the Philadelphia Women's Health Collective soon learned that it had no control over the experimental method used nor the filming of the abortions by a New York TV station. Sixty percent of the women receiving second trimester abortions had serious complications. The article demonstrates the need for women's referral services to watchdog the quality of abortions. Many women still find local doctors or hospitals will not perform abortions, so they must travel to an unfamiliar city where they are vulnerable to quacks and exploitive clinics.

"ABORTION: WOMEN'S FIGHT FOR THE RIGHT TO CHOOSE," Linda Jenness, Caroline Lund, Andrea Morell, Maxine Williams, Pathfinder Press, 410 West St., New York, NY 10010, 1973. 14 pp. $ .35
...contains short articles on the right to abortion, abortion and Black women, and the Supreme Court ruling. Good, reasoned defense of legalized abortion.

CHILDBIRTH

"HOW TO HAVE INTERCOURSE WITHOUT GETTING SCREWED," Lynn K. Hansen, Barbara Reskin, Diana Gray, Associated Students of the University of Washington, University of Washington, Seattle, WA 98105, 1972. 53 pp. ...an unusually thorough guide to birth control and abortion written and distributed by university students. It includes descriptions and diagrams of male and female anatomy, forms of contraception, sterilization, Morning After Pill, pregnancy, abortion, VD and common infections. The Appendix lists local birth control and counseling services and offers two essays on female sexuality. Especially good for student groups.

Other good campus pamphlets are:
"A SPERM AND EGG HANDBOOK," Wayne and Bruce Middendorf, Community Action Corps., 220 Norton Hall, SUNY at Buffalo, Buffalo, NY 14214, 1973. 30 pp.
"HOW TO TAKE THE WORRY OUT OF BEING CLOSE," Marian Johnson Gray and Roger W. Gray, PO Box 2822, Oakland, CA 94618, 1971. 32 pp.
"THE BOULDER BIRTH CONTROL HANDBOOK," Birth Control Information Commission, UMC 178, University of Colorado, Boulder, CO 80302, 1970. 18 pp.
"SEX IN A PLAIN BROWN WRAPPER," Student Committee on Sexuality at Syracuse University, Syracuse University, 7600 Ostrum Ave., Syracuse, NY 13210, 1973. 32 pp.

FILMS

New Day Films, 267 W. 25th St., New York, NY 10001
"It Happens To Us," 30 min. cl. $32 1971 (sale: $325)
Women of different ages, marital status, and race speak candidly about their abortion experiences. Their stories contrast illegal with legal medically safe abortions. One of the best abortion films around.

Newsreel, 26 W. 20th St., New York, NY 10011
"Blood of the Condor," 85 min. b&w (rental is open)
Based on a real occurrence, the film depicts the reaction of an Indian community leader to the forced sterilization of women by US Peace Corps volunteers, the functioning of Bolivian society, the retaliation of the system to the leader's revenge. In Spanish and Quenchua dialect, English subtitles.

Feminist Woman's Health Centers, 746 Crenshaw Blvd., Los Angeles, CA 90005
"Woman Controlled Abortion," 30 min. b&w $30 (sale: $50)
Includes two actual abortions performed at the Women's Choice Clinic (which is completely controlled by women) demonstrating good abortion procedure, and has visual and verbal material on the politics of population control, money, abortion and the women's movement.

The US currently ranks 15th in the world in infant mortality. This is not due to any lack of medical technology, but to poor distribution of doctors, high prices for medical treatment, a shortage of obstetricians, and a lack of other trained personell—including the prohibition of midwifery in some states.

Both the shortage of obstetricians and the predominance of men in this field have helped spark a movement among women to obtain training as midwives. The American College of Nurse Midwifery certifies midwives to work in most states. A Certified Nurse Midwife (CNM) has the equivalent of a Masters Degree in nursing with a specialization in nurse midwifery. She is qualified to prescribe medication, give pre- and postnatal care and participate on a doctor-directed medical team. She performs normal delivery with a doctor on call. In Sweden, the nation with the best record for infant mortality and maternal death, nurse midwives deliver all normal pregnancies.

Another major movement in the area of childbirth is toward prepared or natural childbirth. "Natural childbirth" means bearing a child without such "normal" medical procedures as anesthesia or other drugs. Natural childbirth techniques require exercises to prepare the woman physically for birth, breathing exercises to help ease labor, and education on what to expect during birth. Prepared childbirth refers to births where the mother has gone through the learning and exercises normal to natural childbirth, but with the option of using drugs in case of difficulty or strong pain. In either case, the purpose is to put the mother, or both parents, in control of the delivery, with the doctor playing a much more minor role than usual. With preparation, most women can deliver their children without drugs or anesthesia. This is both physically safer for mother and child, and more emotionally satisfying, since the woman actually experiences the birth rather than going through it in a drug-induced fog. Natural childbirth often includes family-centered maternity care, giving the father access to the delivery room and freeing the entire family to be together as much as desired during the period after birth.

But even women who have a safe and satisfying pregnancy and delivery must face social institutions which have little flexibility in dealing with pregnancy. Women are now working toward pregnancy leave with sick pay for working women and removal of restrictions on pregnant women attending schools. These are elementary, obvious steps in making childbirth a joyful experience for women who have chosen it freely.

BIRTH CENTER...started in 1971 when a group of Santa Cruz women decided to explore the possibility of home delivery. In a two year period they have delivered over 150 babies (all but 20 at home), have learned to provide pre-natal care including urine and blood tests, and have trained fathers to deliver their own children. They serve working class as well as young hip women, and their services are free, although donations are welcome. Birth Center hopes to expand, adding pregnancy and abortion counseling, pediatrics, and classes for new mothers, although they are held back by lack of money and lack of support from area doctors. The six women in Birth Center see pregnancy and childbirth as a potentially joyous experience, all too often ruined by feelings of loneliness and depression. They strive to make the experience of birth exciting and uniting for the entire family. Contact BIRTH CENTER, 208 Escalone Dr., Santa Cruz, CA 95060, 408-423-5632.

AMERICAN COLLEGE OF NURSE-MIDWIVES...is a professional organization consisting of approximately 750 certified nurse midwives (CNM). The college has approved 11 training programs in 8 states and Puerto Rico and certifies graduating Nurse Midwives through a national exam. Certification by the American College of Nurse Midwives is accepted in most states and qualifies the CNM to participate on a medical team headed by a doctor. Under normal conditions of pregnancy, the CNM delivers the baby and offers pre- and post-natal care. CNMs are exploring more comfortable methods of delivery and encouraging hospitals to allow husbands and friends in the delivery room. For more information, including a list of literature and schools offering nurse-midwifery training, contact AMERICAN COLLEGE OF NURSE-MIDWIVES, 50 E. 92nd St., New York, NY 10028, 212-369-7300.

MATERNITY INFANT CARE-FAMILY PLANNING PROJECT (MIC-FPP)...is a program of the City of New York Department of Health. In 1968 MIC-FPP initiated a plan to increase the number of Certified Nurse Midwives in city hospitals by paying 50% of the salary for 20 positions. Approximately one third of the staff is Black and all speak Spanish (non-Spanish speakers are taught the language when they enter the program). Nurse midwives divide their time evenly between the hospital and community-based clinics. MIC-FPP is an example of a positive government program to encourage the use of Allied Health Professionals. Contact MATERNITY INFANT CARE-FAMILY PLANNING PROJECTS, 377 Broadway, New York, NY 10013, 212-966-3828.

AMERICAN SOCIETY FOR PSYCHO-PROPHYLAXIS IN OBSTETRICS (ASPO) . . . is a non-profit, educational organization started in 1961 for the purpose of encouraging the practice of natural childbirth. The more than 20 local chapters, with a total membership greater than 3000, are divided into three subdivisions—doctors, teachers and other professionals, and parents. ASPO is the only organization in the US to train and certify teachers in the Lamaze method of natural childbirth. Occasionally, ASPO has legally forced hospitals to allow men in the delivery room, though they prefer to use persuasion and education. ASPO is financed by dues (doctors -$40; professionals-$25; parents-$7.50), donations, and tuition from childbirth classes. In general very professionally oriented, ASPO is currently seeking to provide more direct services by teaching in homes for single mothers and distribution of literature in Spanish. The national office will help individuals find Lamaze classes in their area, but encourages parents to check locally first as there is often a delay in answering requests. Contact ASPO, 1523 L St. NW, Washington DC 20005, 202-783-7050.

RESOURCES

BOOKS AND PAMPHLET

Birth Book, Raven Lang. Genesis Press, P.O. Box AJ, Cupertino, CA 95014, 1972. 100 pp. $6.00
. . .is written by people who enjoy their bodies and glory in the experience of home birth. This book expresses, through personal accounts, the pleasures and fears of women, their mates and friends participating in home delivery. There are also practical suggestions and warnings of possible problems with local physicians and hospitals. The history of childbirth is summarized, with strong criticism of present attitudes and procedures of childbirth. Amply filled with wonderful photographs, this book is a delight to read.

The Experience of Childbirth, Sheila Kitzinger. Pelican Book, 1972. 280 pp. $1.95.
...sensitive, detailed guide to pregnancy, labor and adjustment after the baby is born. Emphasizes birth as a changing, growing experience for both parents, with chapters on "The Psychology of Pregnancy," "The Parents' Adjustment," and "Childbirth with Joy." Explains the specifics of one technique of natural childbirth, including breathing patterns, muscle exercises, etc. Also covers home delivery (with a strong positive bias) and has five magnificent photos of a mother giving birth to twins. At times the sex-role stereotyping is offensively blatant, but otherwise the information is practical and precise.

"The Cultural Warping of Childbirth," Doris Haire, International Childbirth Education Association, PO Box 5852, Milwaukee, WI 53220, 1972. 35 pp. $ .60
...discusses why the US ranks behind 14 nations in infant mortality. The author shows that birth is much safer (for mother and child) in countries where common practices include the use of midwives, few drugs and more personalized care. Concludes with a checklist of 29 factors in obstetrical care, and explanations of their significance. Factual and forceful.

FILMS

Center for Mass Communication of Columbia University Press, 1365 S. Broadway, Irvington, NY 10533

"All My Babies," 55 min. b&w (sale: $330)
Shows the methods a midwife should follow from the time she takes a case until the baby is taken to its first Well Baby Clinic. Restricted to use by professional audiences and cinema courses.

Susan Kleckner, 117 Waverly Place, New York, NY
"Birth," 35 min. cl. $60 (sale: $350)
No matter whether you've seen films about births already, this is the one to see. A feminist and a lawyer, the mother has her baby at home, and the father is intimately involved. The moment of birth is intensely moving.

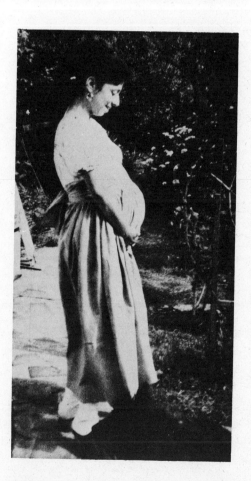

*Give birth to me, sisters, in struggle we transform
ourselves, but how often, how often
we need help to cut loose, to cry out, to breathe!
...This morning we must make each other strong.
Change is qualitative: we are
each other's miracle.*

--Marge Piercy

OCCUPATIONAL SAFETY AND HEALTH

PROBLEM

Sixteen thousand working men and women are killed each year in occupational accidents. Another 2.5 million are seriously injured, and at least 400,000 are stricken annually with serious occupational diseases: coal miners' pneumoconiosis (Black Lung); byssinosis (Brown Lung); silicosis, asbestosis (diseases related to breathing asbestos particles); and many more. Eleven miners a day die from Black Lung. The average life-span of a farm worker is 49 years. These are all only reported figures; as every worker knows, industry takes great pains to cover up as many workplace caused accidents, illnesses and deaths as possible.

One midwestern worker, representative of many, is totally disabled by lung cancer traceable to a six-month work exposure to asbestos. A California welder died after six hours exposure to cadmium fumes in silver solder, while six men in Colorado were hospitalized after breathing mercury fumes when a thermostat ruptured at 600 degrees F. Less blatant but more pervasive is the stress of speed-ups, noise, and generally dangerous and degrading working conditions. One in five US men can expect to have a heart attack in his lifetime; many of these men are blue-collar workers subjected to the physical and mental stresses of unhealthy work conditions. Incidents and statistics like these have made occupational health and safety one of the fastest growing concerns of workers and health activists.

With the passage of the Occupational Safety and Health Act of 1970 (OSHA), workers theoretically have more control over their workplace environment than ever before. The law guarantees certain basic rights (inspection of the workplace at the worker's request, notification of dangerous conditions, access to health records, etc.), protects the worker from retaliation for any action under the law, and states that the safety and health question cannot be removed from collective bargaining. To implement OSHA, the government has created two new agencies: the National Institute of Occupational Safety and Health (NIOSH), which recommends standards, and the Occupational Safety and Health Administration (OSHA), which sets and enforces standards.

But the law has glaring faults, made worse by government indifference and underfunding. Inspectors lack authority to close plants even for the most serious violations of OSHA. Thus, an industry can use the lengthy review proceedings and court action to stall enforcement — in the process, financially draining the union opposing it. In some cases, companies have obtained temporary or permanent variances to government standards. If finally acted against, companies pay negligible fines, averaging $22.50 per violation. The agencies responsible for enforcing the law are crippled by underfinancing and understaffing. OSHA has one inspector for every 7,300 workplaces (more wardens are assigned to our fish and game reserves than inspectors to our workplaces).

To make matters worse, most of the inspectors the government hires are badly undertrained and predominantly business-oriented; the law does not provide for training workers as inspectors. Domination by business also extends to standard-setting agencies like the American Industrial Hygiene Association. Often composed of business hygienists, such agencies recommend and set standards for acceptable levels of exposure to hazardous substances or conditions. Not surprisingly, such standards are often dangerously lax. Many academic resources, too, have traditionally been monopolized by industry. For example, public health schools doing occupational health research often contract with management, and are more sensitive to the company than to the workers' needs.

Provisions of the Occupational Safety and Health Law intended to insure fair employee representation and treatment in inspections have been systematically watered down under industry pressure. Although a "worker representative" may accompany the inspector around the plant, inspectors can block any third-party expert (such as health activists) from participating in inspections. Although advance warning is prohibited, union workers report that inspecting agencies are increasingly lenient in allowing management advance notice of inspection.

Clearly, legislation and litigation are not adequate answers to occupational safety and health problems, though they cannot be discounted as important tools. Reliance on governmental protection cannot take the place of self-education, knowledge, and pressure brought to bear by organized workers.

To complicate the legal picture further, the federal OSH law has provisions for states to take over enforcement of health and safety provisions by 1976. This means that each state theoretically must come up with a plan equal to or stronger than the federal one. This plan must be approved by the state legislature and by the Department of Labor. Passage of state plans has become a significant organizing focus for unions. Most states have even less adequate staff money, and commitment than the federal government in safety and health matters. Unions are fighting against state take-over and the weakening of the law it usually entails.

Miners are not included in the Occupational Safety and Health Act, but are covered under separate acts and amendments, such as the Federal Coal Mine Health and Safety Act. Dealing with safety as well as compensation, this act has the same limitations found in OSHA. Two laws, passed after much struggle initiated by the Black Lung movement, are now in effect covering Black Lung compensation standards. This is the first case of workers winning compensation for an occupational disease (as opposed to injuries). This important gain raises hopes for winning compensation for other occupational diseases as well.

PLATFORM

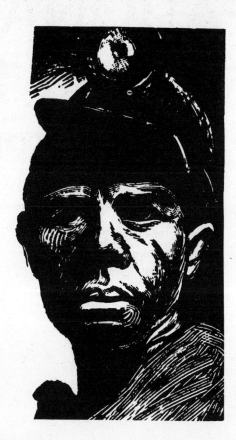

The fight for a decent workplace environment is still in an embryonic stage. Workers are increasingly realizing the importance of strong safety and health positions in collective bargaining; and in some areas they are building coalitions with progressive health, consumer, and environmental groups. An exciting example was the Oil, Chemical, and Atomic Workers' strike against Shell Oil Company in 1973. It marked the first time in recent US labor history that an international union struck over safety and health contract demands. The precedent-setting strike won massive consumer and environmentalist support and provided an invaluable education to many workers and the public in general.

But industry has generally responded to health and safety demands with stop-gap measures (temporary personal safety gear, various degrees of compensation), rather than taking the more expensive route of effective prevention. The medical profession has also failed to respond: occupational health is virtually ignored both in training and research.. And many unions, traditionally more concerned with wage and compensation bargaining, have been reluctant to take up the health and safety fight. The situation is even more difficult for the 60% of US workers who have no union to represent them. They have only the slow and feebly enforced law to rely on, and there is always the risk that the workers bringing a complaint will be fired in spite of the protective provisions of the law. Even when organized workers take strong action they may run up against company threats of shutting down marginally-operating plants rather than spending the money to meet union or government standards. Workers have little protection against such arbitrary decisions. As things stand now, the question often comes down to "your job or your life."

These are basic workers' rights and contract clauses that have emerged from the move towards rank and file control of workplace conditions, and which must be recognized by industry and the government.

WALK-OFF — The right to walk off a particular job if the workers consider the conditions immediately dangerous must be recognized.

HAZARD DEADLINE — Once hazards are identified, specific time limits must be set for their correction.

STANDARD-SETTING — Health and safety standards must be written into contracts so that they are negotiable through grievance procedures. Standards should be in accordance with the Occupational Safety and Health Administration, Environmental Protection Agency, American Conference of Governmental Industrial Hygienists, or (when applicable) other more stringent standard-setting national or international bodies. Workers must have the right to inspect, and if necessary veto any new equipment, machinery, process, or substance introduced into the plant without proper safety and health precautions.

WALK-AROUND PAY — The company must pay any authorized worker-representative for time spent accompanying an inspector around the plant.

RIGHT TO INFORMATION — Worker access to all health and safety records and standards must be guaranteed — including the right to full information about every process and substance used and produced in the plant. Any medical records must be made public except in cases where individual workers request confidentiality.

MONITORING — Workers must be free to bring in their own monitoring equipment and personnel, and be trained to use the company's equipment.

PHYSICAL EXAMS — Each worker must be examined when beginning employment, and at regular intervals afterwards, at company expense. The diagnosis of a private doctor should carry the same weight as that of a company doctor in compensation cases.

WORKER-APPOINTED SAFETY AND HEALTH COMMITTEE — Within each factory on plant, the committee should be empowered to investigate accidents or unsafe working conditions on company time, and to "red-tag" unsafe equipment or areas with the specification that affected employees will not return to the job until the conditions have been corrected to the satisfaction of the committee. Each committee member should receive one paid day a month for independent investigative work with the committee. In addition, each employee must have access to safety and health education with company pay.

BARGAINING AND GRIEVANCE — Specific grievance procedures should be set up to handle safety and health demands. Exclusion of these from collective bargaining must not be permitted.

RIGHT TO STRIKE — Workers' right to strike over safety and health conditions must be insured.

OUTSIDE RESEARCH — Large companies should be required to hire union approved independent health and scientific workers for ongoing independent research to identify hazards

PROGRAM

SURVEY AND RESEARCH YOUR PLANT — Keep a notebook of health hazards, their location, people affected, intervals at which they occur, possible causes, and possible solutions. Know what each health/safety monitoring device is for. Medical tests formerly given by the company can be important clues to hidden health hazards, so be sure to get the records. Check each new substance and operation introduced into the plant, making sure substances are clearly labeled. Keep track of every accident. Contact occupational health groups and health activists for background information and research guides.

INVOLVE OTHER WORKERS — When surveying, have other workers enter their complaints into your notebook. If enough workers have similar symptoms, it is safe to bet that they are a result of plant conditions. Sometimes a questionnaire is helpful. Posting charts of symptoms and the common causes of accidents in the plant is an excellent way to draw hazardous conditions to workers' attention and involve them in the solution.

BEGIN SHOP EDUCATION — Talk about the plant's hazards at informal worker sessions, steward meetings, and union local meetings. Get safety and health issues into the union paper. Health and legal activists can help set up courses to train workers in monitoring techniques, recognizing industrial diseases, and safety and health laws.

FORM A SAFETY AND HEALTH COMMITTEE — The committee can continue and expand your work: research and surveys, education, publicity, tests and inspections, and grievance procedures. It can also take the workers' demands to the local for broader union support.

APPLY PRESSURE AND USE GRIEVANCE PROCEDURES — Make demands specific; know exactly what you want. Look for some success in the beginning, no matter how small; success builds support and confidence. Get cost estimates on correcting unsafe condtions, so management cannot use cost as an excuse not to act. Move forcefully when workers' attention is focused on health and safety problems, such as immediately after accidents or illnesses. Get suggestions from other workers and follow up on them.

GET SAFETY AND HEALTH INTO THE CONTRACT — Contract gains depend on rank and file assertiveness; pressure your local and international unions for strong safety and health clauses. The Platform contains some model contract clauses; others will depend on specific conditions in your plant.

FILE FOR GOVERNMENT INSPECTION — Inspections are carried out under the Occupational Safety and Health Act; but this law is often useless due to inefficiency, delay, and government-company collusion. Unfortuantely, OSHA is the only hope non-union workers have for improved safety and health conditions. For inspection, fill out a written request form from your nearest OSHA office. The law states that NO DISCRIMINATORY OR RETALIATORY PROCEDURES CAN BE TAKEN AGAINST YOU FOR ANY ACTION UNDER THIS LAW. Still, the law remains an inefficent approach to situations requiring worker initiative and unionization. In fact, safety and health can often be key issues in organizing non-union workers.

ALLY WITH OUTSIDE ACTIVISTS — Health workers, engineers, legal activists and environmentalists can provide needed technical research skills, resource materials, and educational projects. Cooperation and coalitions are vital; but remember that the rank and file know the problems of the plant better than any outside activist can.

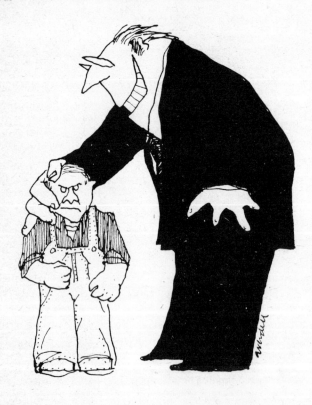

ORGANIZER SUPPORT GROUPS

For many working people, job safety and health cannot become an issue until the more basic one of unionization is taken care of. Unorganized workers lack the clout to bargain for strong safety and health measures. The following are some groups who assist workers in organizing drives.

URBAN PLANNING AID...is a prototype community organizing group which for three years has provided legislative and technical back-up information on occupational safety and health. UPA offers introductory workshops on specific hazards, such as asbestos and other carcinogens; health/safety survey training; lend-out monitoring devices such as noise meters and universal testers; and continuing help in keeping local safety committees informed and operative. Its newsletter, Survival Kit, is an ongoing documentation of workers' fights for their health and lives. UPA's excellent educational manuals and fact sheets spread step-by-step organizing tactics as well as general information on OSHA and plant hazards. UPA prepares pamphlets dealing with particular hazards (Noise and Your Health) and industries (Metal Welding and Cutting) at union request. Contact UPA, 639 Massachusetts Ave., Cambridge, MA 02140, 617-661-9220.

CALUMET ENVIRONMENTAL AND OCCUPATIONAL SAFETY COMMITTEE (CHOKE)...was formed two years ago by a group of young professionals. Realizing that weak and unenforced legislation will not solve health and safety problems, CHOKE provides unions with technical education and skills to survey and monitor plants and to make strong contract demands, especially in the high-risk steel industry. Classes also cover OSHA. In the meantime, CHOKE uses legislation: helping workers prepare for inspection, filing complaints for every thing from respiratory disease conditions to unsafe noise levels and workpeople's compensation. It has also litigated cases, such as a suit against the Environmental Protection Agency for failure to enforce coke emission standards in the steel-dominated Calumet-Gary area. As an offshoot of its health organizing, CHOKE has recently joined forces with Workers for Democracy and the District 31 Demand the Right to Strike Committee, a coalition of caucuses and locals. Contact CHOKE, 433 Locust St., Hammond, IN 46324, 219-937-1800.

OCCUPATIONAL HEALTH PROJECT OF THE MEDICAL COMMITTEE FOR HUMAN RIGHTS...acts as a clearinghouse for information and organizing programs. One main thrust is sponsoring local conferences to bring together workers, health activists, and community people, thus laying the foundation for ongoing local projects. Their publications include tactics and programs for occupational health and safety projects, model contract clauses, fact sheets on specific hazards, and reports on projects around the country. This center is a basic resource for anyone starting out in the occupational health field. Contact Occupational Health Project/MCHR, 688 Capp St., San Francisco, CA 94110, 415-824-5888 or 415-285-4758.

CHICAGO AREA COMMITTEE ON OCCUPATIONAL SAFETY AND HEALTH...is a strong and active coalition that emerged from a conference sponsored by several local unions and the Chicago Medical Committee for Human Rights. CACOSH's main focus is bringing together health personnel and workers to identify workplace hazards and do something about them. Monthly meetings with speakers on specific problems provide one forum for their work. CACOSH will help evaluate problems in the plant, do any kind of research, and secure lab analysis of offending materials. Other important efforts include working with locals and regionals to strengthen OSHA in its letter and enforcement. A company commitment to pay union inspectors has been one main achievement. CACOSH publishes a monthly newsletter. Contact CACOSH, 542 S. Dearborn St., No. 508, Chicago, IL 65607, 312-939-2104.

PITTSBURGH AREA COMMITTEE ON OCCUPATIONAL SAFETY AND HEALTH...grew out of a conference of labor people, health activists (MCHR) and occupational health specialists. The main focus of the group is education. Sessions are held on noise, red-lung, and other occupational diseases, compensation, and OSHA. Labor experts, university people (doctors and scientists), and legal workers, speak, answer questions and join in general discussion. The group would eventually like to get equipment for monitoring. PACOSH is moving in other directions, too. In reaction to the group's strong male and industrial bias, some of the PACOSH women are attempting to collect as much information as possible about occupational hazards related to women workers. This includes service workers, housewives, and other working women, whose problems (such as stress) are less dramatic but still dangerous. The women will push to deal with all areas of occupational health instead of defining the field in narrow industrial terms. PACOSH is now trying to define more clearly its goal and its relationship to workers as a whole; it hopes to sponsor an occupational safety and health conference in the fall of 1974. Contact PACOSH, P.O. Box 7566, Pittsburgh, PA 15213, 412-521-1079.

ENVIRONMENTAL SCIENCES LAB...has been researching chronic occupational diseases for years. Scientists here have done the brunt of the research and exposes on the infamous asbestos-related diseases, such as silicosis and asbes-

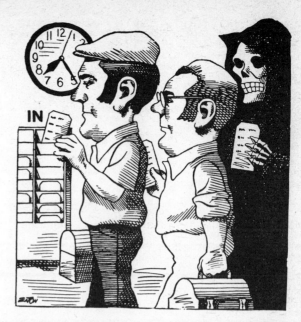

tiosis. The Lab is now concentrating on researching occupational cancers, and heart and pulmonary chronic diseases. Its major new project concerns investigations of polyvinal chloride, thought to cause liver cancer; this chemical is used often in food packaging. Also being studied are the hazards of the printing trades. These studies, like the ones that uncovered asbestos dangers, are based on surveys of causes of death among printing trade workers. The Lab works very closely with unions and locals. Contact Environmental Sciences Lab, Mt. Sinai School of Medicine, 100th St. and 5th Ave., New York, NY 10029, 212-876-1000.

HEALTH RESEARCH GROUP. . .is a Nader-sponsored group researching many areas of health care. It watchdogs OSHA, collects and assesses data on health hazards and exposure levels, and offers technical assistance and consultation to worker groups. HRG aims to provide information on safety and health to workers, and to "encourage public interest activities of scientists, lawyers, and other professionals in the area of occupational health." Contact HRG, 2000 P St. NW, Washington, DC 20008, (202) 872-0320.

BLACK LUNG ASSOCIATION...is a mass-based rank-and-file movement begun in 1968 in reaction to company and government neglect of coal miner's pneumoconiosis. The Association did a massive educational drive through coal mining areas. Miners became aware of the relationship between coal dust and lung failure and that disability and death were not inevitable results of mining. A 23-day wildcat strike in February 1969 which completely stopped coal mining in West Virginia, and a growing interest in the problem outside mining territory, led to state and federal legislation for compensation and safety standards. The BLA is continuing its work to get stronger compensation and safety laws through worker and community organizing (many mining areas have water so contaminated that it must be boiled to be used). Lobbying and running Black Lung afflicted workers for state and union government seats is one tactic used. Another major goal is to get 51% worker representation on Black Lung clinic boards and to force formerly UMW-owned hospitals to put coal miners on their boards. The workers have considerable economic force in this particular conflict, since 85% of the hospitals' income comes from coal miners. BLA is actively fighting the W. Virginia state government's plan to take over coal miners' health and safety laws. One such state plan rules out a federal amendment passed in '72 calling for diagnostic clinics in three states, and replaces them with mobile units, which are inefficient. BLA has been concerned with union democracy for some time. In fact, the rank-and-file Miners for Democracy, which successfully toppled the corrupt UMW leadership after a bloody conflict, was an outgrowth of BLA. A BLA member who has Black Lung was elected as the new President. For more information about state-wide chapters of BLA, contact BLA, c/o Stafford, Box 34, Blackbury City, WV 25664, 304-426-8171.

CUT CANE ASSOCIATES... provides organizing support, research, and technical aid to community and worker organizers throughout the southern and mountain states. CCA has been doing educational work around Brown Lung, including a "Facts About Brown Lung" booklet. This group sees unionization as the first step in cleaning up the workplace environment. They would like to see Brown Lung Organizations, modeled after the Black Lung Movement, carry out the needed educational work on this killer of textile workers. Contact CUT CANE ASSOCIATES, PO Box 98, Mineral Bluff, GA 30559, (404) 374-6611.

CINCINNATI TASK FORCE ON OCCUPATIONAL SAFETY AND HEALTH... began its work in 1973, when it evaluated conditions in a Dayton Foundary on behalf of a UE local facing upcoming negotiations. TFOSH held a mass meeting with men from the plant, discussed hazards (the foundary was found to have high concentrations of dust and silicon) and explained OSHA. The task force helped form a safety and health committee and has written a lengthy report on its findings. It is now investigating two toxic chemicals found in doll manufacturing, and has presented its slide show to high schools and medical schools. It is writing a series of articles for a local workers' newspaper on the history of occupational safety and health struggles, ways to use OSHA, and examples of actions around the country. If contacted by a union, the task force will give assistance in setting up a safety and health committee. Contact TFOSH, c/o Eller, 207 E. University, Cincinnati, OH 45219, (513) 861-2090.

CONNECTICUT OCCUPATIONAL HEALTH AND SAFETY PROJECT... is a group of medical, legal, and scientific workers, some of whom belong to AFT Local 1189, who provide technical assistance to local unions and are affiliated with the New Haven central labor committee. They have done legislative review, sponsored OSH classes, and have been helpful in gaining better working conditions for hospital workers and prisoners in New Haven. Contact OSH Project, c/o Dominski, 473 Elm St., New Haven, CT 16511, (203) 624-4254

UNITED MINE WORKERS FIELD SERVICE OFFICE... was set up to handle Black Lung claims, Social Security Disability and Compensation. The Service Center helps miners understand how to apply for claims, what to do if denied, and how to prepare for hearings. It does not handle individual legal questions, but does test case litigation. The field office puts out important and informative fact sheets and manuals on Black Lung. Contact UMWA, International Field Office, 1723 Kanawha Blvd. E., Charleston, WV 25301, 304-345-1513.

UNIONS
LOCALS

The fight for safety and health is a constant one. It is impossible to give adequate coverage to all the pioneering efforts of workers concerned with this issue. Following is a sketch of some of the activities occuring in shops, locals and internationals throughout the country.

UAW LOCAL 6... is particularly active in health and safety fights, working closely with CACOSH, they do education that includes critiques of Illinois' OSHA and state inspection procedures. Education of stewards and preparation of course manuals on health and safety are high priorities on this local's agenda. The safety and health committee takes an active role in teaching workers how to file complaints, how to get the most from OSHA inspections, and how to best use the grievance procedures. Material describing the local's fight for a safe workplace is available for other unions to share and learn from. Included are documented situations before and after a 1969 strike over safety and health violations, company breach of promise, and the watering down or elimination of fines by government officials. Contact UAW LOCAL 6, 3520 W. North Ave., Stonepark, IL 60615, 312-343-6880.

MEATCUTTERS LOCAL 342... has had a safety program for eight years. As early as 1970, this local negotiated a contract clause granting full-time members a 2½ hour annual safety and health session on company time. Recently, the union decided that in order to deal fairly with and concentrate on the special problems of women in the meat industry, special women's sessions should be held. Due to traditional hiring practices, men usually work heavy equipment and women work the packaging machines and on jobs which require considerable lifting. Since establishing separate sessions, the program is working much more efficiently. Local 342's contract provides for joint labor-management committees which meet every month to work out safety and health problems. Other important work of the union's safety and health committee deals with polyvinal chloride, which composes packaging film. Fumes from this chemical are emitted and inhaled as packaging paper is cut with hot wires. This causes irritation and res-

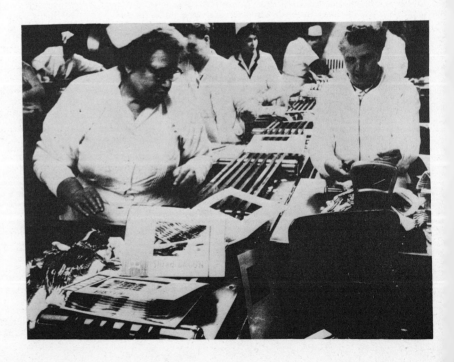

piratory problems ("meatcutters' asthma") and could possibly be linked to liver cancer. The union is planning an extensive study of the ominous hazard with the Environmental Sciences Lab. Because of its successes, the Local's program is being used as a model for other locals, and 342 will soon take on the safety and health program for the Meatcutters' International. Contact MEATCUTTERS' SAFETY AND HEALTH COMMITTEE, 18618 Hillside Ave., Queens, NY 10040.

TUNNEL WORKERS LOCAL 147...has been crusading for safety and health for Tunnel workers for years. Alarmed by the great increase in tunnel accidents and deaths (14 killed in the past two years in New York City tunnels alone), the local has instituted a strong program. Weekly sessions for stewards and rank and file, lasting about an hour each, feature films, teaching of such subjects as first aid, and visual aid devices. During the summer of 1973, the local paid for 10 members to go through an intensive training session of 6 days in the entire field of tunnel safety. After much bargaining and effort, management was forced, under contract, to pay wages for the attendees. The union plans to make good use of the expense and trouble it went to to provide its membership with good safety and health training. Union safety men are present at every job now. Strict enforcement mechanisms and disciplinary procedures have been instituted to get across strongly to membership just how important safety is. Local 147's other major achievement has been its participation in lobbying efforts to get silicosis (lung dust disease) put on the partial disability list for compensation. The effort has been going on for 10 years now, with industry and the insurance company putting their full weight behind efforts to crush the bill. Currently, the bill is stalled in committee "to let it die a slow death." Local 147 and its supporters are fighting to prevent that death. Contact Local 147, Compressed Air and Free Air Tunnel Workers, 175 5th Ave., Rm. 204, New York, NY 10010, 212-AL 4-6770.

STEELWORKERS LOCAL 1865. . .joined with several area universities to sponsor a safety and health conference for the tri-state area of West Virginia, Kentucky and Ohio. Out of this grew an increased safety and health consciousness. Each department in the local has its own safety and health committee, and a joint labor-management committee meets monthly to handle safety and health problems, as stipulated in the contract. Weekly inspection tours cover each department and recommendations go to the union committee. Most problems encountered so far have necessitated large company expenditures. Local 1865 is now trying to establish the exact occurrence rates of "red lung", a condition caused by the inhalation of iron particles; files are being kept on all workers who leave, apply for disability, etc. Hopefully, claims will be established. Upcoming contract demands will include the union's right to determine on the spot whether a condition is unsafe. Contact Local 1865, 734 Carter Ave., Ashland, KY 41101, (606) 325-1950.

Buff (an expert on Black Lung disease) came down hard on the unions for not taking a more active role in campaigns to eliminate occupational hazards. After all, he said, both West Germany and Czechoslovakia have steel mills, and neither country has any Red Lung disease. Are we really free in America, he asked, when medical schools won't diagnose Black and Red Lung disease for fear of losing their jobs?
—Joni Rabinowitz, New American Movement

TEAMSTERS LOCAL 688...has been particularly active in the pursuit of a healthy workplace. Its primary focus has been training stewards in occupational safety and health. Four and five day seminars are given periodically with the University of Missouri Department of Labor Education. The local also participated in the Governor's Safety Conference in 1973, presenting two sessions on health and safety —one to labor and one to management. The significant point was that both management and labor heard about the issues from workers instead of through management's safety officers. The local's educational programs put workers in a position to know the problems and how to deal with them. Local 688 has had several specific successes with area companies in improving safety and health conditions — especially involving large machinery. Through its political arm, the local is trying to insure a strong state OSHA. As for contracts, the local's business agent is presenting clauses stating that health and safety is a mutual endeavor, no longer management's prerogative. Management tends to stick to band-aid approaches like painting warning signs to satisfy thier insurance companies. With labor/management equal responsibiltiy clauses, labor will have to be heard and satisfied in safety and health questions. Local 688 has started to work with other unions and the Joint Council 13; it hopes to act as a safety and health clearinghouse for Teamster shop stewards. Contact LOCAL 688, 300 S. Grand St., St. Louis, MO 63103, 314-289-2489.

INTERNATIONALS

OIL, CHEMICAL AND ATOMIC WORKERS. . .has been the most active international in safety and health matters for over 10 years. It took a pioneering role in exposing asbestos as a killer of workers and an air pollutant. In 1973, the union called a strike against Shell Oil—the first international strike over safety and health in recent US labor history. At issue was Shell's refusal to sign a contract with strong safety and health provisions. Supported by activist health, environmental, labor and community groups, OCAW organized a national boycott of Shell products. The months-long strike ended with Shell signing a contract establishing union safety and health committees in every plant and agreeing to walk-around pay for union safety and health people. Although the victory was partial, OCAW sees this strike as a significant educational tool for consumers and workers, bringing the vital issue of safety and health to the forefront of the labor movement. OCAW has been one of the prime movers in legislation on health and safety, and has sponsored numerous health and safety conferences and courses. The international office in Denver has a paid hygienist chemist on staff to do research in occupational disease and has its own receiving lab for specimens from locals. OCAW is getting into the question of workpeople's compensation, trying to raise benefits, increase accessibility, and broaden the categories covered. OCAW has also assumed a leadership position in pressing OSHA complaints to the highest level of review, supporting locals in participating in review hearings. Contact OCAW, 1126 16th St. NW, Washington, D.C. 20036, (202) 223-5770.

UNITED AUTO WORKERS. . .has taken an active stand on health and safety. In the 1973 contracts it successfully negotiated for labor-designated health and safety representatives—fulltime workers paid by the companies and responsible to the union. They are required to make weekly inspections a and deal with complaints on a weekly basis rather than letting them accumulate. The company also agreed to provide necessary personal protective devices, and to furnish specialized equipment and staff to test workers exposed to specific health hazards. The UAW employs two full-time industrial hygienists and one safety engineer. Their newsletter, "Occupational Safety and Health," carries important information on occupational safety techniques, UAW policy, etc. Contact: UAW SAFETY DIVISION, 1125 15th St. NW, Washington, DC 20005, (202) 296-7484.

Farmworkers are among the most poorly paid working groups in the country, averaging $2,019 per worker for both farm and non-farm work in 1972. A farmworker injured in the field or ill from exposure to pesticide does not receive workmen's compensation. If s/he is sick or cannot find work, s/he does not receive unemployment insurance. Farmworkers are not covered by labor relations laws; they are only partially covered by Social Security and minimum wage laws, and they are often excluded from such programs as general welfare and training programs. They are employed in the third most hazardous occupation in the US.
—Report of the Dept. of Labor Taskforce: "Problems Facing Farmworkers"

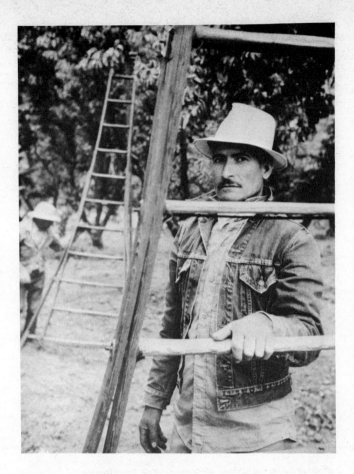

UNITED FARM WORKERS OF AMERICA...has been organizing farm workers since 1962 against incredible odds. This small but active union is pitted against discriminatory NLRB laws that do not protect farmworkers' right to bargain collectively, against the incredibly strong agribusiness lobby, and against other labor unions infringing upon its jurisdiction. The nature of the workplace and the fact that migrants have no strong economic or political base in this country compounds the difficulty of UFW's struggle. Yet this pioneering union has had much success in its short history. It has effectively used strikes in the fields, national boycotts of non-UFW grapes and lettuce, and boycotts against a couple of powerful food store chains to win considerable gains from the growers. These are gains which most workers would take for granted. UFW contracts include provisions for adequate and separate toilet facilities, suitable drinking water, two 10-minute rest periods during the day, protective garments and equipment, a chemical test procedure when organophosphates are used, adequate first aid supplies, and—most importantly—the elimination of certain poisons in UFW-worked fields, including DDT, Aldrin, Dieldrin, and Endrin. Perhaps more than in any other occupation, a farm worker's life is inextricably tied to her/his work. Farm workers (mostly Chicanos and Blacks, with some poor Whites) are paid depression wages. Their seasonal, migratory work makes them dependent on the growers for housing—usually a cold shack with no plumbing or sanitation. Most have no time or money for adequate health care and the conditions in the field add to the problem. Work is literally back-breaking and the indiscriminate use of pesticides has sent many farmworkers and their families to an early death. The only way to mitigate against these conditions and to establish some base of power is through strong organization. But this cannot be done in isolation. Over the past 10 years, UFW's massive educational work has elicited strong support from labor, community, church, and political organizations. Most major cities and migrant stream areas have boycott support committees, and the AFL-CIO recently pledged a $1,000,000 strike fund for an all-out campaign against the Teamsters, who have been undercutting UFW by claiming to represent the farm workers and signing weak contracts with the growers. The UFW has been successful in establishing a medical program with growers paying in 10 cents for every hour a worker labors. The farm workers are also getting three clinics off the ground. These clinics provide a forum for education about safety and health problems as well as general medical problems and preventive medicine. Contact UFW, Box 621, Keene, CA 93531, 805-822-5571.

UNITED RUBBER WORKERS OF AMERICA...was successful in gaining important safety and health language in their present contract. Clauses include provisions for joint union-management research contracts with two major universities to study occupational hazards of rubber workers. Contact URWA, Akron, OH 44308, 216-376-6181.

UNITED ELECTRICAL, RADIO LAND MACHINE WORKERS OF AMERICA. . . works for legislative improvements, trying to get the most out of OSHA' It also acts as a prod for union initiative, giving support to locals in calling OSHA inspections, in using grievance procedures, and, if the companies are still recalcitrant to improve hazardous conditions, in shutting down the offending plant. This independent union, long known for its defense of worker rights and high priority on rank-and-file participation, sponsors district meetings every three to four months, using these as a forum to educate workers about safety and health and what steps can be taken to alleviate hazardous conditions in the plant. With the motto "Knowledge is of value only if it is a guide to practice," UE has long endorsed a national health service plan, as opposed to national health insurance, as the only answer to our health care fiasco that is fair and equitable to workers, as well as the rest of the population. It has extensive information on the nature of the present National Health Insurance bills before Congress and opposed the payroll deduction-based financing as regressive and putting the major burden on working women and men. UE sees important first steps to a national health service as being massive educational campaigns by the unions and active worker organizing. Contact UE, 11 E. 51st St., New York, NY 10022, (212) PL3-1960.

UNITED MINE WORKERS OF AMERICA...ousted a corrupt unresponsive leadership in a classic rank-and-file victory in 1972. Since then it has dedicated itself to ridding the mines of as much danger as possible, and bringing down the average of 20 deaths a month for mining accidents. As one safety worker says, "My job is to keep the men alive so they can get Black Lung." In one significant move, the union successfully demanded the removal of a foreman who repeatedly ordered men into the mines in unsafe conditions—on the grounds that he constituted an "imminent danger" to the men. One of UMWA's first priorities is organizing a structure of safety coordinators at the district level to develop and coordinate safety programs, with each mine having a safety committee of three people. Last summer, the UMW sponsored its first training course at the mine level; another is planned this summer, featuring comprehensive, handbook-sized manuals explaining the safety committee job and how to do it effectively. UMW has begun bringing miners up from the fields to testify at federal regulation hearings. The personal accounts of the rank-and-file say more than reams of testimony from established "experts." UMW has also begun to involve the rank-and-file in administrative repeal procedures and other legal work, hoping eventually to set up a para-legal system within the rank-and-file. In reaction to superficial government training centers set up by the Bureau of Mines, the UMW has begun a pilot project involving eight locals to train its members in the basics of safety control, like studying and monitoring slag piles. The union is also putting together a safety education program for locals featuring movies and presentations. Looking toward contract time, the UMW would like to see a full-time safety committee paid by the company and controlled by the union; in the future, it would like to see a clause similar to the one UAW won for foundry workers: retirement after 25 years with a strong pension plan. Contact UMW SAFETY DIVISION, 900 15th St., NW, Washington, DC 20005, (202) 638-0530, Ext. 76, 77 or 80.

AFL-CIO STANDING COMMITTEE ON SAFETY AND OCCUPATIONAL HEALTH...coordinates legislative activity, training and educational programs and evaluative programs relating to occupational safety and health for the affiliate internationals. It provides speakers and advisors on occupational safety and health, and plans training courses given through the Department of Education of the AFL-CIO, the Labor Studies Institute, and affiliate internationals. Contact AFL-CIO, STANDING COMMITTEE ON SAFETY AND OCCUPATIONAL HEALTH, 815 16th St., NW, Washington, DC 20009, 202-637-5171.

SCHOOLS

Often universities and colleges have skills and technical resources not available elsewhere. For financial and political reasons, these resources are overwhelmingly more available to industry than to labor. However, unions and sympathetic academic resource people are increasingly coming together to share information and skills.

UNIVERSITY OF WISCONSIN EXTENSION PROGRAM SCHOOL FOR WORKERS...has for 50 years provided assistance to workers and unions; health and safety has become one of its major goals. In 1973, the school received a $300,000 grant from OSHA to institute programs around the state of Wisconsin and with internationals on safety and health. The programs included basic courses on the law and compliance procedures, industrial hygiene, identification of health hazards, and industrial disease. Courses last from 1 to 7 days and are aimed at stewards, local representatives and international business representatives. The school has a night school and does initial studies for unions to work out analyses of the dynamics of health and safety fights. Consulting on contract language and grievances, and on-site inspections as part of the courses are other features of the school. Contact School for Workers, University of Wisconsin Extension Program, 432 N. Lake St., Madison, WI 53706, 608-262-2111.

WEST VIRGINIA STATE COLLEGE/URBAN AFFAIRS CENTER...provides excellent technical services to labor unions in West Virginia. The center offers training courses in chemical health hazards and the use of OSHA. Pamphlets on the use of respirators and chemical solvents have been published by the department. In addition, staff people provide consultation in preparations for inspection and in evaluation of safety and health conditions. Contact W. VA State College /Urban Affairs Center, Institute, WV 25112, (304) 766-3216.

LABOR EDUCATION SCHOOL/RUTGERS UNIVERSITY . . .began an occupational safety and health course in 1970. With a strong shop-steward orientation, the curriculum examines the effect of chronic exposure to toxic substances, dust, gases, noise, radiation, etc. The 10 week course deals with ways to incorporate health and safety into collective bargaining and contract demands, and two seminars deal with how to use the law, though dependency on the law for effective change is challenged. Contact Labor Education School, Rutgers University, 1 Lincoln Ave., Newark, NJ 07004, (201) 648-1766.

NEW YORK STATE SCHOOL OF INDUSTRIAL AND LABOR RELATIONS/CORNELL UNIVERSITY...offers an unusually good course in occupational safety and health for trade unions. The course includes an overview of occupational health; specific health hazards; the link between environmental issues and occupational health; some perspectives on other countries; disability and workpeople's compensation; grievance procedures and collective bargaining strategies; and current federal/state OSHA legislation. The course is structured for maximum participation of trade unionists who act as speakers and participants. Course planners act chiefly as coordinators to bring together ideas and people — health and science experts, and workers directly affected by the hazards. The goals are to provide technical assistance in specific problems and to collect resource material so unions can conduct their own safety and health courses. Contact NYSSILR, Cornell University, 7 East 43 St., New York, NY 10017, 212-697-2247.

OCCUPATIONAL HEALTH GROUP/HARVARD UNIVERSITY...is a group primarily concerned with teaching and research in occupational disease. The group gives five-week courses in industrial and occupational health to the students of public health at the university. In addition, they hold sessions for workers, informing them of health hazards and how to get control of occupational health. Committed to the concept of worker control of the workplace environment, the group's goal is to make technical information understandable and to provide workers with the information they need in order to press for change. Contact Occupational Health Group, Department of Physiology, Rm. 1402, 665 Huntington Ave., Boston, MA 02115, 617-734-3300, ext. 2125.

UNIVERSITY OF PITTSBURGH SCHOOL OF PUBLIC HEALTH/DEPARTMENT OF OCCUPATIONAL HEALTH ...researches such areas as the hazardous characteristics of mine dust, physical effects of stresses on miners in emergencies, and the circulatory system reactions of steelworkers exposed to intense heat. Students and staff, acting with the Medical Committee for Human Rights, provide information and courses for unions. The academic program includes training graduate engineers and biologists to identify hazards and to design equipment which will eliminate them. Contact UNIVERSITY OF PITTSBURGH SCHOOL OF PUBLIC HEALTH/DEPT. OF OCCUPATIONAL HEALTH, Pittsburgh, PA 15213, 412-683-1620.

As a form of violence, job casualties are statistically at least three times more serious than street crime . . .
—Ralph Nader

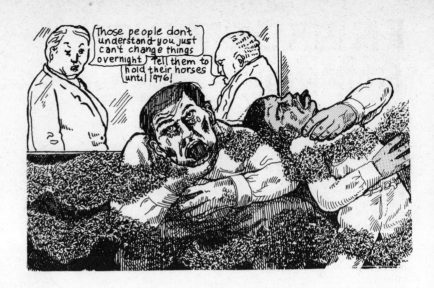

LEGAL GROUPS

Though the law cannot be relied upon as a final goal, it can provide a useful tool to gain control of the workplace environment. Legal workers can provide research and information on the law and contract language necessary for strong labor demands.

MINNESOTA PUBLIC INTEREST RESEARCH GROUP... worked successfully with unions to get asbestos construction waste outlawed in the state. This includes the banning of asbestos used in construction, mining and other industrial production that would pollute the outside environment. MPIRG has proposed a 0 tolerance level to the Department of Labor to do away with asbestos in all production processes. It is now working towards standards for asbestos substitutes, contending that recent studies show it is the size of the fibers, not asbestos itself, that causes cancer. MPIRG was one of the leading forces in winning an unusually strong state OSHA plan. It has gathered and publicized much information on the occupational hazards of farmworkers, hoping to pressure public officials into action. Included in this is a pro-labor environmental impact statement of the effects of pesticide control standards and detailed guidelines for developing such standards. MPIRG has done a detailed study of federal and state job safety and proposed a theoretical model for standards. It has sent bills to Congress to increase appropriations for enforcement, to spread OSHA jurisdiction to miners, and to change OSH procedures to give employees equal jurisdiction with employers in health and safety matters. Manuals and pamphlets deal with how to use OSHA, how to handle pesticides, and information on silicon, iron, and copper. Major concerns in the near future will be further exploration of the effects of pesticides and epoxy resin; studies of prison occupational health (in conjunction with the state Department of Labor and Industry); and investigation of coal and nickel mines. Contact MPIRG, 3036 University Ave., SE, Minneapolis, MN 55414, 612-376-7554.

GUILD LABOR COMMITTEE...is the labor lawyer's group within the National Lawyers Guild. Working closely with rank and file and with newly forming unions, Guild lawyers are now entering the occupational health field as part of an overall labor law strategy. Some Guild chapters have sponsored conferences and training sessions on safety and health in collaboration with workers and health activists. The Committee's Labor Newsletter and the NLG's Guild Notes give a good perspective on their range of activities. Contact GUILD LABOR COMMITTEE, c/o Middleton and Wildorf, 98 Chenery St., San Francisco, CA 94131, 415-647-5008.

NATIONAL HEALTH LAW PROGRAM . . . is a legal services back-up program serving predominantly in the West. Funded through HEW, NHLP provides information to locals on workers' rights, makes sure those rights are protected, and takes court action when they're not. NHLP played a significant role in the recent successful suit to set temporary pesticide standards for farm workers. Two manuals have been prepared by the project listing safety and health laws, regulations, complaint forms and bibliographies for industrial and agricultural workers. Contact NHLP, 10995 Le Conte Ave., Rm. 640, Los Angeles, CA 90024 213-825-7601.

MIGRANT LEGAL ACTION PROGRAM. . .is the OEO-funded legal back-up project that issued the petition and lawsuit that resulted in temporary standards for pesticide control being set last summer. A higher court, however, placed a restraining order on the original standard-setting court order so farmworkers now have no protection from dangerous pesticide levels. The Environmental Protection Agency has proposed a new set of standards which are now under consideration. MLAP holds that OSHA, because of its greater resources, should implement the standards rather than EPA. However, due to bureaucratic governmental infighting, it is unclear who—if anybody—will take over pesticide control. MLAP is also filing suits around other safety and health conditions, including farm machinery safety standards, sanitation, and housing. Their monthly newsletter, covering all legal issues concerning migrants, is free to anyone who cannot afford the suggested donation of $2.50/year. Contact MLAP, 190 "K" St. NW, Washington, D. C. 20006. (202) 785-2475.

BAY AREA LAWYERS' GUILD/OCCUPATIONAL SAFETY AND HEALTH COMMITTEE. . . was begun to assist rank and file caucuses concerned with OSHA. Though still in the infant stages, the committee has begun educational and legislative analysis work and is preparing a pamphlet on California OSHA. Many of the students, legal workers, and lawyers who are affiliated with the group have had previous experience in workpeople's compensation, research on OSHA and standards, and in preparing safety and health complaints. Contact BAY AREA LAWYERS' GUILD/OSHA COMMITTEE, 558 Capp St., San Francisco, CA 94110, (415) 3964.

You may wonder why asbestos workers walk backwards. They don't always walk backwards. It is only going upstairs. They are so short of breath that after two steps they have to sit down. It is easier to go up a flight of stairs backwards than walking up. It is a terrible way to die.

—Irving J. Selikoff, asbestosis expert

ENVIRONMENTAL SUPPORT GROUPS

Groups traditionally concerned with saving the earth's physical environment are increasingly realizing the interconnection between their movement and the environmental battle going on inside the plants. Generally, the same companies that are causing the decay of the whole community's land, air and water, are also causing the decay of the workforce's health.

ENVIRONMENTAL ACTION. . .is the major environmental group working in occupational safety and health. EA led several major environmental groups in support of the recent safety-and-health-centered strike against Shell Oil by the Atomic, Chemical and Oil-Workers Union. Seeing the strike as a rallying point for environmental groups entering the occupational health area, EA published informational material and helped organize strike-support committees around the country. The workplace environment is also discussed in EA's manual, "Earth Tool Kit", and in articles in their magazine, Environmental Action. Contact EA, 1346 Connecticut Ave. NW, Washington, DC 20036, (202) 833-1845.

ENVIRONMENTAL DEFENSE FUND . . . is active in litigation challenging the asbestos standard and in administrative petitions for emergency pesticide standards. In addition, it has been monitoring law enforcement, and lobbying within the Environmental Protection Agency and the Occupational Safety and Health Administration. A full-time noise specialist and biochemist supply backup research for their legal actions. Contact ENVIRONMENTAL DEFENSE FUND, 1525 18th St., NW, Washington, DC 20036, 202-833-1484.

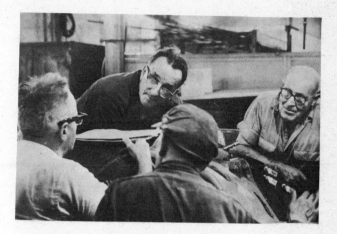

RESOURCES

BOOKS

Work Is Dangerous To Your Health, Jeanne M. Stellman and Susan Daum. Vintage, 201 E. 50th St., New York, NY 10022, 1973. 419 pp. $1.95.
. . . comprehensive, thoroughly useful and action-oriented book combining solid political and economic critique with extensive technical information related to occupational diseases. It is packed with charts, diagrams and tables, and written in language that lay people can understand. Explanations and diagrams of the body systems lay a foundation for dealing with specific occupational diseases and body malfunctions: effects on the body, tests for diagnosis, and treatments. Charts list what chemicals cause which diseases or malfunctions; recommended standards for exposure to many chemicals and to noise, heat, lighting, and other byproducts of industrial processes; the functions of monitoring equipment, and much more. "Low visibility" hazards, such as stress, which pose no immediate, dramatic problems but can in the long run be devastating to a worker's health and life are exposed. The final chapters deal with technical aspects of controlling pollution-measurement, monitoring, keeping health records; they also mention specific tactics for winning health and safety demands. Well-done indexes (general and by substance), a good bibliography, and almost 50 pages listing health hazards by occupation help make this book an invaluable reference guide and manual. The authors state: ". . . our bias favors the worker . . . [we believe that] industry and government must prove that a chemical is safe, not that the workers must prove it is dangerous by developing occupational diseases . . . No essential rights now enjoyed by working men and women were simply bestowed by the government. Rather they were won through struggle."

Bitter Wages: Ralph Nader's Study Group Report on Disease and Injury on the Job, Mary-Win O'Brien and Joseph A. Page. Grossman Publishers, 625 Madison Ave., New York, NY 10022, 1973. 314 pp. $2.95 (all royalties to Center for Study of Responsive Law)
. . .Decrying the "silent violence of occupational disease", this hard-hitting report examines the major health hazards which have turned workplaces into an "invisible arena of violence"; the history of government attempts to deal with job health and safety; the roles played by unions, state agencies, and private groups; the Occupational Safety and Health Act and its implementation; reasons past reform efforts have failed; and specific methods of alleviating the present crisis. The authors honor no sacred cows, but present their findings in a well-documented, highly readable, compassionate yet forceful style. They emphasize the urgent need for workers to control their own lives (using OSHA as a valuable if imperfect legal tool), and demand that labor unions put job safety at the top of their agenda.

Everybody talks about crime in the street, but what about crime committed by industry? Exposing a person to a toxic chemical which shortens his life is tantamount to murder, in my opinion.
—Tony Massachi, OCAW

The American Worker: An Endangered Species, Franklin Wallick, Ballantine Books, Dept. CS, 36 W. 20th St., New York, NY 10003, 1972. 244 pp. $1.60
. . . colorful, yet thoughtful introduction to the occupational safety and health field. Wallick comes down in government, union, scientific, and company indifference to the problems of the workplace environment, presenting good insights into the many levels of bureaucracy and other problems workers must fight to secure their demands. He feels the Department of Labor "swarms with nice guys" who let industry off easy, while industrial scientists are no more than "mercenaries who have peddled a company line on OSH for years . . ." Sprinkled with examples of workers' victories in this important field, the book asserts the need for concerned scientists, students and environmentalists to join in the fight, concluding with a Workers' Bill of Rights and useful suggestions on what can be done to clean up the workplace environment.

The Hazards of Work: How To Fight Them, Patrick Kennersly. Pluto Press, Unit 10, Spencer Ct., 7 Chalcot Rd., London NWL 7LH, Great Britain, 1974. About $3, including shipping. (Allow for delays in shipping)
. . . one of the best handbooks available to workers concerning safety and health. It covers accidents, physical hazards, chemical hazards, toxic substances prevention, and organizing, as well as other subjects. Easy to read and full of practical ideas, it is an excellent complement to Work is Dangerous to Your Health. Because it was written in Britain, the section on law in inapplicable in the US, but the ideas on how to use the law are helpful. Especially important is the focus of the book on things that workers can do directly for themselves to lessen occupational hazards.

"Giving Shell Some Gas: Environmental Issues Reach the Bargaining Table," Cathy Lerza, ENVIRONMENTAL ACTION, Suite 731, 1346 Connecticut Ave., NW, Washington, DC 20036, March 3, 1973, pp. 3-6. $7.50 /year
...an exciting account of the Oil, Chemical, and Atomic Workers' (OCAW) strike against Shell Oil Company. Oil refineries are among the most hazardous of all workplaces. The lead and benzene, among other substances as yet unresearched, can cause serious permanent damage, sometimes death. Shell Oil was the only major oil company which refused to meet OCAW's demands for company-paid medical tests and physical examinations, access to company information on worker morbidity and mortality, and compensation for worker time spent on plant inspection and health committee meetings. Although the struggle ended, after this article was written, in a compromise, it is encouraging to read about environmentalists and oil workers fighting together for mutual benefits.

"FIGHTING NOISE: A MANUAL FOR WORKER ACTION," Industrial Health & Safety Project of the Urban Planning Aid, and Health Research Group, 2000 "P" St., NW, Washington, DC 20036, 1972. 17 pp.
...prepared for the International Printing Pressmen and Assistants' Union of North America, this is an excellent pamphlet on how to tell if your workplace is dangerously noisy, and how to correct the situation. It gives charts on unsafe noise levels, warning signs, such as ringing in the ears, and an account of one union's fight with the WASHINGTON POST to control hazardous noise.

"INFORMATION ON BLACK LUNG," UMWA, International Field Service Office, 1020 Quarrier St., Charleston, WV 25301, 1973. 30 pp.
...gives necessary resources and advice for miners and their widows making Black Lung claims. Tells how to keep a claim open and choose a lawyer, what to do when the claim is denied, and what one needs to know about the Black Lung program of the Labor Department.

PAMPHLETS AND ARTICLES

"HOW TO LOOK AT YOUR PLANT," Industrial Health and Safety Project of Urban Planning Aid, 639 Massachusetts Ave., Cambridge, MA 02139, 1972. 40 pp.
. . . a supremely practical, specific, indispensable tool for locating the obvious and hidden hazards in your plant, and acting on your findings. It proceeds on the assumption that management will do all it can to get off the hook or to make superficial reforms (having workers wear earmuffs to close out noise—unfortunately these also muffle shouts of warning or instructions from fellow workers). This pamphlet advises a no-stones-unturned approach to spotting hazards: noting which medical tests (if any) are given to workers and why; observing which chemicals you can smell that you couldn't if they were present in safe concentrations; asking questions like "Do metal fumes ever make you feel like you have the flu?" or "Do any oils or solvents give you skin rashes?" Stresses the need for workers to unite and push management toward real change; places little faith in the effectiveness of government enforcement of standards. "Legal limits are not necessarily safe limits." The booklet includes a variety of organizing tactics, and suggests health and safety clauses for union contracts. Replete with excellent graphics, checklists, tests, drawings of

monitoring devices that workers can borrow from UPA, helpful pamphlets and books, and groups to contact for information on medical tests, inspections, chemical substances and organizing strategies.

HEALTH HAZARDS IN THE WORKPLACE, MCHR, 542 S. Dearborn St., Chicago, IL 60605, 1972. 70 pp. $3
...describes an MCHR-UAW conference on occupational health. It also gives a good outline of health hazards: dust, gases, radiation and others, as well as an analysis of OSHA and how to organize an occupational health project report.

"A UNIONIST'S GUIDE TO THE OCCUPATIONAL SAFETY AND HEALTH ACT OF 1970, 1971." Industrial Health and Safety Project of Urban Planning Aid, 639 Massachusetts Ave., Cambridge, MA 02139, 1971. 16 pp.
. . . a clear section-by-section review of the recent federal Occupational Safety and Health Act, explaining workers' rights as well as the act's inherent weaknesses. It stresses the fact that only the unions and workers can insure that the law will be enforced and existing hazards abolished. Includes a list of areas covered by OSHA standards, and places to write for copies of the standards.

"Your Job or Your Life," HEALTH-PAC BULLETIN, 17 Murray St., New York, NY 10007, 1973. 16 pp. $5/year for students, $7 for others
...tells how asbestos workers (along with other people working under hazardous conditions) are caught in a "classic bind" — if they keep their jobs and keep quiet, they are risking a painful death at an early age from asbestosis or lung cancer. If they agitate to force companies to meet OSHA standards, the plant may be closed down and they will be left without a job. The issue focuses on the world's largest asbestos producer, Johns-Manville Corporation, and the battle of workers there to eliminate asbestos exposure. It is a shocking and sobering story.

"National Safety and Health Manual for Agricultural Establishments," National Health Law Program. 10995 Le Conte Ave., Rm. 640, Los Angeles, CA 90024, 1974. 53 pp. $2.50
. . . provides valuable information for lawyers doing OSHA litigation. It describes OSHA law and standards comprehensively, ending with sample complaint and statistical forms. It emphasizes the fact that many cases that cannot be litigated under specific OSHA laws and regulations can be litigated under the "general duty" clause. NHELP also puts out an OSHA manual for non-agricultural workers.

"Collective Bargaining for Occupational Health and Safety," Center for Labor Research and Education, Occupational Safety and Health Project, Institute of Industrial Relations, Berkeley, CA 94720, 17 pp. Free
...a useful report on contract clauses and negotiated programs, including a good description of "areas of union interest in supplementing legislative health and safety protection." Safety and health clauses proposed or won by the UFW, UAW, Rubber Workers, OCAW, and Steelworkers are included.

"Contract Clauses for Occupational Health and Safety," UPA, 639 Mass. Ave., Cambridge, MA 15 pp.
...short pamphlet suggesting model contract clauses.

PERIODICALS

UNITED MINE WORKERS JOURNAL, 15th St. NW, Washington, DC 20005, $1.00 for non-UMW members. . .the official organ of the UMW, reports on safety and health issues as well as general miner and worker news. The Journal reflects the rank-and-file attitude of the UMW's new administration.

SURVIVAL KIT, Industrial Safety and Health Project, UPA, 639 Mass. Ave., Cambridge, MA 02140, $2.00 yearly. . .an excellent pro-worker monthly newsletter covering all facets of the safety and health question. It presents first-hand accounts of dangerous and dehumanizing conditions and actions workers are taking to protect their lives. "Survival Kit" contains analyses of legal and legislative action under OSHA, and invaluable material on specific occupational dangers, such as solvents, heat, unsafe machines, noise, and asbestos—what they can do to a worker's health, what symptoms to watch for, and hazard control measures.

HEALTH RIGHTS NEWS, MCHR, 542 S. Dearborn St., Chicago, IL 60605, March, 1972, pp. 6-11. $5/year
...this issue has articles on different aspects of occupational health, most of them centering around the Occupational Safety and Health Act (OSHA) of 1970: the provisions of the law, how it is being enforced, its inadequacies, and how management responds to it. Donald Wharton warns that states are now developing their own plans in lieu of the federal plan; many of them will be even weaker than OSHA, possibly omitting the worker's right to accompany federal inspectors visiting an unsafe plant, and other important provisions of the federal act. Another article is a panel discussion by MCHR and union members on strategies for better health and safety on the job. This issue gives an excellent introduction to the basic problems in occupational health.

HEALTH-PAC BULLETIN, 17 Murray St., New York, NY 10007, September, 1972. 24 pp. $5/year for students, $7 for others
...this issue centers on worker's health and safety: a brief history of occupational health concerns, the bureaucracies that have dealt with the problem, the workings of the OSHA, and a special focus article on byssinosis (Brown Lung), a respiratory disease caused by dust in textile plants. Most of the articles emphasize the attempts of industry to deny the existence of occupational diseases, their cover-ups, and the failure of existing monitoring activities to substantially change hazardous conditions. The OSHA article is especially helpful in pointing out the weaknesses in the act and its management bias.

SPOTLIGHT ON HEALTH AND SAFETY, Industrial Unions Department, AFL-CIO, 815 16th St., NW, Washington, D.C. 20006, free to laborers, $5.00 yearly to others.
. . .is a comprehensive newsletter covering the national OSHA scene. It will keep you up to date on all the political infighting surrounding OSHA.

OCCUPATIONAL SAFETY AND HEALTH PROJECT REPORT, MCHR, 558 Capp St., San Francisco, CA 94110. $2.00 yearly. . .is a valuable resource for occupational safety and health organizers. Reports have included discussions on researching plants, organizing, and using OSHA; how to do a safety and health project on a limited budget; and how to set up a work environment information center. Most recent newsletters have included an excellent national list of safety and health projects and resources, a bibliography of worker-oriented material on OSH, and important information (geared toward the medical and technical assistance sector of the safety and health movement) on how to run an OSH task force.

MOUNTAIN LIFE & WORK, Council of the Southern Mountains, Inc., Old Bank Building, Main St., Clintwood, VA, April 1973, pp. 22-27. $5/year
...this is a special issue on mountain textile factory working conditions, including some personal accounts of the effects of Brown Lung, a fact sheet of common questions and answers, and how to get benefits for Brown Lung victims through Social Security and Workmen's Compensation. A good introduction to Brown Lung.

FILMS AND TAPES

Urban Planning Aid, 639 Mass. Ave., Cambridge, MA 02139

"**Occupational Safety and Health Slide Show**", 30 min. $50 institutions, $35 unions and workers. A solid introduction to safety and health, especially useful for those just beginning to organize a safety and health committee. The show blasts government and management's callous attitude toward safety and health, and gives an overview of major hazards. It ends with a description of worker responses: performing tests themselves, calling in NIOSH and OSHA, forming safety and health committees, strikes and walk-outs.

The Rest Of The News, 306 E. State St., Ithaca, NY 14850

"**Occupational Safety and Health**", 10 min. sale: $6.00 1973. A well-done, brief introduction to the "most neglected environment". Studded with catchy sound effects and powerful statistics, the tape includes short statements by workers about their experiences in the area of safety and health. It describes political problems involved in safety and health, and the pressure workers are bringing to bear on management and government.

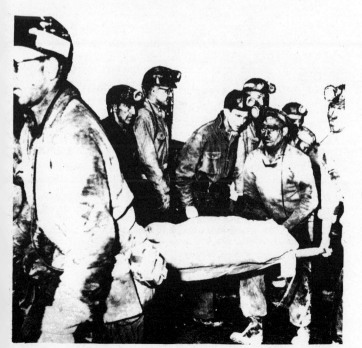

If American coal industry were to lose profits and production in one year, there would be an outcry for reform, correction and financial assistance from the government. But when the industry only has a higher death rate than that of any other major coal producing country, it matters little to owners of industry, the public, or the government.
—Davitt McAteer, UMW Safety Division

ENVIRONMENTAL HEALTH

Mental and physical well-being depend on more than healthy minds and bodies. It requires a healthy environment to support them. Clean air. Pure water. Uncontaminated food. Without them the strongest body will soon weaken; breathing, drinking, eating are silently transformed from the sustainers of life into the agents of death. The full realization of this fundamental connection between the environment and human health was slow in coming to the national consciousness—not really gripping it significantly until the Spring of 1970. On April 22, Earth Day, the environmental movement came of age politically, with budding environmental and ecology groups joining forces with long standing conservation organization to win the environment its fair share of political representation and due process.

Air Pollution: Temperature inversions in heavily polluted cities create health emergencies that shoot up hospital admissions and the death rate. Yet such pollution disasters are only the tip of the iceberg. As a result of chronic low level exposure to air pollution, 80,000 individuals annually follow the advice of their doctors and permanently leave Los Angeles, where cars spew forth close to 80% of the atmospheric contamination. (In a nation where people have been duped by the auto industry and its governmental cohorts to believe that a car in every garage is more important than a mass transit system in every city, automobiles are the number one polluter of air, accounting for 40-60% of pollution on the average in any given area.) In a single decade, deaths attributable to emphysema and chronic bronchitis have more than doubled. Asbestos, beryllium, mercury and lead, all common industrial materials, contaminate the air in some areas and where sufficiently concentrated, cause cancer, lung disease and neurological damage.

Water pollution: From 1961 to 1970, 130 disease outbreaks and approximately 46,000 cases of poisoning were attributed to contaminated water supplies. During the same period, 56% of the public water systems in the US had major deficiencies; 25% contained bacteria or chemicals exceeding safe limits; and additional 16% were distributing water considered dangerous according to Federal drinking water standards.

Pesticides: More than 700 different pesticides have been proved to cause poisoning; 200 people are killed annually from exposure to them. Due to years of massive spraying to control insects, DDT, which is believed to cause cancer in some species of animals, has infected the entire world ecosystem, from mothers' milk (at 4-5 times acceptable levels) to Antarctic penguins.

Solid Waste: Burned, it pollutes the air; buried, it contaminates the soil and infiltrates underground water systems;

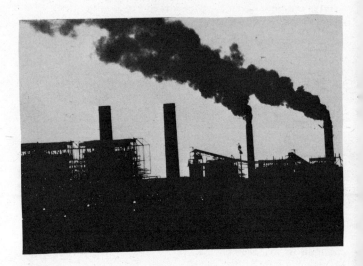

dumped in the ocean, it begins to creep back to shore. In New York City, volatile garbage and trash are the cause of 50% of all reported fires.

Noise: An estimated 16 million people in the US have some hearing loss caused directly by excessive sound. Prolonged exposure can lead to irritability, increased susceptibility to infection, heartburn, ulcers, high blood pressure, heart disease and physical breakdown. While noise surrounds us all, it is the industrial laborer and the construction worker who are exposed daily to the most brutal sonic assaults. (See Occupational Safety and Health).

Radiation: Failure of the Atomic Energy Commission to adequately enforce safety controls on nuclear energy production and armaments as well as waste storage has resulted in instances of dangerous leaks of radioactive material into the environment. Exposure can cause genetic damage, leading to fetal and infant mortality; also leukemia and bone cancer, particularly among the young.

Environmentalists hoped that such dramatic evidence would create a clear cut issue around which all political factions could rally, since we all have to breath the same poisonous air and drink the same dirty water. Politicians were not slow to perceive the political impact and between 1970 and 1973 the nation witnessed a surge of environmental court cases and a rush of legislation. Laws were passed in the areas of water, air, solid wastes, noise, insecticides and more as Congress jumped on the environmental bandwagon in the name of motherhood, applie pie and a clean environment. Industry, quick to recognize the publicity value of the environmental movement made ecology the advertising slogan of the year.

Yet even at the turn of the decade, when the movement was reaching full momentum, some environmentalists already were challenging the basic political and economic assumptions upon which it operated—we do not all drink the same water and breathe the same air. Governmental studies have revealed consistently that the lowest income neighborhoods are in the areas of the worst pollution, amidst the industrial smoke stacks and the greatest concentration of automobile exhaust fumes. Lead, the excessive ingestion of which can lead to seizures, mental retardation, cerebal palsy, and behavioral disorders, is the most heavily concentrated in the air in those urban areas where gasoline consumption is greatest. Yet pollution knows no city limits, and increasingly suburban dwellers are also feeling the effects of inversions, impure waters, etc.

Theoretically, the law places the main responsibility for the clean-up of the environment on the industries that pollute it, although all too often industry-government collusion results in indeterminate delays, bureaucratic negligence and lack of enforcement. And, when business does act on pollution controls, it is the poor and middle class who ultimately bear a disproportionate share of the cost. Industry covers the extra expense by raising the cost of the good or denying workers a salary increase. According to the President's Council on Environmental Quality, the higher prices which result from pollution control will force costs to be borne "disproportionately by those with lower incomes because they spend a larger percentage of their incomes on products such as automobiles—the number one polluter." As one environmentalist said, our society "blesses the rich with profits and the poor with pollution." Truly effective environmental clean-up demands not only stringent pollution control but also radical changes in the life style and economic orientation of our profit and consumption-oriented society.

Although the greatest flourish of activity in the environmental movement occurred immediately following Earth Day, the need for continued political action is far from over. The air, water, pesticides and noise laws that have been enacted are considered strict enough to go a long way toward cutting pollution if only they are properly implemented. However, their enforcement continues to be an on-going battle against a hostile administration, funding cuts and delays—not to mention heavy industry lobbying and the pressure of the so-called energy crisis to gut the existing controls. Groups and organizations across the country are educating, organizing, litigating and lobbying to guarantee the most effective and just enforcement of the pollution laws at the local, state and federal level. Because of time and space constraints, we are only listing groups who are working on a national level; however, many of them are in touch with local projects and can suggest useful contacts. Also, several groups listed in the section on occupational safety and health are working with environmentally related issues.

ENVIRONMENTAL ACTION. . .is an activist group believing that environmental questions must be viewed in a broader context of politics and economics. Their tactics include lobbying, information dissemination and active participation in political campaigns. As a registered lobbying group, EA takes strong stands on solid waste, clean air and energy legislation. The magazine Environmental Action is published bi-weekly and links EA with local citizen activists in its attempt to coordinate citizen pressure. In addition, EA has completed three "Dirty Dozen Campaigns", in which a study is made of the voting records on key environmental issues of the Congresspeople running for election. Those twelve people with the worst voting records are designated the Dirty Dozen and targeted for defeat. EA works with local groups to campaign extensively against them. In the first two election in which EA participated, 11 out of the 24 designated incumbents were defeated. In an important first step toward increased cooperation between environmental groups and labor, EA actively supported the 1973 strike of Shell workers, assisting in the formation of local strike committees. The Environmental Action Foundation (EAF) is the tax-deductible sister/brother organization of EA and is engaged in research and educational work. Most of their work has consisted of education on the present dangers of the nuclear program and development of a fairly impressive solid waste program. EA had conducted conferences and workshops, written a guide to citizen action and is working to set up a citizens' network for action on solid

waste. The Highway Action Coalition, a lobbying coalition of anti-freeway, protransit groups originally created to bust the Highway Trust Fund, was created by EA and remains closely associated with them. Contact: Environmental Action, Inc., Room 731, 1346 Connecticut Ave., NW, Washington, DC 20036 (202) 833-1845.

NATURAL RESOURCES DEFENSE COUNCIL. . . is a public interest environmental law firm, with a staff of lawyers and scientists. NRDC's main thrust is on enforcing existing legislation and standards. This involves closely monitoring and prodding the Environmental Protection Agency and Atomic Energy Commission (AEC), preparing comments on their regulations and taking them to court when necessary. In addition to initiating court cases, NRDC provides legal counsel to citizens, conservation organizations and municipalities seeking to protect the environment. A major criteria in the selection of cases is whether the potential exists for establishing a legal precedent. For example, in May 1971, NRDC filed a lawsuit on behalf of Scientists' Institute for Public Information against the AEC for failing to comply with the National Environmental Policy Act in implementing a specific program. In June, 1973, the court ordered the AEC to prepare a full environmental impact statement review of the program in question. A quarterly newsletter is published. Contact: Natural Resources Defense Council, 1710 N St., NW, Washington, D. C. 20036, (202) 783-5710.

ENVIRONMENTAL DEFENSE FUND. . . is a major environmental law firm paralleling National Resource Defense Council in its philosophy and work, although it is somewhat more issue-oriented and less geared toward enforcing existing standards. The main legal work on pesticide contamination has been done by EDF. In late 1973, following six years of EDF litigation in state and Federal courts, the ban on almost all uses of DDT was successfully upheld. EDF is one of the few environmental groups attacking noise as a broad problem, with one recent law suit resulting in EPA releasing previously restricted information on noise tolerance levels. EDF works in the area of water pollution; it is involved in several lawsuits against the Reserve Mining Company for contaminating Lake Superior with asbestos. A monthly newsletter is published. Contact EDF, 1525 18th St., NW, Washington, DC 20036, (202) 833-1484.

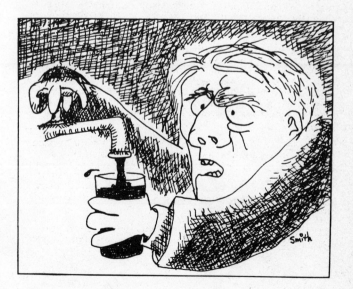

SIERRA CLUB. . . originated in 1892 and has since grown into a broad-based national organization encompassing the whole gamut of environmental concerns: wilderness protection, land use planning, pesticides, air and water pollution abatement and population control. The Club has 43 local organizations and 143,000 members. Of its growing involvement with the urban environment, Sierra Club writes: "The environment of the cities now also needs to be made fit for man. . . Technology must be challenged to do a better job in managing the part of the planet it has already claimed." In 1967, the club lost its tax exempt status when it openly lobbied against the proposed damming of the Colorado River. (Tax exempt organizations are prohibited under the law from spending a "substantial" portion of their time lobbying in Congress.) Although financially hurt by this action, the club chose not to seek renewal of its exemption in order to go all out in its lobbying efforts. One of the major forces behind the enactment of the Clean Air Act of 1970, the Sierra Club has continued to fight against legislative amendments that seek to weaken the law. In addition to lobbying, the Club publishes the Sierra Club Bulletin, "The Weekly Natural News Report", and several books. The club's Legal Defense Fund, with offices in San Francisco and Denver, pursues litigation on environmental issues of national significance. Contact Sierra Club, 1050 Mills Tower, San Francisco, California, 94104 or 324 C St., SE, Washington, D.C. 20003, (202) 547-1144.

THE LEAGUE OF WOMEN VOTERS. . . has a reputation among environmentalists, politicians and bureaucrats for sound research, probing pamphlets, and effective citizen education around the problems of air and water pollution and solid waste management. Since it is not tax exempt, the League's legislative action division has lobbied extensively on behalf of environmental legislation and then followed up the laws in their bureaucratic implementation. The League's vice president and head of its environmental quality program is the only woman sitting on the President's Advisory Council to the U.S. Environmental Protection Agency. Contact: Environmental Quality Program, League of Women Voters of the United States, 1730 M St., NW, Washington, D.C. 20036 (202) 296-1770.

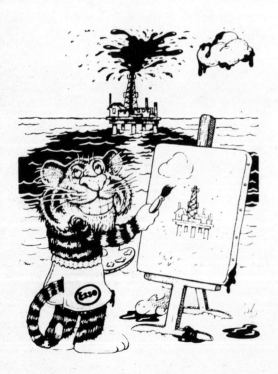

FRIENDS OF THE EARTH. . . a 25,000-member organization which educates and lobbies around environmental issues. Created in 1969, FOE is a broad-based environmental group with activity ranging from saving wilderness and wildlife to coming down hard on big industry polluters. A number of health-related topics have been of major concern to FOE: lobbying against relaxation of the Clean Air Act in the face of the ongoing energy controversy; participating in hearings on pending solid waste legislation; forming a coalition to stop the SST. One of the major anti-nuclear lobbyists, FOE has spoken forcibly against the Atomic Energy Commission and the unresolved safety problems of nuclear plants. Recognizing the dangers of strip-mining (acid runoff and waterway course changes which severely affect area water supplies), FOE created a major anti-stripmining coalition. They put out two regular publications: Not Man Apart, their monthly periodical, and ECO, a series of issue-oriented reports. Contact Friends of the Earth, 620 C St., SE, Washington, D.C. 20003 (202) 543-4312.

HEALTH RESEARCH GROUP/PESTICIDE PROJECT. . . has been under the Nader umbrella since 1969. Presently it is a two-pronged project: advocating for the implementation of the 1972 Pesticide Act, and investigating possibly harmful pesticides and working for their removal. Because the implementation schedule for the 1972 Congressional Pesticides Act goes until 1976, the Pesticide Project is especially active. EPA taskforces are working to formulate the regulations for this act; a large amount of the project's time is spent advising the taskforces, monitoring regulations and offering criticisms and suggestions for improvements. Rather than use litigation, the Pesticide Project prefers the tactic of petitioning (submitting formal requests). Project petitions have requested the banning of various dangerous pesticides, helped to rescind actions taken by EPA, and requested the release of the names of pesticides which have potentially harmful ingredients. The project does some lobbying. Contact HEALTH RESEARCH GROUP/PESTICIDE PROJECT, 2000 P St., NW, Washington, DC 20036, (202) 872-0320.

THE NATIONAL AUDUBON SOCIETY. . . isn't just for the birds. The 225,000 member organization produces a slew of educational services: films, pamphlets, newsletters, the bi-monthly illustrated Audubon magazine, camps and training programs. The Audubon Society has followed pesticides closely and consistently since the late 1940's when it was the first national organization to call for a ban on the use of DDT. Since then, it publicized the dangers of a variety of toxic pesticides, called for natural, biological substitutes, and plugged away at the Federal government for stiff controls on the manufacture and use of pesticides. With the enactment of the 1972 pesticides legislation, Audubon has been among the few environmental organizations to keep close tabs on the Environmental Protection Agency's development of regulations to implement and enforce pesticides control. Contact: National Audubon Society, 950 Third Ave., New York, NY 10022 (212) 832-3200 and 1511 K St., NW, Washington, D.C. 20005, (202) 833-3892.

NATIONAL INTERVENORS. . . calls for a moratorium on the construction and operation of nuclear power plants "until such problems as reactor safety, routine radioactive releases, transportation and diversion of nuclear materials for private atomic weapons are resolved." The coalition of over 100 local groups was originally engaged in lobbying at nuclear-related hearings; however, based on its own experiences, NI has come to see the effectiveness of lobbying as minimal. NI now serves as an information clearinghouse, acting on the belief that a nuclear moratorium will only be achieved through greater public awareness. A newsletter is put out monthly as well as a wealth of reprints on the hazards of nuclear power. Contact: National Intervenors, 153 E St., SE, Washington, D.C. 20003 (202) 543-1642.

NATIONAL CLEAN AIR COALITION. . . is a lobbying group composed of numerous national and local environmental, labor and health organizations including Friends of the Earth, Sierra Club, United Auto Workers, Oil Chemical and Atomic Workers, American Lung Association and American Public Health Association. Formed in 1973 in the face of pending Emergency Energy Legislation which called for a major weakening of the Clean Air Act of 1970, the Coalition is working for implementation and enforcement of the provisions of the Clean Air Act. The Coalition views the Emergency Energy Legislation as only the first of many administration and industrial attempts to weaken the Clean Air Act. By combining the strength of national and local organizations, NCAC has been able to play a significant role in Congressional Committee actions; amendments strengthening the Clean Air Act have been introduced by the Coalition through sympathetic Congresspeople. The Coalition encourages the formation of state level Clean Air Coalitions, informs and helps to coordinate the actions of its member groups and provides up-to-date information on the status of clean air legislation. Contact National Clean Air Coalition, 1609 Connecticut Ave., NW, Washington, D.C. 20009, (202) 462-0660.

CITIZENS AGAINST NOISE. . . is the only national citizens' group concerned with all types of noise pollution. Originally created to substantiate the need for anti-noise ordinances in its native Chicago. CAN currently answers inquiries from local citizen groups concerning noise preventive action, and advises state and city governments as they write laws and ordinances. Municipal groups are assisted in preparation of testimony for noise control hearings. Contact: Citizens Against Noise, c/o Theodore Berland, 2729 W. Lunt Ave., Chicago, IL 60645 (312) 274-0980.

SCIENTISTS' INSTITUTE FOR PUBLIC INFORMATION . . . is a national clearinghouse for information on science-related public issues as well as the national coordinating body for its affiliated local scientist's committees. SIPI believes that it is the responsibility of scientists to share socially important technical information with the general public; toward that end, they strive to inform scientists of the social implications of their work and enlist their support in informing the public. Local affiliated science information committees and special task forces publicize issues in Environment magazine, SIPI's official publication; the SIPI environmental workbooks; occasional special reports; and conferences and workshops. SIPI works in the areas of air, water and soil pollution; the effects of pesticides, radiation, lead, mercury and other heavy metals in the environment; the growth of energy production and resource utilization; alternatives to present utilization of technology. A major part of SIPI's attention has gone to studying and providing widely used information about the civilian nuclear power industry. In a recent lawsuit against the Atomic Energy Commission, the unanimous court opinion confirmed the view held by SIPI that the nation has not yet developed an adequate policy for future energy development. Maintaining that "the development of a rational energy policy for the US is far too important to leave solely in the hands of the AEC," SIPI established a task force to develop and make available to the public the relevant factual information. Contact SIPI, 30 E. 68th St., New York, NY 10021. (212) 249-3200.

Young people today are the first generation to carry strontium 90 in their bones, DDT in their fat, and asbestos in their lungs.
—Science In The Public Interest

CENTER FOR SCIENCE IN THE PUBLIC INTEREST. . . is the 1971 brainchild of four alumni of Ralph Nader's Center for the Study of Responsive Law. Believing that "the myth of objectivity is the worst myth we've got in the scientific profession", they work to spark the social consciences of scientists and establish the legitimacy of scientific advocacy in the public interest. CSPI provides competent witnesses to testify at congressional hearings on science-related legislation, informs consumers about scientific problems and instigates lawsuits on public interest questions. CSPI's team of six scientists focuses on air and water pollution, food additives, energy consumption, solid wastes and more. In recent months, CSPI has joined twelve other environmental organizations in suiing the U.S. Environmental Protection Agency for issuing regulations that fail to remove lead immediately from gasoline, thereby violating the Clean Air Act. It has also cooperated

with environmental groups campaigning for restoration of federal spending in solid waste management and is pursuing research exposing the hazards of nuclear power plants. Recent publications include two extensive reports on the health and environmental effects of asbestos and auto-induced air pollution. A quarterly newsletter records the activities of CSPI and is complemented by an issue-oriented monthly "Public Newsletter". Contact: Center for Science in the Public Interest, 1779 Church St., NW, Washington, DC 20036 (202) 332-6000.

UNION OF CONCERNED SCIENTISTS. . . is a coalition of scientists, engineers and other professionals operating out of the Massachusetts Institute of Technology since 1969. Bringing a high level of technical expertise to their work, UCS is concerned with the impact of advanced technology on society. In the last several years, UCS has put the majority of its energies into an intensive technical study of nuclear power plant safety and other aspects of the nuclear program. Alternative energy resources being studied by UCS and brought to the public's attention. Major objectives of UCS are to confer to the public the results of research, to supply citizen action groups with technical assistance and to participate in pertinent hearings requiring technical testimony. Contact: Union of Concerned Scientists, P.O. Box 289, MIT Branch Station, Cambridge, MA 02139, (617) 253-7584.

RESOURCES

BOOKS

The Environmental Handbook, Garrett De Bell. Ballantine Books, 36 West 20th St., New York, NY 10003, 1970. 367 pp. $.95
. . . compilation of introductory essays by numerous noted environmentalists, originally published for the April 22, 1970 "Earth Day". The book covers possible solutions to the major problems of the ecological crisis, research and educational actions the individual may pursue and political action. Friends of the Earth defend their belief that conservation will have no real power until it becomes a major election issue. Environmental groups must establish themselves as a strong lobbying force and also support politicians from either party who are true conservationalists. The book is a good basic introduction to some of the philosophy, causes and problems that must be dealt with and some solutions that must be taken if Earth and its inhabitants are to survive.

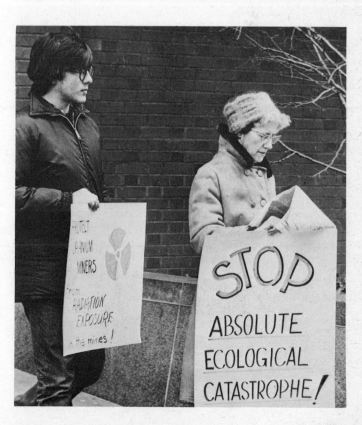

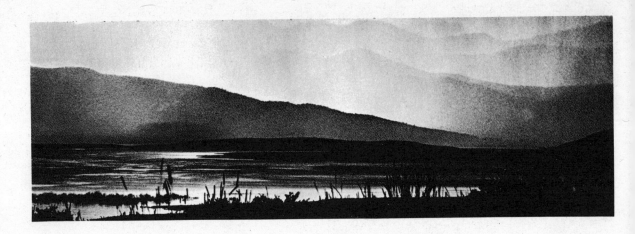

Poisoned Power, John W. Gofman and Arthur R. Tamploin, Rodale Press Book Div. Inc., 33 E. Minoe St., Emmaus, PA 18049, 1971. 368 pp.
. . . well written, rudimentary explanation by two experts on nuclear processes (power plants, fission, reactors) and potential dangers of radiation to human beings and the environment. Discusses in detail the lethal effects of radiation exposure which include injury to the cells leading to cancer or leukemia. The dangers of the growing use of nuclear fission for electrical power production presents no alternative except the development of safe energy sources such as geothermal, solar, and fusion. Provides a sound background to the problem as well as an educational base for political action against the proliferation of nuclear breed reactor construction.

Nixon and the Environment: The Politics of Devastation, League of Conservation Voters Report, Village Voice, 80 University Place, New York, NY 10003, 1972. 179 pp. $2.45
. . ."a reasoned persuasive indictment of a regime that has mastered the theatrics but not the substance of environmentalism." Nixon is a collection of essays written by respected environmental activists on twelve major environmental issues, each examining the role of the (first) Nixon administration to a specific issue. Included are chapters on air pollution, water pollution, energy, pesticides and solid wastes. It focuses on the environmentally crucial years of 1970-72, tracing the role and position of the Nixon Administration on environmental legislation and enforcement of that period. The book documents its basic thesis that Nixon's promises to fight pollution have been little more than rhetoric. For example, the chapter on water pollution illustrates how the Nixon record on new water pollution legislation displays a reluctance to extend the basic principles of law and order to outlaws of the big business variety. Though a bit outdated in regard to recent legislation and administrative action, the book is an excellent expose of the often devastating influence of the powers that be.

Water Wasteland, David Zwick and Marcy Benstock. Bantam Books, Inc., 666 Fifth Ave., New York, NY 10019, 1971. 494 pp. $1.50
. . .a Ralph Nader Task Force Report on Water Pollution, which lays out a devastating critique of federal and state governments' cosmetic attempts at water pollution control between 1948 and 1971. "The major problem in pollution control is the vast economic and political power of large polluters. Water pollution exists, in large part, because polluters have more influence over the government than do those they 'pollute'." This book played a significant role in the subsequent revamping of the federal water pollution control program in the fall of 1972 when Congress overrode Nixon's veto of the Federal Water Pollution Control Act Amendments of 1972. As a result, many of Wasteland's specific criticisms are outdated as the government tries to implement the new law and different problems and obstacles arise. Nevertheless, the report's expose of bureaucratic breakdowns, industry lobbying to undermine the law's administration, funding shortages, and political infighting are still relevant to an appreciation of the ongoing problems that tie up the nation's efforts to clean up its waters. Zwick and Benstock's book is still unmatched as the most penetrating political analysis of water pollution in America.

Conservation Directory 1974, The National Wildlife Federation, 1412 Sixteenth St., NW, Washington, D.C. 20036. 206 pp. $2.
. . .comprehensive directory of governmental and citizen organizations and agencies concerned with the use and management of natural resources. Provides an extensive listing of such groups at the national level plus detailed listings for the individual states.

Highways and Air Pollution, A Citizens' Primer, James B. Sullivan, Center for Science in the Public Interest, 1779 Church Street, NW, Washington, D.C. 20036. 53 pp. $3.00
. . .provides a technical examination of the impact of auto pollution on human health and the environment. The author's purpose is to enable citizens to critically evaluate the environmental impact of proposed highways & prevent the construction of those roadways that pose unacceptable pollution threats. The U.S. Environmental Protection Agency which has concluded that in at least 37 urban areas the volume of traffic and not just the individual auto emissions, must be curtailed if federal air quality standards are to be achieved. In light of this, it is particularly important that citizens fight against the construction of highways which would attract new traffic into an area and further undermine air quality.

"Ecology and Revolutionary Thought," Murray Bookchin, in Post Scarcity Anarchism, Ramparts Press, 1280 Lincoln Ave., Palo Alto, CA 94301. 288 pp. $2.95
. . . one of the earliest, and one of the best political analyses of the implications of ecological disaster. Proposing rather than indicting, Bookchin deftly builds the argument for a decentralized, reconstructive anarchic society which accentuates and develops variety in necessary industries, agriculture, and interpersonal relationships. "Anarchism is not only a stateless society but also a harmonized society which exposes man to the stimuli provided by both agrarian and urban life, to physical activity and mental activity, to unrepressed sensuality and self-directed spirituality, to communal solidarity and individual development, to regional uniqueness and worldwide brotherhood, to spontaneity and self-discipline, to the elimination of toil and the promotion of craftmanship."

Finding Your Way Through EPA, Office of Public Affairs, US Environmental Protection Agency, Washington, D.C. 20460 Free

. . .is a directory to the offices and administrators in the US Environmental Protection Agency. Information on all EPA publications on air, water, solid waste, radiation, noise, and toxic substances can be obtained through this mailing address, or Citizen Information Division, US Environmental Protection Agency, Waterside Mall—West Tower, Washington, D.C. 20460.

"Is the Water Safe to Drink" and two sequel articles, Robert Harris and Edward Brecher, Consumer Reports, June, July and August issues, 1974, $.60 /issue

. . .a series of three articles which comprise one of the few publications on the need to upgrade the drinking water piped into homes and businesses. Although further research on the identification of drinking water contaminants and their health effects is encouraged, the authors urge that such research accompany and follow immediate major improvements in today's drinking supplies. Of special interest to those wishing to launch a community action program is the final article on community water action programs, describing the step by step procedure which was successfully carried out by an Alameda County, California group, People for Better Water.

The Case For A Nuclear Moratorium, Environmental Action Foundation, Suite 732, Dupont Circle Building, Washington, D.C. 20036. 30 pp. $.50

. . .presents three essays supporting a moratorium on the construction and operation of nuclear power plants by Wilson Clark, energy consultant for the Environmental Policy Center, John W. Gofman, Professor of Medical Physics, University of California; and Mike Gravel, U.S. Senator from Alaska. All three have been outspoken critics of the promotion of nuclear power by the Atomic Energy Commission, the reactor manufacturers, and the electric utilities.

PERIODICALS

Environmental Action, Environmental Action, Inc., Suite 731, 1346 Connecticut Ave., Washington, DC 20036. $10/year
. . .comes out bi-weekly on 50 percent recycled paper. Includes "eco notes" and two major stories on the latest political happenings in the environmental movement. The magazine's staff doubles as a political lobbying force organized to focus concern on the environmental crisis.

Environment, Scientists' Institute for Public Information, 438 N. Skinker Blvd., St. Louis, MO 63130. $10/year, ten issues
. . .recommended by most groups we contacted as the best environmental magazine. The official journal of SIPI.

Not Man Apart, Friends of the Earth, 529 Commercial Street, San Francisco, CA 94111. $5/year
. . .is published monthly, featuring news reports on the environment, in-depth issue analyses, and regular columns on "Congress In Action", "Pacific Northwest News", "Farthest North: Alaska Report", and more. Approaches the environment from a multiple perspective focusing on the scientific developments, the political battles and current literature in the field.

Air/Water Pollution Report, Business Publishers, Inc., P.O. Box 1067, Blair Station, Silver Spring, MD 20910. $120/ year
. . . ten page monthly newsletter that covers legislative, administrative, and legal developments in the fields of air and water pollution control plus selected news on industrial issues. Business Publishers also publishes: Energy Resources Report, $120/year, weekly; Noise Control Report, $60/year, biweekly; Solid Waste Report, $70/year, biweekly; and Toxic Materials News, $96/year, twice monthly.

Environmental Update on Solid Waste Management, The League of Women Voters Education Fund, 1730 M St., NW, Washington, D.C. 20036, Free
. . .collection of monthly and bimonthly newsletters providing a running commentary on federal legislative developments in solid waste management.

FILMS AND TAPES

Oil, Chemical and Atomic Workers Union, 1636 Champa, Denver, CO 80202

"By Land, Sea And Air", 31 min. cl. $10.00/day
Effects of pesticides on farm workers and environment.

Impact Films, 144 Bleeker St., New York, NY 10012

"How Safe Are America's Reactors?", 26 min., 1972, $50. (sale: $250.)
Calls attention to the unresolved dangers of this country's nuclear energy program.

McGraw Hill Film Rental, 330 W. 42nd St., New York, NY 10036

"Death Be Not Loud", 29 min. cl., $28, (sale: $340.00)
Produced for ABC news, reviews noise pollution problem and some possible solutions to it.

Cedar
and
jagged
fir uplift
sharp barbs
against the gray
and cloud-piled sky;
and in the bay blown
spume and windrift
and thin, bitter spray
snap at the whirling sky;
and the pine trees lean
one way.

A wild duck calls to
her mate, and the ragged
and passionate tones stagger and
fall, on these stones—are lost
in the lapping of water on smooth, flat
stones.

This is a beauty of disonance, this
resonance of stony strand, this smoked
cry curled over a black
pine like a broken and
wind-battered branch
when the wind bends
the tops of the
pines and curdles
the sky from the
north.

This is the beauty
of strength broken
by strength and
still strong.
—Chevron/LNS

GOVERNMENT

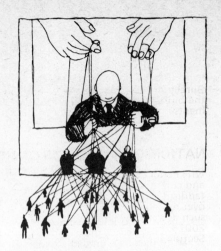

Trying to understand the Department of Health, Education and Welfare, which is the key government agency responsible for health, is an extremely frustrating task. The health structure of the department is constantly undergoing reorganization—agencies appear, disappear, and pop up in new places under slightly different names. Yet for many local projects, sorting out the jumble of departments and agencies is a crucial first step toward receiving funding. Therefore, we are including a section on government to provide an overview of the various health related organizations as well as a brief description of their responsibilities and short-comings.

It is important to understand that the federal government uses social service spending as an economic tool rather than as a means to help low-income people. This means that social and welfare programs are arbitrarily cut to slow down inflation, regardless of their human value, while corporate subsidies and military spending remain constant or increase. When Nixon makes drastic cuts in health care appropriations, he is choosing a poor victim to right a wrong that he, his predecessors and an inflationary capitalist system have created.

President Nixon is an advocate of "New Federalism" which basically means less federal government control over state and local programs. His emphasis is toward getting the government out of direct delivery of health services by subsidizing private industries and giving money to individuals as opposed to public institutions; and by decentralizing the federal government's responsibility and putting more power at the state and local level. As a part of "New Federalism", Nixon has terminated or cut back on health services planning and development programs, health service delivery programs, health service delivery programs, and research training and manpower programs, thus, bringing down the wrath of health professionals, educators, and consumers throughout the country.

Some groups are organizing around federal cuts in an effort to keep public health hospitals and local services open. After all, many federally-funded clinics and hospitals provide crucial services to millions of people. But money and token restructuring alone will not solve the crisis of a dilapidated health "non-system". Among other things, genuine local control and coordinated planning are vitally important.

The following list and description of health-related government agencies should give you some idea of basic organizational structure, who is responsible for what, and which agencies might fund community projects. (These are mainly centered in Health Resources Administration and Health Services Administration). Most of the agencies distribute free pamphlets describing their activities in detail, available on request from their officers of public information. Since there is constant reorganization within this great bureaucracy, groups desiring updated information should contact the government directly. Some of the resources at the end of the section provide an in-depth analysis of administrative and legislative developments in the field.

DEPARTMENT OF HEALTH, EDUCATION, AND WELFARE

Public Health Service

PHS is under the direct authority of the Assistant Secretary of Health, Charles Edwards, a Nixon mouthpiece formerly of the Office of Management and Budget. The five member agencies (National Institutes of Health; Food and Drug Administration; Alcohol, Drug Abuse and Mental Health Administration; Health Resources Administration and Health Services Administration) are responsible for helping states and communities develop local health resources, conducting and supporting medical research, and developing cooperation in health projects with other nations. The Executive Office is located at 5600 Fishers Lane, Rockville, Md 20852, (202) 245-6297.

FOOD AND DRUG ADMINISTRATION

FDA is the federal government's primary consumer protection agency. FDA is responsible for seeing that foods, drugs, and cosmetics on the market are safe and that their manufacturers do not make false claims as to their effectiveness. Unfortunately FDA officials have shown a disturbing tendency to act in the interests of industry rather than protecting the consumer. Twenty-two of the 52 top officials at FDA have worked for industries regulated by the Administration and 37 of 49 recently retired high officials are now working for such companies. FDA's relatively small budget does not allow them to hire enough scientists to adequately research each new drug and and cosmetic; often when they do discover obvious dangers, they keep quiet because of the industries' pressures. See Drugs and Community Health.

Bureau of Biologics regulates biological products shipped in interstate and foreign commerce, such as vaccines and blood.

Bureau of Drugs develops standards and regulations and collects research on drugs.

Bureau of Foods researches and develops standards for the composition, safety and nutritional value of foods, additives, coloring, and cosmetics.

Bureau of Radiological Health protects the public from unnecessary exposure to radiation from such products as color TVs, and X-ray machines.

Bureau of Veterinary Medicine

Bureau of Toxicological Research conducts research to study the biological effects of chemical substances in the environment.

NATIONAL INSTITUTES OF HEALTH

NIH conducts biomedical research into the cause, prevention and cure of disease. A Major criticism is that NIH is prone to faddism, emphasizing spectacular and prestigious diseases over more mundane ones that perhaps affect more people, such as hypertension. 9000 Rockville Pike, Bethesda, MD 20014, (301) 656-4000. See Health Personnel and Training Section on Research.

National Cancer Institute is responsible for coordinating cancer research and seeing that new knowledge is quickly applied.

National Health and Lung Institute researches heart and lung diseases and is responsible for sickle cell anemia work.

National Library of Medicine

National Institute of Arthritis, Metabolism and Digestive Disease

National Institute of Allergy and Infectious Disease

National Institute of Child Health and Human Development researches aging, mental retardation, and infant death.

National Institute of Dental Research fights a continuing valiant battle against the sinister forces of tooth decay.

National Institute of Environmental Health Sciences researches biological, chemical, and physical factors in the environment.

National Institute of General Medical Sciences supports research and research training in the basic medical sciences, especially emphasizing trauma therapy, anesthesiology, and genetics.

National Institute of Neurological Diseases and Stroke researches such diseases as multiple sclerosis, muscular distrophy, and epilepsy.

National Eye Institute

Clinical Center is both a research lab and hospital. "Only people with rare diseases need apply" since the Center only accepts patients useful for Institute studies.

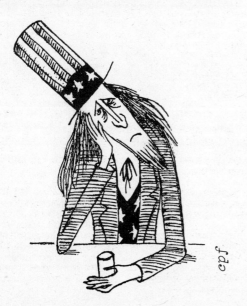

Fogarty International Center is responsible for promoting the development of science internationally as it relates to health.

Division of Computer Research and Technology has a research and service program in computer-related sciences in support of NIH programs.

Division of Research Resources supports research centers and develops special programs in support of health-related research.

Division of Research Services provides needed centralized scientific, technical, and engineering services for biomedical research, medical arts and photographic work.

Division of Research Grants collects statistics on Public Health Service programs, helps formulate policies on research and research training programs, and evaluates NIH grant and award applications.

ALCOHOL, DRUG ABUSE, AND MENTAL HEALTH ADMINISTRATION

ADAMHA has the responsibility for preventing, controling and treating alcoholism, drug abuse, and mental/emotional problems. In the past the Administration attitude toward drug abuse was purely punitive. It now funds primarily methadone maintenance programs.

National Institute on Drug Abuse

National Institute on Alcohol Abuse and Alcoholism

National Institute of Mental Health is responsible for conducting and supporting programs for the development of personnel and services for rehabilitation and the promotion of mental health. It is a focus for behavioral science activities directed at cultural and social problems related to mental health, as well as studying alcoholism, narcotics addiction, and drug abuse.

HEALTH SERVICES ADMINISTRATION

Health Services Administration (HSA) is concerned with the quality, cost, and utilization of health care services. This is where funding for various community health demonstration projects and services comes from.

Indian Health Service (IHS) provides direct care for Native Americans and Alaskans through a system of over 450 hospitals, health centers, health stations and satellite field health clinics. Facilities are very understaffed and over half of IHS hospitals do not meet Joint Commission on the Accreditation of Hospital standards.

Federal Health Programs Service provides care for merchant seamen, Coast Guardsmen and Federal employees with illnesses and injuries related to work. They also operate Public Health Service Hospitals.

Bureau of Community Health Services is developing various models for providing maternal and child clinics, neighborhood health centers and family planning programs; it operates the Migrant Health Program and Regional Medical Programs.

The government bureaucracy shifts so constantly they can't even keep track of themselves. It can take 10 or 15 calls to extract a piece of information from that maze, partly because people are still directing you to call bureaus that no longer exist, etc. Researching this section has shown me that the government is even more (expletive deleted) than I always thought.

—a usually reliable Source

Health Maintenance Organizations and the National Health Service Corps (See Health Personnel and Training) have also been moved to this bureau.

Center for Disease Control (CDC) administers national programs for the prevention and control of disease including lead poisoning, rat control and smoking.

The National Institute of Occupational Safety and Health (NIOSH), which has legal responsibility for enforcement of the Occupational Safety and Health Act is under CDC. See Occupational Health section.

HEALTH RESOURCES ADMINISTRATION

Bureau of Health Services Research is empowered to fund demonstration projects in health services delivery that involve innovative use of personnel.

Bureau of Health Resources Development is responsible for Comprehensive Health Planning (CHP), Hill-Burton activities, manpower programs, health planning, and gives administrative support to Regional Medical Programs (RMP).

National Center for Health Statistics collects, analyzes, and disseminates data on health trends and needs.

End of Public Health Services. Also under HEW:

SOCIAL AND REHABILITATION SERVICE

SRS provides technical, consultative, and financial support through social rehabilitation income maintenance, medical and child welfare services for the disabled, the needy, the aged, and children. 330 "C" St., SW, Washington, D.C. 20203, (202) 655-4000.

Rehabilitation Services Administration was created to administer state and federal programs of vocational rehabilitation for the disabled and developmentally disabled, preparing them for employment, independent living, and self-help. This agency is known to be haphazard and paternalistic. (See Deaf section)

Assistance Payments Administration coordinates federal and state expenditures on public assistance programs.

Community Services Administration assists states in providing social services to welfare recipients, and former and potential applicants or recipients. This includes Aid to Families with Dependent Children, day care, and family planning.

Medical Services Administration administers programs of medical service to the needy and medically needy.

SOCIAL SECURITY ADMINISTRATION

SSA is a national program of contributory social insurance. It covers Medicare and Black Lung benefits, enforcing the Coal Mine Health and Safety Act of 1969. The Administration is reticent to pay benefits, particularly for Black Lung. 1325 "K" St., NW, Washington, DC 20203, (202) 953-3600.

Program Bureaus of SSA:

Bureau of Retirement and Survivors Insurance directs the Social Security Administration (SSA) abroad, and directs the administration of retirement and survivor insurance programs. It deals with all processes and policy issues that are common to all social security programs.

Bureau of Disability Insurance directs the administration of disability and Black Lung benefit programs and with the Social Rehabilitation Service administers the Disability beneficiary rehabilitation program.

Bureau of Health Insurance directs the administration of health insurance programs.

Bureau of Supplemental Security Income for the Aged, Blind and Disabled develops, recommends, and issues policies to direct the Supplemental Security Income program.

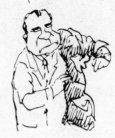

DECENTRALIZE THE POWER STRUCTURE!

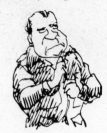

REDISTRIBUTE THE INCOME!

Operating Bureaus of SSA:

Bureau of Data Processing establishes and maintains basic records of the Social Security programs.

Bureau of District Office Operations

Bureau of Hearings and Appeals provides direction and operation instructions for the hearing and appeals process of Social Security programs.

DEPARTMENT OF AGRICULTURE

DOA controls diseases of livestock and poultry transmissable to people, researches food consumption practices and is involved in pest control programs. Independence Ave., between 12th and 14th St., SW, Washington, D.C. 20250, (202) 655-4000.

FOOD AND NUTRITION PROGRAM

It is significant that this program is under the Department of Agriculture rather than under HEW. The priorities are to use up extra food and support the agriculture business rather than to serve hungry people. Theoretically the budget is open-ended (they can spend an unlimited amount of money), but DOA makes little to no effort to encourage the use of Food Programs and turns money back to the treasury each year.

Food Stamp Program is a system of selling eligible people a set amount of food stamps each month for a fee determined by each person's income and expenses. The stamps can then be exchanged for food at most grocery stores. Participants regularly complain of the incredible bureaucracy and inefficiency that characterize this program.

Once when I was getting recertified for foodstamps, I could hear the caseworker in the next booth talking to someone who was apparently there for the first time. He was an old man and had probably been waiting all morning. He didn't understand how the program worked, and he just kept getting more and more confused. He just kept saying he needed food stamps. The caseworker got more and more exasperated and finally almost yelled, "Just because you don't have any money doesn't mean you qualify for foodstamps." And that's the way it is. Just because you don't have any food doesn't mean you're going to get any. It's the rules that count.
—a Washington, D.C. woman

Child Nutrition Programs include the National School Lunch Program, School Breakfast Program, Special Food Program for Children, and the Special Milk Program. The first two are usually operated through public schools. The problem is that they only provide money for food, none for equipment or workers' salaries, so some schools may not be able to afford them. The Special Food and Milk Programs for Children receive the least funding and are not widely used. (See Community Health.)

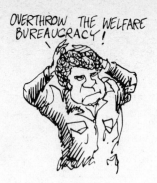

OVERTHROW THE WELFARE BUREAUCRACY!

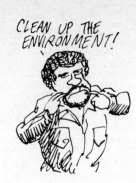

CLEAN UP THE ENVIRONMENT!

DRUG ENFORCEMENT AGENCY

DEA controls narcotic and dangerous drug abuse through enforcement and prevention programs. It conducts domestic and international investigation of illegal drug traffickers, offers training programs for law enforcers, and regulates legal traffic in narcotic and dangerous drugs.

LAW ENFORCEMENT ASSISTANCE ADMINISTRATION

LEAA funnels money into state programs to "combat crime." This has involved funding prison programs that use behavior modification and psychosurgery. On the whole, LEAA concentrates on supporting local police power rather than attacking the roots of crime.

Food Distribution Program distributes surplus food to individuals, to schools, and during disasters. In most states, this program has been replaced by the food stamp program. It is superior to the food stamp program in that it is completely free, but the food comes in bulk and is difficult to transport and store for some people. It is also fairly low in quality and nutritional value.

DEPARTMENT OF LABOR

DOL has information on health careers and assists in limited training for health occupations. The Occupational Safety and Health Administration is under DOL. Constitution Ave., and 14th St., NW, Washington, D.C. 20210, (202) 393-2420.

DEPARTMENT OF TRANSPORTATION

Department of Transportation is concerned with auto and highway safety as well as the safety of workers in highway and tunnel construction. 400 7th St., NW, Washington, D.C. (202) 655-4000.

Rescue and Emergency Medical Services Division designs emergency medical technician training courses and has useful publications on emergency care.

DEPARTMENT OF JUSTICE

BUREAU OF PRISONS

BOP has jurisdiction over all federal prisons and community treatment facilities, but not over state and local facilities which are generally of much poorer quality. The Health Services Division is responsible for medical and dental care of federal prisoners.

VETERAN'S ADMINISTRATION

VA "operates a chain of hospitals for veterans. Some, but not all, are pretty grim." (HEALTH/PAC). VA funds some methadone maintenance programs, and very few drug-free programs. Only vets with honorable or general discharges are guaranteed VA benefits. A general criticism of the VA is its "American Legion mentality." 2033 "M" St., NW, Washington, D.C., 20420, (202) 872-1151.

APPALACHIAN REGIONAL COMMISSION

ARC is a quasi-government agency which gives grants for demonstration health projects and provides supplements to Hill-Burton Funds, as well as doing non-health related funding work in the Appalachian states. 1666 Connecticut Ave., NW, Washington, D.C. 20235, (202) 967-3167.

ENVIRONMENTAL PROTECTION AGENCY

EPA is an independent executive branch agency chartered with the responsibility of protecting the environment against pollution and degradation. Waterside Mall, 4th and M Sts., SW, (202) 755-2673.

These increased enrollment levels (in health training) will lead to large increments in the future number of active physicians, dentists and nurses. If the training capacity continues to increase, as in the past, there is a distinct possibility of an oversupply of medical personnel.
—Nixon's Fiscal 1975 Federal Budget request explaining a $198 million cut in the HEW Health Manpower training funds.

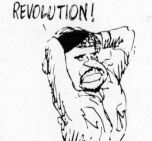

REVOLUTION!

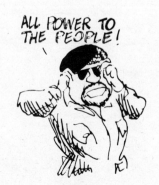

ALL POWER TO THE PEOPLE!

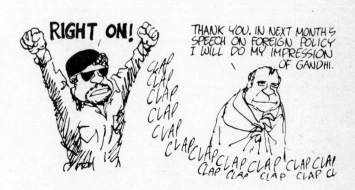

RIGHT ON!

THANK YOU. IN NEXT MONTH'S SPEECH ON FOREIGN POLICY I WILL DO MY IMPRESSION OF GANDHI.

CLAP CLAP CLAP CLAP CLAP CLAP CLAP CLAP CLAP CLAP CLAP CLAP CLAP CLAP CL

HEW Regional Offices

RESOURCES

HEALTH/PAC BULLETIN, 17 Murray St., New York, NY 10007, May, 1973. 28 pp.
. . . this entire issue is devoted to federal health policy according to Richard Nixon. It gives an outstanding analysis of the reasons behind federal health cutbacks, focusing on the specific programs that are being cut and documenting "the repercussions of the Nixon Administration's health budget and cutbacks" on three health institutions in the Bronx. The writers warn health activists against organizing around the issue of cutbacks since Great Society programs have demonstrated that money alone is not the cure for our ailing health system. Especially interesting is the article about Richard Nixon's methods of weakening HEW's resistance to budget cutting: he gradually replaced HEW administrators with people from the Office of Management and Budget "who are imbued with 'budget-mindedness and management capability,'" such as Caspar (Cap the Knife) Weinberger.

U.S. Government Manual 1973/74, Office of the Federal Register, available from the Superintendent of Documents, Government Printing Office, Washington, D.C. 20402, 794 pp. $4.00
. . . brief description of all major government agencies and quasi-government agencies. It is slightly outdated already, but is still a good introduction to how the government is set up.

CONGRESSIONAL QUARTERLY WEEKLY REPORT, 1735 "K" St., NW, Washington, D.C. 20006. $4 00/year for non-government individuals and organizations. Write them for government employees' rates.
. . .discusses important legislative developments in Congress each week and is available in most libraries. The subscription fee includes 52 reports, 3 month indexes, an almanac and access to direct research.

1973 Catalog of Federal Domestic Assistance, Executive Office of the President, Office of Management and Budget, available from the Superintendent of Documents, Washington, D.C. About 800 pp. $7. $9.50 with binder.
. . . a comprehensive listing and description of Federal programs and activities providing assistance or benefits to the public. Lists 1,051 programs of 61 different Federal departments, independent agencies, commissions, and councils. The programs involve grants, loans, scholarships, mortgage loans, insurance and other types of financial assistance.

WASHINGTON REPORT ON MEDICINE AND HEALTH 437 National Press Building, Washington, D.C. 20004. $75/year
. . . this weekly report gives headline news relating to health, although it does not go into any depth. Available in medical school libraries.

MODERN HOSPITAL, 230 W. Monroe, Chicago, IL 60606. $12/year for students, $15 for others
. . . this monthly magazine keeps track of legislative and administratives trends and decisions that affect health. Fairly liberal in its viewpoint.

HEW Budget for 1975
Health Programs—Summary

(Budget Authority in Millions)	1973	1974	1975	Change
Food and Drug Administration	$ 149	165	200	+35
Health Services Administration	1,082	1,176	1,177	+1
Center for Disease Control	160	136	138	+2
National Institutes of Health	1,758	1,781	1,835	+54
Alcohol Drug Abuse and Mental Health Administration	881	833	735	—98
Health Resources Administration	1,249	1,137	574	—563
Assistant Secretary of Health	76	74	97	+23
TOTAL	$5,355	5,302	4,756	—546
TOTAL OUTLAYS	*4,311*	*5,271*	*5,591*	*+320*

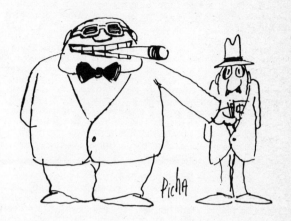

HEALTH FINANCING AND PLANNING

PROBLEM

To understand the health care system in the United States, it is crucial to look at both financing and planning. These two concepts are intricately related. Problems with planning flow directly from the economic base upon which our health care system is founded. Financing of health care is based in the private sector; therefore, planning is geared towards guaranteeing hefty profits and prestige for health care providers and the myriad of satellite industries they support.

At present, health care financing is done primarily through insurance, both private (Blue Cross/Blue Shield, and commercial companies) and public (Medicare and Medicaid). Fundamental problems are inherent in this method of financing. Whether legally "profit" or "non-profit", all the private companies are out to make money and secure their own position in the massive health hierarchy. And no insurance system—public or private—is actively concerned with the quality of care or over-all planning. No amount of money poured into the present system will result in significantly better care.

Blue Cross and Blue Shield were created during the Depression by doctors and hospitals eager to insure payment of bills and their own financial stability. Although technically "non-profit", they receive over $110 million each year in investment returns and spend $300 million on advertising and administrative salaries and costs. Indeed, the only thing distinguishing the Blues from profit making companies is the fact that stockholders do not receive dividends.

The segment of the private insurance industry is the commercial company. Most commercial insurance companies are closely tied to the giant financial powers in this country—and are blatantly in the business for money. Some commercial companies have been documented as having up to a 35% profit margin.

In 1972 private health insurance companies received $21.1 billion in premiums while paying out only $19 billion in benefits. The remaining $2.1 billion, coupled with returns on investment, went to overhead, advertising and profits. Yet, while insurance companies profit from consumer payments, consumers themselves are faced with constantly rising subscriber premiums, deductables and co-insurance. For example, in a two year period in the early 1970's, Blue Cross in Pennsylvania, New Jersey and New York raised their rates by over 40%. It is not difficult to see that the quality and accessibility of health care take second place to the well-being of the insurance industry.

Medicaid and Medicare, once condemned by the AMA as the first step on the rocky road toward socialism, were ostensibly set up to provide adequate health care for the poor, elderly and disabled. They have, however, turned out to be another public subsidy of private industry. Medicare is administered through private insurance companies who receive a comfortable income for their services. Like other government programs, Medicare/caid have been grossly abused and few controls exist. Private doctors have reaped as much as $200,000 annually in medicare/caid payments. Some doctors perform the same procedure twice or call patients in for a second, unnecessary, visit. And it is not uncommon for income from Medicaid/care to be diverted to hospital expansion or other financial adventures rather than improved patient care.

Both private and public sources of financing recklessly pour billions of dollars into health care delivery with no control over where or how that money is used. Hospitals have traditionally used this no-strings attached, cost-plus payment system to expand, buy new equipment, purchase supplies, hike professional and administrative salaries, etc. Most of the decision on how to spend money coming in from insurance payments are not based on a coordinated plan for health delivery, but rather on the financial needs, status and convenience of the particular institutions involved. This combined with the fact that most insurance companies finance (and thereby encourage) in-hospital, rather than ambulatory care, causes massive waste and inefficiency—not to mention a system based on curative rather than preventive care. (See Hospitals).

Rising medical and insurance costs are striking hard at middle, working class, and low income people. In 1972 close to 20% of US citizens under 65 had no hospital or surgical insurance; more than 50% had no medical insurance (outpatient and doctor care). In between those who can (although often with considerable difficulty) afford high insurance payments and those poor enough to receive public insurance, are vast numbers of working people for whom adequate insurance is financially out of the question. With medical costs the number one cause of bankrupcy, one major illness can spell economic ruin for millions of families.

Over the past few years, pre-paid health plans have been heralded as the 'new trend' in providing health care, capable of systematizing services and limiting costs. Developed with an emphasis on primary and preventive care, many offer a full range of services in one or more facilities. Dues are paid in advance with little or no charge at the time of delivery. Thus patients don't have to fear fat bills everytime they pass through the doctor's office. In theory this encourages patients to see doctors regularly rather than waiting for an emergency or until they are sick; with all services often in one building, family-oriented care should become more common. The Committee for National Health Insurance estimates that such group practices can double the number of patients seen by doctors.

Once again, however, private enterprise has stepped in, using the pre-paid concept to bolster bank accounts, rather than to improve the quality of health care. The largest and most successful pre-paid plans are profit making corporations or subsidiaries of the financial giants. Their objective is low cost and high return. Many pre-paid plans do not make the necessary initial outlay of capitol to set up a truly effective preventive health care system and the emphasis on curative care remains. With no one health team responsible for the needs of each individual or family, fragmented, assemblyline care often results. Because the pre-paid corporation receives no payment for in-hospital care beyond the set monthly fee, the emphasis is often on keeping the patients out of the hospital, even when hospitalization is clearly needed. This, combined with the fact that pre-paid plans are largely understaffed and over-enrolled creates a situation in which symptoms are ignored or overlooked to save money and time. Often facilities are difficult to reach and subscribers end up using supplementary services which they pay for out of their own pockets.

Initiating a community-based pre-paid plan or Health Maintenance Organization is a long and difficult process. Raising the money or hassling with government funding with all its red tape and bureaucracy are, at times, insurmountable problems. Yet HMOs not directly controlled by the community are generally more business than service oriented, complete with Public Relations offices and a competitive mentality.

For years the government has had a "hands off" attitude toward the health industry, allowing the private sector to profit at the consumer's expense. In fact, the government has subsidized the industry through such programs as Medicaid/care; contracting with private facilities to provide public services; granting tax exemption to "voluntary" hospitals (many of which perform no charitable or public function); enforcing regulations and granting special privileges to drug, insurance and supply companies; and by its taxation methods, which greatly favor corporations and the wealthy.

Only recently has the government tried to gain control of the monster it helped create. It has instituted new rules and regulations, regulatory agencies, peer review organizations, strict guidelines for federal funding and two new planning programs: Regional Medical Programs (RMP) and Comprehensive Health Planning Programs (CHP). This activity has flourished to the consternation of providers, although many of the more biting policies have been watered down due to industry pressure.

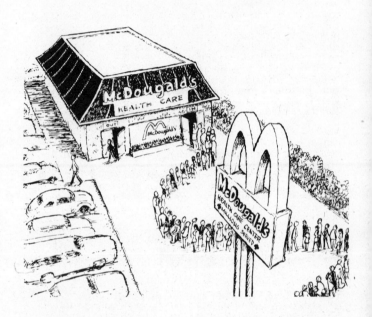

The effect of Regional Medical Programs and Comprehensive Health Planning Boards on government attempts at planning and consumer input has been negligible. Although these two programs have had some success in such areas as regionalizing cancer research and stopping unnecessary expansion, neither program has genuine consumer input (only CHPs are required to have majority consumer representation on the board) and when they do exercise power, it is generally to validate the position of the providers and insure their well-being.

Growing citizen concern over the chaotic and inflationary state of health care is inevitable. Congresspeople, labor leaders, church groups, civic organizations, and even Nixon and the providers themselves are chiming in, calling for: "National Health Insurance". Health insurance is their answer. The great panacea! But let's look a bit closer, remembering the lessons learned from other attempts at private financing and public subsidies. Who is actually being served by National Health Insurance (NHI)? Who is paying for it? Will it improve the quality and accessibility of care? Will the public have a voice in policy? Congress currently has before it over a half dozen bills for NHI and these are some of the questions the consumer must ask in evaluating them. It is imperative that voters know what NHI actually is when election time approaches and candidates lure them with altruistic promises of "quality health care available for all."

No two NHI proposals are alike. They range from Senators Long and Ribicoff's Catastrophic Health Insurance Program to the relatively comprehensive labor-supported Health Security Act (formerly sponsored by Senator Kennedy). Yet, all have a few qualities in common. The NHI bills are basically proposals for systems of financing (often employing the worst elements of the present system) and not for planning health care delivery and quality control. They all serve to keep the health industries happy—at the expense of working people and the poor. While more people receive certain needed services under NHI proposals, most are riddled with limitations: selective coverage, co-insurance, deductables, and regressive payment formulas. To some extent they all subsidize the private insurance and health industry, its profits and excesses.

Most of the proposed NHI plans are clearly set up for the benefit of health care providers: they make no attempt at systematizing services or controlling costs and quality (except through weak HMO models). The Health Security Act is the only one to include an attempt at cost control and planned delivery, although both are based on inadequate financial incentives, playing into the profit motive. None provide effective structures for planned distribution of resources, and provisions for consumer-worker input into policy making are vitually non-existent. Where they do exist, they are in the form of vaguely defined advisory boards. Furthermore, few of the bills mention the role of non-professional health workers; quality review is delegated to professional review boards, loosely structured advisory boards, or not mentioned at all.

Most of the NHI proposals perpetuate a dual system of health care either by omitting certain categories of the poor from coverage or by charging burdensome insurance payments, co-insurance, and deductibles. The Health Security Act, by far the most progressive, promises free health care at the point of delivery. But its financing is based on such inequities as the regressive social security tax and the loop-hole ridden income tax. Relying on these two methods to collect taxes is blatantly unfair.

We cannot hope to have a good, low-cost, accessible health care system without creating a publically financed, planned and controlled health care system. The United States needs a National Health Plan, not National Health Insurance. The power of private enterprise in this country, combined with the negligence of government has resulted in a private sector capable of capturing the financial resources—and therefore the wo/man power and physical resources—from the public sector. This has resulted in the decay of public facilities. As long as this continues, there will be a two-class system with control vested in wealthy providers; health care delivery will not change markedly. Consumers can not have effective input—much less control—without a total restructuring of the health care system.

GLOSSARY OF TERMS:

Out-of-Pocket payment is the amount a person pays for health services at the time of delivery or which s/he pays upon being billed.

Deductible is the fixed amount of money a person must pay for health care before her/his insurance will pay any expenses at all.

Co-insurance is a percent of the cost of an insured service that a person pays her/himself.

Co-payment is a small out-of-pocket payment, such as $2 for a doctor's visit or $.50 for a prescription which is sometimes imposed in an HMO or insurance plan.

Premium is the monthly or yearly amount paid by a person to an insurance company for a policy or to an HMO for enrollment.

PLATFORM

The following is a synthesis of some of the key components of a National Health Plan, aimed at radically changing our system of health care delivery. Some are widely accepted while others have been points of debate among health. The list is neither complete nor static, actually raising more questions than it could hope to answer. But, it is a starting point —and an important one at that.

COST AND FINANCING OF A NATIONAL HEALTH PLAN

—Health care should be free at the point of delivery for all people.
—All private profits coming from the delivery of health services must be eliminated. Under a National Health Plan (NHP), drug and supply companies would be made public; the insurance industry would be abolished. Hospitals and other health care facilities would be publically financed and controlled.
—Financing sound be based on a system of progressive taxation, one in which rich people pay proportionately more than working and low-income people. All forms of income and wealth should be taxed, including savings, inheritance, stocks, bonds and real estate, loopholes should be eliminated.

DISTRIBUTION OF FACILITIES

—Every community (population 10-50,000) will have one or more health centers, plus satellite clinics to provide primary and preventive medical care, dental care, drugs, diagnostic services, lab work and X-rays. Each will have mental health services, drug abuse and alcoholism programs, rehabilitative and social services, out reach work, transportation, home care services, and adult/child day care.
—Training for community members and upgrading of workers will be a regular feature of each clinic or a consortium of several in a given geographic area.
—Each clinic will be linked to a general hospital for in-patient care, consultation, specialized diagnosis and treatment. These hospitals, in turn, will be linked to regional specialized hospitals for rare or difficult cases, such as heart surgery, certain cancers respiratory, renal problems, etc.

TRAINING AND DISTRIBUTION OF HEALTH PERSONNEL

—Clinics and hospitals will have in-house training and upgrading programs to teach skills to community people and workers. In addition, each will offer health education classes for community people.
—Health training centers will replace the fractured system of teaching health sciences which presently exists (i.e., separate schools for doctors, dentists, nurses, pharmacists, etc.). Each will offer a core curriculum with courses for a wide range of health personnel, from aides to doctors. Courses will be geared toward increasing skills along a career ladder and tailored to the students' past training and needs.
—Training in such neglected areas as women's health, geriatric health, occupational health, and the special needs of the incarcerated, will be integrated into regular course work.
—A system to insure adequate distribution of health personnel and resources will be developed. This may mean limiting the number of a given type of personnel in a geographic area or requiring people to practice in the community in which they received training. For the most part, medical training centers will recruit people from the community and region in which they are located to insure the adequate passing on of skills to women, low-income and Third World people, and others who have been denied access to such training and education under our present system.

—Training will be geared to the needs of the patient, rather than those of the researcher and educator, and emphasize a wholistic view of the patient.
—Health science students will work with all patients, not only the poor, thus avoiding a situation where only low income people are used as subjects for training and experimentation.

The issue of control is central to the development of a Health Plan. Both financing and control must be public, with consumers and workers exercising direct power over health policy and facilities. Yet there remain many unanswered questions as to who has final jurisdiction—consumers or workers—in many specific areas. The following outline should act as a stimulus for thought on this important issue.

CONTROL OF FACILITIES

—Each institution will be controlled by a board of consumers and workers.
—Decisions concerning specific departments will be made by all the health workers in that department, while inter-departmental issues will be handled by a committee of workers from each department.
—Decisions involving the expansion of facilities, restructuring of services, or financing will be made by an administrative consumer-worker board. Hopefully, sometimes natural antagonism between providers and consumers which often exists will diminish as more and more workers come from the community in which the facility is located and as the facility begins offering more community-oriented services.
—The administrative board will be the first step in the grievance procedure for workers and consumers.

COMMUNITY HEALTH COUNCILS

—Community Health Councils should be elected by the community, with health workers and consumers from the area represented. At-large representatives would be elected to protect the board from parochial interests and to insure representation of special groups such as the elderly, handicapped, incarcerated, and workers threatened by occupational disease. These councils must truly represent the community served—in terms of race, income, sex, and age.
—Community councils should oversee the needs of the area served, set health policy, and make provisions for the building of needed facilities.
—It will receive funds from the regional planning council and distribute them on a per capita/need basis to neighborhood health centers and satellite clinics.
—The Council would deal with worker and consumer grievances which local facilities were unable to settle.

REGIONAL HEALTH COUNCILS

—Regional Councils should be composed of worker and consumer representatives from community councils, plus at-large members.
—These councils should plan and coordinate resources, allocate funds and work with local and national councils to set overall policy. They will control medical training centers and act as a resource bank for local communities.
—The Regional Council will serve as a third level for consumer and woker grievances.

NATIONAL HEALTH COUNCILS

—The National Health Council would be composed of Regional Council members with at-large representatives.
—It will allocate tax revenue to regional councils according to a formula based on population and special needs of the area.
—The National Council should take an overview of planning and distribution needs, working with local and regional councils to set priorities.
—The Council would set and moniter research policy, and allocate resources for research, both medical and administrative.
—The National Council would develop a resource bank of statistical and technical information to be drawn upon by the regional and community councils.
—It would act as the final grievance step within the health system, with unresolved questions going to the courts.

PROGRAM

I. RESEARCH AND EDUCATE AROUND EXISTING PLANNING AND FINANCING STRUCTURES

A. Research what health financing plans are available in your community, workplace or school.
—what benefits, services or payments are covered by the program.
—what abuses have been perpetrated against members: cutting people off without due process, making people ineligible for benefits on a technicality, raising rates without reason, refusing to authorize a covered service, cut backs in services
—who controls the plan, makes decisions, handles appeals
—what conflicts of interest exist between Boards of Directors and health care providers and financiers.

B. Find out from the local health department who in the area acts as a health planning agency, both private and public, contact the state health department for state-wide agencies, your congressperson for national agencies.
—research the power structure of local agencies for conflicts of interest.
—research where health facilities are located and how locations for facilities have been chosen. For example, are all the major facilities in one area near a medical school?

C. Meet with other community members, workers and students to discuss and publicize the results of your research
—educate others about their rights and existing conditions.

II. BEGIN TO ORGANIZE TO MAKE HEALTH CARE FINANCIALLY AVAILABLE

A. Work to get consumers on policy boards of Blue Cross/Blue Shield (there is now a commitment by Blue Cross to do this—don't let it remain tokenism)
—get workers on Boards who aren't upper rank professionals, for example technicians, aides, LPNs and other allied health personnel
—attend all rate hike hearings in large numbers; make your protests heard
—bring class action suits against waste and mismanagement, refusals to pay full reimbursements, coverage drops, and monopoly and trust building.

B. Educate people about eligibility requirements for Medicare and Medicaid and organize to expand coverage
—do mass sign up campaigns
—fight for consumer and worker representation on Professional Standards Review Organizations, set up by Medicare/caid requirements for quality control
—apply community pressure and take legal and legislative action to change regulations, eliminate bureaucratic red tape and broaden health care coverage to include everything from dental care to hearing aids, abortions to home visits.
—bring class action suits against cuts in federal funding, individual and mass cut-offs, refusals by the states to provide thorough outreach programs and implement regulations
—fight to get Medicare/caid to reimburse for team care, not just individual physician care

C. Educate the public about HMOs and strive to get more representation for consumers and non-professional workers on policy boards
—work for broader services and coverage under the plan
—work to lower monthly payments and membership fees
—do community outreach to get more low-income people on the plan; Medicaid will pay for a pre-paid health plan
—challenge doctors and other health workers with professionalist, sexist, and racist attitudes
—meet with health workers of the plans; their grievances often resemble community members' and they can be important allies in the struggle for better health care delivery

D. Force union officials to bring important health decisions to the rank and file for a vote; union plans cover a significant portion of the population
—agitate for more health care coverage when contract negotiations come up; don't let health care be used as a padding demand that is eventually dropped
—demand that you have a choice of health plans, ranging from insurance to pre-paid plans.

III. BEGIN TO MAKE PLANNING RESPONSIVE TO COMMUNITY NEEDS

A. Attend meetings of local planning agency boards and executive councils

—ask to see your local Comprehensive Health Planning "Master Plan" and review it for defects: are minority groups adequately planned for? are such services as rehabilitation hospitals, half-way houses, health education, drug programs and screening available? If not, it is probably because they are low profit ventures, and no one has bothered to include them

—push for these services at the city and county Health Department or contact the local Tuberculosis Association. Heart, Association, etc. to set up screening and health education

—do advocate planning for your community, helping to set priorities and find resources

—agitate for facility construction in low-income areas and outside of medical empire domination

—file legal suits against those provider members involved in decisions where a conflict of interests exists

—challenge the standing of private corporations as federal agencies and their lack of compliance with federal regulations

B. Organize new channels for obtaining data and statistics relevant to health planning; break the chain of industry-generated, industry-controlled information that supports its desires.

—make use of community organizations and surveys, hospital workers information and advice

C. As informed citizens, demand representation on planning agencies

—keep abreast of decisions

—get community people into public health schools which train planners so that they can get key staff positions on planning boards.

—hold training sessions for consumers and providers on planning boards, educating around community health needs

IV. EXPLORE POSSIBILITIES OF ALTERNATIVE AND COMMUNITY BASED PLANNING AND FINANCING

A. Consider the possibility of setting up a pre-paid community health center, run co-operatively and capable of giving better care, particularly to families

—research state and local laws concerning pre-paid health plans

—investigate the possibility of federal funding, support from local churches and social service agencies

—explore the feasibility of cooperation with area hospitals for back-up services

—recruit doctors and other health personnel willing to accept community control

B. Study the possibility of organizing a non-profit, private planning corporation with representatives from the area communities, progressive health workers and supportive politicians

—demand that the state agency recognize you as the CHP for the region in compliance with federal guidelines

—devise a counter or alternative regional health plan

V. TIE ALL THESE STRUGGLES INTO A FIGHT FOR A COMPREHENSIVE NATIONAL HEALTH PLAN

A. Discuss national health issues and what is needed for an adequate health plan in your workplace, school, church and community

—point out the flaws in the present proposals

—compare them to a National Health Plan and some of the health systems in other countries

—form study groups around the issues and help work out a strategy for meeting your community's health needs

B. Pressure your union, community organization, etc. to make a public statement in favor of a national health plan, putting your group's clout behind the statement

—force legislators to take stands on health issues

—testify on a state, local and national level in favor of a health plan; this can be a good forum for getting issues to the public

C. Remember—building a mass base of power and support in the community and workplace is the first and most important step toward winning a national health service. Changing the institutions and policies that affect people directly and building strong community-controlled facilities and educational resources is vital; as people feel the strength of their own power, they can build the momentum needed to change the direction of health care in this country.

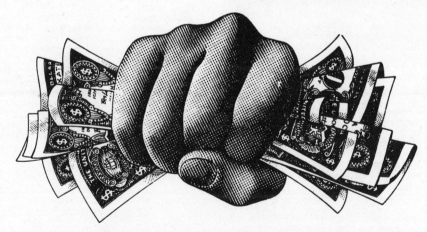

That any sane nation, having observed that you could provide for the supply of bread by giving bakers a pecuniary interest in baking for you, should go on and give a surgeon a pecuniary interest in cutting off your leg is enough to make one dispair.
—George Bernard Shaw

INSURANCE

Blue Cross/Blue Shield, the big names in the health insurance racket, carry slightly under half of all private insurance policies. Because of their central position in the financing structure, the Blues could be very instrumental in controlling hospital and other medical costs, thus significantly influencing the health care system. But 40 years after their creation by doctors and hospitals, the Blues remain faithful to their founders—the health care providers.

Blue Cross and Blue Shield are separate, "non-profit" corporations. Blue Cross, which covers hospital expenses, has 74 plans, over 80 million subscribers and processes the claims of over 20 million medicaid/care enrollees per year. Complementing Blue Cross is Blue Shield, which pays for doctor bills; it claims 72 local plans, 65 million subscribers and responsibility for processing 13 million medicare/caid patients.

Support of health providers by the Blues is manifest in a multitude of ways. Under the cost-plus system of payment, Blue Cross foots the bill for general hospital overhead as well as the cost for the specific treatment performed; this includes unnecessary expansion and purchase of expensive equipment. The Vermont Regional Medical Program reports that a 36% annual rise in X-ray therapy costs will result from the installation of an unnecessary radio therapy unit. This cost could have been avoided if investments by different hospitals had been coordinated. But instead of encouraging such inter-hospital cooperation, Blue Cross underwrites inefficiency and poor planning. Ultimately it is the consumer who must pay in the form of more costly services and higher insurance premiums.

The heavy domination of Blue Cross/Blue Shield boards by providers and businesspeople guarantees conflicts of interest. Although the Blue Cross Association claims that only 45% of Board members are providers, a 1972 study by the Vermont Public Interest Research Group found that for the 17 "general public" members of the Blue Cross/Blue Shield Boards, 18 cases of special interest were found, including insurance, hospital, business and banking connections. Nine of the directors were affiliated with banks and five of those banks held Blues money.

Blue Cross is further strengthening its place in the health care industry by buying into hospitals, nursing homes, and pre-paid plans. And, according to the Blue Cross/Blue Shield Consumer Report newsletter, "Fifty-three of the 74 Blue Cross plans in the US are now providing financial ($1.5 million) and staff support to area-wide planning agencies"—thus extending the Blue's domination to these supposedly consumer-oriented boards.

On an individual level, subscribers find most of the Blues plans are full of deductables, co-insurance payments and limitations. Since plans generally do not cover outpatient services, screening, home health care, and outreach, many subscribers wait until they are acutely sick before seeking care; others go into the hospital for what could normally be taken care of on an out-patient basis. This system of only financing in-patient treatment results in a false need for expensive hospitalization and acute care services, wrongly slanting planning and resource allocation away from out-patient and preventive care. The higher costs of inpatient care are passed on to the consumer in the form of increased health care costs and third party payments. According to the National Health Service Task Force of the Grey Panthers, "Experts estimate that between 1/5 and 1/3 of all patients in a hospital at a given time need not be there but have been admitted. . . because that is the only way they can get insurance coverage and because there are no appropriate facilities available to them." A recent HEW report points out that enrollees in group practice plans are hospitalized about one half as many days as those in the traditional plans provided by the Blues.

Commercial insurance companies (for profit as opposed to the "non-profit" Blues) have been growing in a number for the past 20 years. Covering a large part of union and company-sponsored plans they now control more than half of the insurance policies in the US. The president of the Insurance Company of North America sums up their attitude toward health care delivery better than we could hope to: "All things we desire can come only from profit." Most commercial companies are part of giant Wall Street-based financial empires, with all decisions and policy set forth by corporate executives. There is no pretense of public accountability.

Choosing a commercial insurance plan is even more of a headache than purchasing one from the Blues. Over 1000 different policies exist, some providing better coverage than the Blues and many worse. Most commercial policies and premiums are based on experience rating machanisms, which means that those classified as low risk pay less for the same coverage as those in the high risk category. Thus older people, those with chronic health conditions, and a range of other selected groups bear a heavier burden of insurance costs—not to mention costs incurred while in the hospital.

Short of changing the economic base of health care financing, there is only a limited amount that consumers can do about the present situation. Nevertheless, during the last several years, challenges to the monopolistic powers of Blue Cross/Blue Shield have increased. The public has begun questioning rate increases and the lack of consumer representation on Boards. The Blue Cross policy of pre-setting reimbursement rates has been contested in court as had Blue Cross-hospital collusion resulting in special rates for the Blues which works against competition with other insurance companies. Consumers have sued the Blues for inefficiency in management and bookkeeping. Comprehensive studies have been made by consumer and community groups into the power structure of the Blues. Activity has even reached governmental circles, with the appointment of a public-interest minded insurance commissioner in Pennsylvania who entered office under the motto: "The consumer has been screwed too long!"

Yet, consumer input into the Blues policies will have limited effect on the delivery of health care in the long run. It may bring a degree of financial relief to subscribers and force better monitoring and cost control in institutions, but it does little to make health care more accessible for the millions who cannot afford an insurance policy. It does not take the profit out of health care, nor does it change the two-class system.

For a limited segment of the population a third type of financing, public insurance, is available in the form of Medicare and Medicaid. Medicare, available to anyone over 65 on social security, and the disabled, is financed by federal funds from payroll deductions and is uniform nationally. Part A is universally available and covers basic hospital costs. However, there are many restrictions: the first $84 of expenses each year must be paid by the patient; after 90 days of hospitalization, coverage ends; after 60 days of hospitalization, the patient must start paying $18/day toward cost of care; and psychiatric care, nursing home coverage and home care are all limited. Part B is a supplemental medical insurance plan, available to seniors able to pay $6.30/month. It covers doctors fees; out-patient care; 100 home visits (with some restrictions)

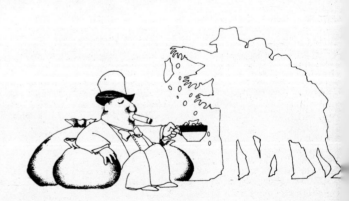

and limited psychiatric care. The consumer must pay the first $60 of annual expenses and only 80% of "reasonable" subsequent charges are covered. Not included in the plan are: check-ups, drugs, hearing aids, glasses and dental care—some of the main expenses of older people. There is no means test for medicare and therefore, no stigma attached to receiving funds.

Medicaid, unlike Medicare, is a joint federal/state-financed program administered by the states (except Arizona which has no Medicaid program) and the District of Columbia. Coverage varies widely from state to state, although there are some minimal federal guidelines. Medicaid has a means test and is considered a poverty program; to qualify an individual (or family) must have an income below 133% of the welfare cut-off level. Recipients fall under two classifications: the categorically needy (those on welfare) and the medically needy (those not on welfare, but unable to afford private insurance).

Many people eligible for medicaid do not have it. Procedures for obtaining medicaid are confusing and dehumanizing, while regulations regarding benefits, eligibility and coverage are constantly changing on a state and federal level. The mandatory three month delay between registration and receipt of benefits under medicaid is a hardship for many poor people. And the Welfare Reform Bill of 1972 permits states to arbitrarily reduce coverage. When states cut medicaid benefits, thousands of families are often left in the middle of therapeutic programs.

Government outreach and education efforts around rights under medicaid and who is eligible for it are negligible. For instance, two years after the passage of legislation providing for the early periodic screening, diagnosis, and treatment of young children covered by Medicaid, the Welfare Rights Organization and other poor peoples' groups had to sue HEW to force them to publish federal regulations and implement the program. Medicaid represents another classic case of the government instituting a program and then discouraging participation in it.

Although Medicare and medicaid have allowed many poor people to receive medical care they would otherwise be unable to afford, neither one comes close to providing a solution to the rising cost and inefficient delivery of health care. Indeed, reckless spending under Medicaid/care have served to encourage inflation and inefficiency. In the first year after Medicare/caid began, hospital costs jumped 19% and doctors' fees 7%. The first six years saw medical prices increase by over 40% compared to an increase of 20% in the previous six years. Given the level of co-payments and premiums, many older people participating in the Medicare program pay more for health care now than they did in 1965 (before the creation of Medicare.) For obvious reasons, many community groups see fighting for better Medicaid/care benefits as an important organizing tool.

NEW JERSEY PUBLIC INTEREST RESEARCH GROUP... has researched and exposed indictive facts concerning Blue Cross/Blue Shield in the wake of an 80% rate increase in a three year period. Conflicts of interest on the Boards of the Blues were rampant, including bankers representing the "general public" while their banks held large accounts for the Blues; as might be expected, the majority of Board members are White businessmen. One public representative told the PIRG office: "I believe Blue Cross is a wonderful organization. . . . It is a long-standing policy of mine not to talk as an individual Board member, but to let the chairman of the Board or the President talk for the Board." Another responded to an appointment request by asking PIRG to get the appointment approved by the Blue Cross president first. As a result of the study, public hearings were held on the past rate increases and demands such as greater public input, an open decision making process and consumer health education workshops were made by NJPIRG. Some changes have resulted: more women and a more diverse cross section of the public have been put on the Blue Cross Board, as well as two strident consumer advocates. NJPIRG will continue monitoring the Board and Blue Cross actions.as well as opposing the size of Blue Cross' retention fund (the amount kept in the bank to guard against an emergency) which currently equals $300 million. Contact NJPIRG, 32 W. Lafayette St., Trenton, NJ 08608, (609) 393-7474.

THE VERMONT ALLIANCE. . . is a research and organizing project formed after a "people's fair' in 1973. Putting out a pamphlet criticizing Blue Cross/Blue Shield and organizing around rate increase hearings were some of its first actions. The Alliance is currently pressuring for an all-consumer Board for Blue Cross and for a moratorium on rate increases until the hospitals cut down costs. Vermont's Insurance Commissioner permitted a rate increase although less than the requested amount, claiming that the Blues were on the brink of bankruptsy and could only cut costs if they were financially solvent; the Alliance contends this action diminishes consumer leverage, but will continue monitering the insurance commissioner and the Blues. The ultimate goal of the Alliance is to build a mass-based movement calling for the institution of a primary health care system including screening, health education, medical care, and training of community members as health workers. Such a system would be financed by a tax on the income of commercial insurance companies. They plan to introduce this proposal in the next session of the state legislature and are working on models for the primary health system. The Alliance views working for free, comprehensive care as a valuable organizing tactic, and, in the long run, politically feasible if the discontent of Vermonters can be tapped and usefully channeled. Contact VERMONT ALLIANCE, 5 State St., Montpelier, VT 05602, (802) 229-9104.

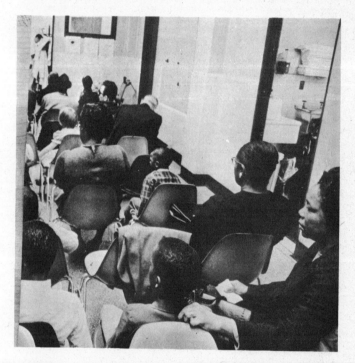

The cost of medicine is one of those expenses that nags endlessly at a poor man. The shots or pills needed to check diabetes, the pills needed for high blood pressure, the nonprescription pills and syrups needed to fight the colds all winter are items which cut unbearable holes in the budget of the black man in the Delta. It is a bitter joke for a tenant farmer to pay ten dollars for an examination that shows he has 'high blood' and must pay four dollars each month of his life for pills. The money is just not there. Rather than follow the doctor's instructions, he will buy, if he is able, a month's supply of pills and make them last six months.
—Our Land Too

NATIONAL WELFARE RIGHTS ORGANIZATION. . . is an umbrella organization for local and statewide groups of welfare recipients and poor people. Working toward "adequate income, dignity, justice and democracy" for all people, NWRO provides information and technical assistance on organizing and welfare laws and regulations. Through national actions, the effectiveness of local chapters is increased. Although facing severe financial difficulties, NWRO serves an important function by putting people in touch with each other and providing valuable informaion on the rights of the poor. Contact NWRO, 1424 16th St., NW, Washington, D.C. 20006, (202) 483-1531.

DUVALL COUNTY LEGAL AID. . . recently won a case against the local welfare department which arbitrarily cut off the $20 monthly drug allowance for medicare recipients. The case was brought when a dying patient could not even afford painkillers. The court ordered the welfare department to reimburse the patient for previous expenses and to institute due process procedures in the future. Recently Legal Aid conducted a survey of doctors and dentists in an effort to correlate the low level of participation by health professionals in Medicaid with the program's inefficiency and bureaucracy. Results of the study are being used to educate and organize people as well as to make a presentation to a state legislative committee on Medicaid. Since Medicaid is legally required to run in an efficient enough manner to attract physicians, Legal Aid feels that it has the grounds for a suit—if Medicaid doesn't reorganize itself. And, in the meantime, Legal Aid is negotiating with doctors and local medical societies to provide care for the indigent. Contact DUVALL COUNTY LEGAL AID, 205 E. Church St., Jacksonville, FL 32202, (904) 356-8375.

CALIFORNIA RURAL LEGAL ASSISTANCE. . . part of the Senior Citizens Law Center, provides legal back up and training on old people's issues on both a state and national scope. CRLA does extensive litigation and legislation in all areas of concern to seniors, including Medicare, Social Security and nursing homes. They were successful in restoring a planned Social Security cut of $140 million by the governor of California and restoring benefits to 10,000 Californians. Although they were unsuccessful in a suit against a Medicare co-payment plan (under which seniors are required to pay a fixed percent of medical costs), their experience may help people in other states who are coming up against the same problem. CRLA drafts model legislation, including a nursing home health and security act which sets up grievance procedures. Extensive resources are available on all aspects of health delivery to the elderly, including a handbook describing the steps involved in setting up a legal services office for seniors and model training programs for paraprofessionals. Other publications include an advocate's handbook and an analysis of the various state and federal programs available to seniors. Contact CLRA, 942 Market St., No. 606, San Francisco, CA 94102, (415) 989-3966.

MICHIGAN LEGAL SERVICES. . . successfully sued the state Medicaid program for failure to institute and publicize an early periodic screening, diagnosis and testing program for children covered by Medicaid. Working with the local Welfare Rights Organization, Legal Services used the suit as a basis for organizing and educating poor people about their rights under Medicaid; training sessions and forums were held by the two groups. Legal Services is actively involved in other welfare and Medicaid issues including the right to day care, education and training for Medicaid workers, and transportation to medical facilities. Recently they brought another class action suit against Medicare for retroactive termination of patients. Contact MICHIGAN LEGAL SERVICES, 468 W. Ferry, Detroit, MI 48202, (313) 577-4822.

WASHINGTON RESEARCH PROJECT. . . originally did general civil rights litigation and is now concentrating on children's law and rights. They have been involved in several Medicaid suits and have good contact with groups organizing around Medicaid thru'out the country. Lawyers with the project have litigated around the use of children in experiments. Contact WRP, 1763 "R" St., NW, Washington, D.C. 10009, (202) 483-1470.

RESOURCES

BOOKS

Blue Cross:What Went Wrong, Sylvia A. Law. Yale University Press, 92A Yale Station, New Haven, CT 06520, 1974. 320 pp. $10.00
. . . carefully documented indictment of Blue Cross. This book covers the history and characteristics of Blue Cross, its status under state laws, its relationship to state regulatory agencies, its role under existing federal health insurance programs as well as the way that Blue Cross has handled reimbursement for hospital services and review of the medical necessity for hospital services provided for subscribers. Law accuses Blue Cross of ignoring consumer input and working to directly further the interests of the corporate elite. Concludes with a proposal for public supervisory boards responsible to patients and the public, not the hospital.

Advocate's Handbook for Pennsylvania's Medical Assistance Program, Health Law Project, University of Pennsylvania Law School, 133 S. 36th St., 6th Floor, Philadelphia, PA 19104, 1973. 132 pp.
. . . prototype guide to one state's medical assistance program. In non-bureaucratic language, it covers who is eligible for Medical Assistance, coverage, how to apply, fair hearing procedures, patients rights and other sources of health care. Respect for the intelligence of the reader and clever graphics help keep this potentially dry handbook a valuable resource and model for community groups.

PAMPHLETS AND ARTICLES

"WHO RULES THE BLUES?" Vermont Public Interest Group Inc., 26 State St., Montpelier, VT 05601, January 1974. 11 pp.
. . . in-depth study of who controls Blue Cross/Blue Shield in Vermont. The pamphlet reviews the findings of a similar study done in 1972, showing the magnitude of change. The Blues made token improvements, presenting them as major changes. Useful model for state-wide surveys.

"Milling Around Medicaid," HEALTH/PAC BULLETIN, 17 Murray St., New York, NY 10007, July/August 1972, pp. 1-4
. . . describes the health centers which "derive a substantial income exclusively treating patients on Medicaid." Doctors working these "Medicaid mills" either pay a flat rent or a percent of income, often to a health professional who owns the building. Although this arrangement superficially resembles a group practice, it is in fact a far cry from this concept. To begin with, most centers do not have a regular group of doctors present each day. Rather, a doctor may spend only a day or two at the center each week and a different doctor may occupy his space on other days." The list of indictments is long: few back-up services (hospitals), superficial care, patients shuffled from one doctor to another and excessive testing and treatment. One New York City "mill," Manhattan Uptown Medical Center in East Harlem, included "one doctor, a confessed junkie, who purchased his own narcotics from his addict patients. . . filthy floors, blood stained instruments, fallen plaster and broken liquor bottles in the bathroom." Nevertheless, Medicaid mill doctors are virtually alone in venturing into poor neighborhoods and offer the only alternative to hospital-based care.

"YOUR MEDICARE HANDBOOK," HEW. Government Printing Office, Washington, D.C. 20402, 1973. $.55
. . . clear explanation of all rights under Medicare, both hospital insurance and medical insurance plans. Covers benefits offered, how to make claims, and common questions asked. Practical guide well worth distributing at Senior Citizen Centers, hospitals and nursing homes.

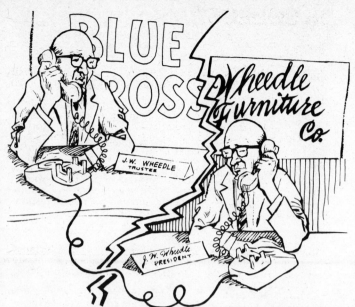

"WHEEDLE? ... WHEEDLE HERE... SEND ME A BUILDING FULL OF YOUR MOST LUXURIOUS OFFICE FURNITURE."

"VERMONT BLUE CROSS, HOW OUR HELPERS HELP THEMSELVES," Vermont Alliance, 5 State St., Montpelier, VT 05602, 1973. 16 pp. $.10
... handy little guide to Vermont's Blue Cross plan, covering a background of the plan and an analysis of the current situation. Documents the exorbitant rate increases of Blue Cross plans recently: "43% in New York, 25% in Connecticut, 44% in New Jersey, 33% in Rhode Island, and a 27% boost in New Hampshire." A clear reason for steep rate increases in the prevalence of conflicts of interest. "Among the seventeen members of the Board of Directors who were representatives of the 'general public', eighteen cases of special interest were found" in Vermont in 1972. The authors realize that comprehensive health planning (and not just financing) is imperative yet make several interim suggestions: 1. no conflict of interest on the Board should be allowed, 2. Blue Cross should force hospitals to lower rates, 3. hospitals should be forced to stay within a set budget, 4. generic drugs should be used whenever possible, 5. public hearings should be held throughout the state to encourage consumers to participate actively.

"Blue Cross Pays the Bills," Joel Seldin, available from Louise Rice, 65 Chestnut St., Cambridge, MA, 02139, July 1969. 5 pp. $.27
... provocative discussion of how insurance companies, medicare and medicaid help finance hospital union-busting campaigns. "When a hospital elects to oppose the unionization of its employees, the costs of the campaign are incurred in a number of ways. There can be greater than usual pay increases to convince the workers that the union is unnecessary. The costs of meetings, leaflets, direct mail and similar 'informational' activities are also frequently substantial. Such expenditures are usually listed as personnel expenditures." These expenses are then passed on to insurance companies and the consumer in the form of increased overhead costs. The author of this unusual article uses Roosevelt Hospital (New York City) as an example of the devious and expensive tricks used by management to thwart unionization.

For years I have been a union representative on the Blue Shield Board and sat at board meetings and watched the doctors bargain with themselves.

—Heal Yourself

"MEDICAID SERVICES STATE BY STATE," HEW, Government Printing Office, Washington, D.C., September 1972. 1 p.
... in chart form, shows what services are available in each state under local Medicaid programs. Services range from Arizona (which has no Medicaid program) and Wyoming (which only covers institutional services in intermediate care facilities) to Washington, New York, North Dakota, Nebraska, Minnesota, Massachusetts and Kansas (whose services include eye glasses, dental care, family planning, clinic services and more.)

"Health-care Delivery System Reform Via Blue Cross Hospital Contracts," Herbert S. Denenberg and James M. Mead, HOSPITAL TOPICS, 6525 N. Nashville, Chicago, IL 60631, December, 1972
... annotated list of 30 point program to reduce insurance costs and improve hospital care. The program is a model Blue Cross-Hospital contract, calling for the elimination of hospital subsidies of unsafe and substandard beds; use of generic drugs; increased use of pre-admissions testing; graded care and short procedure units; required disclosure of all costs of the hospital and more. The article accurately concludes "The 30 point program is not meant to be a panacea for all the problems of the health care system. It is, however, a major step forward in combatting the rising costs of care through Blue Cross-Hospital contracts." Although the recommendations are less extensive than desired, the program may be an important first step for state-wide action.

"The Blue Cross Double Cross," Andrew Bajonski, CHICAGO JOURNALISM REVIEW, 192 North Clark St., Chicago, IL 60601, February 1972, pp. 3-7
... expose of Illinois Blue Cross/Blue Shield program with an emphasis on who controls the Blues and who profits. This article offers several examples of banks receiving large interest-free deposits at the same time that one of their executives is made a Board member of the Blues. "Take the case of John Mannion, a vice-president of the Continental National Bank of Chicago. When he joined the Illinois Blue Cross Board in 1947, Blue Cross had less than one million dollars on deposit at the Continental. By 1954, the plan's balances at Continental had risen to $2 million and Mannion's position at Continental had risen to senior Vice President. And in 1963, when Mannion became chairman of Illinois Blue Cross, the plan's balance at Continental passed $7 million... The curious thing about Blue Cross's deposits at Continental is that Continental hasn't paid a cent in interest on them since Mannion joined the Blue Cross Board." Points out that legally the Blues are non-profit membership organizations and all consumers have a right to vote for the Board of Directors.

"Medicaid Lessons and Warnings," SOCIAL POLICY, Suite 500, 184 Fifth Ave., New York, NY 10010. Jan/Feb 1971,
... focuses on the inherent failings of the Medicaid program. Points out the lack of consumer participation in decision-making, subtle obstructions placed in the way of patients (endless forms, changing regulations, hassled and incooperative personal) and double standard for health care. This article is, essentially, a good description of justified anger at the Medicaid program.

"BIOGRAPHICAL STUDY-DIRECTORS OF PENNSYLVANIA BLUE SHIELD," available from DC PIRG, George Washington University, 2121 "I" St., NW, Washington, D.C. 20037
... lists the names, occupations, sex, age, and residence of the 32 members of the Board of Directors of the Pennsylvania Blue Shield, as well as an analysis of possible conflict of interest. This revealing survey shows that there is only one woman on the Board, the mean age is 61.9 and there is a heavy domination of Doctors, college administrators and past officers of the Blues. Model research job.

"MEDICAL ASSISTANCE (MEDICAID) FINANCED UNDER TITLE XIX OF THE SOCIAL SECURITY ACT," HEW, Government Printing Office, August, 1972. 28 pp.
... good statistical guide for groups researching Medicaid. Charts show payments by states, for a variety of Medicaid programs. Available for every month.

PRE-PAID PLANS

A prepaid health plan (with the exception of Medical Foundations) is a substitute for the usual pay-as-you-go method of financing health care. Instead of paying for each visit to the doctor or hospital, a person or family pays a set sum each month and makes use of health services as often as necessary. Sometimes there is a small charge for each visit. Generally a wide range of services are offered including specialists, laboratory tests and X-rays; most plans do not cover such important areas as maternity and dental care, which the patient must pay out of her/his pocket.

From this common denominator a number of different types of pre-paid health plans have evolved: private, profit-making corporations; private, non-profit-making corporations; cooperative corporations where consumers own the company; group practices by MDs; foundations for medical care by medical societies; and Nixon's pet project, the health maintenance organization. Each is slightly different; some supply all services including home care; some simply pay the doctor like an insurance plan; and some supply only office visit care.

Health Maintenance Organizations (HMO) are those prepaid plans which include both outpatient and inpatient care under the same prepayment. Since outpatient care is less expensive than inpatient, the doctors are assured of better salaries, more year-end bonuses (surplus revenue is divided among the doctors at the end of the year), etc., if they can prevent hospitalization as often as possible—thus the term "health maintenance."

Foundations for Medical Care, one type of HMO, also deserve special mention. As an administrator of the American Association of Foundations for Medical Care has unabashedly said, they are the doctors' way of preserving free-for-service health care. A Foundation for Medical Care (FMC) is somewhat like a group practice formed through the local medical society. People enroll with the foundation, pay a monthly fee, and choose any of its doctors as a personal physician. The FMC pays the doctor on a fee-for-sevice basis and the doctor retains her/his autonomy, private office and secretary, and the knowledge that the more patients s/he sees, operations s/he performs, and services s/he renders the more money s/he will make. All the problems of medical professionalism, fragmented care, and lack of preventive care are accentuated as doctors see patients as rapidly as possible, attending to only the obvious symptoms, in order to make as much money as possible. Under the FMC, doctors preserve the sacred "doctor-patient" relationship rather than switch to a team approach; the only quality control is through peer review; they are not subject to federal 'snooping' or regulations; and payment is guaranteed.

The corporate, pre-paid approach to health care supposedly offers great advantages. Not only are health care payments set, so that the worry of a whopping bill for some unforeseen medical emergency is reduced, but also preventive and diagnostic care are easier to give. Health personnel are on salary, and therefore they are more likely to keep track of preventive care because it will reduce their workload in the long run. The administrative paperwork that is included in figuring each bill is reduced, helping to keep costs down. Doctors in common specialities such as internal medicine, pediatrics, obstetrics and gynecology, surgery and psychiatry are hired by and work in the clinic. Others work on a contract basis, treating patients from the pre-paid plan when their particular specialty is needed. Thus, oftentimes patients do not have to make trips to two different doctors' offices when special care is required. This arrangement facilitates the accessibility of care. And, since doctors are paid a salary, they are less likely to abuse patients for the purpose of making more money, and will have less reason to carelessly rush through visits. If the corporation is a community group this means that the community has more control over its health workers and services.

However, in the hands of a capitalist system, the pre-paid health plan corporation has many drawbacks. Many corporations labeled "non-profit" are subsidiaries of, or have common Boards of Directors with profit making companies from which they buy supplies and equipment. Many well-known pre-paid plans such as Kaiser-Permanente, Rhode Island Group Health, and HIP in New York have simply produced an alternative for the relatively healthy and wealthy while grossing huge profits without solving the crisis in health care at all. Those without money still cannot pay the monthly health plan fee. And since few cities have more than one pre-paid plan, enrollment is competitive allowing plans to accept only the healthiest. Those few low-income people enrolled frequently live far from the central facility and have limited access to transportation; thus, they often end up paying extra to see doctors in their neighborhood, or go without care.

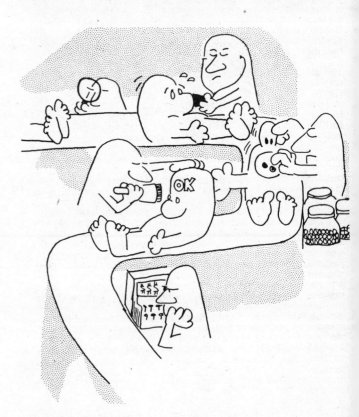

Recently the government has suggested that Medicaid patients be cared for by pre-paid plans. The idea was to have private corporations set up HMOs on the border of low income areas, in the hopes of making them available to both the wealthy and the poor. The plan would then enroll a certain percentage of low income people and the govenrment and payments by the wealthy would subsidize the monthly payments of those who could not afford them. But the rich won't enroll in a plan on the edge of a low-income district. Thus, fewer and fewer medically indigent people can be enrolled, as Medicaid only covers a limited range of the services provided by pre-paid plans.

Past experience shows that many problems exist. For example in California, a corporation had to pre-enroll a certain number of people before it could be permitted to start an HMO by the state. Medicaid patients were enrolled in pre-paid plans before they had functional clinics; they then found themselves tricked, ignored, and ordered around. Many were sent to hospitals outside the plan from treatment. Although they had no money, the plan would not pay for them, and because the plan held their Medicaid card to show the state as proof of enrollment, the hospital could not bill Medicaid. Many of these people had enrolled under duress since the plans solicited welfare recipients on a door-to-door basis, threatening their welfare status when people showed reluctance. Afterward, people had no idea in what they had enrolled or how to get care. When they did understand the program, it did not help them much: the plans provided little transportation, meager pharmacy facilities, and few evening, week-end or emergency services.

Even for the well-off the promises of pre-paid plans are often unmet. Starting a program of preventive rather than curative care calls for a great deal of testing and physical examinations—but most corporations would rather have quick returns from the plan and refuse to spend the necessary money for a large staff. Instead they overwork staff and never really set up a system of preventive care. Many plans are over-enrolled and much of the money that should be going into health care goes into advertising—which just aggravates the over-enrollment problem further. Patients who enroll in a plan thinking that they will have input into policy decisions soon find otherwise. A big corporation is a mechanical place; one voice is easily ignored in the chain of bureaucracies and red-tape. And because membership is not based on a geographic community, trying to organize other dissatisfied patients is difficult. This is true whether the plan is a cooperative, where members buy a piece of the corporation, or a private corporation. When Group Health of Puget Sound had only 200 members, it is possible that they all had a voice in decisions. With 171,000 members, this is utterly impossible.

The alternative to large, impersonal corporations is a community-founded, community-controlled pre-paid health plan or HMO. This option has been increasingly considered by communities and, in a few places, such plans have been established. In many cases formerly OEO clinics have become government funded HMOs, although it has meant a reduction in services as government funding for HMOs covers only a limited number of services. For community groups wishing to set up pre-paid plans, the problems are enormous. First, establishing a community health plan operating out of a centrally located building is an expensive project. In a low-income or working class community amassing the capital to found a community corporation of this type takes a great deal of effort and backing from at least one large outside organization such as a church or social welfare agency. In the case of an HMO the government may be a source of funding, but to obtain any money the plan will have to agree to provide specified services which may not be of top priority in the community. Federal funds are limited and many have already been snatched up by the big, corporate HMOs; and those community groups wishing to comply with regulations must prove "fiscal responsibility", which means obtaining the support of a wealthy organization such as a bank. All in all, it takes about $2-4 million just to start an HMO, an impossible sum for most communities to raise. Federal guidelines for HMOs are so strict and rigid that it is virtually impossible for community groups to comply with all the details while still maintaining autonomy. Nevertheless, many community groups are obtaining federal "feasibility" grants which enable them to hire one or two full-time people and get something started, although on a smaller scale.

The second obstacle that a community health group usually encounters is becoming incorporated. In Texas two Chicano HMOs found their incorporation blocked by laws that said only doctors could incorporate to deliver health services, a law existing in many states; officials claimed that non-doctor groups incorporating would be providing medicine without a licence. Laws like these and others that the city and state can find may be used against community efforts to control its own health. The best recourse presently available is a good lawyer and the support of all the social welfare agencies in the area. Other obstacles invariably crop up—finding doctors willing to work for a salary and accept community control locating hospitals willing to contract for in-patient care; establishing a policy board that truly represents the community; getting certified to collect Medicaid/care benefits; and getting community people to accept and join the plan. Taking more money from an already poor community is not the answer to the problem of financing health care; most community corporations cannot buy and run a hospital and many cannot even collect enough money to remain open unless they enroll patients from outside the community. Although there are a myriad of problems facing communities trying to set up HMOs, those able to overcome the obstacles have found them to be a positive alternative.

TWO HARBORS COMMUNITY HEALTH CENTER, INC . . . is a unique and long-standing pre-paid health plan. In 1944 two doctors who were providing medical care for employees of the local railroad company decided to retire, selling their clinic to a group of railroad employees, local unions, and community civic associations. Various community residents subscribed to the new Community Health Center which then contracted with three doctors to staff the Center as a group practice. The subscriber-members elected the Board of Directors and became, essentially, the controllers of CHC. CHC has grown and now provides medical services for almost half of the Two Harbors area residents, including local Medicaid/care recipients and employees of a variety of companies. Monthly rates are fairly low and membership fees can be paid annually. No drugs, appliances (glasses, hearing aids, braces, artificial limbs), or dental care are covered. The center has a Home Health Nursing Service for homebound patients to keep them out of nursing homes and is joint-owner of the local hospital. It has had many run-ins with the local AMA because of its stand on group practice, pre-paid health services, and community consumer oriented health plans: all these are major objectives of the Association. Contact CHC, 4th and 11th Ave., Two Harbors, MN 55616, (218) 834-2171.

LEE COUNTY CO-OPERATIVE CLINIC . . . was set up by the community with the assistance of HEW, OEO, and a neighborhood action council. Although members of this clinic pay a membership fee and, therefore, own and control the clinic, in the past federal funding regulations have limited the membership to those eligible for service under the OEO poverty guidelines. The set-up will probably change drastically in the near future due to the demise of OEO, but the clinic hopes to continue as a pre-paid health plan. As with other OEO clinics forced to find alternate funding, this will mean a considerable cut-back in services and number of patients able to be seen. The services now provided cover a wide range of out-patient care, including dental, pharmaceutical, outreach and transportation programs. Vision, hearing, and other problems not covered in the clinic are referred to outside physicians or agencies, with transportation provided in some cases. While the clinic seems to be dominated by the federal professionals at the East Arkansas Community Action Agency, it is a definite step forward for Lee County. Contact LEE COUNTY CO-OPERATIVE CLINIC, 530 Atkins Blvd., Marianna, AR 72360, (501) 295-5225.

GROUP HEALTH COOPERATIVE OF PUG ˉ SOUND . . . is one of the oldest co-operative pre-paid plans in the US. It was begun in 1947 by physicians and consumers and had 200 members, all of whom had a voice and vote in the nonprofit operation. Today the enrollment is 171,000 individuals; more than 55% of the 28,400 Co-op families have paid the $200 entrance fee, membership fees and capital dues, and are, therefore, full-fledged members of the co-op. Many others are simply part of a group plan through a workplace or union (they do have the option, for a fee, of becoming co-op members), choosing from two lists of services and two sets of prices depending on the form of coverage affordable. The Co-op has recently begun to enroll a limited number of Medicaid/care patients on a trial basis, although the price of membership is prohibitively expensive for most low-income and working people, thus perpetuating a two class system of health care. The Co-op description brochure boasts that members and enrollees pay no charge at point of delivery for doctors' services, X-rays and lab services, prescribed medicines, outpatient mental care, eye examinations and 80% of the cost of a kidney machine (up to $10,000/year). However, some very basic exclusions and limitations exist: contraceptives, eye glasses, artificial appliances, dental care, and mental h health care requiring hospitalization or special care. Maternity coverage is included only if conception occurs 30 days after enrollment and the family or individual must still pay a Maternity fee ($200 for members). The plan operates its own hospital and has an emergency line and services available 24 hours a day. Although enrollment is large, 7 district medical centers and one main center allow for greater accessibility of care. Contact GHC, 200 15th Ave. East, Seattle, WA 98002, (206) 325-9400.

MARICOPA COMMUNITY HEALTH NETWORK. . . plans to operate three primary health care centers in urban areas and two in rural areas. One center is now open. Their membership was originally drawn from the poor and near-poor, with part or all of the premium paid by HEW and other government programs. They now have full-paying members as well. Feeling that HEW funding will only last for a limited time, they hope that increased full-paying membership will help subsidize the services for poor people. The 25-member Board of Directors, elected by the subscribers, includes 16 poor people and representatives of the poor, 5 providers, and 4 others (labor leaders, business men and women, etc.). Contact MCHN, Greater Arizona Savings Bldg., Suite 700, 112 North Central Ave., Phoenix, AZ 85004, (602) 252-7541.

G3003 of 524
NORTHEAST VALLEY HEALTH CORPORATION. . . serves a racially and economically mixed area. They currently have one medical center of their own and are planning to build others. The Board of Directors, made up largely of community people who helped start the project, has equal White, Brown and Black caucuses. However, there is no set percentage for low-income members. They have approximately 4,000 enrollees (around half fully-paying, others subsidized by Medicare, Medi-Cal or HEW). Besides standard benefits, they provide such services as interpreters, transportation and child care for low-income subscribers. They seem unusually committed to reaching the whole community—at least some of their publicity material is in Spanish as well as English. NEVHC is trying to move towards self-sufficiency through recruiting fully-paying members, and through contracts with the state to provide care for Medicare and Medi-Cal patients. Contact NEVHC, 14935 Rinaldo St., Suite 603, Madison Hills, CA 91340, (213) 365-0861.

RESOURCES

"THE KAISER PLAN," Health/PAC, 17 Murray St., New York, NY 10007, November 1973. 18 pp. $.60
. . . dynamite resource for anyone trying to get a grasp on the HMO industry. In an objective yet critical manner, it covers Health Maintenance Organizations (HMOs), the Kaiser-Permanente Plan (K-P) and Prepaid Health Plans, offering both an explanation of services and an analysis of the inherent drawbacks. "Whether Kaiser physicians or subscribers like it or not, Kaiser-Permanente is part of the Kaiser Industries empire and is largely controlled by it. Kaiser Industries consists of about 100 active companies including Kaiser Aluminum and Chemical, Kaiser Steel, Kaiser Cement and Gypsum, Kaiser Engineers and Kaiser Aerospace and Electronics." Profit is a key concept here. "Whether for profit or technically 'non-profit', private corporations have always committed themselves to maximizing their income, reducing their expenditures, and using the surplus for expansion. The profit incentive leads private HMOs to limit services by hiring an inadequate number of physicians and other personnel so that patients will be discouraged from seeking care. In this way, expenses go down and surplus goes up." To insure increased profit, K-P insures growth. "Most subscribers don't even know that 4 percent of their premium plus a minimum of 15 cents per member per month is budgeted for expansion." This article points out that "Many Californians think Kaiser's not good, but it's the best around." However, it is critical of the way K-P treats workers, ignores the medically indigent, minimizes taxable income and functions internally.

The Kaiser-Permanente Medical Care Program, Anne R. Somers, ed., The Commonwealth Fund, 1 East 75th, New York, NY 1971. 232 pp.
. . . text of speeches given by officers and leading doctors of the largest and best known prepaid health plan to the Association of American Medical Colleges. Its value lies in the detailed explanation of how the Kaiser-Permanente plan functions: members pay a flat fee per year, receiving total coverage in Kaiser-Permanente facilities (exceptions made for emergency care). Unfortunately the book is very pro-Kaiser and ignores common criticisms of the plan such as the fact that surplus revenue is given as a bonus to doctors, not consumers, and the overenrollment of patients resulting in long delays before treatment.

PLANNING AGENCIES

Health planning encompasses everything from allocating money for health facilities and services to guaranteeing that enough workers will be available to staff them. Before the last two decades planning for health care was practically non-existent. But, with the realization in the late 1950's that poverty and ill-health are not isolated phenomena, both private and public agencies began working to make health care facilities more available to communities—the first steps in making health care an organized system. Unfortunately, however, the system was not designed to serve the public, with most of the private health planning agencies founded by health professionals—and remaining professional organizations to this day. The communities they purport to serve are rarely represented on decision-making bodies and when a policy board does have a consumer majority, those consumers come from the well-to-do where health care providers abound. The interests private planning agencies represent are usually those of the health industry: hospitals, construction companies, equipment, data processing and drug firms, insurance companies, banks and doctors.

In 1966 the federal government moved to insure that services provided for in Medicaid and Medicare existed. To do this, it entered the health planning field with two programs: Regional Medical Programs (RMP) and Comprehensive Health Planning (CHP). The Regional Medical Programs were originally designed to encourage the regionalization of facilities, equipment, personnel, and research in the areas of cancer, heart, lung and kidney disease. Their major function was to coordinate, select, and fund proposals sent to them in these areas. Subsequent legislative changes watered down the Act. Emergency care and post-graduate medical education became the main priorities. This shift is emphasized by the fact that in almost all areas RMPs were formed by a medical school or schools, who use the program to provide funding for their research staff. Medical schools, in essence, divide up the turf, with each school obtaining RMP money for a particular research specialty. Consumer and community input have been limited to an advisory committee which is appointed by the provider-dominated board and has no power to enforce recommendations.

The creation of RMPs by medical schools was not done without reluctance. Originally the medical industry was wary of government interference in any form—even money—and almost every year the funds allocated for RMPs have been underused. As a result, almost every year the funds allocated for RMPs have grown smaller. Although there have been a few successful programs funded by RMP (midwifery, para-professionals, training, rural clinics), by and large programs are provider-dominated and plagued by professional reluctance to create health care delivery centers which give control to community groups at the expense of medical schools. What was originally envisioned as a comprehensive network of regional centers for the treatment, research, and diagnosis of four killer diseases has deteriorated into piecemeal projects that bring money into meidcal schools and add to their prestige. RMPs are more geared toward fancy library systems, research projects and technique classes than serving the people needing immediate and direct services as was their original intention.

In contrast to the provider domination of RMP, the Comprehensive Health Planning Agencies were intended to have consumer majorities on the Boards. Yet, CHPs have fallen far short of being consumer advocates. CHPs were designed to coordinate, and in many ways, compliment the already existing private planning agencies created by hospitals and providers. Therefore, when CHP legislation was enacted, it was not surprising that in many cities private, non-profit planning corporations added token consumer representatives to their Boards and applied to be recognized as CHP agencies. Presently, almost 75% of the 218 regional CHPs are private, non-profit corporations. The legislative guidelines for CHPs state that membership must "include representatives of public, voluntary and non-profit agencies, institutions and or-

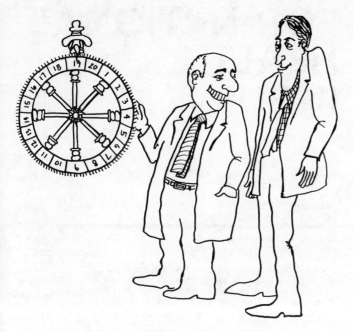

"WE HAVE A VERY SCIENTIFIC MEANS OF SELECTING PRIORITIES"

Another department of the government can fund the proposal. Or, an institution can simply ignore a negative CHP decision, building an extra wing or buying expensive specialized equipment on its own. Only recently was a law enacted whereby a facility must submit all proposals exceeding $100,000 to the CHP for a "certification of need" or lose its Medicare certification.

Gaining any degree of consumer control of CHPs has been a difficult task. Because consumers lack technical training in the intricacies of health planning, they can be easily intimidated or co-opted by professional providers and planners. Furthermore, much of the data which the CHP must use in planning is generated and controlled by the health industries.

In a provider-controlled planning agency, backing decisions with force is no problem—industry, professional organizations and medical schools can all threaten to cut off support and services to an offending institution. Consumer-controlled CHPs have no such voice or power. Blocking a proposal favored by the health industries can result in the industries forming a consolidated force against the CHP. In such situations, health planning for a whole region is blocked, enabling the state and local government to form a new CHP with business interests in control. For example, in Chicago, the Daly political machine took over a CHP that made decisions against its interests; however, members from the original CHP then formed a new planning agency to advocate for consumer needs.

Because of the entrenched power of health care providers, CHPs with consumer majorities have a difficult time exerting their power. It is important for communities to train people in planning skills when they do manage to elect members of the Board.

It seems that RMPs and CHPs may not be around much longer. The National Health Policy and Health Development Act of 1974, now pending in Congress, would do away with CHPs RMPs, and the Hill-Burton Hospital Construction Act. Development and planning would be done by the Health Services Agencies on the local level, State Health Commissions on the state level, and a presidentially appointed National Council for Health Policy on a national level. Unfortunately, many of the bad elements of both RMPs and CHPs are incorporated into this act, including non-profit private corporations with only one-third consumer representation, and location of Health Services Agencies in the areas with medical schools or other academic health centers. The capacity of this health planning network to enforce its decisions is still limited to threats of slashing federal funds. While the hope for CHPs or RMPs becoming progressive forces in the health field is low, efforts could be made to improve them or introduce better bills to compete with present legislation or those before Congress.

Ultimately, no rational plan for health care delivery can be effective until all aspects of health care (from the community health center to the drug industry, national health financing to medical education), lie in the hands of representatives of the community served.

ganizations concerned with health, representatives of the interests of local government, of the RMP for the area, and of consumers of health services." As in the case of RMPs, this strong role of the providers has extended the potential monopoly in delivery of health care for these groups. When it is to the benefit of member organizations (be they hospitals, universities or industry) the CHP has been found to "protect inefficient firms, restrict price competition, and subsidize uneconomic activities" (Community Health, Inc. HEALTH PLANNING ISSUE PAPER, June 1973).

Lack of resources has also plagued CHPs since their inception. The program has neither the money nor the power to implement decisions. Most CHPs have only been able to hire a couple of staff people and have not been able to develop "master plans" for community-wide health needs (although they are legislatively mandated to do this). Most CHPs do no more than react to other people's plans, either accepting or rejecting them in a piecemeal fashion.

Regional CHPs are subordinate to state CHPs (represented by the state health department in most states) which in turn are subordinate to a National CHP Advisory Board at the Department of Health, Education and Welfare. All proposals for such diverse programs as Hill Burton Hospital Construction, Migrant Health Services, HMOs, and Community Mental Health Centers or those seeking HEW funding must be reviewed by the regional CHP. This requirement appears to give the CHP considerable power. However, after the regional CHP reviews a proposal, the state CHP and then the National Advisory Board review the proposal. The decision of the regional CHP can be overturned at any of these points, thus greatly reducing the impact of local agencies. And, the rejection of a proposal does not necessarily mean the proposal is stifled.

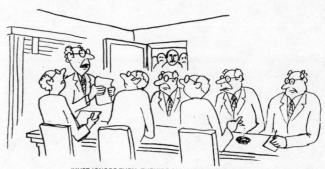

"JUST IGNORE THEM. THEY'RE ONLY THE 'COMMUNITY'"

RESOURCES

"Ho Jo Of Health Care," HEALTH/PAC BULLETIN, 17 Murray St., New York, NY 10007, March 1972, pp. 1-7
. . . critical evaluation of Health, Inc., a new Massachusetts based "Franchise health care center" using the Howard Johnson concept of modular design. . . in the clinic set-up. The goal of Health, Inc. is to provide primary care in neighborhood clinics, back-up services in hospitals, nursing homes, etc. all on a prepaid basis at a reduced cost to the consumer. In actuality few of the promotional promises have been met (at writing of the article): patients see many doctors and receive little continuity in care; the clinic is open fewer hours than scheduled; preventive care and health education are virtually non-existent; there is no consumer input into decision-making and cost to the patient is not lower than area facilities. The originator of Health, Inc., Dr. Leonard Cronkhite, "has built his career on finding management solutions to medical institutional problems. The failures of Health, Inc. to provide effective health care testifies to the limitations of this approach."

HEALTH POLITICS: A QUARTERLY BULLETIN, Committee on Health Politics, New York University, 547 La Guardia Place, New York, NY 10003. Free
. . . "designed to serve the needs of social scientists, especially political scientists, interested in the political dimensions of health care." These bulletins are extremely informative in their coverage of health issues, such as the re-organization of HEW, consumer participation in Comprehensive Health Planning, and Nixon's National health strategy. They are presented in an objective manner, with excellent bibliographies.

HEALTH PLANNING ISSUE PAPER, Community Health Institute, 55 W. 44th St., New York, NY 10036
. . . factual material put out monthly on comprehensive health planning and other community health issues.

Social Security is paid for from an equal employer/employee tax of 5.85% each. The average wage of a worker in manufacturing is $168.42/week. The cost of Social Security to such a worker comes to $604.40/year. Yet, due to Federal and State tax credits, the employer of that worker will pay out only $245.85 in Social Security tax/year.

—Information taken from a speech by a United Electrical, Radio, and Machine Workers of America (U.E.) Vice-President

PROPOSALS FOR NATIONAL HEALTH INSURANCE

Following are brief descriptions of the major National Health Insurance bills before Congress.

President Nixon's bill for National Health Insurance, Comprehensive Health Insurance Program (HIP), is comprised of three distinct plans. The first two plans must be enacted by state legislation, with no provisions made for federal pick-up if states do not initiate programs.

Plan I, Employees Health Insurance Program (EHIP), requires employers (with the exception of small companies which pay low wages) to provide coverage to full-time employees. It is expected that employers would contract out to the major insurance companies and, when available, HMO and Medical Foundation enrollment must be offered. Employees must pay a flat percentage of the cost of insurance and their participation is voluntary. Plan II, Assistance Health Insurance Plan (AHIP), supplements EHIP while replacing Medicaid. It provides for those under 65 and not covered by EHIP such as part-time and seasonal employees, the unemployed, disabled, low income, employees of small, low-wage employers, and high risk self-employed individuals. Medicare would stay intact for seniors with benefits conforming to those of EHIP and AHIP.

HIP includes a $150 deductible /individual (families pay a maximum of $450 in deductibles) for medical expenses and a $50 drug deductible. In addition, consumers must pay 25% of medical costs, with the government assuming full responsibility when a family has paid $1500 in less than a year. Clearly this plan presents a hardship for most consumers.

Under the Nixon plan financing is through private insurance companies—thus greatly strengthening the role of the private insurance industry. Financing is extremely regressive, with all participants paying a flat premium for coverage. Low-income and working class people, therefore, will pay proportionately more of their income for health insurance than the wealthy. Besides, many employers pass on these fringe benefit expenses to workers in the form of denying pay increases;

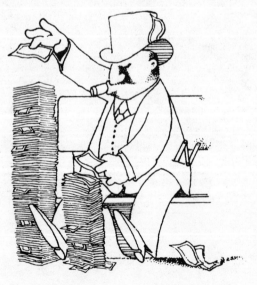

in addition, employers receive tax credits for their portion of payment.

The administration further heralds its plan as saving the government money by not using tax revenues—it fails to note that premium payments to private insurance carriers amount to a tax paid directly to private industry.

Controls on industry in the Nixon plan are virtually worthless. With quality control in the hands of peer review boards, there is little reason to believe that doctors will be seriously challenged. Cost control is a joke and amounts to encouraging consumers not to use medical services. Out-of-pocket payments and premiums would be imposed on most consumers, with the circular reasoning that it would keep costs down by discouraging superfluous use of facilities—unfortunately, it may discourage use when clearly needed also.

It is estimated that under HIP 10 to 12 million people who are currently employed will be without coverage. Because many states provide only minimal Medicaid money, it would be against their financial self-interest to have to assume the extra financial burden of AHIP, thus leaving the poor and unemployed in those states without insurance. Since employers are not required to provide insurance until an employee has worked 90 days, others will receive sporadic coverage at best because they are temporary or seasonal workers. Workers who are laid off or unemployed have only 90 days of partially paid coverage and would have to pay a whopping $50/month to receive it for an additional 90 days. Still others will be unable to afford premiums payments or opt not to join the program. Furthermore, this system has built-in employment disincentives. HIP would promote the hiring of part-time and seasonal employees for whom the employer would not have to make payments; and, because insurance companies charge on the basis of experience ratings, it would discourage the hiring of high risk persons such as seniors, women and the disabled.

All in all, HIP is a provider's dream come true. Private insurance companies are guaranteed income by a tax on employers and employees, which, in turn, insures doctors and hospitals will get their payments, which in turn guarantees the income of drug and supply companies. In fact, the only income not protected is that of the consumer. The hoax of cost control rests on the natural competition principle of capitalist industry and on inefficient governmental regulatory agencies. This system of "control" has always been a disaster. The only mention of more efficient delivery of health care is the administration's pitch for HMOs and prepaid plans, which may limit cost and inefficiency somewhat, but do nothing to challenge the role of the private sector in health care. All in all, the only consistency evident in the administration's bill is Nixon's ability to cover up its limitations and   to industry with fancy words.

The Health Security Act (S3), until April, 1974, sponsored by Senator Kennedy, is by far the most comprehensive bill before Congress. It was drafted by and has the influential support of organized labor. Services covered by Health Security include full physician and hospital care coverage, 120 days of skilled nursing home care (unlimited if the nursing home is owned or managed by a hospital); home health services; and approved drugs and devices. The two most progressive features of S3 are the abolition of private insurance companies and the fact that consumers pay nothing at the time of delivery; there are no deductibles or co-insurance payments with S3.

Health Security is way ahead of other proposals now before Congress, but it too has serious flaws. Health insurance companies would be eliminated but other profit-making sectors of the health care delivery system would remain in tact (i.e., private doctors, hospitals, supply and drug companies). Financing, although an improvement over Nixon's formula, is still 50% based on the regressive Social Security Tax (which taxes income by a fixed percent, not proportionately or on a

sliding scale) and the more progressive income tax. Because of the loopholes taken advantage of by the wealthy, professionals and corporations under federal income tax guidelines, an unfair burden of tax payment is placed on wage earners.

Attempts at distribution and cost control are written into the Health Security Act. However, both are based on weak financial incentives. A budget for institutions and individual providers would be arranged in advance, with the providers obligated to stay within that budget.

Control of the budget—who decides how financial resources are spent—is ill-defined. More money would be put into health personnel training, yet a workable plan for distribution of facilities and health workers is not adequately spelled out. Health Security Act would depend on financial incentives to encourage team practices, HMOs and Medical Foundations.

Unlike the other proposals, S3 at least mentions consumer input: ". . . consumer organizations would be encouraged to make health care a high priority in their overall activities and to sponsor and develop comprehensive, community-wide health care organizations." However, adequate means of participation—much less control—are not insured. Consumer input is relegated to advisory boards, which usually have little power to enforce ideas. As with all the NHI proposals, no mention is made of the decision-making power of non-professional health workers.

Although Health Security would provide comprehensive care for millions who could otherwise not afford it, the proposal still falls short of tackling the roots of the health care delivery problem in this country.

In April 1974, Kennedy reneged on his support of the Health Security Act and proposed a compromise bill with Congressman Mills, claiming that only a more moderate bill will pass in Congress. The Mills-Kennedy bill abandons some of the more progressive features of Health Security. For instance, private insurance companies would still exist, acting as fiscal intermediaries for the financing of a Comprehensive National Health Insurance Act through Social Security Taxes and federal and state subsidy of low-income people. Because deductibles and co-insurance would be imposed on families making

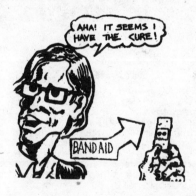

$4,800 or more. Private insurance could continue selling billions of dollars worth of insurance policies to cover deductable costs. Virtually no attempts at cost control are made, and an open-ended budget is in store for hospitals. Quality review is relegated to peer review boards, and benefits are not as extensive as under the Health Security Act.

The Catastrophic Health Insurance Plan, sponsored by Senators Long and Ribicoff, is being pushed by the fiscally conservative wing of the Congress. They reason that a bill covering only catastropic illness will be less expensive for the government than more comprehensive legislation. But, what is less expensive for the government is a greater burden for the consumer! Catastrophic Health Insurance Plan (CHIP) completely bypasses primary needs. Financed by an employee & employer payroll tax and covering only those on Social Security, CHIP contains a 60 day deductible and considerable co-insurance payments. ($12.50/day after the first 60 days.)

Each family would pay the first $2,000 of medical expenses each year and a 20% co-insurance on medical bills over $2,000. No dental work, eyeglasses or drugs are paid for under CHIP. In no way does it challenge the structure of health care delivery, making no provisions for cost control, distribution, training, quality control, or diminishing the two class system. It is a good PR gimmick for those politicians who capture votes by keeping down federal spending, but want to

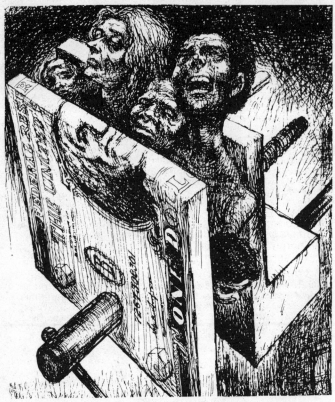

ride the tide of national health insurance sentiment. It supports the belief that health care is an individual responsibility with the government aiding only in extreme emergencies.

Medicredit, the AMA-sponsored proposal, is also chock-full of limitations. Benefits include 60 days of inpatient care, plus all physicians services (small wonder!). A $50 deductible on hospital charges, plus 20% co-insurance (up to $500) on hospital and doctor charges are imposed. Medicredit, once again, is a financing system guaranteeing the flow of money to providers, especially doctors; it does not change the health care system at all. Individuals pay private insurance carriers for policies in exchange for federal income tax deductions: low income people's (defined as those falling below income tax base) insurance is paid for by the government. Providers' roles stay the same and quality review is based on peer review. No provisions for consumer or non-professional worker input nor organizational changes are made. Coverage is voluntary. Medicredit is firmly entrenched in a capitalist system of health care, and the only clever thing about it is its name.

As of this writing, some form of National Health Insurance has a possibility of being passed in 1974, although because of congressional infighting and the heavy influence of big business, the 60 year fight for this significant piece of legislation seems to be ending with a less-than-adequate, watered-down compromise. All speakers for the major providers, the AMA, AHA, Health Insurance Institute, etc., have introduced their own biased proposals. Everyone keeps changing their position, looking for the safest alliance. Politicians have been playing public opinion and legislative wheeling-dealing to the utmost. Nixon, once opposed to NHI, has made urgent appeals for the passage of his bill—perhaps as a deterrent to criticism of the reckless slashing of federal social welfare funds. Kennedy, the major Congressional spokesperson for health care, compromised some of his basic demands for political expediency. And some of the major financial empires in the country, once strong supporters of NHI as a subsidy of private industry, have come out against it, claiming that another major

piece of social legislation would ruin our balance of payments —funny that they don't seem worried about balance of payments when it comes to defense spending. . . .

Yet even if some form of NHI is passed, it is not difficult to see that the health needs of the public would easily be lost in the money-making, bureaucratic inefficiencies and loose structure imbedded in these proposals. The way towards improving the quality and accessibility of health care is not to put more money into the system (the US already pays more per capita in health care than almost any other country), but to institute a full-public system of health care delivery that will be responsive to the health needs of the people, not the financial needs of the providers.

COMMITTEE FOR NATIONAL HEALTH INSURANCE. . . is the United Auto Workers-initiated spokesperson for the Health Security Act. Although biased toward the legislation that they wrote and support in Congress, CNHI puts out good factual material and statistics on all the Congressional proposals and other national health issues. Local committees exist in many states and municipalities. Contact CNHI, 821 15th St., NW, Washington, D.C. 20005, (202) 737-1177.

HEALTH PROFESSIONALS FOR POLITICAL ACTION. . . acts as a focal point for health professionals in the drive for comprehensive health insurance as well as working with citizen's groups in Massachusetts to organize support for the Health Security Act (one of the proposals before Congress on National Health Insurance). HPPA has researched HMOs, PSROs, the role of private health insurance companies in the inflation of health costs, and the AMA's regressive influence on health legislation. They hope to develop a litigation component to aid their work. Contact HPPA, Box 386, Kenmore Station, Boston, MA 00215, (617) 232-2900.

RESOURCES

"WHO WILL PAY YOUR BILLS," Health/PAC, 558 Capp St., San Francisco, CA 94110, 1973. 31 pp. $.50
. . . a concise, low-key introduction to national health insurance, so well-written that it will catch the interest of the most casual reader. Gives a good, basic list of questions that consumers should ask about any NHI proposal, as well as a brief analysis of the main proposals before Congress. The report ends with MCHR's model proposal for a locally-controlled public system of health care.

"CRISIS IN HEALTH CARE: DECENCY DEFEATED, VILLAINY REWARDED AND MISCELLANEOUS OBSERVATIONS," Michael Ross. Commission on Voluntary Service and Action, 475 Riverside Drive, New York, NY 10027. 10 pp. $.50
. . . overview of the health system, with a focus on the need for national health insurance. "To give credit where credit is due, the AMA has a track record of 50 years of successful political obstruction or decades-long delay of necessary social changes and scientific advances in medical service, education, organization and financing." In a brief review of Nixon's national health plan, with its reliance on private insurance companies, the author reminds us: "the neglect of preventive medicine, the concentration on expensive hospital beds and the resulting unnecessary surgery and admissions have been the unique contribution of insurance leadership to the present health crisis." The article doesn't go into much detail, but the analysis of the health system is sound and the writing style delightful. Good general resource.

"The Nixon RX for Health Care," THE WASHINGTON POST, 1150 15th St., NW, Washington, D.C. 20005. Mar 10, 1974. Section B, Page 1
. . . current critical discussion of Nixon's national health plan. "The Administration's system would be one of complexity, confusion, inefficiency and inequity. . . The myth that competition among the private health insurance companies results in greater efficiency than is found in the Social Security Ad-

ministration is simply not supported by fact." Good up-to-date analysis of Nixon's latest effort to trick the taxpayer into subsidizing yet another private industry.

"A CONSUMER CRITIQUE OF NATIONAL HEALTH INSURANCE," Beth Cagan, HEALTH/PAC, 17 Murray St., New York, NY 10007, 8 pp. $.07 for orders of 5 or more.
. . . good introduction to national health insurance: pending proposals, inherent shortcomings and who pays for it. This pamphlet compares three leading bills (Catastrophic Illness Insurance, Senator Long; National Health Insurance Partnership and Family Health Insurance Program, Nixon; and Health Security Act) in terms of who is eligible, benefits provided, financing, administration and breadth of scope. It also discusses the inevitable problems with a program that changes financing without changing the basic structure. The clarity of style, simplicity and conciseness of this pamphlet make it an excellent resource for educating people on what to look for in a health insurance proposal. Somewhat dated.

"Dr. Strangelove Joins Alice-in-Wonderland in Quest of a National Health Plan," Herbert S. Denenberg, THE PROGRESSIVE, 408 W. Gorham St., Madison, WI 53703, May 1973, 17-22 pp.
. . . identifies three major problems in the health system: lack of quality control, lack of price consciousness and secrecy on the part of the medical establishment. The author names three vital components in creating a good, humane system: consumer control, cost control and quality control. In evaluating pending national health insurance legislation, Denenberg finds all miserably lacking in the above, with the Health Security Act the least offensive. The article is good, offering an overview of the health system with specific examples drawn from the Pennsylvania experience in reform.

"The Politics of American Health Care," Godfrey Hodgson, THE ATLANTIC, 535 Fifth Ave., New York, NY 10017, Vol. 5, 1973, pp. 45-61.
. . . articulately condemns the health care system for linking healing with monetary rewards and providing services inequitably. Dramatically traces the history of nation health insurance legislation in the US, beginning in the 1930's with a highly financed AMA lobby "to fight 'the enslavement of the medical profession.'" Offers a factual indictment of the present system, a realistic appraisal of how Congress and the Nixon administration view national health insurance and a pessimistic conclusion. Highly informative reading.

HEW annual funding dropped from $5.5 million in 1972 to $3.3 million in 1973, and will drop even farther this spring. If current Administration Policies prevail, within two years 86,000 poor people will be without dependable out-patient medical care.—
—Wayne Clark, Southern Regional Councils' Governmental Monitoring Project

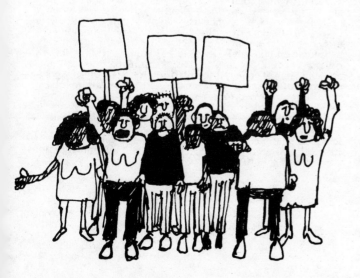

NATIONAL RESOURCE GROUPS

HEALTH POLICY ADVISORY CENTER. . . began its fine work in research and analysing the health care system following a 1967 expose of the New York city municipal hospital system. It has been going strong ever since, serving as a national educational, technical, and organizing resource for communities, workers, and student groups, spearheading radical change in the health system and society as a whole. Always spunky, sometimes brash, HEALTH/PAC BULLETINS present astute analyses of current health issues, focusing on such topics as institutional organizing, health training, the trend of public facilities turning private, women's health, community clinics, federal health, prison health, and more. Staff and associates conduct seminars and workshops and aid in urban and rural organizing efforts. A series of Health/PAC special reports discuss the national health insurance proposals now before Congress and call for an alternate proposal involving radical change in the financing, planning and delivery of health care, a health service free from profit and controlled by the workers and community. Contact HEALTH/PAC, 17 Murray St., New York, NY 10007, (212) 267-8890; 588 Capp St., San Francisco, CA 94110, (415) 282-3896.

MEDICAL COMMITTEE FOR HUMAN RIGHTS. . . is a national organization of activist health workers, professionals, community people, and patients, with local chapters spread throughout the country. Started in 1964 when scores of doctors and nurses went South to provide medical assistance to the civil rights movement, MCHR's most important current projects focus on local health needs, with chapter members taking active organizing roles within their communities. Such issues as patients rights, mental health, women's health, community-controlled clinics, the elderly, prison and occupational health have been prime concerns. National Task Forces serve as resources and clearinghouses in these areas. MCHR has also been giving support to the organizing efforts of hospital workers and providing medical presence (supplies and medical personnel) at Wounded Knee, Attica and other liberation struggles. A recent $10,000 grant will go toward the creation of a nationwide patients' rights clearinghouse. With the fiasco of current health planning and financing a major national concern, MCHR devoted much of its April 1974 convention to refining its 1971 proposal for a national health plan to counter pending reformist and inadequate proposals before Congress. The MCHR plan is based on a belief in comprehensive, accessible and preventive health care, free at the point of delivery, financed through a progressive taxation on all wealth, and controlled by those who use and work in health facilities. Contact MCHR, P.O. Box 7155, Pittsburgh, PA 15213, (412) 682-1200.

NATIONAL HEALTH LAW PROGRAM. . . provides supportive work in the area of health law, assisting legal aid offices and community groups around the country. Operating through an OEO grant, NHLP responds to specific requests from consumers for legal assistance, encourages local attorneys to take cases (especially when NHLP is over-loaded), and supplies them with the necessary technical back-up. Its range of activities covers all fields of health, focusing on problems of the poor. NHLP does extensive work around Medicaid, petitioning for regulation changes and bringing suits against unfair practices; it was instrumental in obtaining a ban on door-to-door selling of HMOs to Medicaid recipients in California and in blocking Medicaid cut-offs. It assisted Eastern Kentucky Welfare Rights Organization and other poor people's groups in challenging the legality of Hill-Burton money going to tax-exempt hospitals which were not serving the poor. NHLP has also done fine work in occupational safety and health and patients rights; has argued against over the counter drug practices, environmental pollution on Indian reservations and much more. The Program puts out a fine monthly newsletter which provides consumers and lawyers with an on-going analysis in the broad field of health law and policy, and keeps them up to date on political happenings. In addition, NHLP periodically publishes manuals covering such issues as occupational safety and health, patients rights, national health issues, and model HMO contracts. Contact NHLP, 10995 Le Conte Ave., Rm 640, Los Angeles, CA 90024, (213) 825-7601.

HEALTH LAW PROJECT... operates out of the University of Pennsylvania Law School with OEO funding. Composed of lawyers, health workers, researchers and students, HLP emphasizes providing consumers with the information and technical resources to help them "develop the capacity to make health systems and institutions publically accountable." The Project has successfully forced Medicaid to provide early periodic screening, diagnosis and testing for children covered by Medicaid. With consumer groups, it has successfully pressured for changes in the health program on federal, state and local levels, as well as establishing the rights of patients. In the area of nursing homes they have set up an ombudsperson program and are working with patients to participate in and enforce quality standards. As a result of its comprehensive survey of health care and conditions in eight state prisons, the governor has commissioned a task force to implement recommendations of HLP and plans to hire a prison health planner to develop a program of comprehensive care. Although oriented toward research and working with local groups to pressure and negotiate for change, HLP is not adverse to using litigation. Consumer-oriented publications and handbooks cover implications of the Health Security Act for the poor, and nursing home organizing as well as a wide range reviewed in this catalog. Materials on the expansion of Medicaid eligibility and family planning for poor women are in preparation. Teaching material on health law is distributed to local legal services. Contact HEALTH LAW PROJECT, University of Pennsylvania Law School, 133 S. 36th St., Rm 310, Philadelphia, PA 19104, (215) 594-6951.

CHURCH HEALTH ACTION COMMITTEE... began in 1971 to work on the health issue in an effort to develop consumer support for a national health service. CHAC originally intended to provide data and other resources for local church and lay organizing efforts around a national health service, but soon discovered that local groups needed organizational skills in order to build a new power base. CHAC now helps local communities do grassroots organizing by helping them understand the issues in the national health crisis, and the underlying political questions. They offer basic organizing and technical skills (such as how to conduct a survey, gather statistical data and publicize work) and help groups plan strategies and develop tactics. The committee is now working directly with about five local groups as well as putting out valuable literature and fact sheets on national health issues. CHAC speaks to community groups and has helped organizations such as the Gray Panthers sponsor symposiums on the health issue. Composed of health professionals, teachers, writers, social workers, clergy, etc., the Committee sees its main point of entry into the community as through Christian churches, although it would like to expand its constituency and influence; it was recently approached by a labor union to do work. Contact CHAC, Box 793, Peter Stuyvesant Station, New York, NY 10009, (212) 674-3215.

RESOURCES

BOOKS

The American Health Empire: Power, Profits, and Politics, A Health/PAC book prepared by Barbara and John Ehrenreich. Vintage Books, 201 E. 50th St., New York, NY 10022, 1970. 279 pp. $1.95
... the classic, biting analysis of a health care system once centered around the family doctor and now controlled by a huge medical/industrial complex. Using New York City as a case in point, the book develops the concept that the

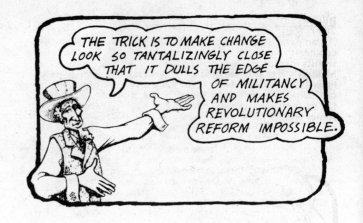

prestige and profits of providers and financiers with the support of government policies—not the needs of consumers—determine the policies and priorities of our health care system. Covering the role of hospitals, the drug industry, planning agencies, insurance companies and the role of banks, construction companies and other support industries, the book concludes with three accounts of workers/ student/community revolts. Though concentrating on New York City, the American Health Empire provides a solid understanding of the political and economic forces which have made the health care industry what it is today. An important resource.

Your Money or Your Life, Richard Kunnes. Dodd, Mead & Co., 79 Madison Ave., NY, NY 10016, 1971. 199 pp. $5.95
... an indictive and challenging book. Kunnes exposes the Medical Industrial Complex (MIC) for what it is: Profit-seeking, racist, elitist and sexist. Believing that doctors can not satisfy both their own greed for money and the physical and emotional needs of their patients, Kunnes documents efforts by the Medical Establishment (AMA) to encourage mystification and professionalism, fight legislation granting the government greater involvement in the health care system, and maintain medicine as a White, male profession. The connection between the Medical Industrial Complex and the Military Industrial Complex is the next subject of Kunnes' wrath. Using specific examples of New York City hospitals, he shows how individuals and corporations made wealthy by Defense Department contracts now control city hospitals. Chapter 4 lists demands for "A People's Health Service," the book ends with the story of the take-over of St. Luke's Hospital in East Harlem by the Medical Liberation Front, local Blacks, Latinos, and Whites (including the author).

The Exploitation of Illness in Capitalist Society, Howard B. Waitzkin and Barbara Waterman, Bobbs-Merrill Co., Inc., 4300 W. 62nd St., Indianapolis, IN 46268, 1974. 132 pp
... an intriguing sociological analysis of "existing institutional structures in the American health system, as well as an appraisal of theory in medical sociology," from a Marxist viewpoint. Although written in an academic style, the book brings up some important concepts, such as the idea that people often play the "sick role" to "relieve strains which otherwise could become a focus of dissatisfaction, conflict and change." The way this role functions as a means of social control is examined in the context of prisons, mental hospitals, the armed forces, and the family. Also discussed are the stratification of the health system along class lines, the doctor-patient relationship, and problems of professionalism. The authors conclude that a humane health care system is impossible in a capitalist society and call for an end to the exploitation of illness, with some solid recommendations on how this should happen.

Billions for Bandaids, Bay Area Chapter, MCHR, P.O. Box 7677, San Francisco, CA 94119, 1972. 128 pp. $2.00
. . . an excellent political and economic analysis of the American health industry. Easy to read, the books forceful analysis hits insurance, drug companies, HMOs, Foundations for Medical Care, and the 'hoax of national health insurance.' How the health industry is tied to the rest of corporate America is exposed throughout the book, as well as how our whole tax system works against the middle and low-income consumer and in favor of the wealthy.

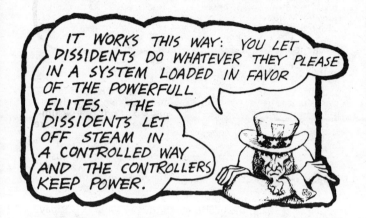

The World Institute Guide To Alternative Futures For Health, Michael Marien. World Institute, 777 United Nations Plaza, New York, NY 10017, 1974
. . . compiled to correct the imbalance in health knowledge which presently concentrates on researching specific diseases rather than on studying general health conditions and alternatives. The guide aims to serve a catalytic educational function—for policymakers, researchers, librarians, teachers and citizens—by piecing together the "heretofore disparate parts" of the health care delivery system. Marien observes that the US spends 5-6 billion each year on national security yet fails to view threats to the health of the people as a threat to security. It includes an incredibly comprehensive range of materials—612 books, articles and reports in all—most of which are annotated (some in great depth) and rated by the author according to quality and audience written for. The volume has a strong scholastic emphasis and summarily comments on each of the various subsections the books fall under. Conscientiously written with an eye towards presenting all sides of the picture, the policyguide is a fine reference tool for anyone concerned about health care in this country—past, present or future.

CIDOC Antologia, Medicina, Centro Intercultural de Documentacion, APDP 479, Cuernavaca, Mexico. $50.00 set of 8 books
. . . although we were unable to see copies of the books, it seems like a valuable resource for libraries and institutions able to afford it. Includes two bibliographies and three books of selections on alternative health care, as well as books on the limits of therapy, and the effectiveness of health services. Covers the work of Thomas Szasz, Ivan Illich and others known for their radical perspective.

PAMPHLETS AND ARTICLES

"THE POLITICS OF HEALTH CARE: A BIBLIOGRA-PHY," Ken Rosenberg and Gordon Schiff. New England Free Press, 60 Union Square, Somerville, MA 02143, 1972. 24 pp. $.30
. . . an annotated compilation of major books, articles, and periodicals that present or support a radical analysis of the

health care system and proposals for its change. Presented in outline form, this impressive list includes general readings, as well as readings on the powers behind the health industry, health capitalism, health workers and professionalism; consumer/community control of services; women and the health system, mental health, occupational health, health and the environment; health and war; systems in other countries; and strategies for change. The resources included in this fine bibliography are especially useful for study groups or courses in health politics and as an actual organizing tool.

"Radicals in Health," WORKFORCE, Vocations for Social Change, 5951 Canning St., Oakland, CA 94609, May to June 1974. 64 pp. $.50-$1.00 per copy
. . . this issue has an introduction to major health issues (occupational, women's, health planning, professionalism) and articles by people from Emma Goldman's Free Clinic, THE PEOPLE'S HEALTH, (a newspaper), and Urban Planning Aid, (an occupational safety and health group). There is also an article about the Health Education Media Project. The issue gives some good insights into how these groups operate and how they've dealt with problems. For instance, the interview with the staff people from Emma Goldman's tells how the women tried to overcome the professional mystique as they learned more advanced paramedical skills. Especially useful for people just getting involved in health.

"YOUR HEALTH CARE IN CRISIS: A HEALTH/PAC SPE-CIAL REPORT", 17 Murray St., New York, NY 10007, 1972. 17 pp. Free
. . . introduction to the failures of the US health system in delivering adequate, low-cost care. Covers insurance companies, medical empires and a brief description of how people are fighting for change. Good for clinic waiting rooms.

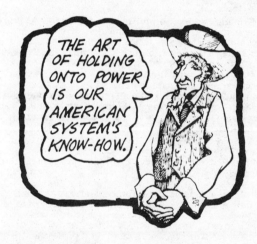

"The Politics of American Health Care," Godfrey Hodgson, THE ATLANTIC, 535 Fifth Ave., New York, NY 10017, 1973, pp. 45-61
. . . articulately condemns the health system for linking healing with monetary rewards and providing services inequitably. Dramatically traces the history of national health insurance legislation in the US, beginning in the 1930's with a highly financed AMA lobby "to fight 'the enslavement of the medical profession.'" Offers factual indictments of the present appraisal of how Congress and the Nixon administration view national health insurance and concludes pessimistically. Highly informative reading.

"PEOPLE'S GUIDE TO HEALTH CARE: HEALTH CARE COST FACTS," Terry Demchak, Legal Aid Society, 2108 Payne Ave., Cleveland, OH 44114, January, 1972. 22 pp. $.25
. . . a guide to all the present health plans (Kaiser, Blue Cross, Medicaid), the AMA and Nixon proposals for National Health Insurance, as well as the MCHR National Health Plan proposal. Also has good diagrams of health expenditures and who pays how much, broken down into private and public percentages. Concise and factual, although some of the material is dated.

OTHER COUNTRIES

PERIODICALS

HEALTH RIGHTS NEWS, Medical Committee for Human Rights, 542 S. Dearborn St., Chicago, IL 60605. $5/year
. . . provides on-going documentation and general analysis of events and trends in the health movement. This monthly newspaper offers an important radical perspective on health issues related to women, prisoners, workers, Third World people, the retarded, and more. It has up-to-date information on events in various cities and keeps up on government involvement in health. A fine resource for health organizers.

HEALTH LAW NEWSLETTER, National Health Law Program, 10995 Le Conte Ave., Room 640, Los Angeles, CA 90024. Free
. . . a great monthly newsletter to keep consumers and legal workers abreast of whats happening in health law, federal health policy, and consumer/community challenges. Covers Hill-Burton, Medicaid&care, abortion, occupational safety and health, health maintenance organizations, federal legislation, and much more. This along with HEALTH/PAC BULLETIN should give any community enough fire and inspiration to challenge their local health power structure.

FILMS AND TAPES

American Friends Service Committee, New England Action Research Project, 48 Inman St., Cambridge, MA 02139

"Behind the Crisis in Health Care," 30 min. slide show, write for information on purchase or on rental
A slide show (with script) critiquing the corporate structure behind our health care system. It focuses on the medical-industrial complex in general and the drug industry, medical technology, and medical empire in particular. Alternatives such as preventive care and community and worker control are proposed.

Great Atlantic Radio Conspiracy, 2743 Maryland Ave., Baltimore, MD 21218

"Health Care in America," 30 min. cassette tape, $2.50 for individuals, $5.00 for institutions (also available in tape reel).
. . . takes you into hospitals, doctors offices and drug company boardrooms—a world where death and disease are profitable. This excellent radical overview of health care combines grim humor, dialogues and factual indictments to get its message across. Begins with a conversation between a self-righteous doctor and an "overdemanding" patient who has been lying in her hospital bedfutilely ringingfor help for four days. It then covers the profits of the drug industry, the realities of our two-class system of health care, and the oppression of women by the health industry. This captivating tape is by far one of the best introductions to the realities of our health care system which dares to fraudulantly proclaim itself "the best in the world".

AFL/CIO, 815 Sixteenth St., NW, Washington, D.C. 20006

"A Nation's Promise: Health Security," 22 min. cl. 1970 $3.00
Case histories of citizens testifying before a Senate Subcommittee conducting hearings on health care document the severity of the problem. Rep. Martha Griffiths discusses the failures of private insurance.

"Don't Get Sick in America," 56 min. b&w 1969 $7.50
Presents facts on the health care crisis in the first reel (28 min.) and concentrates on the causes of our inefficient delivery of health care services in the second reel. (28 min.) Lacks radical perspective, but good information

As we in the United States try to construct a humane and workable model for a national health plan, it is important to draw on the experiences of other countries. This section describes a few examples—it does not pretend to be comprehensive. The health systems of Cuba and China are part of a socialist economy, brought about through armed revolution. Canada, Sweden, and Great Britain have socialized medicine that came about by gradual, legislative change within a basically capitalist economy. The national standard of living, urban/rural population, cultural attitude toward health care and extent of medical resources also varies from country to country. And even in nations experiencing socialist revolutions, serious problems still exist. Nevertheless, the following descriptions and resources are meant to help place the US health care system in some perspective and provide some models for change.

CANADA

Federally subsidized, provincially controlled and administered health plans in Canada offer a wide range of services and benefits. For the majority of the population they increase the availability of health care by minimizing the financial burden.

Because health insurance plans are controlled by the provinces, financing and coverage vary considerably. For instance, in Newfoundland, Prince Edwards Island, New Brunswick, Quebec and the Yukon health care is paid from general tax revenue; in Ontario, premiums of $132 for single people and $264 for couples and families are levied. Likewise, coverage ranges from extensive in Saskatchewan (home, office and hospital visits, surgery, obstetrics, psychiatric care outside mental hospitals, anesthesia, laboratory and radiological services, preventive medicine, certain dental services, and eye glasses) to more limited in Ontario (only emergency care and physical therapy are covered on an out-patient basis). Some provinces include oral surgery and eye glasses. Generally, each province sets a ceiling on how much a doctor can charge for a visit, although they can charge more if they can get the patient to agree to pay the additional expense.

Regional regulations specify to whom coverage is available (residents, non-residents), special assistance and additional programs for the poor. Provincial financing is supplemented by a 50% contribution to each province from the federal government. The federal government also has primary responsibility for research, environmental health and other areas of national concern.

Canada's program is health insurance, not a health plan, and possesses all the limitations of that system. This means that resources are not necessarily equitably distributed, and doctors remain a well-paid privileged class. The two-class system of health care still thrives through the public and private sectors. Nevertheless, Canada has gone a long way toward making health care accessible to all.

GREAT BRITAIN

Great Britain is a good model of a western country with comprehensive, universal, free health care. The National Health System (NHS) was created in 1948 and offers virtually totally socialized medicine.

Coverage is extensive: family doctor services, dental services, hospitalization (in-patient and out-patient), medical treatment for drug addiction, psychiatric care, pre- and post-natal care, home nursing, nursing home, health education and preventive care are all free. Drugs and eye glasses are partially covered with total subsidy for the poor. However those who choose to go to private doctors pay the total cost themselves.

With the exception of a limited number of doctors in private practice, all health workers are paid by the national government. Doctors are paid on the basis of patients treated. The country is divided into regions and the number of doctors permitted to practice in each region is limited. Thus, the NHS hopes to encourage more equal distribution of doctors.

The British system goes a long way toward making health care accessible for all. Medical care is free, and includes preventive care and education. Consumers have input into decisions through representation on regional hospital boards. Domestic help for the elderly and chronically ill is free, thus reducing the number of people in nursing homes. Expectant and nursing mothers and young children receive free or reduced cost milk. And, the British only contribute 4.5% of their GNP to health care, compared to 8% in the US.

As with any complex system, there are difficulties. NHS does not tackle the problems of access to health care, training, professionalism, sexism, racism or classism. Doctors claim that they are over-burdened, and mobility within the system is restricted. Long waiting lists exist for non-urgent surgery. (Though this still looks better than the US, where some die waiting and some don't wait at all.) The construction of Health Care Centers has been retarded by insufficient funds. Bureaucratic inefficiencies exist and patients' complaints are ignored or lost in confusion; their representation on Hospital Boards is limited by lack of medical knowledge and an elitist attitude on the part of the doctors.

Although the shortcomings are evident, the US can certainly learn from Britain's public financing system and its attempts at planning.

SWEDEN

Socialization of health care in Sweden has been a gradual process, although the 1955 enactment of the National Compulsory Health Insurance Plan marked a major step. Subsequent legislation has expanded coverage and integrated health care with other government programs.

Health care in Sweden is decentralized and facility oriented. Each of the 23 counties owns and controls several hospitals whose services are virtually free at the point of delivery. 75% of the nation's doctors are paid by the government with salaries based on position and tenure; the remaining 25% are in private practice. People in hospitals or using outpatient facilities pay a token fee (usually less than $1) while those using private physicians are partially reimbursed.

Funding for health care is shared by the patient (15%), the national government (31%) and the county and municipal governments (54%). As in many countries, cost is rising rapidly, claiming 9% of the GNP.

Strong features of the Swedish health care systems are maternity, infant, and home care. Sweden has the lowest infant

mortality rate and one of the lowest maternal mortality rates. Extensive pre- and post-natal care are standard, with 99% of births performed in hospitals, often by midwives. Parenthood Benefits Insurance offers both mother and father special coverage for the 6 months following birth; in addition, parents are compensated when forced to miss work to care for a sick child.

Home care benefits allow "a person who is ill over a long period and receives home care. ... under certain circumstances (to) be granted an allowance from the county to pay for an attendant, for instance a relative". This decreases the need for long term facilities and enables the patient to be cared for by someone trusted.

Major deficiencies of Sweden's health care system lie in the shortage of personnel and their poor geographical distribution; emphasis on hospital care and research over ambulatory care and preventive measures; poor coordination of mental health and other services; and inadequate communication between hospital services and private physicians. Currently 8.8% of doctor's positions are vacant and 2.1% for nurses, although the shortage is much more severe in the far north.

Despite the nation's shortcomings, Swedes are among the healthiest people in the world. Life expectancy is higher than other western countries and infant mortality is lower. The fact their health care is regionally controlled, available for all and relatively comprehensive puts them miles ahead of the U.S.

CUBA

Medical care in Cuba has vastly improved since 1959, despite the fact that 2,583 of the 6,300 MDs left the country by 1967, the early part of the revolution. Health care is better now due to revolutionary priorities of 1. equitable distribution of doctors within the country; 2. increased number of doctors trained every year; 3. increased appropriations for health; and 4. education and preventive care.

To combat a pre-revolutionary trend of doctors to concentrate in Havana (doctor-patient ratio of 1/310 in Havana compared to 1/2,475 for the rest of the country), the government now requires all interns to spend two years in a rural area, spends disproportionate amounts for rural facilities and offers salary incentives to rural doctors. The number of doctors trained annually has risen from 300 in 1959 to 800 in 1968; 42-50% are women. It is no surprise that the Ministry of Health budget has increased from 25 million pesos in 1958 to 220 million in 1968.

For the average citizen this means more and better treatment. The basic unit of health care is the polyclinic. Providing out-patient care for 25,000-30,000 people, the polyclinic provides diagnosis and treatment of most ambulatory illnesses, follow-up on hospitalization, dental care, classes in hygiene and sanitation and general health education. Generally the staff consists of a General Practitioner, an OB/GYN, pediatrician, dentists, nurses, aids, social workers, lab and X-ray technicians, field nurses and sanitation workers. Although there is no structure to guarantee community control, patients are encouraged to voice their feelings and participate actively in the polyclinic.

Regional hospitals serve as back-up facilities to the poly-clinic, offering a wide range of in-patient services. The only national facilities are a psychiatric hospital and a few specialty institutes engaged in research. The Cuban government pays for all medical care including drugs.

Problems and contradictions still exist. Doctors' salaries are ten times what a janitor earns; the system is hierarchical with no guarantee of consumer input. There are not enough polyclinics in the cities and not enough doctors in the country. Mental illness is given low priority. But these things are inevitable in a poor country that is trying to make such sweeping changes in a short period of time.

The revolution has brought a far better health system to Cuba. The number of hospital beds have doubled since the revolution while the frequency of serious and fatal diseases continues to drop. There are 170 hospitals now, compared to 57 before. Workers are trained on the job and experience considerable upward mobility; nearly 50% of the medical students are women and Blacks, and rural people are encouraged to attend. Medical education is free and emphasizes preventive care.

And compared to other nations of the Americas, Cuba ranks high. "Infant mortality in Central America is currently 67 per thousand live births and in South America 79; in Cuba it was 33.09 (as of 1967). Alianza publications acknowledge that it will not be possible to obtain 5.8 doctors per 10,000 inhabitants in South American by 1980; Cuba had 8.8 by 1966. Maternity mortality in Havana is 30.2 per 100,000 births, and for all of Cuba 43.5; Louisiana has 42 white, 73 non-white." (Ramparts)

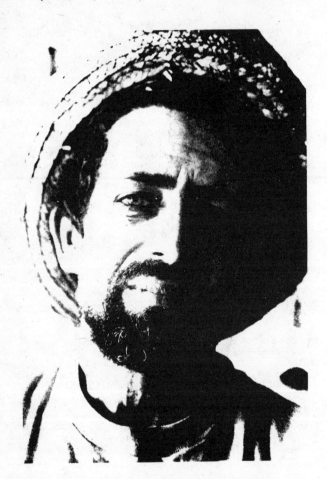

CHINA

More than any other country in the world, health care in the People's Republic of China has improved radically in the past 25 years. VD, prostitution and opium addiction have been virtually eliminated, millions of peasants have seen doctors for the first time and health care has truly become a right, not a privilege.

Prior to the revolution, China was rightfully known as the "sick man of Asia." In 1943, the General Secretary of the Chinese Medical Association gave a statistical profile of some of China's major health problems. The general mortality rate was 25 per 1,000; the maternal death rate was 15 per 1,000 births; and the infant mortality rate was 200 per 1,000. Over one-third of the population were estimated to have dangerous eye diseases while the number of lepers was given as one million. Eight per cent of the population had pulmonary tuberculosis and ten percent syphillis or gonorrhea. In 1949 there were 1200 doctors trained in Western medicine and 500 hospitals to serve a population of over 400,000,000.

Following the revolution, two national health congresses were called, establishing the following priorities: 1. the health system should serve the working people, including peasants and soldiers; 2. emphasis should be placed on preventive care; 3. Western trained and traditional doctors should work together and; 4. when possible, health work should involve mass campaigns and active citizen participation.

For the first fifteen years of the revolution, medical care was primarily urban oriented, although mass campaigns against VD, opium addiction, snails and other common diseases were conducted. In 1965 Mao Tse-Tung gave a speech on health care, which changed this trend substantially: "The Ministry of Health is not that of the people and it is better to rename it as the Ministry of Urban Health or the Lords' Health Ministry or the Urban Lords." Responding to a call by Chairman Mao, medical teams of doctors, nurses, and health personnel left for the countryside to provide basic services and train 1,000,000 barefoot doctors—peasants who have been trained to provide basic health care in 4-5 month sessions (offerred during the winter) for three consecutive years. These doctors are still peasants, receive no extra pay and do not aspire to move to urban areas. They are committed to remain in rural areas, offering a critically needed service to hundreds of millions of medically starved peasants.

Preventive care has meant a two-pronged approach: an attack on those diseases which effect large segments of the population (as snails and TB once did) and the creation of a framework for long term care. Such common diseases as "smallpox, cholera, plague. . . have all been eliminated, and malaria, which afflicted millions in South China has declined sharply." And, the services of rural medical teams and barefoot doctors offer a basis for future preventive and curative care.

The encouraged unity between western trained and traditional doctors is both a response to the crucial doctor shortage and a desire to respect the skills of both. Rural medical teams seek out traditional doctors to learn of herbal cures and other remedies. Medical research teams include traditional and western trained scientists. As a result of this cooperation, "China today stands at the world forefront in the treatment of severe burns, the re-attachment of severed limbs and fingers (critical problems of industrial health), the cure of some of the deaf, dumb and blind by new acupuncture techniques, and the use of electric acupuncture in place of anesthesia."

But the major factors in improved health in China are social, political, and economic. People no longer starve to death, nor must they support themselves through prostitution and drug pushing. Village water supplies have been cleaned up and disease carrying insects exterminated. Medical care is virtually free, increasingly accessible, and aimed at prevention and education. Treatment is routinely done by health teams, actively involving the patient as well as all levels of health personnel in decisions. The paraprofessional concept has certainly been well used in China through the training of the barefoot doctors. These changes have not come about in a vacuum; the health of the Chinese people has improved because China has become a healthier nation.

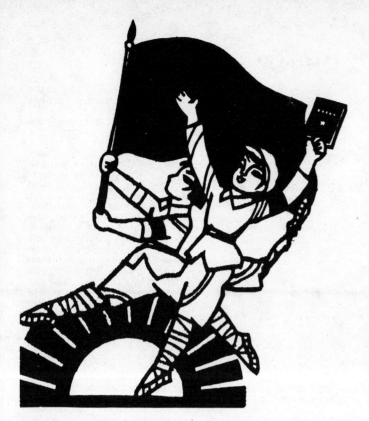

RESOURCES

BOOKS

<u>Away With All Pests</u>, Dr. Joshua S. Horn. Modern Reader, New York and London, 1969. 192 pp. $2.45
. . . explains the basic ideology behind the health delivery system in the People's Republic and then uses specific incidents to show how it actually functions. One excellent example of how the Chinese health system works is seen in the fight against VD. "To find the millions of cases of latent syphilis scattered throughout the country was an immense undertaking which could not be tackled along orthodox lines. . . In a county in Hopei province, after prolonged discussions between political and medical workers, a form was drawn up asking ten questions, an affirmative answer to any one of which would suggest the possibility of syphilis. Propaganda posters were put up in the village streets, one-act plays performed in the market place, talks given over the village radio system and meetings big and small, held night after night at which the purpose of the questionnaire was explained and the co-operation of the peasants gradually won. . . All those having clues were given blood tests and it was found that one in twenty of them actually had syphilis. . . The campaign went on for two months, covering not only syphilis, but also such diseases as ringworm of the scalp, leprosy and malaria." The writing style is warm and simple, and the pictures give a useful insight into life in China. This book is a pleasure to read and strongly recommended.

<u>Medical Workers Serving the People Wholeheartedly</u>, Foreign Languages Press, Peking 1971. 114 pp.
. . . a joy to read. This book, showing the Chinese medical system in action, is full of pictures of barefoot doctors, rural medical teams and happy, cured peasants. Reflecting the Chinese bias towards rural areas, most of the emphasis is on the work of the "Advanced Health Section Serving the People Wholeheartedly" of the People's Liberation Army, which trains peasant medical teams. Example after example of successful operations of seemingly incurable ailments. Shows the removal of a ninety pound tumor from one peasant's stomach, restoration of sight/hearing to previously blind/deaf children and more. Very inspiring, although quite rhetorical.

PAMPHLETS AND ARTICLES

"Public Health Care in Cuba", <u>SOCIAL POLICY</u>, Jan-Feb 1971, pp. 41-46, available from Louise Rice, 65 Chestnut St., Cambridge, MA 02139, Jan 1971. 6 pp. $.23
. . . covers the basics of medical care in Cuba, with a focus on how the system has changed since 1959. Many of the statistics compare pre-revolutionary and current conditions, indicating dramatic progress. "In 1958, Cuba had 25,000 beds in 54 hospitals, providing 3.9 beds per 1,000 people; in 1968, there were 47,000 beds in 180 hospitals, or 5.9 beds per 1,000 people. . . . Corresponding to this steady increase in services, government expenditures on health have risen from $3.50 per person in 1959 to over $20 at present." Shows the emphasis placed on preventive care, education and demystifying the medical profession.

"China: Revolution and Health," <u>HEALTH/PAC BULLETIN</u>, 17 Murray St., New York, NY 10007, Dec. 1972. pp. 2-18
. . . traces the development of health care delivery in China from pre-revolutionary days to the present. "Unfortunately many articles in the popular media emphasize advances in techniques and technology rather than improvements in health care delivery, and the social and political origins of all these are virtually ignored. . . Chinese achievements in eradicating syphilis and opium addiction are reported, but the very basis of their approach is neglected: that the treatment of such diseases cannot be isolated from the socio-economic context in which they arose." This article attempts to correct these concepts, integrating the socio-political and the medical changes in China, thus providing a balanced view of the new health care delivery system. Includes a special section on "Health Care for Women" and many personal observations. Worthwhile introduction to health care in China and a real up to read.

PERIODICALS

BULLETIN OF CONCERNED ASIAN SCHOLARS, Committee of Concerned Asian Scholars, Building 600T, Stanford, CA 94305. students $4/yr., regular rate $6/yr, institutions $10/yr
. . . "The Committee of Concerned Asian Scholars seeks to develop a humane and knowledgeable understanding of Asian societies and their efforts to maintain cultural integrity and to confront such problems as poverty, oppression, and imperialism. We realize that to be students of other peoples, we must first understand our relations to them." The articles are definitely scholarly, but frequently offer valuable insights on China.

TAPES

Radio Free People, 133 Mercer St., New York, NY 10012

"Life and Medicine in Revolutionary China," 90 min. Cassette or reel to reel. $6. $10 for institutions. Includes some of the same material as <u>Away With All Pests</u>. Joshua Horne tells China's story.

"Revolution is Preventive Medicine," 30 min. cassette or reel to reel. $6. $10 to institutions
This tape provides a general overview of the Cuban health care system—its basic tenets and priorities—and of socialist medicine, with great stress placed on the need for preventive care. Cuba is described as "the example of the future. . . in medical care and . . . in humanization." On a broader scale, the tape outlines the 3-level process—national, regional and local—through which a revolution in health care must happen in this country. Urging action towards vast socio-economic political change in the U.S., this material is probably most helpful for initiates to the concept of socialist medicine and what it entails.

SUBJECT INDEX

The Roman Numeral following the page numbers indicate the column.

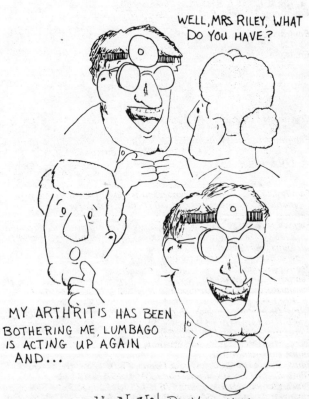

WELL, MRS RILEY, WHAT DO YOU HAVE?

MY ARTHRITIS HAS BEEN BOTHERING ME, LUMBAGO IS ACTING UP AGAIN AND...

NO, NO, NO! DO YOU HAVE BLUE CROSS, MEDICARE, MASTER CHARGE, BANK AMERICARD OR....

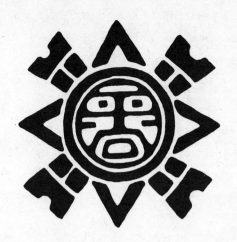

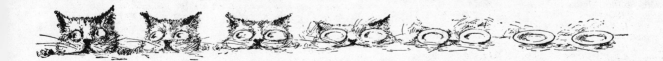

GROUP INDEX

Those numbers without asterisks indicate the pages where the group is written up or mentioned; those with asterisks designate written resources by or about the group; "f" indicates a film.

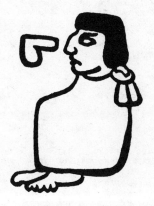

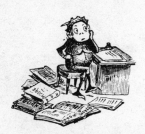

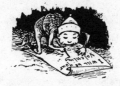

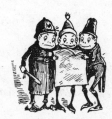

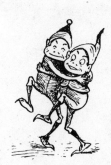

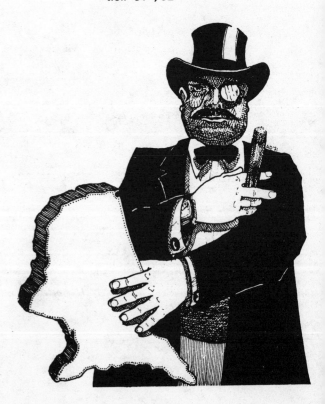

GEOGRAPHIC INDEX

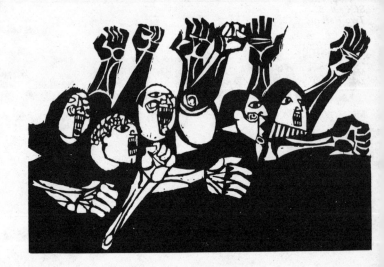

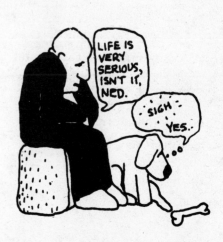

PICTURE CREDITS

Front cover by Jo Ann Moore

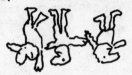

p.3, Michael Abramson
p.3, Daily Kent Stater/LNS
p.3, North East Neighborhood Association
p.4, Cleveland Legal Aid
p.4, Southern Regional Council
p.5, Chip Berlet
p.6, CPS
p.7, LNS/United Farm Worker
p.8, Oliphant/LNS
p.9, AYCE/CPF
p.10, LNS Women's Graphics Collective
p.11, North East Neighborhood Association
p.12, AKWESASNE NOTES
p.12, LNS/La Clinica del Pueblo de Rio Arriba
p.13, Chip Berlet
p.14, Northwest Passage/LNS
p.14, Chip Berlet
p.15, Chip Berlet
p.16, North Carolina Anvil/LNS
p.17, Larry Frank
p.18, Chip Berlet
p.19, "LA ALIANZA HISPANA"
p.20, Chip Berlet

p.49, "LA ALIANZA HISPANA"
p.50, LNS
p.51, LNS
p.52, LNS
p.52, CPS
p.53, CPS
p.54, CPS
p.55, Asian Women
p.56, Health/PAC
p.57, Bay Area MCHR
p.58, LNS
p.59, 1199
p.60, October 4th Organization

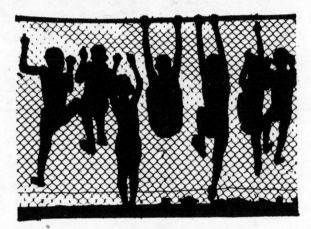

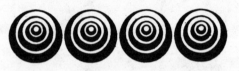

p.22, Ken Light/LNS
p.23, Post American/LNS
p.24, LNS
p.25, LNS
p.26, Michael Abramson/LNS
p.27, Abraxas/LNS
p.27, CPS
p.28, CPS
p.30, Department of Transportation
p.31, Cleveland Legal Aid
p.32, Cleveland Legal Aid
p.33, "MEDICAL CADRE"
p.35, LNS/Michael Abramson
p.36, GAY LIBERATOR
p.37, LNS Women's Graphics Collective
p.38, Utah Migrant Council
p.39, Dorothea Lange/LNS
p.40, Paul Conklin
p.40, LNS/Human Love In Action
p.41, LNS
p.42, LNS Women's Graphics Collective
p.43, Triple Jeopardy/LNS
P.44, NCHO Newsletter
p.44, "LA VOZ DEL PUEBLO"
p.45, NCHO Newsletter
p.46, Michael Abramson
p.48, "LA ALIANZA HISPANA"

p.61, October 4th Organization
p.61, October 4th Organization
p.63, CPF
p.63, Cleveland Legal Aid
p.65, Oliphant/Daily Collegian/LNS
p.66, October 4th Organization
p.68, CPF
p.69, TRANSFUSION
p.71, 1199
p.72, DAYTON WORKERS VOICE
p.73, THE PEOPLE'S HEALTH
p.74, Grape/LNS
p.77, Johns Hopkins University
p.78-79, CPF
p.80, Paul Fusco/LNS
p.82, USCB/Nexus/LNS
p.83, Urban Planning Aid
p.84, CPF
p.85, Michael Abramson
p.85, Nurses NOW
p.86, CPF
p.87, CPF
p.89, "THIS IS YOUR LIFE"
p.89, LNS
p.90, Eileen Whalen/LNS
p.91, "COMPREHENSIVE HEALTH CARE: A SOUTHERN VIEW"
p.93, Cleveland Legal Aid
p.94, Chip Berlet
p.95, "LA ALIANZA HISPANA"
p.97, HEALTH RIGHTS NEWS
p.98, SYNAPSE
p.99, Paul Conklin
p.101, Dept. of HEW
p.103, Scarlet Letter/Rough Times
p.104, Rough Times
p.105, "FORCED TREATMENT EQUALS TORTURE"

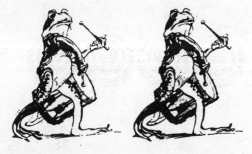

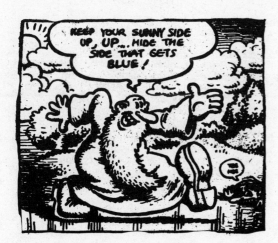

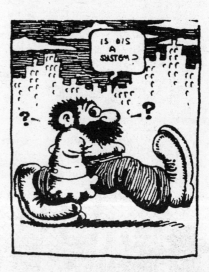

SOURCE STORY

OUR BEGINNINGS . . . were with a bus, the Educational Liberation Front (ELF). This project organizing information center and media-bookmobile traveled 20,000 miles visiting 50 campus communities in '69-'70. After a year's experience, the ELF crew concluded that too much information had been collected for one bus to pass on. From this realization came SOURCE, whose original concept of one catalog quickly expanded to others.

SOURCE OPERATES . . . as a living working collective of 6-8 full time people plus the energy of 5-10 part-time people. The collective doesn't receive salaries, but all housing, food and other necessities are provided. Decisions on work, priorities, and catalog content are made by consensus at weekly meetings. We rotate coordinators weekly: they are responsible for group process and work overview, including getting meetings going, handling business dealings, errand running, etc. House and Office work are shared equally with the intention of transfering skills. We work most of the time though we try to save late evenings for political studies, skills learning or play.

CATALOG RESEARCH . . . starts with group researchers locating and contacting organizations by phone during the day. Nights are spent combing periodicals, etc. for additional groups and working with part-time "writers" to complete descriptions and narrative. Simultaneously a publications researcher, using libraries and bibliographies, assembles the resources. The material is then placed on large mock up sheets for initial editing and criticism by the whole group. Confusing sections and "holes" go back to the researchers while the rest goes on to a rewriter(s) for flow, style and better wording. Pictures and quotes are added to the section for a second editing and then scrutiny by a person from a local project organizing around that issue. Finally it's off to production to be designed, typeset, proofread, and pasted up.

FUNDING

Our funding comes from publisher's advances, catalog sales, outside jobs, churches, small foundation grants, and donations. We are a subsistance collective.

SOURCE SPIN-OFFS

The Organizers' Book Center is a distribution and publishing project for practical organizing materials: from Saul Alinsky and Ralph Nader to the NACLA Research and Methodology Guide, and The New Women's Survival Catalog. Write for their brochure: Organizers' Book Center, P.O. Box 21066, Washington, D.C. 20009.

Resources for Community Change is a recent outgrowth of Source. Its purpose is to answer specific requests for information. It has extensive files to serve the tactical and "how-to" needs of individuals and groups. RCC has published one booklet, Demand for Daycare, and hopes to do more. Contact Resources for Community Change, P.O. Box 21066, Washington, D.C. 20009, (202) 387-1145.

OTHER PUBLICATIONS

COMMUNICATIONS: Source Catalog No. 1, Swallow Press, 1971, 120 p. $1.75
. . . describes over 500 media groups initiating and spreading social change, listener controlled radio, film coops, radical librarian projects, people's presses. . . . It also includes an annotated list of 400 communications resources: a pamphlet on how to start an underground newspaper, books on political theater, films on advertising as social control, bibliographies of non-sexist children's books, articles on community controlled cable and more.

COMMUNITIES/HOUSING: Source Catalog No. 2, Swallow Press, 1972, 254 p. $2.95
. . . an extensive guide to housing organizing, emphasizing pragmatic tactics and visions of new social/political/economic systems. The catalog describes over 700 political and community groups working in the housing struggle that are backed up by an excellent array of book, pamphlet, and film reviews. The catalog covers tenants' unions, model legal aid programs; non-profit housing development corporations: urban homesteading; rural housing; public housing organizing; and housing resources for Blacks, Chicanos, Puertoriquenos, Native Americans, Asian Americans, women and gay people. The concluding section is a thorough indictment of government policy.

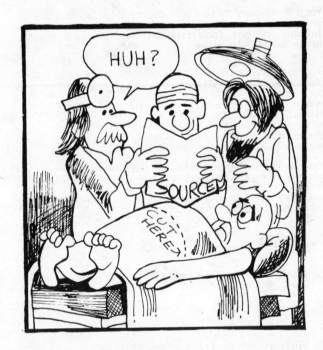

DEMAND FOR DAY CARE: an introduction for campus and community, ed. Resources for Community Change, 1974, 45 p. $1.50
. . . covers varying aspects of developing day care programs—parent involvement, cooperatives, day care's relationship to women's liberation, bi-lingual centers, funding and legal problems, etc. Campus day care is especially emphasized, through articles and an annotated listing of campus centers. The last seven pages list and describe other resources and resource groups. Order from Source or Organizers Book Center.

For bulk orders of Source I and II at the standard bookstore/retailer discount (40%), contact SWALLOW PRESS, 1139 S. Wabash Ave., Chicago, IL 60605. Order Source III in bulk from Beacon Press, 25 Beacon St., Boston, MA 02108. Order single copies from us, SOURCE, P.O. Box 21066, Washington, D.C. 20009, (202) 387-1145.

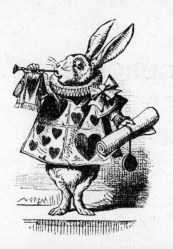

THANKS TO . . . all the projects who sent us information—sometimes taking time out for long conversations and letters; special thanks to Health/PAC and MCHR; to the people who read and criticized the different sections for us; friends in the DC community, especially those who worked part-time with us; people who gave us funding; also the many authors, pamphleteers, and photographers, from whom we drew so much of the catalog.

DOES SOURCE SERVE YOUR NEEDS?

We did not come to Source as professionals, researchers or journalists, but as people interested in community and institutional organizing, and feeling the need for these resources in our own communities.

To serve your community we need to know your needs. Your suggestions and criticisms are essential to improve Source as an organizing tool: prototype groups that weren't included, rip-off ones that were, misrepresentations, out of date material...especially analysis of the general format and section introductions. Books, films, facts you want others to know about, let us know.

Your suggestions have already been the basis for the updating of the **Communications** catalog in the second printing and the format and content change in the second catalog. We need your help as we set future priorities and directions. Send us this questionnaire or make up your own.

1. What is the most helpful to you: groups, resources, or narrative?

2. What would you like us to emphasize more? less?

3. Do you find the problem-platform-program format useful?

4. What is the strongest part of the catalog? weakest?

5. In light of the rising cost of paper, would you rather see us do more catalogs or put out packets with more thorough coverage of smaller areas, such as occupational safety and health or prisons?

6. General comments:

Send to Source, P.O. Box 21066, Washington, D.C. 20009, (202) 387-1145.

249

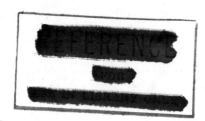